MCAT VERBAL:

108 PRACTICE PASSAGES
for the new
CRITICAL ANALYSIS and
REASONING SKILLS SECTION

Printed in the United States of America

Second Printing, 2017

ISBN 978-1-511766-69-2

Next Step Pre-Med, LLC
4256 N Ravenswood Ave
Suite 303
Chicago, IL 60613

www.nextstepmcat.com

ABOUT THE AUTHORS

Bryan Schnedeker is Next Step Test Prep's Vice President for MCAT Tutoring and Content. He manages all of our MCAT and LSAT instructors nationally and counsels hundreds of students when they begin our tutoring process. He has over a decade of MCAT and LSAT teaching and tutoring experience (starting at one of the big prep course companies before joining our team). He has attended medical school and law school himself and has scored a 44 on the old MCAT, a 525 on the new MCAT, and a 180 on the LSAT. Bryan has worked with thousands of MCAT students over the years and specializes in helping students looking to achieve elite scores.

Anthony Lafond is Next Step's MCAT Content Director. He has been teaching and tutoring MCAT students for nearly 12 years. He earned his MD and PhD degrees from UMDNJ - New Jersey Medical School with a focus on rehabilitative medicine. Dr. Lafond believes that both rehabilitative medicine and MCAT education hinge on the same core principle: crafting an approach that puts the unique needs of the individual foremost.

To find out about MCAT tutoring directly with Anthony or Bryan visit our website:

http://nextsteptestprep.com/mcat

Updates may be found here: http://nextsteptestprep.com/mcat-materials-change-log/

If you have any feedback for us about this book, or if you find an error, please contact us at mcat@nextsteptestprep.com

Version: 2017-01-01

FREE ONLINE MCAT DIAGNOSTIC and

FULL-LENGTH EXAM

Want to see how you would do on the MCAT and understand where you need to focus your prep?

TAKE OUR FREE MCAT DIAGNOSTIC EXAM.
Timed simulations of all 4 sections of the MCAT
Comprehensive reporting on your performance
Continue your practice with a free Full Length Exam

These two exams are provided free of charge to students who purchased our book.

To access your free exam, visit:
http://nextsteptestprep.com/mcat-diagnostic/

CONTENTS

Introduction

Hello and welcome to Next Step's practice book for the MCAT Critical Analysis and Reasoning Skills section. Since that name is quite the mouthful, we're just going to keep it simple and call it "the CARS section".

The book you're holding contains the most extensive practice and explanations available for the CARS section, and presents that practice in the most effective format possible – full 90-minute timed sections. Let's start with just a quick introduction to the CARS section itself.

The CARS section will consist of 53 questions which you'll have 90 minutes to answer. Those 53 questions will be presented as a series of questions associated with a reading passage (much like the old Verbal Reasoning section of the prior MCAT). The section will include approximately 9 passages with four to seven questions with each passage. The AAMC may continue to make adjustments to the CARS section as they administer more of the new-format MCATs, and we will update this book as the AAMC releases new information.

Each section will have roughly 50% of the questions drawn from Humanities topics and 50% from Social Sciences topics. You will not be required to have any prior knowledge of any of the topics discussed. Within those broad categories, the AAMC estimates that the questions will break down as 30% comprehension-based, 30% inference-based, and 40% extrapolation-based (applying the passage reasoning to new situations or incorporating new information into the passage).

The disciplines discussed in a CARS passage can be drawn from any of the following areas:

Humanities: architecture, art, dance, ethics, literature, music, philosophy, pop culture, religion, theater

Social Sciences: anthropology, archaeology, cultural studies, economics, education, geography, history, linguistics, political science, population health, psychology, sociology

As with the science sections, the key to mastering this new section involves taking a step-by-step approach, starting with untimed practice to master your technique, then short timed work on a few passages, and finally full timed sections. If you have not yet gotten the untimed practice you need to establish your best method, I *very strongly recommend* you do so, using a resource such as Next Step's CARS Strategy and Practice book.

Everyone here at Next Step would like to wish you the best of luck with your studies!

Thank you,

Bryan Schnedeker

Co-founder

Next Step Pre-Med, LLC

STOP! READ THIS FIRST!
How to Use This Book

To get the most out of your CARS practice you'll want to follow a few simple guidelines:

• Use the performance tracking sheet in Appendix A to keep track of how you're doing.

• Try different approaches to find your best method. Some people like highlighting; others prefer note-taking; some like to just skim the passage. You may not like a particular approach at first, but be sure to give it a good effort. You may find that it works well despite initial concerns.

• When reviewing your work, *read the explanation for every single question*, not just the ones you got wrong. I cannot emphasize this enough. In my 15+ years of MCAT teaching experience, this is the most common mistake I've seen made by students. You should take just as long to review and analyze a section after you're done as you did to take the section initially.

While you can certainly use the passages in this book in any way that will best benefit your prep, keep in mind that this book has been designed with a single, focused purpose: full *timed* section practice. As such, this book should not be your first resource when it comes to improving your CARS performance.

Doing your best on Test Day requires first that you do untimed work and experiment with different methods. Your CARS practice should begin with a resource (a book, a class, tutoring, etc.) that will give you a simple step-by-step introduction to various approaches to the passage. Be wary of any resource that tells you that there's only one "right way" to do the verbal passages – that's total nonsense!

Instead, you should work to find *your* best method. A book like Next Step's CARS Strategy and Practice book is one way to do this initial work. Once you've tried out several different methods and understand how they work, it's time to use this book to practice those methods.

To get the most out of the dozen sections that follow, you should use the sections in this book as follows:

Sections 1-3: Practice highlighting techniques

Sections 4-6: Practice note-taking techniques

Sections 7-8: Practice skimming techniques

Sections 9-10: Practice main idea techniques

Sections 11-12: Try alternative approaches that combine different methods

When reviewing the explanations to the passages, you will see we've provided a full analysis of each passage with three different forms of annotation. First, in the text itself we use **bold text** as a way to show you which terms and ideas are worth highlighting. Next, between each paragraph you will see notes providing an analysis of that paragraph. These notes are meant as a guide to the sorts of things that are worth jotting down in note-taking techniques. Finally, at the end of each passage we have included a **Main Idea**. If you're using a technique that involves reading briskly and only jotting down the Main Idea, you can compare your Main Idea to ours to see how you did.

After reviewing your understanding and analysis of the passage, read through the explanations to the questions and be sure you understand why each answer choice was right or wrong.

Finally, if you hit a big roadblock and think that you could use extra one-on-one MCAT help, contact Next Step to ask about our tutoring services at 888-530-NEXT.

Good luck with your CARS practice and good luck on Test Day!

SECTION 1
53 Questions, 90 Minutes
Use an answer grid from the back of the book to record your answers

Passage 1 (Questions 1-7)

The movement of art away from representation of things (paintings of people, places, events, etc.) into a wholly abstract presentation undoubtedly reached its zenith in the work of the color field painters. Exemplified by the work of Mark Rothko, color field painting sought to present color in its pure state. This purity made the color itself the subject of the painting, rather than a tool used to express something else. The cubists, surrealists, and other abstract expressionists working earlier in the 20th century may have distorted, mocked, and radically reduced representation (respectively), but it was the color field artists alone who completely stripped out any pretense of painting *something* other than the painting itself. Rothko's works consisted of little more than several large squares of contrasted colors, in various proportions and arrangements.

Those artists who become best known for representing a school of art – and indeed to those outside the highly specialized world of academic high art become the only known example of the school, their name synonymous with the school itself (Pollack and "Drip Painting", Picasso and Cubism, Michelangelo and high Renaissance fresco, etc.) – achieve their notoriety through no more remarkable means than pursuing a certain artistic idea to its very core. The stripping away of every extraneous thought and impulse guided by history and habit leaves the core truth of the movement. One cannot help but wonder, then, why no artist in the millennia before Rothko sought to pursue color itself as the subject of painting. Certainly artists the world over had experimented with how color was represented in their work. Japanese calligraphy paintings often reserved color for a single slash near the edge of the scroll. Zen Buddhist ensō eschew color altogether – using the purity of a single black circle on white background to represent the empty, open mind that has reached enlightenment. The fauvists, on the other hand, used a riot of colors in vibrant, jarring juxtaposition.

In each case, the color (or lack thereof) merely enhanced or commented on the representational efforts of the rest of the composition. Every work we find still relied on line, form, movement, space, perspective, and all the usual tools of a painter to represent a particular thing or idea.

Rothko and the rest of the color field artists broke away from every one of these conventions by removing more and more until only color remained. The typical color field composition has few if any lines or forms, and what forms there are – the boundaries between the different colors – are typically blurred and incoherent. This total lack of form permits no interpretation by the viewer of the painting as being "of something".

And yet when the literature around color field art was being written in the 1970's and 1980's, we consistently see that both erudite critics and casual observers spoke of Rothko's work in terms of representations beyond color itself. The painting *No. 61 (Rust and Blue)* is simply three horizontal rectangles of color – rust red, light blue, and navy blue. The colors are mottled, a result of the staining technique used. The boundaries between the rectangles are blurred and inconsistent. No painting could more clearly be about the colors themselves. However, in instance after instance, observers wrote of *No. 61* as evoking the ocean at sunset, the haze over a lake, the pre-dawn light seen through closed eyelids, etc.

Perhaps pure color is an ungraspable phantom. Even when presented in its purest form, it seems that most observers are unable to accept the work as it is, and ever seek for representation.

1. The author seems to think that when viewing a painting, seeing the painting as representing something is:

   A. an artifact that most avoid when seeing the painting as an example of pure color.

   B. a nearly inevitable part of interpreting the painting, whether the interpreter is a casual observer or an art scholar.

   C. a result of the kind of painting first popularized by Rothko.

   D. a fashion that went out of style in art critic circles after the runaway success of the color field painters.

2. The author's main point in the passage discussion is that:

   A. abstract painters such as Buddhist monks painting their ensō still retained form and thus representation.

   B. it is impossible for any human to view a painting solely as a representation of pure color, but instead we constantly look to interpret paintings as representations of things.

   C. color field artists created a new type of painting that was, for the first time ever, able to wholly leave behind the elements of representation and focus on color itself as the subject of the painting.

   D. the history of art is full of various uses of color, from mere emphasis to the total absence of color.

3. The author's discussion about painters prior to Rothko using color to comment on representation indicates that before Rothko:

    A. painters had not attempted to use color as the sole subject of painting.

    B. the aesthetic value of black and white abstract paintings was in doubt.

    C. artists were afraid to surrender representation entirely and thus used line, form, and color to make paintings that were "of something".

    D. color itself could be the subject of representation.

4. The passage assertion that a single artist can come to represent an entire movement of art in the minds of the public is:

    A. only mentioned in passing and assumed to be true, with the author providing no support.

    B. patently absurd because it cannot, in principle, be empirically investigated.

    C. supported by specific examples of the phenomenon.

    D. an axiomatic statement upon which the main thesis of the passage relies.

5. The passage suggests that Rothko became the foremost example of a color field artist because he:

    A. more than other prior or contemporary artists, was able to pursue the effort of non-representation to its logical conclusion leaving only color itself as the subject of painting.

    B. was the artist most successfully able to meld traditional art techniques of color oil painting with the new artistic notion of removing all elements of representation.

    C. took the notion of representing color itself to the highest possible level, tying color into traditional notions of form.

    D. was by far the most commercially successful and his art was depicted in a number of important cultural contexts.

6. Suppose a museum curator discovers a heretofore unknown collection of paintings by a German artist working in the early 19th century and the paintings are little more than large blobs of color, with no discernable objects or forms. This discovery would most weaken the author's assertion that:

    A. Rothko had set aside previous artistic habits and history when creating his color field works.

    B. Rothko and the color field artists working in the mid-20th century were the first to totally divorce color and painting from representation of objects.

    C. color field art is continually misinterpreted since viewers seem to insist on seeing the color blobs as being paintings "of something".

    D. audiences prior to those present in mid-20th century America were unwilling and unable to embrace color field art as an accepted art movement.

7. An experimental filmmaker in the 1980's began creating compositions that entirely removed any traces of the plot or narrative structure that had, up to that point, always been present in both film and television and created works that were little more than meditations on movement and form. The author would likely assert that such films would garner which of the following reactions from audiences?

    A. Most observers would express strong distaste for the work.

    B. Audiences would speak about the progression of the various images in terms of narrative structures that were familiar to them from earlier film and television.

    C. Such works would be well-received in film studies circles but would never achieve any large commercial success.

    D. Nearly all audience members would mistakenly draw parallels between this work and the works of famous color field painters such as Rothko.

Passage 2 (Questions 8 – 12)

The usual story about the invention of paper gives credit to Cai Lun, an official of the imperial court in Han Dynasty China. Cai Lun's credit as the inventor of paper rests on claims that he was the first to significantly improve and standardize paper-making, turning it into a product that could be produced in massive quantities at low cost. Certainly paper-like substances long predate Cai Lun (and even both the Han and Qin dynasties), as Egyptians were writing on papyrus two to three thousand years before the Qin dynasty.

Cai Lun began his service as a court eunuch in 75 AD, and was promoted in 89 AD to the official in charge of the manufacture of instruments and weapons. After the death of his patron, Empress Dou, in 97 AD, Cai Lun is said to have set about working at a feverish pace to craft some invention that would win him the favor of the Emperor and return him to a position of influence in the court. It would seem that he achieved this in 105 AD upon completing his paper-making technique.

As historian Will Durant explains, Cai Lun perfected a recipe consisting of bark, hemp, silk, and even chunks of fishing net. The fibers were laid out in sheets and suspended in water. Removing the water, compressing the fibers, and allowing them to dry created a thin matted sheet of paper, which could then be cut into any desired size.

The relative simplicity of the craftsmanship in Cai Lun's method seems to speak against it requiring any special learning or great insight. Simple experimentation would have sufficed to produce the paper used throughout China in the centuries following Cai Lun's death. Historian Thomas Carter posits that one of Cai Lun's subordinates of a lower craftsman class is much more likely to have developed the technique for which Cai Lun takes credit or that Cai Lun simply re-discovered an older technique.

Carter's support for his revisionist view of the invention of paper rests on several observations. In 1986, an excavation at the Fangmatan site near Tianshui in the Gansu province uncovered a tomb including fragments of a paper map. Dating of artifacts surrounding the tomb led researchers to assume the paper map was from early 2nd century BC. The quality of the paper itself, as well as the ink used, show a craftsmanship very nearly similar to Cai Lun's method. Second, Carter discusses the huge number of journeyman and apprentices working under a highly ranked official like Cai Lun. With nearly a hundred journeymen, and double that number of apprentices, the odds that Cai Lun himself was the one to make a particular discovery seem slim.

Finally, Carter notices a remarkable dearth of other writings or innovations in Cai Lun's own personal notes or even in the hagiography that grew up around the man in later years (he became a subject of ancestor worship in the following centuries, with temples dedicated to his honor). A man with the mind of an experimenter must have hit on at least some other developments in the arts, or at least left behind records of failed attempts in his personal notes. Yet none such seem to exist.

On this final point, Carter may reach too far. After all, one may be struck by a single great insight, or have a single great stroke of luck but leave behind no other great inventions. Not all innovators need be an Edison or a Da Vinci. On the structure of Cai Lun's workshops, we routinely give credit to inventors and artists who have many working underneath them. The artist Andy Warhol even called his studio a "factory", so repetitive and machine-like was the production of works. Yet we don't worry about the authenticity of such a work being a "real" Warhol, since we recognize and give credit to the master's guiding hand and insight.

8. Based on the passage, the level of technical skill necessary to develop the paper-making techniques discussed was:

    A. low enough that the paper could have been invented by any number of craftsmen.

    B. so low that any uneducated peasant could have developed it.

    C. remarkably high, as is demonstrated by the fact that Chinese paper-making was a feat not duplicated elsewhere for a millennium.

    D. about the same as would have been needed to be accepted as a journeyman under Cai Lun's service.

9. Based on the passage, it is most likely true that Durant and Carter would disagree about which of the following?

    A. Whether there were an unusually large number of craftsmen working under Cai Lun

    B. Whether a work made by one of Andy Warhol's assistants in The Factory can properly be credited to Andy Warhol

    C. Whether Cai Lun was definitely the one to develop the recipe of bark, hemp, silk, and fishing net and the technique of compressing and drying it

    D. Whether the absence of any other great insights by Cai Lun proves that he must not have had the one insight into paper-making for which he is given credit

10. The author would most likely agree with which of the following?

    A. The presence of paper with similar qualities to Cai Lun's paper that predates Cai Lun's innovation by centuries speaks strongly to the fact that Cai Lun should not get sole credit for inventing paper.

    B. When examining the intellectual history of developments in a certain field, one can make strong inferences from the absence of information about a particular thinker.

    C. The usual story about the invention of paper is largely correct.

    D. The sophistication of Egyptian papyrus merits giving credit to the Egyptians for inventing paper, even if the structure and method for papyrus-making differs substantially from contemporary paper-making.

11. The passage implies that Carter would believe which of the following about a work conceived by and created by an apprentice working in Andy Warhol's Factory?

    A. Andy Warhol should be credited as the artist for that work.

    B. Andy Warhol should not be credited as the artist for that work.

    C. The artist who created the work should get to decide whether to take credit for the work or to let Warhol sign the work and claim it as his own.

    D. Credit should be shared among all working in a given workshop for any invention that comes out of the shop, since it is the collective work of everyone that allows the workshop to function.

12. Which of the following would most weaken the theory that Cai Lun did not invent paper?

    A. Because he was a very highly ranked imperial official, special care was taken to preserve Cai Lun's personal notes and correspondence after his death.

    B. It was standard practice in Han Dynasty China for the most highly-ranked member of a household or government office to take credit for any good works done by those in that household or office.

    C. Several broad surveys of both well-known and obscure inventors have shown that any inventor who had at least one major breakthrough engaged in extensive trial-and-error towards various inventions and techniques.

    D. When it was built, the tomb at Fangmatan was filled with artifacts from several hundred years earlier to honor the noble who was buried there.

Passage 3 (Questions 13 – 18)

In 2013, two Colorado men brought a discrimination suit against the Masterpiece Cakeshop, saying that the bakery refused to make their wedding cake because the couple was gay. The baker, Jack Phillips, claimed that as a private businessman, he had the right to choose whom he would or would not serve. However, a Colorado state judge ruled that Phillips would have to provide wedding-related services to same-sex couples, even though he objects to gay marriage on religious grounds. "At first blush," Administrative Law Judge Robert Spencer wrote, "it may seem reasonable that a private business should be able to refuse service to anyone it chooses." Yet this view, Spencer said, does not take into account the cost to society and the hurt caused to persons who are denied service "simply because of who they are."

A similar discrimination case arose in New Mexico, when photographers Elaine and Jonathan Huguenin refused to photograph a lesbian couple's commitment ceremony in 2006; the New Mexico Supreme Court ruled that state law made their refusal discriminatory. The Huguenins' lawyers cited their clients' First Amendment rights: as artists, they had a right to free expression, and they should not be obligated to create work that is in contrast with their beliefs. Forcing the photographers, lawyers claimed, to photograph the commitment ceremony is tantamount to requiring them to express a message with which they don't agree.

Both of these cases have brought to the fore the complex legal issues of whether individual businesspeople are required to provide wedding-related goods or services to same-sex couples. Gay rights advocates say that the cases are in line with public accommodation laws, which ban discrimination based on sexual orientation. Many religious-liberty advocates, however, assert that state public accommodation laws – which originated in the 1960s to prevent discrimination based on race but have grown to include discrimination based on gender and marital status – were not designed with same-sex marriage in mind.

Some conservatives have tried to take a spurious "middle ground," asserting that the private businesspeople, such as baker Jack Phillips and photographers Elaine and Jonathan Huguenin, are not refusing to serve gay people per se, but are taking a stand against gay marriage. In an interview, Phillips said that he would have "no problem" baking cupcakes for a gay person's birthday party, or serving gay customers who come into his Denver-area shop. The issue, he claims, is not discriminating against gay people – it's about being forced to support marriage equality. And these, Phillips claims, are two different issues.

Yet advocates for the LGBTQ community say that such thinking represents a moral and legal "slippery slope." Discrimination is discrimination, one gay-rights advocate said; saying that it's OK to refuse to make a wedding cake or take wedding photos might lead to efforts to refuse housing to same-sex couples or to terminate gay, lesbian or transgender employees. So far, the courts seem to largely agree, and as of May 2014, more than half of Americans express support for marriage equality. As same-sex marriage becomes more familiar, perhaps fewer businesspeople will claim their questionable right to refuse service to gay customers by any rationale.

13. According to the passage, a "religious-liberty advocate" might agree that:

    A. religious organizations face similar issues as arts groups.

    B. religious groups should be allowed to discriminate against groups that violate their beliefs.

    C. public accommodation laws do not apply to the case of same-sex marriage.

    D. same-sex couples should be protected by state public accommodation laws.

14. An analogy to the belief that taking a stand against same-sex marriage is not akin to discriminating against individuals might be:

    A. asserting that opposing inter-racial marriage does not constitute racism.

    B. believing that same-sex marriage should be legal is not the same as encouraging it.

    C. arguing that having ageist attitudes doesn't preclude fair hiring decisions regardless of age.

    D. taking a stand against same-sex marriage but supporting inter-racial marriage.

15. Which of the following might be another example of the "First Amendment rights" argument mentioned in Paragraph 2?

    A. A schoolchild who refuses to recite the Pledge of Allegiance

    B. A property owner who neglects to pay real estate taxes

    C. A same-sex couple that chooses to marry

    D. A taxi driver who refuses service to a same-sex couple

16. Which of the following best captures the author's point of view?

    A. While it is not morally permissible to discriminate against gay people, individuals should be allowed to refuse to support same-sex marriage.

    B. Although the "private business exemption" is not valid, the First Amendment should protect individuals from any obligatory speech or expression of beliefs.

    C. Public accommodation laws need to be expanded to include discrimination based on sexual orientation.

    D. Private businesspeople do not have the right to discriminate against same-sex couples.

17. The passage states all of the following relating to same-sex marriage EXCEPT:

    A. the possibility that allowing individuals to refuse services related to same-sex marriage might lead to other forms of discrimination against gay people.

    B. the courts differ from the majority of Americans in their stance towards same-sex marriage.

    C. refusing wedding-related services to same-sex couples discriminates against people "simply because of who they are."

    D. refusing services to individuals because of who they are comes at a cost to society.

18. Which of the following best summarizes the "private business exemption" argument put forth in Paragraph 1?

    A. Private business owners are protected by First Amendment rights.

    B. Although private business may not discriminate in their hiring practices, they may do so in their serving policies.

    C. Privately owned businesses are required by law to serve all individuals who seek service.

    D. Because a business is privately held, the owner should be allowed to choose whom he or she serves.

Passage 4 (Questions 19 – 25)

Aristotle was a student of Plato and he always remembered it, as the best students do, in order to oppose him. For some years he taught Philip's son, the future Alexander the Great, and for many years he taught in Athens. After Alexander's death, he became the target of the eternal accusation of impiety that plagues so many great minds, so he retired to Chalcis, where he died. Before all else, Aristotle was an educated man. He desired to embrace the entirety of the knowledge of his time, which at that time was actually possible, albeit with prodigious effort, and he succeeded, his countless works being a testament.

His works are the summa of all the sciences of his epoch, but here, we shall occupy ourselves primarily with his philosophical ideas. To Aristotle, and just as it was to Plato, but more precisely, man is composed of body and soul. The body is a well-made machine, consisting of organs, and the soul is its final purpose. Together, the two form a continuous harmony. The body results in the soul, and in turn, the soul acts on the body, and is not its end but its means of acting upon things. The faculties of the soul are both its diverse aspects and its diverse methods of acting, for the soul is indivisibly one.

Reason refers to the soul being able to conceive what is most general, and therefore it is the intermediary between ourselves and God. God is unique, eternal, and from all eternity gave motion to matter. He is purely spiritual and all else besides him is purely material. Unlike Plato, Aristotle believes that God does not have ideas, or immaterial living personifications, residing in his bosom. It is here that we may note, from Plato to Aristotle, progress towards monotheism: Plato's Olympus of ideas was still a kind of polytheism. Aristotle's work contained no such polytheism.

Aristotle's moral system sometimes approaches Plato's, like when he claims that supreme happiness is the supreme good, and that the supreme good is the contemplation of thought by thought, this being completely self-sufficient. This is approximately the imitation of God recommended by Plato. Sometimes, on the contrary, it is very practical and nearly mediocre, like when he claims morality to be a mean between extremes, a certain tact, an art rather than a science, being of practical science rather than of conscience.

His political philosophy is very confused, perhaps because the volume containing it was likely composed after his death from passages and fragments of different lectures. In general, it is a review of the divergent political constitutions that existed in his time throughout the Greek world. His tendencies in political philosophy, for there are no conclusions in this work, are notably aristocratic, but less so than those of Plato.

Because of his universality, his clarity, and because he frequently dogmatizes instead of discussing and collating, Aristotle had a greater authority throughout antiquity and the Middle Ages than Plato. In fact, this authority became despotic and nearly sacrosanct, except on matters of faith.

By the time of the sixteenth century, he was relegated to his due esteem: lower than sacrosanct, but still quite high, for he is often regarded among the geniuses of widest range, if not of greatest power. Even today, he is far from having lost significance. For some, he functions as a bridge between the subtle yet always poetic Greek genius and the Roman genius, more positive, more plain, more practical, more attached to reality, and more grounded in pure science.

19. Based upon the passage, what exactly is reason?

   A. The soul viewed in a particular way

   B. A particular part of the soul

   C. The meeting of body and soul

   D. Divinity disguised in human form

20. Based upon the passage, which of the following is the most likely reason why the author constantly compares Aristotle with Plato?

   A. Because he believes Plato and Aristotle to have been equally valuable philosophers, especially in morality

   B. Because he believes Aristotle to be entirely derivative of Plato, especially in morality

   C. Because he believes both philosophers are important in the context of Aristotle's work

   D. Because he believes Aristotle's desire to oppose his teacher informed all of his work

21. If the author were alive today, which of the following statements would he be most likely to believe, given the passage?

   A. Aristotle's conception of monotheism was important to scholars in the Middle Ages.

   B. Aristotle's conception of morality is more influential now than it was in the Middle Ages.

   C. Aristotle's conception of political philosophy was more influential in antiquity than it is now.

   D. Aristotle's conception of God was less influential during the Middle Ages than Plato's conception.

22. Based upon the context of the passage, which of the following is the most likely meaning for the Latin word "summa?"

   A. Greatest

   B. Collection

   C. Pinnacle

   D. Summary

23. Say you are a scholar of Aristotle in the sixteenth century. As the Renaissance continues to develop, you begin to realize certain things about your subject. Based upon the passage, which of the following might be one of those things?

   A. Aristotle's philosophy is ultimately less praiseworthy than the full range of his pursuits.

   B. Aristotle's conception of monotheism was actually hugely influential on scholars since.

   C. Aristotle's take on morality has increased in influence while the rest of his work has lessened.

   D. Aristotle's philosophy bridges the more succinct practical Greek genius to the more lyrical Roman genius.

24. All of the following are similarities between Plato and Aristotle EXCEPT:

   A. the duality of body and soul.

   B. the high esteem assigned to contemplation of thought by thought.

   C. the high esteem assigned to the golden mean.

   D. there is one God who may or may not possess within him "ideas".

25. Based upon the passage, which of the following statements are true of Plato?

   I. He espoused a pantheon of Gods.

   II. His writing on body and soul was more vague than Aristotle's.

   III. His moral system was superior to Aristotle's.

   A. I and II only

   B. I and III only

   C. II and III only

   D. I, II, and III

Passage 5 (Questions 26 – 30)

James Olney's discussion of two distinct forms of autobiography is useful in order to distinguish between Hemingway's and Gaines's writings. On the one hand, Olney describes a particularly Western tendency "to take the life of the self to be the true self, the real self, the life about which an autobiography should be written" ("Value" 53). This form of autobiography Olney calls "autoautography." Hemingway seems to be an especially strong representative of this form of life-writing. Even though not strictly autobiographical, his works, even *For Whom the Bell Tolls* in spite of Robert Jordan's transformation, remain focused on the individual. Hemingway can therefore be said to represent the Western tradition that takes the self to be at the center of life. Stressing the singularity of each character's life, Hemingway's works reflect renewed attempts to portray his own struggle, to give expression to his own inner confusion.

Certainly, Olney's definition of the autobiographical act applies to Hemingway: "The autobiographical act . . . [is] a perpetually renewed attempt to find language adequate to rendering the self and its experience, an attempt that includes within itself all earlier attempts" (Memory 9). Read as such, Hemingway's miscellaneous works, his short stories, novels, autobiographical writings, and travel accounts provide us with intriguing insights into the man behind the pen, as they "bring forth ever different memorial configurations and an ever newly shaped self" (Memory 20). If we read Hemingway's works as instances of life-writing, we thus arrive at a composite picture of one man, starting with the fear of night and mortality as a boy in "Three Shots," continuing with his attempts as a man to create an identity in various countries, while always attempting to come to terms with the father, and ending with the old fisherman's proven heroism even as he loses the prize (marlin). Always the focus is on one individual's struggle— the man himself behind the pen.

In this context, Michel de Montaigne, who writes of the "consubstantial" process of self creation and book creation, comes to mind: "I have no more made my book than my book has made me—a book consubstantial with its author, concerned with my own self, an integral part of my life" (504). We can therefore ask whether Hemingway's writing about his own experiences and the concomitant public myths he created also "made" him in the same way. Did not Hemingway in writing about his various exploits— as a wounded war hero, as a skilled hunter, as an expert fisherman—"fashion and compose" himself so often that "the model itself has to some extent grown firm and taken shape," as it has in Montaigne's case (504)? Was he not afterwards trying to live up to the myths that he created with the thinly disguised self-portrayals in his works? Are not the agonizing and sorrowful thoughts of Nick Adams in "Fathers and Sons" the writer's own with regard to his alienation from his father and his sons?

These questions seem to be bound up with the pervasive emphasis on the self and the cyclical view of life that we see manifested in Hemingway's work and life. Hemingway's writings are an "involuted and reflexive exercise," as the writer constantly looks inward, toward his own self (Olney, "Value" 53). Whereas Hemingway's writings are firmly situated in the Western tradition of autoautography, Ernest Gaines's works can be seen as representing a more African notion of autobiography. Referring to the Sonjo people in Tanzania, John Mbiti explains that "the individual is united with the rest of his community, both the living and the dead, and humanly speaking nothing can separate him from this corporate society" (117). Reminiscent of Jefferson's "lowly as I am, I am still part of the whole" in *A Lesson Before Dying* (LBD 194), the Sonjo exclaim, "I am because we are, and since we are, therefore I am" (Mbiti 117).

26. Given the different emphases between Western and African autobiography, which of the following motifs would be handled differently by Hemingway and Gaines?

I. Independence

II. Identity

III. Memory

A. I and II only

B. I and III only

C. II and III only

D. I, II and III

27. Later in the passage, the author states "If one considers the pervasive father-son relationship and other recurring themes in both Hemingway's and Gaines's oeuvres, it furthermore seems as if their narratives are never finished within the cover of a single book, but that the writers have to continually go back where they have left off and wrestle with the same issues again, under a different light, with changing scenarios." This is an example of which concept from the passage?

A. The "consubstantial" process

B. The autobiographical act

C. The Western tradition of autobiography

D. The African tradition of autobiography

28. Based on the information in the passage, which of the following claims about Hemingway's works would the author agree with LEAST?

A. Hemingway's Nick Adams stories are the closest Hemingway comes to writing true autobiography as Nick Adams can be regarded as Hemingway's alter ego.

B. Hemingway's works must be considered collectively in order to understand the author as a whole.

C. Hemingway's works can all be considered instances of life-writing, created out of his own experiences in the war, traveling, etc.

D. Hemingway's works are static depictions of his life and had very little influence on his later life and works.

29. Of the following examples from Gaines's work, which is the best example of the Sonjo people's beliefs concerning community?

A. In *A Lesson Before Dying*, Jefferson's understanding that he is "part of the whole" when the entire community pays him a visit in jail

B. In *The Autobiography of Miss Jane Pittman*, neighbors and friends helping Miss Jane remember her life, which is not only her life, but the life of a whole people who have survived from the Civil War to the civil rights movement

C. In *In My Father's House*, Philip Martin learning about his son's suicide and applying the lessons he learns regarding his own past to the future

D. In *A Lesson Before Dying*, Jefferson's diary assuming a central place as it sums up his belief in the interdependence of the individual and the community and speaks the words of love and support that will serve as a powerful script for the community's future

30. Which of the following claims' implications would contradict the author's argument?

A. Hemingway's works, including the character Nick Adams, are works of fiction.

B. Gaines was heavily influenced by Hemingway's writing.

C. Gaines's early writing focuses primarily on the individual.

D. Neither Hemingway nor Gaines explicitly intended their writing to be autobiographical.

Passage 6 (Questions 31 – 36)

The organ is more than a single instrument. It is an orchestra, a collection of the pipes of Pan of every size, from those as small as a child's playthings to those as gigantic as the columns of a temple. Each one corresponds to what is termed an organ-stop. The number is unlimited. The compass of the organ far surpasses that of all the instruments of the orchestra. The violin notes alone reach the same height, but with little carrying power. As for the lower tones, there is no competitor of the thirty-two-foot pipes, which go two octaves below the violoncello's low C. Between the *pianissimo* which almost reaches the limit where sound ceases and silence begins, down to a range of formidable and terrifying power, every degree of intensity can be obtained from this magical instrument. The variety of its timbre is broad. There are flute stops of various kinds; tonal stops that approximate the timbre of stringed instruments; stops which serve to imitate the instruments of the orchestra. Then we have the innumerable combinations of all these different stops, with the gradations that may be obtained through indefinite commingling of the tones of this marvelous palette.

Let us have the courage to admit, however, that these resources are only partly utilized as they can or should be. The organ places before the organist extraordinary means of expressing himself. The organ is a theme with innumerable variations, determined by the place in which it is to be installed, by the amount of money at the builder's disposal, by his inventiveness, and, often, by his personal whims. As a result time is required for the organist to learn his instrument thoroughly. After this he is as free as the fish in the sea. Then, to play freely with the colors on his vast palette, there is but one way—he must plunge boldly into improvisation.

Under the pretext that an improvisation is not so good as one of Sebastian Bach's or Mendelssohn's masterpieces, young organists have stopped improvising. That point of view is harmful because it is absolutely false; it is simply the negation of eloquence. Consider what the legislative hall, the lecture room and the court would be like if nothing but set pieces were delivered. We are familiar with the fact that many an orator and lawyer, who is brilliant when he talks, becomes dry as dust when he tries to write. The same thing happens in music. As one touches the organ, the imagination is awakened, and the unforeseen rises from the depths of the unconscious. It is a world of its own, ever new, which will never be seen again, and which comes out of the darkness, as an enchanted island comes from the sea.

Instead of this fairyland, we too often see only some of Sebastian Bach's or Mendelssohn's pieces repeated continuously. The pieces themselves are very fine, but they belong to concerts and are entirely out of place in church services. Furthermore, they were written for old instruments and they apply either not at all, or badly, to the modern organ. Yet there are those who think this belief spells progress.

I am fully aware of what may be said against improvisation. A mediocre improvisation is always endurable, if the organist has grasped the idea that church music should harmonize with the service and aid meditation and prayer. If the organ music is played in this spirit and results in harmonious sounds rather than in precise music which is not worth writing out, it still is comparable with the old glass windows in which the individual figures can hardly be distinguished but which are, nevertheless, more charming than the finest modern windows. Such an improvisation may be better than a fugue by a great master, on the principle that nothing in art is good unless it is in its proper place.

31. In paragraph 1, the author uses the word "compass" to mean:

    A. sound.

    B. value.

    C. range.

    D. size.

32. Which of the following best describes the author's attitude towards the compositions of Sebastian Bach and Mendelssohn?

    A. They are fine pieces, but they do not express the organ's compass.

    B. Although they are excellent as compositions, they are rarely played with passion.

    C. While they are fine compositions, they are more suited to concert hall than to church.

    D. Unlike improvisations, they are difficult to play well.

33. The passage describes all of the following qualities of the organ EXCEPT:

    A. its suitability for improvisation.

    B. the wide breadth of its timbres.

    C. its tremendous range of volume.

    D. its difficulty for musicians.

34. In the final paragraph, which of the following does the author suggest is the problem leveled by critics of improvisation?

    A. Improvised music rarely inclines church audiences toward prayer.

    B. Improvised music is often mediocre.

    C. Compared to Bach's and Mendelssohn's compositions, improvised music is dry as dust.

    D. Improvised music does not display the organ's full potential of tone and timbre.

35. Why does the author raise the example of the orator who is "dry as dust" in paragraph 3?

    A. To argue that improvisation is rarely as good as the music of Bach and Mendelssohn

    B. To draw an analogy between brilliant improvised oration and inspiring improvised music

    C. To assert that composed music, like composed writing, is mostly dull and uninspired

    D. To posit that improvised speaking, unlike improvised music, is rarely rousing to audiences

36. Suppose a church organist improvised a composition that was technically flawed but spiritually uplifting. What would the author's attitude towards the performance most likely be?

    A. Critical, because he believes that such compositions should be both technically and spiritually inspiring

    B. Critical, because it reveals that the music is not "in its proper place"

    C. Accepting, because he reveres organ music of any sort

    D. Accepting, if it aids in prayer and is "in its proper place"

Passage 7 (Questions 37 – 42)

Salmonella bacteria infects over a million people in this country each year; more Americans die from its effects than from any other food-borne illness. Salmonella is shockingly prevalent in our food: a recent study by the U.S. Department of Agriculture found that nearly a quarter of all packaged chicken parts are contaminated by some form of it. But if you thought that such a high degree of contamination would be in violation of federal food safety laws, you would be mistaken. There is no set standard for the amount of allowable salmonella contamination in cut up chicken parts, for example, or for numerous other meats, such as lamb chops and pork ribs. This means that one hundred percent of these products may be contaminated, with no penalty to the producer. Some products do have performance standards, but few consumers would find them reassuring: the allowable percentage of salmonella contamination in ground turkey, for example, is 49.9 percent.

The oversight mechanisms for food safety are somewhat arcane. Fifteen different agencies are responsible for the safety of our food. The two most important of these are the U.S. Department of Agriculture's Food Safety and Inspection Service, or FSIS, and the Food and Drug Administration, or FDA, which is a division of the federal Department of Human Services. Adding to the problem are the limitations on the two agencies' authority. Even when an agency finds that the allowable limits of contamination are exceeded, the only option it has is to request that the producers remove the product voluntarily. Moreover, the agencies may only do this when they have proof, usually in the form of a genetic match, that a particular product is making consumers sick. If a consumer has eaten the tainted chicken (for example) and discarded the packaging, it is nearly impossible for the oversight agencies to request a recall.

One particular outbreak of salmonella contamination illustrates this. Over the course of 17 months in 2013 and 2014, over 600 people reported severe illness that was linked to chicken tainted with salmonella Heidelberg, an especially virulent strain of the bacterium. Although the FSIS tracked down over a hundred patients who had eaten chicken from one producer, Foster Farms, and had become ill, they were unable to make a genetic match until a year after the outbreak began. The match allowed the government to request that Foster Farms recall chicken produced in certain facilities. Foster Farms complied – but only withdrew chicken produced in a six-day period. The rest remained in the market. Since some scientists estimate that for every reported case of salmonella, 29 go unreported, it is likely that the tainted Foster Farms chicken had sickened nearly 18,000 people.

Food safety advocates and lawyers say that the system is clearly broken, but that relatively simple changes in the production process would vastly improve the safety of our food. They point to Denmark, where after a spate of salmonella cases in the 1980s, the Danish government enacted changes in processing that were extremely effective. The new regulations dictate that poultry workers are required to wash their hands before entering the plant, and to perform extensive microbiological testing. More important, though, is that as soon as a pathogen is found, recalls are imposed on the producers. As a result of these changes, less than two percent of poultry in Denmark is contaminated with salmonella.

It would be relatively simple for the United States to follow Denmark's example, as have several other European countries, to great effect. But for this to happen, the USDA would have to emphasize its regulatory function and role as protector of the people, and de-emphasize its current focus, which is to advance the interests of big agriculture. Unless that happens, millions will suffer needlessly.

37. Which of the following best captures the meaning of "arcane" in paragraph 2?

 A. Effective

 B. Nonsensical

 C. Unclear

 D. Disturbing

38. Suppose that following a salmonella outbreak, a clear genetic match could be made between lamb processed by a particular producer and individual consumers of that product. Which of the following represent options the USDA and/or FDA might take to protect consumers from this strain of salmonella?

 A. They could require the producer to recall meat that was proven to be tainted.

 B. They could insist upon microbiological testing at the processing facility.

 C. They could request that the producer recall the tainted meat.

 D. The agencies do not have the authority to take any action.

39. Which of the following best reflects the author's opinion regarding food safety?

 A. The food safety system in our country is woefully ineffective and needs to be revamped in order to protect consumers.

 B. While most of our food is safe, careless production methods in a small number of facilities give the impression that food-borne illness is more prevalent than it actually is.

 C. Food-borne illness is among the most pressing public health issues worldwide.

 D. Educating consumers about food safety is key in preventing the spread of food-borne illnesses.

40. Of the following, which represents the most significant difference between anti-salmonella measures taken by the United States and those enacted in Denmark?

 A. Denmark requires microbiological testing in production plants, but the United States does not.

 B. While the U.S. does not force producers to recall tainted products, Denmark requires mandatory recall.

 C. Denmark has a single regulatory agency overseeing food safety, while the U.S. has fifteen.

 D. U.S. regulatory agencies advocate for the interests of the producers, but Danish agencies act in the interests of consumers.

41. According to the passage, what percentage of a given quantity of food is permitted to be tainted by salmonella?

 A. 49.9%

 B. Up to 100%

 C. None

 D. It depends on the particular food.

42. Why does the author describe the case of Foster Farms chicken in paragraph 3?

 A. To illustrate the difficulty of containing a salmonella outbreak under current regulations

 B. To underscore the prevalence of salmonella-tainted food

 C. To criticize Foster Farms for its unwillingness to take effective measures to recall its unsafe product

 D. To emphasize that certain strains of salmonella can cause particularly severe illness

Passage 8 (Questions 43 – 47)

The health care services sector is a large and growing segment of the economy. The share of GDP devoted to health care services has doubled over the past 25 years, to 16 percent in 2005. Looking ahead, this growth is expected to continue, as aging baby boomers continue to increase the share of elderly in the population, a segment of the population that accounts for a disproportionately high level of expenditures on health.

These rising health care costs have raised questions about whether these medical expenditures are, in some sense, worth it. A natural starting point is to ask how much of the rising costs represent increases in real services vs price inflation, a question that can be addressed using price deflators or indices. However, studies in the health economics literature have raised questions about the use of standard price indices for this purpose and their empirical findings suggest that some of what is currently recorded as price increases actually represents increases in services.

Currently-available price indices define the "good" or the "output" of health care as the treatment (i.e., an office visit or prescription drug) and track the prices of those treatments over time. Health economists have long advocated an alternative definition of output as the bundle of treatments received by a patient for the treatment of some condition. The existing empirical evidence suggests that how one defines the good matters. Detailed case studies of important diseases show that, for these conditions, the price indices that health economists advocate show slower price growth than standard indices. This result is consistent with the view that indices that track the prices of individual treatments tend to miss any shifts towards lower-cost treatments that may occur over time. For example, in the treatment of depression, there has been a shift away from talk-therapy and towards (the lower cost) drug therapy that has reduced the cost of treating depression. Because standard indices track prices for these two types of treatments separately, they miss this substitution and overstate the cost of treating depression.

These studies also account for changes in the quality of health care by measuring the health outcomes associated with treatment. For example, Cutler, in his study of heart attacks, found that the substitution pattern there was towards more costly treatments. But, because the costlier treatments provided better outcomes in terms of health improvements the quality-adjusted price still showed slower growth than standard indices.

To explore the sources of those cost savings, we develop an algebraic expression for the contributions of shifts in different treatments to the cost savings by linking the preferred index to one that tracks fixed baskets of treatments, the type of index typically produced by statistical agencies. In our empirical work, the decomposition confirms the presence of treatment substitution for several important disease classes: shifts from office visits towards drugs in many psychiatric conditions, shifts from care at hospitals towards care at ambulatory surgical centers for orthopedic and gastroenterological conditions, and similar shifts in endocrinology (a disease class that contains diabetes and obesity). However, the decomposition also reveals other patterns associated with these cost savings. In cardiology, for example, the data literally show a large decline in the use of inpatient care with little change in the intensity of other treatments. We take this to mean that although patients appear to do as many office visits and purchase as many prescriptions as they did in 2003, perhaps the treatments they receive in 2005 are better, obviating the need for inpatient care and, thus, giving rise to cost savings. Finally, there are disease classes where the cost of treating conditions rises faster than the prices of the underlying treatments. Two notable cases are obstetrics and neonatology; where the increased intensity of treatment is associated with complications while normal pregnancies and uncomplicated neonatal management show little to no cost savings, respectively.

43. What is the purpose of the author's citation of the fact that more drug therapy than talk-therapy is now being used to treat depression, compared to earlier times?

   A. To illustrate that the form of medical treatment is ever-changing, making accurate cost assessments difficult

   B. To illustrate that medicine in the United States is leaning more towards cheaper drug therapies

   C. To give an example that illustrates how the cost of certain medical treatments might be overstated

   D. To reiterate that depression treatments are now more available to the general public

44. Which of the following is NOT an assertion made in the passage?

   A. When determining price indices, it is better to track prices of treatment separately than to account for the entire bundle of treatments received by patients.

   B. There has not been a decrease in treatment of cardiology patients over the past few years.

   C. Quality adjusted prices for modern medicine will tend to show estimates lower than current price indices.

   D. Currently available price indices probably overestimate price growth.

45. Which of the following are arguments that the author makes to show that standard price indices are inflated?

   I. That standard price indices don't use quality adjusted prices

   II. That standard price indices do not consider the price of treatment to the consumer

   III. That standard price indices only consider the prices of individual treatments

   A. I only

   B. I and II only

   C. I and III only

   D. II and III only

46. Which of the following are assumptions that the author makes?

   I. The elderly spend more on health care.

   II. The rate of complications in pregnancies is increasing.

   III. The percentage of people with heart health problems is rising.

   A. I only

   B. I and II only

   C. II and III only

   D. I, II, and III

47. A patient comes in to his doctor's office complaining of chest pains. In assessing the cost of treating this patient, what would the author of the passage believe is the appropriate way to analyze the good or service delivered?

   A. Look to the sum total of the office visits, drugs and other therapies prescribed, hospital visits, etc. and bundle the costs of all these treatments together

   B. Determine what course of treatment is considered the appropriate standard of care and calculate the cost of those treatments, regardless of the actual services delivered to this patient

   C. Calculate costs separately for each service or good as it is delivered to the patient for any condition needing treatment

   D. Look to the sum total of the office visits, drugs and other therapies prescribed, hospital visits, etc. and bundle together the costs of all these treatments for this condition and then adjust the cost based on the outcome the patient experiences

Passage 9 (Questions 48 – 53)

Shirley functions as an oddity in Charlotte Brontë's oeuvre: sandwiched between *Jane Eyre* and *Villette*, masterpieces of psychological realism and interiority, Shirley is, instead, fragmented in terms of plot and purpose. Much of this fragmentation may be ascribed to Brontë's employment of an industrial plot: the novel begins with the attack of loom breakers on flinty industrialist Robert Moore's factory, and concludes only after the end of the Napoleonic wars allows him to return to trade and thus propose to the woman of his dreams, Caroline Helstone. Critics have generally persisted in reading these plot elements as a misstep of some sort: Catherine Gallagher writes that "industrial conflict in *Shirley* is little more than a historical setting and does not exert any strong pressure on the form" while Rosemarie Bodenheimer notes the "virtual abandonment of the industrial issue" in the text.

But in *Shirley* the historical is irreducible from the psychological. In his recent article, Peter Capuano suggests we stop reading the novel in terms of "displacement"; instead "we really should pay attention to the industrial element in Shirley" focusing on "obvious textual features that critics have overlooked." Capuano focuses on the connection between surplus hands in the mill and surplus "female handiwork in the novel's middle-class homes" a connection that chronicles "the ways in which new modes of relation arose within the middle-class household." I argue in the opposite direction, suggesting that in the novel the romantic, seemingly contained within the middle-class household, inevitably gestures out to the social and, particularly, the industrial. This diversion suggests that the energies of erotic love can be read as similar to those of industrial forces.

Louis reveals his desire for Shirley late in the novel in what he admits are a series of "metaphors," ones that jumble the romantic and industrial. Musing on his attraction to Shirley, Louis states:

I worship her perfections; but it is her faults, or at least her foibles, that bring her near to me, that nestle her to my heart, that fold her about with my love, and that for a most selfish but deeply-natural reason. These faults are the steps by which I mount to ascendency over her. If she rose a trimmed, artificial mound, without inequality, what vantage would she offer the foot? It is the natural hill, with its mossy breaks and hollows, whose slope invites ascent, whose summit it is pleasure to gain.

This metaphor also invokes the industrial in two key ways: the language of manufacture and, more broadly, the idea of "wild" resources.

Louis seems to dismiss manufacture here, disdaining the "trimmed, artificial mound" in favor of "the natural hill." Yet it is the "steps," or artificially constructed tools, that he finds so attractive in Shirley's willfulness. Thus we can argue that it is the possibility of construction and alteration that Louis finds so attractive. This metaphor of manufacture circulates throughout the text, and is remarkable for how well it adapts itself to different situations. When Louis and Shirley finally declare their love for each other, he invokes her "lands and gold," metonymically picturing her as a series of materials for manufacture. While he boasts that he "care[s] not for them," he suggests that Shirley becomes the driving engine for his own transformation: "What change I underwent I cannot explain, but out of her emotion passed into me a new spirit." Thus Shirley serves multiply as a space on which manufacture can take place, a source of the raw materials of manufacture, and as a machine itself, whose "emotion" sets into motion Louis's own transformation. Louis pictures Shirley as the various modes of manufacture in an almost Marxist sense, envisioning a series of circulating and transforming energies that both please him erotically and profit him emotionally.

48. Based on the passage, it can be assumed that a Marxist reading is primarily concerned with:

   A. the division of classes displayed in mills and factories.

   B. how commodities move through and affect a system.

   C. how the domestic substructure reflects capitalism.

   D. the connections between the erotic and the industrial.

49. The author discusses Jane Eyre and Villette in order to:

   A. establish Brontë's importance as a writer in the nineteenth century.

   B. highlight the ways in which Shirley does not fit into expectations.

   C. argue that industrial plots can lead to fragmentation.

   D. establish the importance of publication order in reception.

50. Which of the following terms would the author NOT use to describe the focus of Shirley?

   A. Manufacture

   B. Erotic Power

   C. Psychological Realism

   D. Domesticity

51. Suppose that a section of Shirley contained a detailed description of a picnic lunch packed by Caroline Helstone. Which critic would be most likely to analyze it?

   A. Capuano, because of the focus on specific textual details

   B. The passage's author, because of the focus on middle-class homes

   C. Gallagher, because of the refusal of the industrial

   D. None, because of its focus on Caroline rather than Shirley

52. Based on the passage, all of the following might be metaphors Louis uses to describe Shirley EXCEPT:

   A. a cotton mill.

   B. a barnyard.

   C. virgin timber.

   D. a quiet stream.

53. The writer of this passage opposes the opinion of all of the following EXCEPT:

   A. Gallagher.

   B. Capuano.

   C. Marx.

   D. Bodenheimer.

This page intentionally left blank.

SECTION 1
Answer Key

1	B	12	D	23	A	34	B	45	C
2	C	13	C	24	C	35	B	46	A
3	A	14	A	25	C	36	D	47	D
4	C	15	A	26	D	37	C	48	B
5	A	16	D	27	B	38	C	49	B
6	B	17	B	28	D	39	A	50	C
7	B	18	D	29	B	40	B	51	A
8	A	19	A	30	C	41	D	52	D
9	C	20	C	31	C	42	A	53	C
10	A	21	C	32	C	43	C		
11	B	22	D	33	D	44	A		

Passage 1 (Questions 1-7)

The movement of art **away from representation** of things (paintings of people, places, events, etc.) into a wholly abstract presentation undoubtedly reached its **zenith** in the work of the **color field painters**. Exemplified by the work of Mark **Rothko**, color field painting sought to present **color in its pure state**. This purity made the **color itself the subject** of the painting, rather than a tool used to express something else. The cubists, surrealists, and other abstract expressionists working earlier in the 20th century may have distorted, mocked, and radically reduced representation (respectively), but it was the color field artists alone who **completely stripped out** any pretense of **painting** *something* other than the painting itself. Rothko's works consisted of little more than **several large squares of contrasted colors**, in various proportions and arrangements.

Opinion: author thinks that art's movement away from representing things hit its high point with color field and Rothko

Cause and effect: because Rothko painted things like large squares of color he was able to completely remove any representation and make color itself the painting's subject

Those artists who become **best known** for representing a **school of art** – and indeed to those outside the highly specialized world of academic high art become the only known example of the school, their name synonymous with the school itself (**Pollack** and "Drip Painting", **Picasso** and Cubism, **Michelangelo** and high Renaissance fresco, etc.) – achieve their notoriety through no more remarkable means than pursuing a **certain artistic idea to its very core**. The stripping away of every extraneous thought and impulse guided by history and habit leaves the core truth of the movement. One cannot help but wonder, then, why **no artist** in the millennia **before Rothko** sought to pursue **color itself as the subject of painting**. Certainly artists the world over had experimented with how color was represented in their work. Japanese **calligraphy** paintings often reserved color for a single slash near the edge of the scroll. Zen Buddhist **ensō** eschew color altogether – using the purity of a single black circle on white background to represent the empty, open mind that has reached enlightenment. The **fauvists**, on the other hand, used a riot of colors in vibrant, jarring juxtaposition.

Key terms: Pollack, Picasso, Michelangelo, calligraphy, ensō, fauvists

Cause and effect: taking one idea and stripping it down to its essence is what makes an artist best known for a certain school of art

Opinion: author wonders why nobody before Rothko made color itself the subject of the painting

In each case, the **color** (or lack thereof) **merely enhanced or commented** on the representational efforts of the rest of the composition. Every work we find still relied on line, form,

movement, space, perspective, and all the **usual tools of a painter** to **represent** a particular thing or idea.

Opinion: author thinks in works before Rothko, color "merely" enhanced a work that was still basically about representing something else

Rothko and the rest of the color field artists **broke away from every one of these conventions** by removing more and more until **only color remained**. The typical color field composition had **few if any lines or forms**, and what forms there are – the boundaries between the different colors – are typically blurred and incoherent. This total lack of form permits **no interpretation** by the viewer of the painting as **being "of something"**.

Cause and effect: color field painters stripped away line, form, etc. to create a painting that was only about color and could not be a painting "of something"

And yet when the **literature around color field art** was being written in the 1970's and 1980's, we consistently see that both **erudite** critics and **casual** observers spoke of Rothko's work in terms of representations beyond color itself. The painting *No. 61 (Rust and Blue)* is simply three horizontal rectangles of color – rust red, light blue, and navy blue. The colors are mottled, a result of the staining technique used. The boundaries between the rectangles are blurred and inconsistent. **No painting could more clearly be about the colors themselves.** However, in instance after instance, **observers** wrote of *No. 61* as **evoking** the ocean at sunset, the haze over a lake, the pre-dawn light seen through closed eyelids, etc.

Contrast: author thinks color field art, especially *No. 61* is purely about color, but other observers always talked about the painting representing other things like the ocean

Perhaps **pure color is an ungraspable** phantom. Even when presented in its purest form, it seems that most observers are unable to accept the work as it is, and **ever seek for representation**.

Opinion: author speculates that people may need to see representation in artistic works and that we can't accept a painting that is only about color

Main Idea: Color field painters, especially Rothko, were the first in the history of art to make paintings that were solely about color itself, rather than an attempt to use color to represent something else; they did this by stripping away line, form, and all the other tools normally used by painters; despite these efforts observers continue to see color field paintings as being paintings that represent something.

1. B is correct. The author tells us in the final two paragraphs that, even in the case of paintings the author sees as unambiguously about nothing more than color itself, viewers still wanted to see the paintings as representing something else. Rothko's blue squares were interpreted as the ocean or the light over a lake, etc. The author suggests at the end that we always seem to look for representation in our paintings.

   A: Given that color field art is relatively new in the art world, it's much more likely that most painters are painting representation, not pure color like the color field artists.

   C: Rothko painted pure color, not an attempt to represent something.

   D: Even the color field artists are still being interpreted as representations of something.

2. C is correct. The author introduces the main theme in the first paragraph, telling us that color field artists focused on creating paintings in which color itself was the subject of the painting. He then emphasizes further down the passage that the color field artists were unprecedented in that regard.

   A: The passage only mentions the Buddhist painters in passing as a supporting detail.

   B: The author himself seems to think he can interpret Rothko's work as pure color, so it is too extreme to say that it is impossible for "any human" to view a painting as pure color.

   D: While the author does discuss the history of art, the focus is strongly on the color field artists and Rothko in particular.

3. A is correct. Throughout the passage the author emphasizes that the color field painters were unique in breaking wholly with any traditional representation or the tools of representation (line, form, etc.). Thus, before Rothko and the other color field painters, other artists were not making paintings that were solely about color itself.

   B, C: Neither of these statements are found anywhere in the passage.

   D: This is the opposite of the passage, as it was Rothko's breakthrough to make color itself the sole thing that the painting was an image of.

4. C is correct. After stating that a single artist could come to serve as the symbol of an entire movement, the author provides a series of three specific examples.

   A: The author provides support in the form of examples.

B: The claim is given support in the passage and that support could, in theory, be empirically investigated (by, for example, asking members of the public to name the artist who worked in a given field of art).

D: The main thesis could still be true even if Rothko was not the most famous color field artist; the author is more concerned with color field art in general than whether or not Rothko was, in fact, the best example.

5. A is correct. The author tells us that artists can gain their fame simply by pursuing a particular artistic idea to its extreme, final conclusion. Thus, in the case of abstract art and a focus on color, Rothko succeeded by totally stripping away all historical ties to representation – shedding line, form, etc., leaving behind pure color.

   B: Nothing in the passage suggests that Rothko was using traditional oil painting techniques.

   C: Rothko got rid of line and form; he didn't meld it into his work.

   D: The passage never discusses other cultural contexts.

6. B is correct. Part of what the author finds so remarkable is that no artists in the millennia preceding Rothko simply created painting that was about color itself, and that it was left to the color field artists to make paintings that were solely about color itself. If a new trove of paintings showed that other artists in the prior century had done just that, then the author's contention would be wrong.

   A: Since this collection of works was recently rediscovered, it would not have been part of the art history that Rothko would have known about and set aside. Thus the new discovery is irrelevant to this statement.

   C, D: Nothing in the passage or the question tells us how audiences in Germany reacted to the newly-discovered works.

7. B is correct. The passage tells us that viewers insisted on seeing Rothko's color field paintings as being paintings of something when the author (and presumably Rothko himself) sees the work as being meditations on pure color and not of anything. Similarly, a film that has no plot at all and no narrative would likely be incorrectly interpreted by the audience as attempting to present some sort of narrative.

   A, C: We have no idea if audiences would like the work.

   D: We're being asked to extrapolate the author's reasoning beyond the passage and nothing suggests that the films described would actually be like Rothko's paintings.

Passage 2 (Questions 8 – 12)

The **usual story** about the **invention of paper gives credit to Cai Lun**, an official of the imperial court in Han Dynasty China. Cai Lun's credit as the inventor of paper rests on claims that he was **the first to significantly improve and standardize paper-making**, turning it into a product that could be produced in massive quantities at low cost. Certainly paper-like substances long predate Cai Lun (and even both the Han and Qin dynasties), as Egyptians were writing on papyrus two to three thousand years before the Qin dynasty.

Opinion: the usual story gives the credit for inventing paper to Cai Lun

Cause and effect: because Cai Lun significantly improved paper-making and standardized the method, he gets credit for the modern invention of paper

Cai Lun began his service as a court eunuch in 75 AD, and was promoted in 89 AD to the **official in charge of the manufacture of instruments and weapons**. After the **death of his patron**, Empress Dou, in 97 AD, Cai Lun is said to have **set about working at a feverish pace to craft some invention that would win him the favor of the Emperor** and return him to a position of influence in the court. It would seem that he achieved this in 105 AD upon completing his paper-making technique.

Key terms: official in charge of the manufacture of instruments and weapons

Cause and effect: Cai Lun had a connection with the empress, and after she died he worked hard to come up with a new invention that would return him to power at court

As historian Will **Durant** explains, **Cai Lun perfected a recipe** consisting of bark, hemp, silk, and even chunks of fishing net. The fibers were laid out in sheets and suspended in water. Removing the water, compressing the fibers, and allowing them to dry created a thin matted sheet of paper, which could then be cut into any desired size.

Key terms: Durant

Opinion: Durant believe that Cai Lun perfected a certain recipe and the technique to using it

The relative **simplicity** of the craftsmanship in Cai Lun's method seems to **speak against it requiring any special learning** or great insight. **Simple experimentation would have sufficed** to produced the paper used throughout China in the centuries following Cai Lun's death. Historian Thomas **Carter** posits that **one of Cai Lun's subordinates** of a lower craftsman class is much more likely to have **developed the technique** for which Cai Lun takes credit or that Cai Lun simply **re-discovered an older technique**.

Opinion: Carter thinks Cai Lun re-discovered an older method or took credit for the work of his underlings

Cause and effect: because the paper-making technique credited to Cai Lun was pretty simple, any craftsman doing basic experimentation could have come up with it

Carter's support for his revisionist view of the invention of paper rests on several observations. In 1986, an excavation at the **Fangmatan** site near Tianshui in the Gansu province uncovered a tomb including **fragments of a paper map**. **Dating of artifacts surrounding the tomb** led researchers to assume the paper map was from **early 2nd century BC**. The quality of the paper itself, as well as the ink used, show a craftsmanship very nearly similar to Cai Lun's method. Second, Carter discusses the **huge number of journeyman and apprentices** working under a highly ranked official like Cai Lun. With nearly a hundred journeymen, and double that number of apprentices, the **odds that Cai Lun himself** was the one to make a particular discovery seem **slim**.

Opinion: Carter thinks that odds are one of the journeymen or apprentices discovered paper-making since there were hundreds of them and only one Cai Lun

Cause and effect: because the artifacts in the tomb pre-date Cai Lun by several hundred years, Carter thinks that paper fragment present also pre-dates Cai Lun

Finally, **Carter notices a remarkable dearth of other writings or innovations in Cai Lun's own personal notes** or even in the hagiography that grew up around the man in later years (he became a subject of ancestor worship in the following centuries, with temples dedicated to his honor). **A man with the mind of an experimenter** must have hit on at least **some other developments** in the arts, or at least left behind records of failed attempts in his personal notes. Yet none such seem to exist.

Opinion: Carter thinks the kind of mind that would experiment and discover paper must've also done work on other projects, and the absence of records about such projects implies that Cai Lun wasn't of the inventor mindset

On this final point, **Carter may reach too far**. After all, one may be struck by a single great insight, or have a single great stroke of luck but leave behind no other great inventions. Not all innovators need be an Edison or a Da Vinci. Similarly on the structure of Cai Lun's workshops, **we routinely give credit to inventors and artists who have many working underneath them**. The artist Andy **Warhol** even called his studio a "factory", so repetitive and machine-like was the production of works. Yet we don't worry about the authenticity of such a work being a "real" Warhol, since we recognize and **give credit to the master's guiding hand and insight**.

Opinion: author seems to disagree with Carter on Carter's final two points: a person may legitimately have only a single great innovation or invention, and there's no problem giving credit to the master for the work done in a workshop by various underlings

Main Idea: Although Cai Lun is usually given credit for the invention of paper, some historians challenge this story on the basis of archaeological and other evidence, although the author disputes the validity of this other evidence.

8.   A is correct. In the fourth paragraph we read that the craftsmanship was relatively simple and that Cai Lun's technique could have been found with simple experimentation. Later in the passage, we read that at least one historian thinks that it was one of the craftsmen working under Cai Lun that developed the technique.

B: While the passage calls the technique simple, we're never told that an entirely uneducated person could do it.

C, D: Neither of these ideas are mentioned anywhere in the passage.

9.   C is correct. The third paragraph tells us that, according to Durant, "Cai Lun perfected a recipe". Later in the passage we're told that Carter disputes that Cai Lun was the one who developed the recipe and technique for which he is given credit.

A: Nowhere in the passage is it mentioned that anyone thought Cai Lun's number of craftsmen was unusually large.

B, D: These are points on which the author seems to disagree with Carter. We're not told what Durant would think.

10.   A is correct. In the final paragraph, the author seems to dispute two of the three points that Carter brings up. Since he doesn't dispute Carter's primary archeological evidence, we can infer that the author accepts Carter's basic theory – that Cai Lun should likely not get sole credit for inventing modern paper (after all, paper just like Cai Lun's was found that was hundreds of years older than Cai Lun).

B: The author explicitly shoots down the idea that the absence of other inventions from Cai Lun counts as proof that Cai Lun did not invent paper.

C: Given the time the author devotes to discussing how Carter disputes the usual story, and that the author brings up a piece of archaeological evidence that seems to directly counter that Cai Lun invented paper, it is unlikely that the author disagrees with this view.

11.   B is correct. Carter thinks that Cai Lun should not get credit as the sole inventor of paper, and one of his points is about how it is very likely that one of the craftsmen working under Cai Lun actually developed the new paper-making technique. Thus, generally, it seems that Carter thinks that the person who actually discovers or creates a thing should get credit for it, rather than credit being taken by the master of the workshop.

A: This is the opposite of Carter's view.

C, D: These ideas are never presented in the passage.

12.   D is correct. The passage tells us that archaeologists dated the artifacts in the tomb to several hundred years before the life of Cai Lun. From there we are to suppose that the paper they found was also that old. But if the artifacts were already hundreds of years old before being placed in the tomb, then it is possible that the paper was made after it had been invented by Cai Lun.

A, B, C: These would all strengthen the notion that Cai Lun did not himself invent paper.

Passage 3 (Questions 13 – 18)

In 2013, two **Colorado** men brought a discrimination suit against the **Masterpiece Cakeshop**, saying that the bakery **refused to make their wedding cake** because the couple was **gay**. The baker, Jack **Phillips**, claimed that as a **private businessman**, he had the **right to choose** whom he would or would not serve. However, a **Colorado state judge** ruled that Phillips would **have to provide wedding-related services** to same-sex couples, even though he objects to gay marriage on religious grounds. "At first blush," Administrative Law Judge Robert **Spencer** wrote, "it may seem reasonable that a private business should be able to refuse service to anyone it chooses." Yet this view, Spencer said, does not take into account the **cost to society** and the **hurt caused to persons** who are denied service "simply because of who they are."

Key terms: discrimination suit, same-sex couples, private business, refuse service

Opinion: a private business owner said he had the right to refuse wedding-related services to same-sex couples; judge said cost to society and hurt to gay couples means they would have to provide such services

A similar discrimination case arose in **New Mexico**, when photographers Elaine and Jonathan **Huguenin** refused to photograph a lesbian couple's commitment ceremony in 2006; the New Mexico Supreme Court ruled that state law made their **refusal discriminatory**. The Huguenins' lawyers cited their clients' **First Amendment rights**: as artists, they had a **right to free expression**, and that they should not be obligated to create work that is in contrast with their beliefs. Forcing the photographers, lawyers claimed, to photograph the commitment ceremony is tantamount to **requiring them to express a message with which they don't agree**.

Key terms: similar discrimination case, First Amendment rights, free expression

Cause and effect: the photographers said that forcing them to provide service to a same-sex couple was in violation of their First Amendment rights

Both of these cases have brought to the fore the **complex legal issues** of whether **individual businesspeople** are required to provide **wedding-related** goods or services to same-sex couples. Gay rights advocates say that the cases are in line with **public accommodation laws**, which ban discrimination based on sexual orientation. Many religious-liberty advocates, however, assert that state public accommodation laws – which originated in the 1960s to prevent discrimination based on race but have grown to include discrimination based on gender and marital status – **were not designed with same-sex marriage in mind**.

Key term: public accommodation laws

Opinion: religious liberty advocates say public accommodation laws don't apply

Some conservatives have tried to take a **spurious "middle ground**," asserting that the private businesspeople, such as baker Jack Phillips and photographers Elaine and Jonathan Huguenin, are not refusing to serve gay people per se, but are **taking a stand against gay marriage**. In an interview, Phillips said that he would have "no problem" baking cupcakes for a gay person's birthday party, or serving gay customers who come into his Denver-area shop. The issue, he claims, is not discriminating against gay people – it's about being **forced to support marriage equality**. And these, **Phillips claims, are two different issues**.

Cause and effect: the photographers claim they are taking a stand against gay marriage, which is not the same as discriminating against gay people

Opinion: the author says this is "spurious"

Yet **advocates for the LGBTQ community** say that such thinking represents a moral and legal "slippery slope." **Discrimination is discrimination**, one gay-rights advocate said; saying that it's OK to refuse to make a wedding cake or take wedding photos might lead to efforts to refuse housing to same-sex couples or to terminate gay, lesbian or transgender employees. So far, the **courts seem to largely agree**, and as of May 2014, more than half of Americans express support for marriage equality. As same-sex marriage becomes more familiar, perhaps fewer businesspeople will claim their **questionable right to refuse service to gay** customers by any rationale.

Cause and effect: gay rights advocates say allowing any discrimination may lead to more discrimination

Opinion: author is coming down pretty clearly in favor of the position of the LGBTQ community, calling the right to refuse service to such people "questionable"

Main Idea: Two cases are presented that challenge private business owners' obligation to provide services to same-sex couples using two different rationales, but the author seems to strongly express that neither is valid.

13. C is correct. The arguments against same-sex marriage put forth by "religious-liberty advocates" appear in paragraph 3; the thought is that the public accommodation laws that protect against discrimination based on race, gender, and marital status do not apply to the case of same-sex marriage.

14. A is correct. In paragraph 4, we hear the argument that taking a stand against gay marriage is not the same thing as discriminating against gays. Choice A is analogous in saying that taking a stand against inter-racial marriage is not the same thing as discriminating against people of other races.

   B: The contrast between what's legal and what's encouraged is not discussed by the author.

   C: This gets it backwards by saying that the person is prejudiced but may not act in a prejudiced way.

   D: The analogy in the passage only relates to differing attitudes about a single class of people, not attitudes across different groups of people (gay couples vs inter-racial couples).

15. A is correct. The First Amendment rights alluded to in Paragraph 2 center on freedom of expression; in this case, refusing to express that which one does not believe. A schoolchild refusing to say the Pledge of Allegiance is a similar situation.

   B, C: These choices don't relate to First Amendment rights.

   D: The taxi driver is discriminating against a same-sex couple, but this is more related to the private business exemption situation than the First Amendment case.

16. D is correct. You have to dig a little bit to get the author's opinion, but you can find it in Paragraphs 4 and 5: in 4, the author calls the "middle ground" point of view "spurious," or false. And in Paragraph 5, the last two sentences express the author's view that the right to refuse service for any reason is "questionable."

   A: No evidence is presented that the author supports this under any circumstances.

   B: Neither private business nor First Amendment arguments are supported.

   C: Proponents of same-sex marriage say these laws already do prohibit discrimination.

17. B is correct. The only choice that is not mentioned in the passage is choice B; in fact, the last paragraph says that both the courts and the majority of Americans support marriage equality.

18. D is correct. The private business exemption argument says the owner of a private business has the right to choose whom he or she serves.

A: First Amendment rights is another argument, pertaining to the case of the photographers in Paragraph 2.

B: The passage doesn't mention any exemptions in hiring practices.

C: This choice gives the ruling that the private business owners are rebelling against.

Passage 4 (Questions 19 – 25)

Aristotle was a student of **Plato** and he always remembered it, as the best students do, in order to oppose him. For some years he taught Philip's son, the future **Alexander the Great**, and for many years he taught in **Athens**. After Alexander's death, he became the target of **the eternal accusation of impiety** that plagues so many great minds, so he retired to Chalcis, where he died. Before all else, Aristotle was an educated man. He desired to embrace **the entirety of the knowledge of his time**, which at that time was actually possible, albeit with prodigious effort, and he succeeded, his **countless works** being a testament.

Key terms: Aristotle, Plato, Alexander the Great, Athens

Cause and effect: because he pursued his desire of embracing the entirety of the knowledge of his time with prodigious effort, he succeeded, and his countless works are proof

His works are the **summa** of all **the sciences** of his epoch, but here, we shall occupy ourselves primarily with his **philosophical ideas**. To Aristotle, and just as it was to Plato, but more precisely, man is composed of **body** and **soul**. The **body** is a well-made **machine**, consisting of organs, and the **soul** is its **final purpose**. Together, the two form a continuous harmony. The body results in the soul, and in turn, the soul acts on the body, and is in not its end but its means of acting upon things. The **faculties of the soul** are both its **diverse** aspects and its diverse methods of acting, for the soul is indivisibly one.

Cause and effect: the body is not the end of the soul (what the soul wants), but rather, the soul's means of acting upon things

Contrast: the soul is one but the faculties of the soul are diverse

Reason refers to the **soul being able to conceive what is most general**, and therefore it is the intermediary between ourselves and **God**. God is unique, eternal, and from all eternity gave motion to matter. He is **purely spiritual** and all else besides him is purely material. Unlike Plato, Aristotle believes that **God does not have ideas**, or immaterial living personifications, residing in his bosom. It is here that we may note, from Plato to Aristotle, **progress towards monotheism**: Plato's Olympus of ideas was still a kind of polytheism. Aristotle's work contained no such polytheism.

Contrast: God is purely spiritual vs all else is purely material, Plato's notion of God having ideas within him vs Aristotle not

Cause and effect: because Aristotle does not believe in Plato's "Olympus of ideas," Aristotle represents progress away from polytheism and towards monotheism

Aristotle's **moral system sometimes approaches Plato's**, like when he claims that supreme happiness is the supreme good, and that the supreme good is the contemplation of thought by thought, this being completely self-sufficient.

This is approximately the imitation of God recommended by Plato. Sometimes, on the contrary, **it is very practical and nearly mediocre**, like when he claims morality to be a **mean between extremes**, a certain tact, an art rather than a science, being of practical science rather than of conscience.

Contrast: when Aristotle claims that supreme happiness is the supreme good and that the supreme is contemplation of thought by thought, his moral system approaches Plato's; when Aristotle claims morality to be a mean between extremes, his moral system can be quite practical and nearly mediocre

His **political philosophy** is very **confused**, perhaps because the volume containing it was likely **composed after his death** from passages and fragments of different lectures. In general, it is a review of the divergent political constitutions that existed in his time throughout the Greek world. His **tendencies** in political philosophy, for there are no conclusions in this work, are notably **aristocratic**, but less so than those of Plato.

Cause and effect: because the volume containing his political philosophy was likely composed posthumously from different sources, Aristotle's political philosophy is very confused

Because of his **universality**, his **clarity**, and because he frequently dogmatizes instead of discussing and collating, Aristotle had a **greater authority throughout antiquity and the Middle Ages** than Plato. In fact, this authority became despotic and nearly sacrosanct, except on matters of faith. By the time of the **sixteenth century**, he was relegated to his **due esteem**: lower than sacrosanct, but still quite high, for he is often regarded among the **geniuses of widest range**, if not of greatest power. Even today, he is far from having lost significance. For some, he functions as a **bridge** between the subtle yet always poetic **Greek** genius and the **Roman** genius, more positive, more plain, more practical, more attached to reality, and more grounded in pure science.

Key terms: antiquity, Middle Ages, Greek genius, Roman genius

Cause and effect: because of Aristotle's clarity, and propensity for dogmatization, he had a greater authority up to the Middle Ages; because of his range and the nature of his work, he serves as a bridge between the Greek genius and the Roman genius

Opinion: author thinks Aristotle should be highly esteemed but that he was *too* highly esteemed in the past

Main Idea: The author gives us a brief summary of Aristotle's life and work, paying attention mainly to his philosophical work; Aristotle is often compared with his famous teacher, Plato; the author leaves us with a description of Aristotle's legacy, lessened from its zenith, but still very significant.

19. A is correct. As the author writes at the beginning of the third paragraph, "Reason refers to the soul being able to conceive what is most general . . ." And, as the soul, in Aristotle's conception, is indivisible, this is not a part of the soul, but rather, the soul viewed in a particular way.

    B: Soul cannot be divided up.

    C, D: These are never said. Rather, it is a meeting point between the divine and the human.

20. C is correct. The very first words of the passage are: "Aristotle was a student of Plato." For the purposes of studying Aristotle, and though he does diverge, one must view him as following in Plato's footsteps. Within the context of Aristotle's work, we study Aristotle, but also Plato. Within the context of Plato's work, we study Plato and Socrates (who is, admittedly, harder to study, as he never wrote anything).

    A: Rather, the author writes that Aristotle's moral system "sometimes approaches Plato's," implying it is not as thoroughly sound.

    B: Certainly Aristotle is not entirely derivative, and definitely not in morality, for his golden mean approach to philosophy differs from Plato's. There are enough differences between the two to say that Aristotle is not totally derivative of Plato.

    D: Though he does account for Aristotle wanting to oppose his teacher, it does not seem the author believes this to be the case for all of Aristotle's work.

21. C is correct. As the author writes, Aristotle's authority became despotic and nearly sacrosanct in antiquity and the Middle Ages, except in terms of religion. This implies that all of his pursuits, save religion, were taken very seriously. This then would include his political philosophy, even though the author regards it as confusing. By the sixteenth century, his influence was tamped down a bit, and politics would be included in this as well.

    A: The key phrase here is, "except on matters of faith." The author undermines only Aristotle's take on religion in terms of the influence during the Middle Ages.

    B: Rather, less.

    D: Well, even though Aristotle's conception of religion was not very influential in the Middle Ages, it was likely more influential than Plato's polytheism.

22. D is correct. At the end of the first paragraph, the author tells us that Aristotle sought to embrace all the known knowledge of his time, and he succeeded, with his works being the testament. Therefore, these works contain at least some mention of all the known knowledge of his time. He did not create this knowledge, he rather took it in, learned about it, and wrote about it. Therefore, his work was a summary of the knowledge of his time.

    A: The author concedes that Aristotle is considered as being among geniuses with the widest range, and not necessarily with the greatest power. Therefore, summary is more appropriate than greatest.

    B: Collection more assumes that Aristotle took all the known work in the world and put it together. More apt to say he summarized it.

    C: This is similar to Choice A. Since two answer choices can't both be right, you could eliminate both A and C as being nearly synonymous.

23. A is correct. Again, Aristotle is considered "among the geniuses with the widest range, if not of greatest power." So, the more impressive of the two is his range, not his power in any one subject, philosophy included.

    B: We know that Aristotle's writings on religion were not influential.

    C: Rather, it has all lessened in influence.

    D: The descriptions of Greek and Roman genius are reversed here.

24. C is correct. The author never claims this as a similarity between the two. In fact, he considers it one of the areas where Aristotle's philosophy is actually mediocre in comparison to Plato's.

    A, B, D: These are all true. Choice D may be the most confusing of the three, but both believe in one God, though in Plato's conception, that one God contains "ideas" which constitute a polytheism.

25. C is correct. II: This is true because, as the author writes, "To Aristotle, and just as it was to Plato, but more precisely, man is composed of body and soul." Therefore, Aristotle's conception was more precise and Plato's more vague. III: This is true because, as the author writes, "Aristotle's moral system sometimes approaches Plato's." This implies that Plato's was greater overall.

    I: This is false because Plato does not espouse a pantheon of Gods as much as one God who contains "ideas."

Passage 5 (Questions 26 – 30)

James **Olney's** discussion of **two distinct forms of autobiography** is useful in order to distinguish between **Hemingway's** and **Gaines's** writings. On the one hand, Olney describes a particularly **Western** tendency "to take the life of the **self** to be the true self, the real self, the life about which an autobiography should be written" ("Value" 53). This form of autobiography Olney calls "**autoautography**." **Hemingway** seems to be an **especially strong representative** of this form of life-writing. Even though not strictly autobiographical, his works, even *For Whom the Bell Tolls* in spite of Robert Jordan's transformation, remain **focused on the individual**. Hemingway can therefore be said to represent the Western tradition that takes the self to be at the center of life. Stressing the singularity of each character's life, Hemingway's works reflect renewed attempts to portray his own struggle, to give expression to his own inner confusion.

Opinion: the author thinks that Hemingway's writing is an example of Olney's autoautography

Contrast: there is a difference between Hemingway and Gaines's writing – they are different forms of autobiography; Western autobiography's focus on the individual is different from autobiography in other parts of the world

Certainly, Olney's definition of the **autobiographical act** applies to Hemingway: "The autobiographical act . . . [is] a perpetually renewed attempt to **find language adequate to rendering the self** and its experience, an attempt that includes within itself all earlier attempts" (Memory 9). Read as such, **Hemingway's miscellaneous works**, his short stories, novels, autobiographical writings, and travel accounts provide us with intriguing **insights into the man** behind the pen, as they "bring forth ever different memorial configurations and an ever newly shaped self" (Memory 20). If we read Hemingway's works as instances of life-writing, we thus arrive at a **composite picture of one man**, starting with the fear of night and mortality as a boy in "Three Shots," continuing with his attempts as a man to create an identity in various countries, while always attempting to come to terms with the father, and ending with the old fisherman's proven heroism even as he loses the prize (marlin). Always the focus is on one individual's struggle— the man himself behind the pen.

Opinion: the author of the piece thinks Hemingway's writing provides readers with insights into his life

Cause and effect: if looked at as life-writing, then Hemingway's works can tell us a lot about the man

In this context, Michel de **Montaigne**, who writes of the "**consubstantial**" process of **self** creation and **book creation**, comes to mind: "I have no more made my book than my book has made me—a book consubstantial with its author, concerned with my own self, an integral part of my life" (504). We can therefore ask whether Hemingway's writing about his own experiences and the concomitant public myths he created also "made" him in the same way. Did

not Hemingway in **writing about his various exploits**— as a wounded war hero, as a skilled hunter, as an expert fisherman—"**fashion and compose**" himself so often that "the model itself has to some extent grown firm and taken shape," as it has in Montaigne's case (504)? Was he not afterwards trying to live up to the myths that he created with the thinly disguised self-portrayals in his works? Are not the agonizing and sorrowful thoughts of Nick Adams in "Fathers and Sons" the writer's own with regard to his alienation from his father and his sons?

Opinion: the author of the piece thinks that Hemingway's writing both shaped who Hemingway was and influenced Hemingway's actions

Cause and effect: Michel de Montaigne's consubstantial process of self creation is one of cause and effect moving in two directions; the creation of the book affects the creation of self, and the creation of self affects the creation of the book

These questions seem to be bound up with the pervasive emphasis on the self and the cyclical view of life that we see manifested in Hemingway's work and life. Hemingway's writings are an "involuted and reflexive exercise," as the writer constantly looks inward, toward his own self (Olney, "Value" 53). Whereas Hemingway's writings are firmly situated in the Western tradition of autoautography, Ernest **Gaines's** works can be seen as representing a more **African** notion of autobiography. Referring to the **Sonjo** people in Tanzania, John **Mbiti** explains that "the **individual** is united with the rest of his **community**, both the living and the dead, and humanly speaking nothing can separate him from this corporate society" (117). Reminiscent of Jefferson's "'lowly as I am, I am still part of the whole'" in *A Lesson Before Dying* (LBD 194), the Sonjo exclaim, "'**I am because we are**, and since we are, therefore I am'" (Mbiti 117).

Opinion: the Sonjo people of Tanzania think individuals cannot be separated from the larger society which consists both of the living and the dead

Contrast: Gaine's works reflect African autobiographical practices which are more focused on the group, as opposed to Hemingway's works which reflect the Western tradition's focus on the individual

Main Idea: Olney describes two forms of autobiography, one by Hemingway in the Western tradition in which autobiography is about the individual, and one by Gaines in the African tradition in which autobiography includes the community; Hemingway's process of writing meant that he was creating a book at the same time as he was creating himself, as described by Montaigne's consubstantial process.

26. D is correct. We must consider: would the Western focus on the individual mean independence is handled differently or similarly than the motif would be handled in the African traditions' focus on the community? The correct choice is choice D because the Western and African traditions would likely approach each of these motifs differently, so the authors, following their

traditions would handle them differently. A focus on the individual would mean different things in terms of independence (I), identity (II), and memory (III) compared to a focus on the community. Each of these motifs would be tied to the community.

27.   B is correct. In the passage, the autobiographical act is defined as the "perpetually renewed attempt to find language adequate to rendering the self and its experience, an attempt that includes within itself all earlier attempts." The repetition of the wrestling with the same issues in changing scenarios is an example of renewed attempts to find language to render the self and its experiences.

   A: In the passage the consubstantial process is defined as process of self creation and book creation. This concept does not necessarily include revisiting the same issues under different lights and changing scenarios.

   C, D: The author indicates that Hemingway is writing in the Western Tradition (C. of autobiography, with its focus on the individual, and Gaines is writing in the African tradition of autobiography, with its focus on the community. The correct answer has to be a concept that both authors are employing in their writing.

28.   D is correct. It is incompatible with the author's claims about the consubstantial process, specifically the claim that Hemingway was trying to live up to the myths that he created with the thinly disguised self-portrayals in his works.

   A: The author claims the agonizing and sorrowful thoughts of Nick Adams in "Fathers and Sons" are the writer's own with regard to his alienation from his father and his sons, which would be compatible with choice A.

   B: The author claims that reading "Hemingway's miscellaneous works, his short stories, novels, autobiographical writings, and travel accounts provide us with intriguing insights into the man behind the pen." Although the author might not claim that the works must be read as a whole, this claim is still more compatible with the author's existing claims than choice D.

   C: The author claims, "If we read Hemingway's works as instances of life-writing, we thus arrive at a composite picture of one man," and "Did not Hemingway in writing about his various exploits— as a wounded war hero, as a skilled hunter, as an expert fisherman," which are compatible with the claim in choice C.

29.   B is correct. It best illustrates the Sonjo belief that the individual is united with the rest of his community, both living and dead, and nothing can separate him from this corporate society.

   A: This choice does not incorporate the aspect of the Sonjo belief that Jefferson is united with both the living and the dead. In this example, Jefferson only realizes his connection to the living community.

   C: This choice does not incorporate the aspect of the Sonjo belief that Philip Martin is part of a corporate society. While this example addresses the past and the future, the focus is on Philip Martin himself and not the community or his connection to it.

   D: This choice does not incorporate the aspect of the Sonjo belief that the community consists of the living AND the dead. In this example, the diary only serves to influence the future community, and there is no mention of the past community.

30.   C is correct. The implication of this claim is that Gaines was writing in the Western tradition of autobiography rather than in the African tradition of autobiography, which would contradict the author's claim that Gaines wrote in the African tradition.

   A: The claim does not contradict the author's argument. Certainly Hemingway's novels and characters are fictional, but that doesn't stop them from being a form of an autobiographical work as described in the passage.

   B: The claim, and any of its implications, do not necessarily contradict the author's argument. It could be possible for Gaines to have been influenced by Hemingway and for the author's claim that Gaines wrote in the African tradition of autobiography to still be true.

   D: The claim, and any of its implications, are irrelevant to the author's argument. It would not be necessary for the writers' to have intentionally written autobiographically. The author claims that if we look at their writings as instances of life-writing (autobiographical) we can make the following argument, so the argument is not contingent on whether the authors intended their works to be read this way or not.

Passage 6 (Questions 31 – 36)

The **organ** is more than a single instrument. It is an **orchestra**, a collection of the pipes of Pan of every size, from those as small as a child's playthings to those as gigantic as the columns of a temple. Each one corresponds to what is termed an **organ-stop**. The number is unlimited. The compass of the organ far surpasses that of all the instruments of the orchestra. The violin notes alone reach the same height, but with little carrying power. As for the lower tones, there is no competitor of the thirty-two-foot pipes, which go two octaves below the violoncello's low C. Between the *pianissimo* which almost reaches the limit where sound ceases and silence begins, down to a range of formidable and terrifying power, **every degree of intensity** can be obtained from this magical instrument. The **variety of its timbre** is broad. There are flute stops of various kinds; tonal stops that approximate the timbre of stringed instruments; stops which serve to imitate the instruments of the orchestra. Then we have the **innumerable combinations** of all these different stops, with the gradations that may be obtained through indefinite commingling of the tones of this marvelous palette.

Key terms: organ, organ-stop, timbre

Opinion: the organ has the range and timbre of the entire orchestra; it is virtually limitless in its potential

Let us have the courage to admit, however, that these **resources are only partly utilized** as they can or should be. The organ places before the organist extraordinary means of expressing himself. The organ is a theme with innumerable variations, determined by the **place** in which it is to be installed, by the amount of **money** at the builder's disposal, by his **inventiveness**, and, often, by his personal **whims**. As a result **time is required for the organist to learn his instrument** thoroughly. After this he is as free as the fish in the sea. Then, to play freely with the colors on his vast palette, there is but one way—he **must** plunge boldly into **improvisation**.

Opinion: improvisation would allow the organist to take full advantage of the organ's innumerable resources

Cause and effect: Despite its huge potential, the organ is rarely utilized as it could be; the organ's function can vary based on place, money, inventiveness, and whim of the player

Under the pretext that an **improvisation is not so good** as one of Sebastian Bach's or Mendelssohn's masterpieces, young organists have **stopped improvising**. That point of view is harmful because it is absolutely false; it is simply the negation of eloquence. Consider what the legislative hall, the lecture room and the court would be like if nothing but set pieces were delivered. We are familiar with the fact that **many an orator** and lawyer, who is **brilliant when he talks**, becomes **dry as dust** when he tries to **write**. The same thing happens in **music**. As one touches the organ, the **imagination is awakened**, and the unforeseen rises from the depths of the unconscious. It is a world of its own, ever new, which

will never be seen again, and which comes out of the darkness, as an enchanted island comes from the sea.

Opinion: many people think that improvisation is inferior to playing works of great composers

Contrast: while written music (and words) can be dry, improvisation is new and thrilling

Instead of this fairyland, we too often see only some of Sebastian **Bach's** or **Mendelssohn's** pieces repeated continuously. The **pieces** themselves are very fine, but they **belong to concerts** and are entirely out of place in church services. Furthermore, they were **written for old instruments** and they apply either not at all, or badly, to the modern organ. Yet there are those who think this belief spells progress.

Opinion: Bach's and Mendelssohn's compositions are good, but suitable for concerts, not church

I am fully aware of what may be said against improvisation. A **mediocre improvisation is always endurable**, if the **organist** has grasped the idea that church music should harmonize with the service and **aid meditation and prayer**. If the organ music is **played in this spirit** and results in harmonious sounds rather than in precise music which is not worth writing out, it still is comparable with the old glass windows in which the individual figures can hardly be distinguished but which are, nevertheless, more charming than the finest modern windows. Such an improvisation may be **better than a fugue by a great master**, on the principle that nothing in art is good unless it is **in its proper place**.

Opinion: improvisation is good enough if it results in harmonious sounds that aid in prayer

Contrast: precise music is less important than the spirit of the music

Main Idea: The organ is an instrument with amazing possibility, but to be player properly the organist must engage in improvisation of work in a way that fits with the meditation and prayer of a church service, rather than simply repeating the old fugues of the great masters.

31. C is correct. Use the context to get the meaning of "compass," as used in the first paragraph. Immediately after using the word, the author describes the high notes of the violin and the low tones of the thirty-two-foot pipes – meaning, how high the high notes are, and how low the low notes.

32. C is correct. In paragraph 3, the author makes the point that the compositions of Bach and Mendelssohn are "very fine," but more suited to a concert hall than to a church.

A: This is tricky; clearly the author thinks that it is through improvisation that the organ truly displays its gifts. But he never criticizes the works of these two composers for failing to express the organ's compass, or tonal range.

B, D: How the pieces of these masters are played is never an issue.

33. D is correct. Paragraph 1 describes the organ's suitability for improvisation (choice A), its breadth of timbres (choice B), its range of volume (choice C). The only quality NOT mentioned in the passage is its "difficulty".

34. B is correct. Look at the first two sentences of the paragraph 5. First, the author says he knows what critics find problematic with improvisation. Then, he immediately admits that mediocre improvisations are always endurable, given certain conditions. What can you surmise, then, that critics find faulty with improvisation? That it's often mediocre.

35. B is correct. In paragraph 2 the author draws a parallel; just like a preacher or lawyer might speak brilliantly but produce an uninspired written work, so might the organist shine in improvising, but lose his or her "magic" in trying to commit music to the page.

  A: Quite the opposite – the author argues that improvised music can, in its appropriate setting – be as captivating as the music of the masters.

  C: This distorts the point the author is making through the analogy: it's that SOME orators and SOME musicians do better winging it – not that all sorts of composed materials are necessarily dull.

  D: Actually, the author is making the point that improvised speaking and improvised music can both be rousing.

36. D is correct. Look to paragraph 5 for the answer to this one. There, the author says that even if the music is not precise – not technically perfect – it may still be suitable if it harmonizes with the church service and aids in meditation and prayer. Furthermore, the passage's final sentence notes that all good art is "in its proper place."

Passage 7 (Questions 37 – 42)

Salmonella bacteria infects over a million people in this country each year; more Americans die from its effects than from any other food-borne illness. Salmonella is **shockingly prevalent** in our food: a recent study by the U.S. Department of Agriculture found that nearly a **quarter of all packaged chicken parts** are contaminated by some form of it. But if you thought that such a high degree of contamination would be in violation of **federal food safety laws**, you would be mistaken. There is **no set standard** for the amount of allowable salmonella contamination in cut up chicken parts, for example, or for numerous other meats, such as lamb chops and pork ribs. This means that one hundred percent of these products may be **contaminated**, with **no penalty** to the producer. Some products do have performance standards, but few consumers would find them reassuring: the allowable percentage of salmonella contamination in ground turkey, for example, is 49.9 percent.

Key words: salmonella, prevalent, federal food safety laws

Cause and effect: much of our food is contaminated by salmonella; a million people are sickened by its effects each year; due to lack of standards there is no penalty for salmonella contamination

The **oversight mechanisms** for food safety are somewhat **arcane**. Fifteen different agencies are responsible for the safety of our food. The two most important of these are the U.S. Department of Agriculture's Food Safety and Inspection Service, or **FSIS,** and the Food and Drug Administration, or **FDA,** which is a division of the federal Department of Human Services. Adding to the problem are the limitations on the two agencies' authority. Even when an agency finds that the allowable limits of contamination are exceeded, the **only option** it has is to **request** that the producers **remove** the product voluntarily. Moreover, the agencies may **only** do this when they have proof, usually in the form of a **genetic match**, that a particular product is making consumers sick. If a consumer has eaten the tainted chicken (for example) and discarded the packaging, it is nearly impossible for the oversight agencies to request a **recall**.

Key words: oversight mechanisms, FSIS, FDA, recall

Contrast: while many agencies oversee food safety, such agencies cannot actually force producers to recall tainted food

Opinion: the author thinks the oversight mechanisms are unclear

One particular outbreak of salmonella contamination illustrates this. Over the course of 17 months in 2013 and 2014, over 600 people reported severe illness that was linked to chicken tainted with salmonella **Heidelberg,** an especially **virulent strain** of the bacterium. Although the FSIS tracked down over a hundred patients who had eaten chicken from one producer, **Foster Farms,** and had become ill, they were unable to make a **genetic match** until a year after the out-

break began. The match allowed the government to request that Foster Farms recall chicken produced in certain facilities. Foster Farms complied – but **only withdrew chicken produced in a six-day period**. The rest remained in the market. Since some scientists estimate that for every reported case of salmonella, 29 go unreported, it is likely that the tainted Foster Farms chicken had **sickened nearly 18,000 people**.

Key words: Foster Farms, genetic match

Cause and effect: FSIS was able to trace over a hundred cases of food-borne illness to Foster Farms and make a genetic match, thereby allowing a request for a recall

Food safety advocates and lawyers say that the system is clearly broken, but that relatively **simple changes** in the production process would **vastly improve the safety** of our food. They point to **Denmark**, where after a spate of salmonella cases in the 1980s, the Danish government enacted changes in processing that were extremely effective. The new regulations dictate that poultry workers are required to wash their hands before entering the plant and to perform extensive microbiological testing. More important, though, is that as soon as a pathogen is found, **recalls are imposed** on the producers. As a result of these changes, **less than two percent** of poultry in **Denmark** is **contaminated** with salmonella.

Key words: food safety advocates, Denmark, recalls are imposed

Opinion: food safety advocates see a big problem in the oversight system

Contrast: in Denmark, oversight agencies can require recalls if contamination is found, but U.S. officials may only request voluntary recalls

It would be relatively **simple** for the United States to **follow Denmark's example**, as have several other European countries, to great effect. But for this to happen, the USDA would have to emphasize its **regulatory function** and role as protector of the people, and de-emphasize its current focus, which is to advance the interests of big agriculture. Unless that happens, millions will suffer needlessly.

Key words: Denmark's example, regulatory function

Opinion: the author thinks that the USDA needs to focus more on consumer safety and less on the interest of big producers

Main Idea: Because regulations regarding food safety and salmonella contamination are complicated and ineffective, salmonella contamination is a much bigger problem in the US than it is in Denmark and other countries that have followed Denmark's example, and these regulations need to be changed to protect the health of consumers.

37. C is correct. Use the context to get the meaning here. We're told there are 15 different oversight agencies,

different acceptable levels of contamination for different foods, and some situations – but not others – in which agencies can call for recalls of tainted food.

38. C is correct. In paragraph 2, we're told that if a clear genetic match can be made between tainted food that's gotten a consumer sick and a specific producer, the best option the regulatory agencies have is to request that the producer recall the product.

   A: According to the passage, there are no circumstances in which a producer is required to recall tainted meat.

   B: The passage notes that this is required in Denmark – but not in the U.S.

   D: The agencies can request a voluntary recall.

39. A is correct. The author is overtly critical of the food safety system in the US, and calls for change (quite clearly in the passage's final paragraph).

   B: No, the author seems to think that food-borne illness is widespread, due in part to lax safety regulations.

   C: This is beyond the scope of the passage, as the author is concerned with US food safety, not the whole world.

   D: While the author probably thinks educating consumers is important, this passage focuses on regulatory agencies.

40. B is correct. The key difference is that Denmark requires a mandatory recall of tainted food, but the U.S. merely requests that the producer of tainted food recall the food in question.

   A: We don't know whether or not the U.S. requires microbiological testing.

   C: We also don't know how many regulatory agencies are active in Denmark.

   D: Nor do we know whether Danish agencies consider the interests of the producers – it's not mentioned in the passage.

41. D is correct. The first paragraph tells us that some foods have performance standards, and some don't.

42. A is correct. The case of the tainted chicken produced by Foster Farms is an example of how hard it is to control an outbreak because of problems with the current regulations. Notice how the paragraph regarding Foster Farms starts, by the way – telling us it is an example of the problem discussed in the previous paragraph.

Passage 8 (Questions 43 – 47)

The **health care services sector** is a large and growing segment of the economy. The share of GDP devoted to health care services has doubled over the past 25 years, to **16 percent** in 2005. Looking ahead, this growth is expected to continue, as **aging baby boomers continue to increase the share of elderly** in the population, a segment of the population that accounts for a disproportionately high level of expenditures on health.

Key terms: health care services sector, 16 percent, baby boomers

Cause and effect: health care expenditures are expected to be increasing due to aging baby boomers

The rising health care costs have raised questions about whether these medical expenditures are, in some sense, worth it. A natural starting point is to ask how much of the rising costs represent increases in **real services** vs **price inflation**, a question that can be addressed using **price deflators** or **indices**. However, studies in the health economics literature have raised questions about the use of standard price indices for this purpose and their empirical findings suggest that some of what is currently recorded as price increases actually represents increases in services.

Key terms: real services, price inflation, price deflators, indices

Opinions: the author believes that current price indices are not accurate

Contrast: the author starts by asking how much of rising health care costs are due to inflation and how much is the cost increase a result of improved treatments (real services)

Currently-available price indices define the "**good**" or the "**output**" of health care as the **treatment** (i.e., an office visit or prescription drug) and track the prices of those treatments over time. Health economists have long advocated an alternative definition of output as the **bundle of treatments** received by a patient for the treatment of **some condition**. The existing empirical evidence suggests that how one defines the good matters. Detailed case studies of important diseases show that, for these conditions, the **price indices that health economists advocate show slower price growth** than standard indices. This result is consistent with the view that indices that track the prices of individual treatments tend to miss any shifts towards lower-cost treatments that may occur over time. For example, in the treatment of **depression**, there has been a shift away from **talk-therapy** and towards (the lower cost) **drug therapy** that has reduced the cost of treating depression. Because standard indices track prices for these two types of treatments separately, they miss this substitution and overstate the cost of treating depression.

Contrast: the price indices currently available are often overestimates of the reality; they are contrasted to the price indices advocated by health economists

Cause and effect: the new price indices are better because they account for the bundle of treatments available and in what proportion they are actually used instead of the individual prices of treatments; depression treatments are given as an example of this

These studies also account for changes in the quality of health care by measuring the health outcomes associated with treatment. For example, **Cutler**, in his study of **heart attacks**, found that the substitution pattern there was towards more **costly treatments**. But, because the costlier treatments provided better outcomes—in terms of health improvements—the **quality-adjusted price** still showed slower growth than standard indices.

Key terms: Cutler, quality-adjusted price

Contrast: quality adjusted prices are contrasted to price increases used by standard indices

Cause and effect: quality adjusted prices will often be lower than earlier prices because the quality of medical treatment is growing faster than the prices of treatment

To explore the sources of those cost savings, we develop an algebraic expression for the contributions of shifts in different treatments to the cost savings by linking the preferred index to one that tracks fixed baskets of treatments, the type of index typically produced by statistical agencies. In our empirical work, the decomposition confirms the presence of treatment substitution for several important disease classes: shifts from **office visits towards drugs** in many **psychiatric** conditions, shifts from **care at hospitals towards care at ambulatory surgical centers** for **orthopedic** and **gastroenterological** conditions, and similar shifts in **endocrinology** (a disease class that contains diabetes and obesity). However, the decomposition also reveals other patterns associated with these cost savings. In cardiology, for example, the data literally show a large decline in the use of inpatient care with little change in the intensity of other treatments. We take this to mean that although patients appear to do as many office visits and purchase as many prescriptions as they did in 2003, perhaps the treatments they receive in 2005 are better, obviating the need for inpatient care and, thus, giving rise to cost savings. Finally, there are **disease classes** where the **cost** of treating conditions **rises faster than the prices of the underlying treatments**. Two notable cases are **obstetrics** and **neonatology**; where the **increased intensity** of treatment is associated with complications while normal pregnancies and uncomplicated neonatal management show little to no cost savings, respectively.

Cause and effect: several relationships are discussed in this paragraph; there is a shift from office visits to drug usage, a shift from hospital visits to ambulatory site visits, a decline in inpatient care for cardiology without a decrease in treatment, and increase in treatment without an increase in price

Main Idea: The passage is a treatment of some aspects of the economic side of health care; the author discusses price indices and how to accurately measure whether price increases relate to improved care.

43. C is correct. The author introduces the idea at the end of the third paragraph and states that "indices that track the prices of individual treatments tend to miss any shifts towards lower-cost treatments". He or she then gives the example in question.

    A: The "ever changing" part of this choice is too strong since the passage is only giving an example of a single shift in treatment modality.

    B, D: These are not main themes discussed in the passage nor the function of this specific example.

44. A is correct. The passage states that it is better to track the entire bundle of treatments instead of the prices of individual treatments. Depression treatment is given as an example of this.

    B: The passage implies that this is true.

    C, D: These are true and stated in the passage.

45. C is correct. The author argues in the third and fourth paragraphs about bundling treatments and quality adjusted prices. This means that I and III are true.

    II: This is exactly how the current standard price indices work – just considering the price tag on a given treatment.

46. A is correct. The author states that as the baby boomers age, increasing the number of elderly people, expenditures on healthcare will increase. This assumes that the elderly are spending more money on healthcare.

    II: There is no assumption made here; the author doesn't say that there are more pregnancies with complications, only that the intensity of treatment available for complicated pregnancies is increasing.

    III: The author cites a shift in care for cardiology patients but does not assume an increase in number of patients.

47. D is correct. The passage suggests that the "good" in healthcare should be defined as the entire bundle of services used to treat a particular condition. Later in the passage, the author also brings up the fact that the costs should be adjusted by how successful the outcome was.

Passage 9 (Questions 48 – 53)

Shirley functions as an oddity in **Charlotte Brontë's** oeuvre: sandwiched between *Jane Eyre* and *Villette*, **masterpieces** of psychological realism and interiority, **Shirley** is, instead, **fragmented** in terms of plot and purpose. Much of this fragmentation may be ascribed to Brontë's employment of an **industrial plot**: the novel begins with the attack of loom breakers on flinty industrialist Robert Moore's factory, and concludes only after the end of the Napoleonic wars allows him to return to trade and thus propose to the woman of his dreams, Caroline Helstone. Critics have generally persisted in reading these plot elements as a misstep of some sort: **Catherine Gallagher** writes that "industrial conflict in Shirley is little more than a historical setting and does not exert any strong pressure on the form" while **Rosemarie Bodenheimer** notes the "virtual abandonment of the industrial issue" in the text.

Key terms: *Shirley*; Charlotte Brontë; *Jane Eyre; Villette*;

Opinion: Gallagher and Bodenheimer both argue that the industrial setting of the novel is not a major factor in its plot or structure

Contrast: *Shirley's* fragmentation vs *Jane Eyre* and *Villette's* psychological realism and interiority

But in *Shirley* the **historical is irreducible** from the **psychological**. In his recent article, **Peter Capuano** suggests we stop reading the novel in terms of "displacement"; instead "we really should **pay attention to the industrial** element in Shirley" focusing on "obvious textual features that critics have overlooked." Capuano focuses on the connection between surplus hands in the mill and surplus "female handiwork in the novel's middle-class homes" a connection that chronicles "the ways in which new modes of relation arose within the middle-class household." I argue in the **opposite direction**, suggesting that in the novel the romantic, seemingly contained within the **middle-class household**, inevitably **gestures out** to the social and, particularly, the **industrial**. This diversion suggests that the energies of erotic **love** can be read as **similar** to those of **industrial** forces.

Opinion: Capuano argues for focus on industrial element and how it shows up in household

Contrast: Capuano's focus on industrial within household vs author's on romance within the industrial

Cause and effect: focusing on romantic and erotic love in the novel connects to social and industrial issues

Louis reveals his desire for Shirley late in the novel in what he admits are a series of "metaphors," ones that jumble the **romantic** and **industrial**. Musing on his attraction to Shirley, Louis states:

I worship her perfections; but it is her faults, or at least her foibles, that bring her near to me, that nestle her to my heart, that fold her about with my love, and that for a most selfish but deeply-natural reason. These faults are the steps by which I mount to ascendency over her. If she rose a trimmed, artificial mound, without inequality, what vantage would she offer the foot? It is the natural hill, with its mossy breaks and hollows, whose slope invites ascent, whose summit it is pleasure to gain.

This metaphor also invokes the industrial in two key ways: the language of **manufacture** and, more broadly, the idea of **"wild" resources**.

Opinions: Louis says he loves Shirley for her faults because they give him power over her

Contrast: trimmed artificial mound vs natural hill

Cause and effect: because he has to conquer Shirley, Louis finds pleasure in having power over her

Louis seems to dismiss manufacture here, disdaining the "trimmed, artificial mound" in favor of "the natural hill." Yet it is the "steps," or artificially constructed tools, that he finds so attractive in Shirley's willfulness. Thus we can argue that it is the **possibility of construction and alteration that Louis finds so attractive**. This metaphor of manufacture circulates throughout the text, and is remarkable for how well it adapts itself to different situations. When Louis and Shirley finally declare their love for each other, he invokes her "lands and gold," metonymically **picturing her as a series of materials for manufacture**. While he boasts that he "care[s] not for them," he suggests that Shirley becomes the driving engine for his own transformation: "What change I underwent I cannot explain, but out of her emotion passed into me a new spirit." Thus Shirley serves multiply as a space on which manufacture can take place, a source of the raw materials of manufacture, and as a machine itself, whose "emotion" sets into motion Louis's own transformation. Louis pictures Shirley as the various modes of manufacture in an almost **Marxist sense**, envisioning a series of circulating and transforming energies that both please him erotically and profit him emotionally.

Key terms: Marxist sense

Cause and effect: because he focuses on artificial steps, Louis shows he values transformation and manufacture; Shirley serves as a metaphor for the space of manufacture, the raw materials of manufacture, and the machine that manufactures

Main Idea: The passage argues that *Shirley* uses metaphors of romantic love to explore industrial images and issues, opposing this reading to many other critics' ignoring of either the industrial or the romantic elements of the novel.

48. B is correct. The fourth paragraph states that Louis imagines Shirley "in an almost Marxist sense, envisioning a series of circulating and transforming energies that both please him erotically and profit him emotionally." Thus an emphasis on how goods circulate and are transformed, as in choice B, is the credited answer.

A: Neither class, mills, nor factories are invoked when the author discusses "Marxist" issues.

C: The domestic is not discussed in this section of the passage.

D: There is no indication that Marxist readings require a connection between the erotic and the industrial, though the author does suggest that industrial energy pleases Louis erotically.

49. B is correct. The passage on the whole is focused on Shirley and begins by stating that it is "an oddity in Charlotte Brontë's oeuvre" and discusses the ways in which it is not like Jane Eyre or Villette. Thus the two novels are introduced to demonstrate how Shirley differs from them.

    A, D: The passage does not focus on either Brontë's reputation or publication order.

    C: It is suggested that because *Shirley* is an industrial novel it is fragmented, but *Jane Eyre* and *Villette* are offered as a contrast to that.

50. C is correct. Psychological realism is used to describe Jane Eyre and Villette, which are contrasted to Shirley, so the author would not describe it thusly.

    A, B, D: These are all used in the passage to describe elements of *Shirley*.

51. A is correct. Capuano argues that "we really should pay attention to the industrial element in Shirley" focusing on "obvious textual features that critics have overlooked." A detailed description of a picnic lunch would fall in that category.

    B: It is Capuano, not the passage's author, who focuses on middle-class homes.

    C: Gallagher argues that the industrial is not a major element of the novel, but does not say it refuses the industrial, as in choice C.

    D: There is no discussion of any critic focusing on one character over another.

52. D is correct. The passage states that "Shirley serves a metaphor for the space of manufacture," such as the barnyard, where things are made, as in choice B, "the raw materials of manufacture," such as the timber in choice C, "and the machine that manufactures," such as the cotton mill in choice A.

53. C is correct. In the final paragraph the author states that Louis envisions Shirley in an almost Marxist sense, suggesting agreement with Marx's ideas; thus the author agrees with Marx.

    A, D: Gallagher and Bodenheimer argue that the industrial is not a major part of the novel, whereas the author argues that it is.

B: The author states that while "Capuano focuses on the connection between surplus hands in the mill and surplus 'female handiwork in the novel's middle-class homes' ... I argue in the opposite direction."

SECTION 2

53 Questions, 90 Minutes

Use an answer grid from the back of the book to record your answers

Passage 1 (Questions 1-6)

The San Francisco Ballet (SFB), the oldest professional ballet troupe in the US, is lauded the world over for its masterful execution of ballet in the neoclassical "Balanchine aesthetic". The San Francisco Ballet School (SFBS) is one of the most competitive dance programs in the world, with even the Level One program (for dancers aged 7-8) rejecting over 85% of auditioners. Certainly the raw athleticism, coordination, and grace of the dance students in the SFBS is remarkable, although in this regard the SFBS does not stand out from its peer institutions in New York, Moscow, Tokyo, and elsewhere around the word. But what makes the SFB and the SFBS unique is its especially strong adherence to the uniformity of body type demanded by the Balanchine aesthetic.

George Balanchine was at the forefront of the neoclassical emphasis on movement itself as the key expressive element of ballet as a medium. He stripped away props, sets, and even costumes and haircuts. Dancers wore plain leotards, kept their hair in a tight bun, and were encouraged to have no facial expression at all – nothing to distract from the pure expression of movement. In his later years, Balanchine continually revised his works to simplify everything but the movement and music, and demanded ever more rigorous uniformity in the look and bodies of the dancers themselves. To those who continue the Balanchine approach into the 21st century, classical ballet all but demands a dancer have a height as near as possible to 5' 8", an exceptionally slim build, a small head and bust, and long, willowy arms and legs.

An adherence to this look landed the SFBS in hot water in 2001 when it found itself subject to a lawsuit by Krissy Keefer on behalf of her 8 year-old daughter, Fredrika Keefer. Krissy is herself a classically trained dancer and knows, better than most, the rigors of a classical ballet education. Several members of the SFBS faculty suggested to her that it would not be worth Fredrika's time to audition as she would be unlikely to be selected. Nonetheless, Krissy persisted and the school permitted Fredrika to audition. Afterwards, when 18 of the 22 auditioners were rejected, Fredrika found herself as one of them.

This would normally be the end of the story, but for a then very-recently enacted municipal statute in San Francisco which barred employer discrimination on the basis of height or weight (expanding the existing statute covering usual things like race, gender, sexual orientation, etc.) Given the ridiculously overbroad language in the statute, even a privately-funded school selecting dance students on the basis of bona fide occupational qualifications (the usual legal test for discriminatory action) would fall under the rule's purview.

The media attention the case received has, unsurprisingly, prompted a large response from across the spectrum in both the dance and legal communities.

Many correctly point out that it seems long past time to move beyond the strictures of neoclassical ballet and Bal-anchine's increasingly-outdated 1930's worldview about what makes for an exceptional ballet dancer. Critics point out that even companies doing revivals of Balanchine classics like The *Firebird* or *Swan Lake* always include embellishments in the sets or costumes that would have made Balanchine himself livid. In a world where Alvin Ailey's *Revelations*, with its dancers of various shapes and sizes, commands more respect, bigger audiences, and more imitation than any neoclassical work, it is time we free ourselves from the shackles of a 111 year old Russian's view as to what comprises ballet. This view is limiting and in dancers' efforts to achieve some perfect look they often end up with eating disorders and doing long-term damage to their bodies.

Yet is it appropriate to put this eight year-old girl in the crosshairs of this debate? And is the legal system the appropriate venue for ballet to carry out this necessary soul-searching? If the San Francisco ballet, of anyone, cannot make its own decisions about who is and who is not qualified to meet its own particular artistic requirements, one fears for a future in which any institution must keep a federal district judge on staff to guide its artistic decision-making.

1. Balanchine would most likely approve of which of the following artistic works?

    A. A modern dance depicting the effect that technology has had on social isolation, using modern lighting and projection techniques to provide context for the dancers' movements

    B. The sculpture *Bird in Space* renowned for its elegance in evoking the puffed chest and upward movement of a flying bird while stripping away elements extraneous to the expression such as the tail and wings

    C. A revival of a classic Greek dance in which the story-telling of the chorus is replaced by a group of dancers using only movement to express the dramatic beats of the narrative

    D. A combine in the style of Rauschenberg that manages to masterfully evoke the paintings of Kirchner and the sculpture of Donatello

2. The author would most likely disapprove of which one of the following as a basis for a lawsuit?

    A. A modern dance company refuses to hire black dancers as a part of its debut season.

    B. A highly respected sculpture school refuses to admit any student who is unwilling to invest six months in reproducing at least one work of a Renaissance master as part of the application process.

    C. A new clothing store that seeks to appeal primarily to wealthy white suburban teenage girls refuses to hire homosexual or transgender employees for any position that involves customer contact.

    D. An artist of Mexican nationality who grew up as an undocumented immigrant in Tucson sues the Phoenix Art Museum for excluding works by Latino artists in its "Voices of the Arizona Territory" special exhibit.

3. The passage suggests that:

    A. had Fredrika been rejected from a similar program in another city, no lawsuit would have followed.

    B. George Balanchine's aesthetic views were informed by his political orientation.

    C. Alvin Ailey pursued a similar aesthetic to George Balanchine.

    D. the author believes that tort law in the U.S. has gotten out of hand.

4. The author would most likely agree with which one of the following statements?

    A. The lawsuit against the SFBS is a good thing because it will decrease the likelihood of future dancers damaging themselves in an effort to achieve a certain look.

    B. It is inappropriate to place children as young as 7 or 8 into rigorous classical ballet programs.

    C. More cities ought to enact laws like the one Krissy Keefer used to sue to SFBS.

    D. The view of ballet established by George Balanchine is outdated and merits significant revision.

5. Which of the following arguments most closely parallels the main argument presented by the passage author?

    A. A hospital administrator believes that a pharmaceutical company has been engaging in price gouging towards urban hospitals and organizes a class-action lawsuit.

    B. A government contractor has a slow, cumbersome appeals process that provides a formal mechanism for censuring employees, and one manager at the company requires every disciplinary action against his subordinates to go through this process rather than a simpler informal discussion.

    C. A software development company discovers that a competitor has engaged in corporate espionage to beat them to market with a new piece of software and decides to sue for patent infringement.

    D. A school official argues against instituting a formal dress code with rules and punishments even though she agrees that some students currently dress in a manner that is unsuitable and that these students' behavior should change.

6. Which one of the following statements, if made by the author in another publication, would most contradict the views expressed here?

    A. Balanchine's view of ballet is outdated and should be revised by lawsuit or threat of lawsuit.

    B. Both ballroom dance and jazz dance, as media with more variety and fewer restrictions than classical ballet, are ultimately more expressive art forms.

    C. Dancers who join specialized troupes such as The Rockettes are often required to have even more strict physical uniformity than SFB dancers.

    D. Alvin Ailey was a much less prolific choreographer than George Balanchine, but he produced works of higher merit.

Passage 2 (Questions 7-12)

The German Empire existed for only 47 years and yet in that time did more to shape the nature of the 20th century than any other state in Europe (or possibly, the world). While most will only remember the end of the Empire – starting World War I and then being dissolved upon losing it – the German Empire should instead be remembered for its startling internal contradictions. It was a nation of impressive social, electoral, and economic advances but also a strictly authoritarian place. It is in this tension that Germany embodied much of the zeitgeist of the subsequent century.

In 1871, the newly-minted Empire enacted universal male suffrage. At a time when poll taxes and literacy tests were being aggressively used to disenfranchise black voters in the U.S. and while the U.K. still had property requirements for suffrage, the German Empire permitted every single male the right to vote. Germany also created Europe's first social welfare system, providing old-age pensions, sickness benefits, and accident and disability insurance for its industrial workers. The model set by the Empire saw increases in worker health and productivity that would not be rivaled for over a century (with the dawn of the information economy). This combination of expanding political participation, capitalist welfare systems, and freedom of the press set the tone for much of the political progress of the 20th century.

In addition to these social reforms, the Empire experienced an unprecedented industrial and military expansion. Germany can rightly claim to be the first truly "urbanized" nation in the world. In 1870, Germany had almost no rail system to speak of and yet by 1913 had the largest rail network in the world, after the U.S. Germany's dye and chemical industries grew exponentially in the decades prior to 1900, and expanded into pharmaceuticals, electrochemistry, and agricultural chemicals. This rapid industrial expansion had two significant corollaries: the development of the first class of industrial managers in the world – bureaucrats in the classic Song Dynasty sense who also embodied the scientific and technical know-how that created a strongly practical world-view; and second the research and development needed to drive this industrial expansion created a scientific Renaissance in German universities – over 1/3 of all Nobel prizes issued during the German Empire's existence went to German scientists.

The strong investment in industrial and scientific expansion was not without a significant dark side. The authoritarianism that quickly built an impressive industrial base also lent itself to disastrous social policies. Extending the vote to every adult male meant that suddenly, repressed Catholic and Polish minorities had a voice in the government. In response, Bismarck carried out two campaigns: the kulturkampf and Germanization. In the former, the Imperial government attempted to seize control of all Catholic churches. Over the course of a decade, every single Catholic bishop was imprisoned and as many as 1/4 of parishes found themselves without a priest. In line with government efforts to spread Lutheranism were the efforts to get every single person in the Empire to speak German. Significant minorities spoke French, Polish, and Lithuanian and efforts to force such groups to adopt German backfired spectacularly. In one province, the percentage of German-speaking citizens actually dropped by over 10% in the decade during which Germanization was being most aggressively pursued. The authoritarianism that failed so markedly in social policies had an even more impressively negative effect in foreign policy . . .

This set of contrasting, yet complementary, approaches to authoritarianism is best revealed by the incident which led to Chancellor Bismarck's resignation. Near the end of 1889, a group of coal miners in the German region of Silesia went on strike. Bismarck's reaction was swift: he began mobilizing the Army to go in and crush the strike. Emperor Wilhelm, however, stopped him and sent an official to negotiate with a delegation from the miners. The strike ended without violence and Bismarck resigned months later. Wilhelm is reputed to have said, "I do not wish to stain my reign with the blood of my subjects." Yet such measured non-violence obviously did not stay the Emperor's hand in dealing with the Empire's colonies.

7. The author would most likely approve of which one of the following policies enacted by the German Empire?

    A. Shortly after enacting universal male suffrage, the empire enacted a policy requiring any legislation passed by elected members of the Reichstag to be approved by the Bundesrat, a legislative body consisting of un-elected landowning nobles.

    B. The imperial treasury paid companies for expenses incurred providing free housing to workers.

    C. Males living in Kingdoms, Grand Duchies, and Duchies of the Empire could vote, but those living in Principalities and Free Cities could vote only in local politics and had no representation in Imperial assemblies.

    D. Areas which embraced Germanization and had near-100% adoption of the German language for schools and businesses saw significant improvements in quality of life due to subsidized investments by large industrial firms.

8. The passage suggests that the Empire's violent authoritarianism in foreign policy was:

    A. primarily due to Emperor Wilhelm.

    B. primarily due to Chancellor Bismarck.

    C. crafted by Chancellor Bismarck and executed by Emperor Wilhelm.

    D. an outgrowth of policies of worker support and control in domestic policy.

9. The author of this passage is most likely:

    A. a social conservative who favors limiting entitlement spending.

    B. a historian discussing his area of expertise.

    C. a journalist who specializes in studying the after-effects of European colonialism.

    D. a Catholic scholar who examines the suppression of the Catholic faith around the world.

10. The passage suggests that Chancellor Bismarck's role in aggressive domestic policies like the kulturkampf and Germanization was:

    A. at least passive approval, if not active support and direction.

    B. ignorance, as the Chancellor was only concerned with foreign policy.

    C. one of active disapproval, with the Chancellor using his political influence to oppose the Emperor.

    D. nonexistent, as Bismarck was not Chancellor of the German Empire during those two initiatives.

11. The author discusses the rail system in order to:

    A. demonstrate the superiority of the German industrial base as compared to its continental neighbors.

    B. provide proof that had the German Empire continued into the twentieth century, it would soon have out-stripped even the U.S. in its advancement.

    C. compare Germany's successes at expanding its rail system with its failure to develop other technologies.

    D. provide supporting detail about the swiftness of Germany's industrial expansion.

12. The author's respect for the achievements of the German Empire is:

    A. founded in an ideological respect for the top-down organization of the various Germanic kingdoms into a single quasi-federal Empire.

    B. unreflective and thoughtlessly positive, suggesting that the author himself is a German nationalist.

    C. tempered by an appreciation for the negative consequences that came with achievements made possible by strong authoritarian control.

    D. balanced by his awareness that the authoritarian style of German governance paved the way for the atrocities of World War II.

Passage 3 (Questions 13-18)

Olav Hammer's scathing critique of anthroposophy centers primarily on his assertion that anthroposophy is not science, but scientism – the inappropriate application of the methods of empirical science to all areas of life and the assertion that the only true knowledge or facts that can be discovered are those revealed through typical scientific methods. Both in subsuming the natural sciences under the umbrella of spiritual "science" and in its unjustifiable defense of fringe sciences such as biodynamic agriculture, anthroposophy places itself firmly in the realm of the delusional, holds Hammer.

Anthroposophy is a philosophy founded at the start of the 20th century by Austrian philosopher and social reformer Rudolf Steiner. The core mission of anthroposophy is to help individuals develop imagination and intuition, and to study the spiritual world with the same objective rigor as the natural sciences. People were expected to develop a super-sensory consciousness which could then be used to study the spiritual realm and report back in a way intelligible to those who had not yet developed such consciousness. Steiner believed that the spiritual realm was real, and had the same objective existence as our material one.

Steiner defined human nature as existing of four different components – a physical body that is created from and returns to the inorganic world; an etheric body (similar to all living things); an astral body (similar to all sentient beings); and a unique self-aware component called the ego. Humans reincarnate as part of a karmic cycle and are a higher life-form because they are less specialized. This last point reflects anthroposophy's odd view of evolution: a single unspecialized archetype was the progenitor of all animal life and organisms are devolved from this state, rather than evolved towards increasing complexity as in Darwinism.

It was in this discussion of anthroposophical evolution that Steiner's work drew the attention and ire from so many in both philosophical and scientific circles. Steiner's defenders in the middle and later parts of the 20th century emphasized that such criticism ultimately missed the point. While any number of esoteric traditions flourished at the end of the 19th century (most prominently the Theosophy from which anthroposophy derived), none of them come in for the same criticism as anthroposophy. Defenders such as Herbert Hahn counter that we ought to look at the practical application of anthroposophic ideas and judge the philosophy not on its rarefied esoteric principles, but on its effect in the real world. "Christianity is not to be judged through a meditation on the paradox of how a being, Jesus, could be both fully man and fully God, but rather on the great works and good charity actually demonstrated by Christians," held Hahn. "We only ask the same."

Hahn points out the Waldorf schools around the world which focus on holistic, developmentally-appropriate education for students at all levels. Waldorf schools typically produce young adults that are far more well-rounded and creative, and who excel at lateral thinking and problem solv-ing, they assert. Biodynamic agriculture, developed in the early 1920's, laid the foundations for both modern organic farming and what would eventually become Integrated Pest Management, the gold standard in sustainable agriculture. Finally, Steiner's ideas about socially responsible financial associations set the framework for Social Finance that began with the *Gemeinschaftsbank* in Germany in the 1970's.

Both critics and defenders of Steiner's work have valid points, so far as they go, but ultimately end up speaking past one another.

13. Had Steiner's writings never addressed the concept of evolution, which one of the following would likely have occurred?

    A. Organic farming would never have been developed.

    B. Anthroposophy would have received less criticism from some scientists and philosophers.

    C. Anthroposophy would have developed a view of humanity as consisting of three components instead of four.

    D. Biodynamic agriculture would have developed along different lines.

14. Which of the following would be an example of scientism, as the word is used in the passage?

    A. A behavioral economist thinks the best way to assess how effective a product's packaging is as a marketing tool is to empirically observe actual shoppers and whether they look at or reach for a type of package, rather than through surveys or focus groups.

    B. A psychic claims he is able to channel the spirit of Albert Einstein because he is able to relate minor details about Einstein's life and able to answer questions about physics that he would otherwise not know.

    C. A psychologist believes cognitive behavioral therapy is the most effective therapy technique for treating a certain mental illness based solely on data about reduced need for medication rather than any subjective feedback from patients.

    D. A researcher believes the only true way to measure the value of poetry is to do brain scans of people while they read the poem and measure the level of activity in the brain's pleasure center.

15. Hahn and Hammer would most likely disagree about which of the following?

    A. Anthroposophy has had at least some positive impact on the world through its effective education.

    B. Biodynamic agriculture laid the groundwork for subsequent developments in organic farming.

    C. The methods and worldview of empirical science should remain tightly confined to the ambit of the classic natural sciences such as physics, chemistry, and botany.

    D. When evaluating a certain intellectual position, one should consider only the principles and assumptions of the position itself.

16. The author would describe which of the following as an example of people who are "speaking past one another"?

    A. A parent and teenager fight over whether the teenager should get to drive the family's car, with the teenager pointing out how many of her peers get to drive their family car.

    B. Two political candidates discuss foreign policy in a debate, with one candidate focusing on the political interests of U.S. allies overseas and the other candidate emphasizing the need to spend more government money on solving domestic issues.

    C. Two chemists have different theories about a proposed mechanism for a chemical reaction and are each able to produce and publish data supporting their hypotheses.

    D. Two children on the playground get in a fight about whether one superhero could beat up another superhero, each supporting his argument with reference to the super-powers possessed by the superhero.

17. The passage mentions Christianity in order to do which of the following?

    A. Provide an example of one means used by defenders of anthroposophy to bolster their position against critics.

    B. Prove that anthroposophy is not an example of scientism.

    C. Demonstrate that anthroposophy's positive effects through Waldorf schools and organic farming make anthroposophy a valuable philosophy.

    D. Imply that Christianity itself is an example of scientism and point out the hypocrisy of those attacking anthroposophy.

18. Those who defend anthroposophy rely on each of the following EXCEPT:

    A. Reasoning by analogy based on other worldviews

    B. A demonstration of apparent hypocrisy by critics

    C. A proof that scientism is irrelevant to the good works done based on a view

    D. A utilitarian argument about positive outcomes

Passage 4 (Questions 19 – 23)

Political ideals must be based upon ideals for the individual life. The aim of politics should be to make the lives of individuals as good as possible. There is nothing for the politician to consider outside or above the various men, women, and children who compose the world. The problem of politics is to adjust the relations of human beings in such a way that each severally may have as much of good in his existence as possible. And this problem requires that we should first consider what it is that we think good in the individual life.

We may distinguish two sorts of goods, and two corresponding sorts of impulses. There are goods in regard to which individual possession is possible, and there are goods in which all can share alike. The food and clothing of one man is not the food and clothing of another; if the supply is insufficient, what one man has obtained is at the expense of some other man. This applies to material goods generally, and therefore to the greater part of the present economic life of the world. On the other hand, mental and spiritual goods do not belong to one man to the exclusion of another. If one man knows a science, that does not prevent others from knowing it; on the contrary, it helps them to acquire the knowledge. If one man is a great artist or poet, that does not prevent others from painting pictures or writing poems, but helps to create the atmosphere in which such things are possible. If one man is full of good-will toward others, that does not mean that there is less good-will to be shared among the rest; the more good-will one man has, the more he is likely to create among others. In such matters there is no possession, because there is not a definite amount to be shared; any increase anywhere tends to produce an increase everywhere.

There are two kinds of impulses, corresponding to the two kinds of goods. There are possessive impulses, which aim at acquiring or retaining private goods that cannot be shared; these center in the impulse of property. And there are creative or constructive impulses, which aim at bringing into the world or making available for use the kind of goods in which there is no privacy and no possession.

The best life is the one in which the creative impulses play the largest part and the possessive impulses the smallest. This is no new discovery. The Gospel says: "Take no thought, saying, What shall we eat? or What shall we drink? or, Wherewithal shall we be clothed?" The thought we give to these things is taken away from matters of more importance. And what is worse, the habit of mind engendered by thinking of these things is a bad one; it leads to competition, envy, domination, cruelty, and almost all the moral evils that infest the world. In particular, it leads to the predatory use of force. Material possessions can be taken by force and enjoyed by the robber. Spiritual possessions cannot be taken in this way. You may kill an artist or a thinker, but you cannot acquire his art or his thought. You may put a man to death because he loves his fellow-men, but you will not by so doing acquire the love which made his happiness. Force is impo-

tent in such matters; it is only as regards material goods that it is effective. For this reason the men who believe in force are the men whose thoughts and desires are preoccupied with material goods.

What we shall desire for individuals is now clear: strong creative impulses, overpowering and absorbing the instinct of possession; reverence for others; respect for the fundamental creative impulse in ourselves. A certain kind of self-respect or native pride is necessary to a good life; a man must not have a sense of utter inward defeat if he is to remain whole, but must feel the courage and the hope and the will to live by the best that is in him, whatever outward or inward obstacles it may encounter. So far as it lies in a man's own power, his life will realize its best possibilities if it has three things: creative rather than possessive impulses, reverence for others, and respect for the fundamental impulse in himself. Political and social institutions are to be judged by the good or harm that they do to individuals. Do they encourage creativeness rather than possessiveness? Do they embody or promote a spirit of reverence between human beings? Do they preserve self-respect?

19. Which of the following would the author most likely classify as a mental or spiritual good?

    A. Time

    B. Love

    C. Money given to charity

    D. Food

20. Which of the following statements would the author be LEAST likely to make?

    A. Institutions, and especially economic systems, have a profound influence in molding the characters of men and women.

    B. It is not a separate ideal for each separate man, but one ideal reality for all men, that has to be actualized if possible.

    C. Those who realize the harm that can be done to others by any use of force will be very full of respect for the liberty of others.

    D. Few men can succeed in being creative rather than possessive in a world which is wholly built on competition.

21. Which of the following claims would most likely follow directly after the end of the passage?

    A. In all these ways the institutions under which we live are very far indeed from what they ought to be.

    B. The possessive impulses, when they are strong, infect activities which ought to be purely creative.

    C. There is in human beings, as in plants and animals, a certain natural impulse of growth, and this is just as true of mental as of physical development.

    D. We see that men's political dealings with one another are based on wholly wrong ideals.

22. Which of the following would be the most surprising discovery?

    A. That the author is a politician

    B. That the author is a philosopher

    C. That the author believes all people are born with a desire for competition and power

    D. That the author believes all people are born with an innate capacity for creative impulses

23. What is the purpose of the author's reference to the Bible?

    A. To illustrate the benefits of putting others first over oneself

    B. To give further evidence to the claim that creative impulses are preferred over possessive impulses

    C. To show that it is more socially acceptable to indulge creative impulses than possessive

    D. To demonstrate the benefits of cultivating artistic and musical ability because they cannot be stolen

Passage 5 (Questions 24 – 29)

During most of the post-World War II era, Japan's economy experienced a remarkable and, to many, enviable period of rapid economic growth. Between 1965 and 1980, nominal gross domestic product grew from $91 billion to $1.065 trillion. In the 1980s, Japan had the highest productivity of any country in the world. Many Westerners of the time were not only envious but curious. What had produced such a dramatic Japanese expansion and economic boom? Attempts were made to study the factors which had turned the "Land of the Rising Sun" into such a brightly shining economic star. Many of these observers had the specific, ideal end goal of determining whether this good fortune could be replicated in the United States and other Western countries.

One attempt to discern the reasons for Japan's economic success focused on attitudes in the workplace. One such approach focused on the differences between the so-called Theory X and Theory Z. Theory X, created by management professor Douglas Murray McGregor, refers to the viewpoint that workers are inherently lazy, dislike their jobs and their careers, and aren't likely to apply themselves to their jobs without the use of constant supervision and prodding. Many observers believed that American workplaces of the era contained a high percentage of people who subscribed to this theory about their workers. But in 1981, a book by Dr. William Ouchi described an alternative viewpoint called "Theory Z". The book stated that the attitudes in Japanese workplaces promoted employee satisfaction and morale by focusing on the employee's well-being, on and off the job, which was conducive to productivity and other positive economic benchmarks. For many, this provided an explanation of why Japan had become the world's most productive country.

Other theories, more based in macroeconomics than in management theory, saw Japan's success as less a consequence of the employer-employee dynamic and more a consequence of serendipitous and not particularly complex economic trends which, in the era studied, overlapped with one another. One of these factors was low worldwide oil prices, translating into lower prices for gasoline and other essentials of a growing economy such as energy. Another factor related to the speed of technological advancement. In economic supply-and-demand theory, newly introduced technological developments can shift the curve of aggregate supply. When this occurs, production increases, causing economic growth, and there is downward pressure on prices, keeping inflation in check. Postwar Japan could advance very rapidly simply by importing advanced technologies from other countries without having to invest in costly research and development. After a few decades, though, Japan had essentially caught up to the rest of the world in terms of technology. Once Japan reached technological parity with the world's other advanced countries, the playing field was level again – Japan could no longer simply import technological advancement, and was now able to advance technologically only by creating its own advances through expensive investment in research and development.

By the late 1990s, trouble in the Japanese economy had started to reach a tipping point. Consumer spending and investor spending were simultaneously dropping, and Japan's traditionally low unemployment rate was on the rise. Concern about weak aggregate demand led to both domestic and international pressure to fix the issue, as Japan's economy was the world's second-largest at the time and there was fear that Japan's economic troubles could affect business cycles in other countries. Facing this, the government decided to apply the dual fiscal stimuli of cutting taxes and increasing government spending. Other measures over the next several years followed, none fully effective. Deflation, which was re-aggravated in some ways by the government's attempts at structural reform, dampened both production and consumer demand, and led to legitimate fears of a disastrous deflationary spiral. After experiencing what many call a "lost decade" in economic growth, Japan might now be entering a second one.

24. Suppose monetary policymakers in the Japanese government were to implement a policy of increasing the money supply in the Japanese banking system, which would likely alleviate deflation while carrying the risk of excessively increasing inflation in the long term. In this case, the author would be most likely to:

A. support the policy, because if Japan experiences a second "lost decade" of growth, it may never again develop a strong economy.

B. support the policy, because of how severe the cost of deflation would be if allowed to continue.

C. oppose the policy, because inflation needs to be held in check for an economy to have any chance at success.

D. oppose the policy, because Japan's inability to import advanced technology is the only factor limiting economic growth, and it cannot be solved by increasing the country's money supply.

25. The author's purpose in discussing Theory X and Theory Z is to:

A. show how Japanese culture is healthier for workers than the way workers are usually treated.

B. show how employer attitudes can become self-fulfilling prophecies.

C. show that an outside perspective can improve results compared to traditional ways of thinking.

D. show how attempts were made to form connections between management theory and the postwar economy.

26. According to the passage, which of the following has been theoretically associated with Japan achieving a degree of technological sophistication which matched those of other countries?

A. The elimination of aggregate supply-based advantages

B. The reduction of an impetus to focus national efforts on research and development

C. Low worldwide prices for oil, gasoline and energy

D. An economic situation that prevents inflation from rising excessively

27. What conclusion might be drawn from the effects described in the last paragraph of the government actions to respond to Japan's weak economy?

A. Efforts to fix economic problems may lack success even if sufficient motivation exists.

B. International economic cooperation to fix a weak economy cannot prove effective.

C. Structural reform might be one of the best techniques there is to limit inflation.

D. Weak aggregate demand of one country will significantly affect the business cycles in other countries.

28. With which of the following statements would the author be LEAST likely to agree?

A. Structural reform may be theoretically helpful, but has a chance of falling short if actually used.

B. Many Western countries probably believe that economic contagion can cross national borders.

C. Consensus is lacking in regard to both the achievement of Japanese postwar circumstances, and how Japan might emerge from its present-day situation.

D. Japan can be counted on to find a way out of its current economic problems.

29. How does the author characterize the people described in the passage who believed it was a good idea to determine how Japan had achieved its economic success?

I. Altruistic

II. Purposeful

III. Inquisitive

A. I and II only

B. I and III only

C. II and III only

D. I, II and III

Passage 6 (Questions 30 – 35)

Titian, Velasquez, and Rembrandt are generally acknowledged to be the greatest masters of painting the world has known, and to each of them, we happily and fittingly apply the word genius. Of all the definitions of that abused word, there is one that states that genius comes not from seeing more than other people, but from seeing differently. In this way, we acknowledge a painter as genius when he is able to, beyond his masterly technical skills, present to us a view of life or nature that we have never seen, but that we are deeply and immediately convinced is a product of deeper vision than our own. The painter has seen it: only because of our shortcomings, and the dimness or narrowness of our outlooks, is it that we do not see it also.

A great painter writes us a letter, filled with details of the things he has seen and heard and felt, giving us a look into the world in which he lives. A great painter bares his personality to us, and personality in art is of inestimable value. We love Corot's *Arcadia* landscape because it is the vision, heart, and character of the personality of the artist, distilled and presented directly to us. A Rembrandt may express personality abundantly. A Velasquez, on the other hand, may express personality negatively.

In judging a painter, we must be vigilant to carefully distinguish between his own personality and the personality of those who interpret him. The more that we give of ourselves to a painter, or any other kind of artist, the more his work returns our giving with appeal and interest. Cleave the wood of your brain and you find the artist reaching out with communications. Raise the stone of your imagination and the artist is revealed.

There was a certain critic who had devoted his life to the study of Reynolds. Once, while lecturing upon the great achievements of his subject, the critic put a large subject-picture upon the screen: this was not one of Reynolds's happier efforts, but rather, an unattractive and obviously labored design which we know gave Reynolds a sea of troubles. This critic's analysis of the picture was so scientific, so interesting, so absorbing, that many of the audience were persuaded that they were looking upon a masterpiece. In reality, they had been hypnotized by the subtleties of this critic's personal approach to Reynolds.

On the other hand, some criticism has tended towards depreciation, due to the predilection of some critics for objective as opposed to subjective criticism. As P.G. Hamerton once wrote of Rembrandt, "The chiaroscuro (treatment of light in a drawing or painting) of Rembrandt is often false and inconsistent, and in fact he relied largely on public ignorance. But though arbitrary, it is always conducive to his purpose."

"Conducive to his purpose!" Those four words contain much virtue. Perhaps more than anybody, Rembrandt knew that his style of lighting was not a facsimile of nature, that it did not represent the chiaroscuro seen by the average eye. He had an aim, a vision before him, and he never hesitated

to interpret that particular vision in his own particular way. So, who dares to say Rembrandt was disloyal to nature?

Our concern ought to be not what he should have done, but what he did, seeing with his own eyes. These are the questions we should ask ourselves: Is his interpretation of the world beautiful, profound, stimulating, and suggestive? Does the imprint of his personality in paint add to our own knowledge and hone our aesthetic perception? Does his work extend our horizons by showing us visions that our imperfect eyes and minds cannot see except through him?

30. Which of the following artists does the author most closely compare with Rembrandt in terms of ability to distill and present personality in a painting?

   A. Titian

   B. Corot

   C. Velasquez

   D. Reynolds

31. Which of the following is most likely the reason why the author introduced the anecdote about the critic who devoted his life to studying Reynolds?

   A. In order to provide another example of an artist distilling and presenting personality in his paintings

   B. In order to demonstrate how some critics have a notable penchant for objectivity over subjectivity

   C. In order to prove the importance of distinguishing between the personalities of the painter and the critic

   D. In order to set up the argument that we ought not to judge what artists should have done, but what they did

32. Based upon the passage, it can be implied that the author would most agree with which of the following statements?

   A. A masterly painter need not necessarily be technically skilled.

   B. A masterly painter is always remembered more than an average one.

   C. A masterly painter must necessarily be highly technically skilled.

   D. A masterly painter often hides secrets about his personality in his work.

33. Based upon the passage, which of the following most accurately describes how Rembrandt's chiaroscuro affects the author?

   A. It allows him to have a view of life that he doesn't have regularly.

   B. It allows him to appropriate an element of Rembrandt's personality.

   C. It allows him to fully realize the genius of Rembrandt's work.

   D. It allows him the ability to sift through overly positive or negative criticism.

34. Suppose there is a painter who is frustrated by the fact that he is not considered great. Though he has master level technical proficiency, he is still not considered to be a great painter. According to the passage, which of the following might be a reason why this painter is frustrated?

   A. The critics that review his work favor objectivism and tend to depreciate him.

   B. The critics that review his work favor subjectivism and tend to overly appreciate him.

   C. The critics find that his work lacks a sense of his distinctive personality.

   D. The critics find that his work is too unrealistic and unrepresentative of life.

35. According to the passage, all of the following statements about great artists are true EXCEPT:

   A. they are always technically proficient.

   B. their work is typically underappreciated.

   C. they share their personalities through their work.

   D. they show us different ways of looking at the world.

Passage 7 (Questions 36 – 40)

The codes of ethics of all health care professionals include a duty to provide care to patients even at some risk to themselves. In the Veterans Health Administration (VHA), staff who are not clinicians also have a duty as VA employees to contribute to the mission of VHA in supporting the delivery of health care services. The duty to provide or support the provision of care is strong, but is not absolute and has certain justifiable exceptions. Those exceptions become relevant in circumstances when caring for patients imposes a disproportionate risk on the health care providers and staff providing that care.

The experience in West Africa and elsewhere indicates that caring for patients with Ebola (EVD) may involve personal risk to health care providers and others, including the risk of infection or death, burden to their families, and possible quarantine or isolation, if exposed. Caring for patients with EVD may also involve a risk to an entire health care system if first-line providers become ill or die, leaving the health care system without vital resources to treat EVD as well as other illnesses. Caring for patients with EVD may also involve a risk to other patients if providers become infected and then serve as vectors for transmission. To date, the experience in the U.S. has demonstrated that health care providers' exposure can be mitigated by the proper use of personal protective equipment (PPE), that actions can be taken to ensure that an exposed or infected health care provider will not transmit the virus to others, and that an infected health care provider has a good chance of clearing the virus.

In its Framework for Ebola Preparedness and Response, VA leadership is initially asking health care providers and staff to indicate their willingness to volunteer for Ebola Response Teams at Tier 1 VAMCs. VA has also issued guidance on the Use of Telework or Authorized Absence in Cases of Suspected Exposure to Ebola, and is committed to providing PPE and training for its proper use. Those health care professionals and staff who volunteer out of a sense of altruism, compassion, or duty personify the highest values of the VA and their professions. In deciding whether to volunteer to care for patients with Ebola, clinicians and staff should consider their professional role-based obligations as well as other obligations to their own health, to colleagues, friends, and family. As a health care organization, VA has ethical obligations toward its employees, known as the duty of reciprocity. VA is committed to supporting employees who would bear a larger burden of risk in caring for patients with EVD by reducing the risk of exposure as much as possible through PPE and training in its proper use, maintaining as physically safe and secure a work environment as possible, organizing and delivering care consistent with the best evidence available, and allowing flexibilities such as telework and authorized absence for any employee who is asked to be isolated or quarantined.

Should the public health situation evolve to a point where there are not adequate volunteers to care for patients with EVD, VA is committed to ensuring that principles of solidarity and a transparent, fair process will be utilized to assign appropriately trained and qualified employees to work with patients with EVD. Excluding any group of health care providers from reasonable duties in support of EVD response should be made on the basis of a fair and consistent decision-making process to specify the limits or exceptions to employees' duty to provide care.

36. Where would the passage most likely be found?

    A. A training manual for a private institution

    B. A government publication

    C. A textbook on infectious diseases

    D. A radio program

37. Which of the following best describes one of the author's intentions?

    A. To educate the public on the dangers of Ebola

    B. To propose a policy change

    C. To inform people of enacted policies

    D. To train health care workers in the use of PPE

38. The "duty of reciprocity" can best be described as the duty that:

    A. healthcare workers have to care for their patients and protect themselves from danger.

    B. patients have to protect their health care providers just as health care providers protect their patients.

    C. an organization has to protect those who are at the greatest risk of being infected.

    D. an organization has to protect those who are employed by it.

39. Which of the following would be the best title for the passage?

    A. Ethical Issues in Ebola Virus Disease Preparedness and Response

    B. Ebola Preparedness and Response Procedures for VHA

    C. Issues Facing Health Care Workers in the Treatment of Ebola Virus Disease

    D. Issues Facing the Public in an Ebola Virus Disease Outbreak

40. Suppose it were discovered that EVD has a rate of recovery of 90%. How would this affect the author's information?

    I. Healthcare workers treating EVD patients would be expected to take fewer precautions with their patients.

    II. Healthcare workers would be expected to more readily treat EVD patients.

    III. The risks mentioned in the second paragraph would not be considered as grave.

    A. I only

    B. II only

    C. II and III only

    D. I, II, and III

Passage 8 (Questions 41 – 47)

Specialists in non-epidemiological public health will tend to advocate for carrying out medical testing that can, if performed correctly, lead to early detection of conditions that have substantially lower morbidity and mortality rates when early treatment is indicated as opposed to treating the patient after the condition has progressed further. A medical test known as a Pap smear is one such example. Many experts recommend that women of age 21 and above should begin to have this test conducted on a regular basis as a method of checking for a few different types of developing medical conditions. Dysplasia and cervical cancer, as well as related conditions such as the presence of human papilloma virus (HPV), are conditions which fall into this category. Often, if a Pap smear is conducted and leads to a positive test result – carcinoma in situ and ASCUS/AGUS are two such examples – further testing will be recommended in order to determine whether a hazardous medical condition is or is not present in the patient.

However, there are certain demographic groups for whom Pap testing is not recommended due to the potential for elevating the patient's anxiety level, extra expense, and the risk that a false positive will lead to unnecessary and invasive follow-up procedures such as colposcopies or biopsies of the patient's cervix. This is particularly the case for women under age 21, for whom cells detected by a Pap smear and/ or a cytology exam can be expected to disappear on their own rather than develop further. In general, false negative results of a Pap test are not cause for concern if testing is done regularly, because the cells missed by this initial Pap test will divide and grow over time, reaching the point where a follow-up Pap test will detect them. Another reason why certain demographic groups are being dissuaded from Pap testing under current guidelines is that a false positive would probably lead to the patient's treatment provider recommending additional Pap smears, and these could likely lead to consequences analogous to those of the initial test.

Interestingly, a combination of a "better-safe-than-sorry" attitude in the medical community, as well as inadequate data regarding effectiveness of Pap testing, affected Pap testing guidelines in ways that, in all likelihood, led to excessive testing of most demographic groups in past years. More recent guidelines, based on new data taken from organized population-based studies conducted in a number of different countries, indicate that little to no benefit accrues when Pap testing is done every year as opposed to every three years. The guidelines in the United States, promulgated by the American Cancer Society and others, have been updated to reflect this. Additionally, the guidelines now reflect that testing every five years is adequate if a Pap test is combined with a separate test for HPV, as this virus is one of the most frequent causes of cervical cancer.

In examining these guidelines, it is worth noting the harmful effects of conducting excessively frequent Pap smears, not only for patients but for the wider health care system. The medical literature has indicated that, due largely to

follow-up testing, Pap test-related visits can cost over $1,000, despite the fact that a Pap test itself will typically cost only $25 or so. As a result, the new guidelines not only can prevent invasive and possibly damaging medical procedures or follow-up procedures, but they can prevent the unnecessary use of scarce resources that our health care system can ill afford to waste. In this way, more harmful solutions, such as the rationing of care, can be avoided through the intelligent use of evidence-based medicine to determine the true effectiveness of testing, and allowing for the revision of previous assumptions.

41. Which of the following would the author most likely view as an example of evidence-based medicine?

   A. Population-based studies

   B. Use of screening tests to detect dangerous conditions at early stages

   C. Lower morbidity and mortality rates due to Pap testing

   D. Studies which show why cervical cancer is connected with human papilloma virus

42. Based on the passage, which of the following would the author be most likely to view as an ethical issue relating to Pap testing?

   A. Informed consent

   B. Efficient utilization of resources

   C. Fully sharing information with the patient

   D. Prioritizing mortality reduction over lesser considerations

43. All of the following viewpoints are represented in the passage EXCEPT:

   A. the previous set of Pap testing guidelines was affected by a medical community which prioritized caution.

   B. follow-up testing following a positive Pap test result is associated with the possibility that both the patient and society as a whole will experience undesirable effects.

   C. demographics are an important component of the decision whether to recommend a certain category of screening test.

   D. prevention of epidemiological diseases is preferable to the prevention of diseases that only occur in certain demographic groups.

44. Which of the following will probably NOT change the analysis in the passage of whether the guideline recommendations for testing frequency are appropriate?

   I. New data showing that detected carcinoma in situ can grow much faster than previously thought under certain conditions

   II. New data showing that certain lifestyle choices can prevent disappearance of cells detected by Pap testing or cytology testing

   III. New data showing that tests for other conditions, such as HIV, can save more lives than Pap smear testing and yet they are conducted less frequently

   A. I only

   B. II only

   C. III only

   D. I, II and III

45. What is one of the main concerns of the author in writing this passage?

   A. Highlighting the connection between HPV and cervical cancer

   B. Discussing the extent to which physicians can use positive test results, such as carcinoma in situ and ASCUS/AGUS detection, to lower morbidity and mortality rates

   C. Investigating the issues surrounding the collection of evidence necessary to revise Pap testing guidelines

   D. Demonstrating how application of recent evidence can provide benefit and prevent harm

46. The second paragraph mentions analogous consequences. What are some of the consequences to which this language refers?

   I. Excessive psychological distress

   II. Unnecessary cervical biopsies

   III. False negative test results

   A. I only

   B. II only

   C. I and II only

   D. II and III only

47. The author assumes which of the following when discussing the recent revisions of Pap testing guidelines?

   A. That the reduction in recommended frequency of Pap smear testing does not, itself, qualify as rationing of health care

   B. That large-scale studies have been carried out relating to Pap testing

   C. That early-stage screening can detect conditions which are in the early or middle stages of development

   D. That a patient's anxiety level will be elevated whenever the patient sees a positive test result

Passage 9 (Questions 48 – 53)

In the late 1960s, following the success of the civil rights movement for African Americans, Mexican-Americans began to form and develop the Chicano movement. The origin of the word Chicano is debated: it may be from a transcription of the Nahuatal word "Meshico," (Nahuatal was the primary language of the Aztecs) which denoted one from the Meshica Pueblo (eventually a shift in the Spanish language led to using an "he" for previous "sh" sounds, denoted by an "x": thus some proponents prefer the spelling "Xicano" to reflect the etymology), or it may be a bastardization of the Spanish word "Mexicano." While it served as a derogatory term for Mexican-Americans in the first part of the 20th century, suggesting that their identity was lost by living in the U.S. rather than Mexico, it was reclaimed by activists in the latter half, much as "Black" was in the African-American movement. The term was meant to reclaim both ethnic and political identity (another term, "la raza," or "the race," also serves a similar function). As actor and activist Cheech Marin writes: "Hispanic is a census term that some [governmental worker] made up to include all Spanish-speaking brown people. It is especially annoying to Chicanos because it is a catch-all term that includes the Spanish conqueror. By definition, it favors European cultural invasion, not indigenous roots." Thus Chicano was meant to evoke a particular identity: a Spanish-speaking person with indigenous roots (such as the Aztec heritage evoked by "Meshico"), rather than a person of European descent who came to Mexico after Columbus's European discovery of the New World. People with indigenous blood had lower social, and thus economic, status in colonial Mexico; politically, then, the Chicano movement addressed these inequalities as well as questions of ethnic identity. Today some Mexican-Americans steer away from the term because of its politicized element: Nahuatal; Latino identifies all Spanish-speaking inhabitants of the New World, stressing their indigenous heritage in a way that "Hispanic" does not.

The Chicano movement's political origin was spurred on by labor activists such as Cesar Chavez and Delores Huerta; its roots, therefore, gave models of both male and female participation. The academic, side, however, arose from more solely masculine models. Mexican writers such as Octavio Paz and José Vasconcelos, both of whom had lived in America for part of their careers and wrote of a cosmic race made up of people of Mexican descent, were the primary influences in academic Chicano studies. It was this tradition that shaped much of early academic Chicano studies, and indeed the masculine ending of the word reflects this focus.

In 1987, Gloria Anzaldúa's Borderlands/La Frontera: The New Mestiza addressed the issue of gender in Chicano studies particularly by ushering in an era of Chicana studies. In 1981, she and Cherrie Moraga had edited This Bridge Called My Back: Writings by Radical Women of Color, but Borderlands/ La Frontera more specifically addressed the heritage of Mexican American women. Anzaldúa begins the work with an "autohistoria," or personal history. She draws upon the experiences of her family, who had lived for many years in the Rio Grande Valley, first a part of Mexico, then ceded to Texas and the United States. Originally landowners, the Anzaldúa family were displaced and had to work as laborers on their own land. Anzaldúa extends her analysis by tracing the history of the Native Americans who migrated from the Bering Straits down to Mexico, passing through the American Southwest on their way. Anzaldúa writes that "our Spanish, Indian, and mestizo ancestors" returned to "the U.S. Southwest as early as the sixteenth century ... thus making Chicanos originally and secondarily indigenous to the Southwest. Indians and mestizos from central Mexico intermarried with North American Indians. The continual intermarriage between Mexican and American Indians and Spaniards formed an even greater mestizaje." Anzaldúa's terms her work "the new Mestiza." The translation of mestiza is "a woman of mixed parentage" (particularly Spanish and Native American), but for Anzaldúa the term mixed extends to the many "border crossings" she encountered in her daily life, reaching out to disenfranchised women of all races and sexualities. While Mestiza has not caught on as a descriptive term, Anzaldúa's work raised attention to gender disparities in academic studies of Mexican-American identity, so that practitioners commonly refer to Chicano and Chicana studies or, typographically, as Chican@ studies.

48. It can be inferred from the passage that Anzaldúa would refer to a male Mexican American as a:

   A. Chicano.

   B. Mestiza.

   C. Mestizo.

   D. Mestizaje.

49. The author assumes which of the following when asserting that the term "Latino" stresses heritage in a way that "Hispanic" does not?

   A. Language is not the only identity marker to which Latin Americans ascribe.

   B. Stressing the original root of a language results in a clearer sense of identity.

   C. No Mexican-American is willing to be identified as Hispanic.

   D. Gender identity is more important than ethnic or social identity.

50. With which of the following statements would the author be most likely to agree?

   A. The naming of a movement sends important cues about its political, ethnic, and gender-based concerns.

   B. The Aztecs were the original inhabitants of the Rio Grande valley.

   C. Gloria Anzaldúa is most important for her coining of the term "Chican@."

   D. Writers such as Octavio Paz and José Vasconcelos do not reflect the concerns of Mexican-Americans.

51. Suppose it was discovered that the current Spanish word "jalapeno" comes from the Nahuatal "xalapeno." The author would suggest that:

   A. many words for indigenous food groups come from the original Nahuatal.

   B. the change reflects language shifts in post-colonial Mexico.

   C. Mexican-Americans deliberately employ the term to honor their Aztec heritage.

   D. jalapenos are most likely grown in the Rio Grande valley.

52. Which of the following terms is LEAST like the others?

   A. Hispanic

   B. Latino

   C. La Raza

   D. Mestiza

53. Suppose that it was discovered that the ancestors of the Anzaldúa family had lived, during the early 1500s, in what is now Mexico. The author would most likely:

   A. question the timeline that allowed migration from the Bering Strait to Mexico in such a short time period.

   B. accept that such information lessened the claim her family had on its ancestral lands in the Rio Grande Valley.

   C. point out that it would be impossible for mestizaje in Mexico to intermarry with North American Indians.

   D. point out that the forbearers of Chicanos and Chicanas returned the Rio Grande Valley as early as the 16th century.

This page intentionally left blank.

SECTION 2
Answer Key

1	C	12	C	23	B	34	C	45	D
2	B	13	B	24	B	35	B	46	C
3	A	14	D	25	D	36	B	47	A
4	D	15	D	26	A	37	C	48	C
5	D	16	B	27	A	38	D	49	A
6	A	17	A	28	D	39	A	50	A
7	B	18	C	29	C	40	C	51	B
8	A	19	B	30	B	41	A	52	A
9	B	20	B	31	C	42	B	53	D
10	A	21	A	32	C	43	D		
11	D	22	C	33	A	44	C		

Passage 1 (Questions 1-6)

The **San Francisco Ballet** (SFB), the oldest professional ballet troupe in the US, is lauded the world over for its masterful execution of ballet in the neoclassical "**Balanchine aesthetic**". The San Francisco Ballet School (SFBS) is one of the **most competitive** dance programs in the world, with even the Level One program (for dancers aged 7-8) rejecting over 85% of auditioners. Certainly the raw athleticism, coordination, and grace of the dance students in the SFBS is remarkable, although in this regard the SFBS does not stand out from its peer institutions in New York, Moscow, Tokyo, and elsewhere around the word. But what makes the SFB and the SFBS unique is its **especially strong adherence to the uniformity of body type demanded by the Balanchine aesthetic**.

Key terms: San Francisco Ballet, Balanchine aesthetic, San Francisco Ballet School

Opinion: author thinks the SFBS stands out for its especially strict requirements about body type

George Balanchine was at the forefront of the neoclassical emphasis on **movement itself as the key expressive element** of ballet as a medium. He stripped away props, sets, and even costumes and haircuts. Dancers wore plain leotards, kept their hair in a tight bun, and were encouraged to have no facial expression at all – **nothing to distract from the pure expression of movement**. In his later years, Balanchine continually revised his works to simplify everything but the movement and music, and **demanded ever more rigorous uniformity in the look and bodies of the dancers themselves**. To those who continue the Balanchine approach into the 21st century, classical ballet all but demands a dancer have a height as near as possible to 5' 8", an exceptionally slim build, a small head and bust, and long, willowy arms and legs.

Opinion: Balanchine thought movement itself was the way dance was expressed and that to focus solely on movement required stripping away everything else, and having dancers with a strict, uniform body type

An adherence to this look landed the SFBS in hot water in 2001 when it found itself subject to a lawsuit by **Krissy Keefer** on behalf of her 8 year-old daughter, **Fredrika Keefer**. **Krissy is herself a classically trained dancer** and knows, better than most, the rigors of a classical ballet education. Several members of the SFBS faculty suggested to her that it would not be worth Fredrika's time to audition as she would be unlikely to be selected. Nonetheless, Krissy persisted and the school permitted Fredrika to audition. Afterwards, when 18 of the 22 auditioners were **rejected, Fredrika found herself as one of them**.

Key terms: Krissy Keefer, Fredrika Keefer

Cause and effect: SFBS's rejection of Fredrika Keefer led to her mother filing a lawsuit

This would **normally be the end of the story**, but for a then very-recently enacted **municipal statute in San Francisco** which **barred employer discrimination on the basis of height or weight** (expanding the existing statute covering usual things like race, gender, sexual orientation, etc.) Given the **ridiculously overbroad language in the statute**, even a privately-funded school selecting dance students on the basis of bona fide occupational qualifications (the usual legal test for discriminatory action) would fall under the rule's purview.

Cause and effect: under other circumstances, Fredrika's rejection would be the end of the story, but San Francisco had a law that let Krissy sue

Opinion: the author doesn't like this law

The **media attention** the case received has, unsurprisingly, **prompted a large response** from across the spectrum in both the dance and legal communities.

Cause and effect: media attention created a large response

Many correctly point out that it seems long past time to **move beyond the strictures of neoclassical ballet** and Balanchine's increasingly-outdated 1930's worldview about what makes for an exceptional ballet dancer. Critics point out that even companies doing revivals of Balanchine classics like *The Firebird* or *Swan Lake* always include embellishments in the sets or costumes that would have made Balanchine himself livid. In a world where **Alvin Ailey's *Revelations*, with its dancers of various shapes and sizes**, commands **more respect, bigger audiences,** and more imitation than any neoclassical work, it is time we free ourselves from the shackles of a 111 year old Russian's view as to what comprises ballet. This view is limiting and in dancers' efforts to achieve some perfect look they often end up with eating disorders and doing long-term damage to their bodies.

Contrast: Ailey uses dancers of various body types and gets more respect and bigger audiences than Balanchine-style ballet

Opinion: author agrees that it is time for ballet to move past the Balanchine look

Cause and effect: trying to fit into the strict Balanchine look makes many dancers damage their bodies

Yet is it appropriate to put this eight year-old girl in the crosshairs of this debate? **And is the legal system the appropriate venue for ballet to carry out this necessary soul-searching?** If the San Francisco ballet, of anyone, cannot make its own decisions about who is and who is not qualified to meet its own particular artistic requirements, **one fears for a future in which any institution must keep a federal district judge on staff to guide its artistic decision-making.**

Opinion: author thinks that the legal system is the wrong way to tackle the issue

Main Idea: The San Francisco ballet's strict adherence to the Balanchine look for its students and dancers led one rejected student's mother to sue the program; while the author agrees that the Balanchine look is something we should move past, he thinks the legal system is the wrong way to go about it.

1. C is correct. In the passage, Balanchine is said to have stripped away everything but movement itself as the expressive medium.

    A: Using extraneous elements such as lighting or projection would be antithetical to Balanchine's view.

    B, D: We don't know what Balanchine thought of sculpture or painting.

2. B is correct. The author seems to disapprove of using the legal system to resolve disputes related to artistic sensibility or aesthetic. He even sarcastically comments that artistic institutions would need to hire a federal judge to help their decision-making.

    A, C: The author explicitly mentions race and sexual orientation as the "usual" things protected by law.

    D: Nationality or immigration status is never mentioned.

3. A is correct. In the fourth paragraph, the passage tells us that Fredrika's rejection would normally be "the end of the story" and points out that San Francisco was special in having its statute relating to height and weight.

    B, D: The passage never discusses these concepts.

    C: We're specifically told that Ailey's *Revelations* includes dancers of various shapes and sizes, in contrast to Balanchine's work.

4. D is correct. In the next to last paragraph, the author speaks in a strong, negative way about the Balanchine aesthetic and our need to move past it.

    A, C: In the final paragraph the author disapproves of the lawsuit.

    B: The author never suggests that ballet education should wait until children are older.

5. D is correct. The argument structure presented in the passage is "this thing is generally bad and outdated and should be reformed, but using official government channels to do so is a bad idea."

    A, C: The author argues that a lawsuit isn't the way to solve the problem.

    B: The author argues against a formal system like a legal proceeding as a way to deal with problems in the classical ballet community.

6. A is correct. Near the end of the passage, the author strongly expresses the view that Balanchine's view of ballet should be revised, but that a lawsuit is very much the wrong vehicle by which to carry out such revision.

    B, C, D: The author never expresses opinions about these facts and so they would not contradict the author's views.

Passage 2 (Questions 7-12)

The **German Empire** existed for only 47 years and yet in that time did more to **shape the nature of the 20th century** than any other state in Europe (or possibly, the world). While most will only remember the end of the Empire – starting World War I and then being dissolved upon losing it – the German Empire **should instead be remembered for its startling internal contractions**. It was a nation of impressive social, electoral, and economic **advances** but also a **strictly authoritarian place**. It is in this tension that Germany embodied much of the zeitgeist of the subsequent century.

Opinion: the author thinks that the German Empire was an authoritarian place marked by internal contradictions

In 1871, the newly-minted Empire enacted **universal male suffrage**. At a time when poll taxes and literacy tests were being aggressively used to disenfranchise black voters in the U.S. and while the U.K. still had property requirements for suffrage, the German Empire permitted every single male the right to vote. **Germany also created Europe's first social welfare system**, providing old-age pensions, sickness benefits, accident and disability insurance for its industrial workers. The model set by the Empire **saw increases in worker health and productivity** that would not be rivaled for over a century (with the dawn of the information economy). **This combination of expanding political participation, capitalist welfare systems, and freedom of the press set the tone for much of the political progress of the 20th century.**

Key terms: universal male suffrage

Cause and effect: expanding the welfare programs available to German workers helped increase their health and productivity

Opinion: the author thinks that these positive German reforms set the tone for much of the 20th century

In addition to these social reforms, the Empire experienced an **unprecedented industrial and military expansion**. Germany can rightly claim to be the **first truly "urbanized" nation** in the world. In 1870, Germany had almost no rail system to speak of and yet by 1913 had the largest rail network in the world, after the U.S. Germany's dye and chemical industries grew exponentially in the decades prior to 1900, and **expanded into pharmaceuticals, electrochemistry, and agricultural chemicals**. This rapid industrial expansion had two significant corollaries: the development of the first **class of industrial managers in the world** – bureaucrats in the classic Song Dynasty sense who also embodied the scientific and technical know-how that created a strongly practical world-view; and second the research and development needed to drive this industrial expansion created a scientific **Renaissance in German universities** – over 1/3 of all **Nobel prizes** issued during the German Empire's existence went to German scientists.

Key terms: Nobel prizes

Cause and effect: the industrial expansion carried with it the development of a new class – industrial managers – and an increase in scientific achievement

The strong investment in industrial and scientific expansion was not without a **significant dark side**. The authoritarianism that quickly built an impressive industrial base also lent itself to **disastrous social policies**. Extending the vote to every adult male meant that suddenly, repressed **Catholic and Polish minorities** had a voice in the government. In response, Bismarck carried out two campaigns: the *kulturkampf* **and Germanization**. In the former, the Imperial government attempted to seize control of all Catholic churches. Over the course of a decade, **every single Catholic bishop was imprisoned** and as many as 1/4 of parishes found themselves without a priest. In line with government efforts to spread **Lutheranism** were the efforts to get every single person in the Empire to **speak German**. Significant minorities spoke French, Polish, and Lithuanian and efforts to force such groups to adopt German **backfired** spectacularly. In one province, the **percentage of German-speaking citizens actually dropped by over 10%** in the decade during which Germanization was being most aggressively pursued. The authoritarianism that failed so markedly in social policies had an **even more impressively negative effect in foreign policy** . . .

Contrast: while the German Empire was successful in some ways, its ways of dealing with Catholics and non-German-speaking citizens were bad

Opinion: the author thinks the kulturkampf and Germanization efforts were a disaster; the author also thinks the authoritarian approach had even worse outcomes in foreign policy

This set of **contrasting, yet complementary, approaches to authoritarianism** is best revealed by the incident which led to Chancellor Bismarck's resignation. Near the end of 1889, a group of coal miners in the German region of **Silesia** went on **strike**. Bismarck's reaction was swift: he began mobilizing the Army to go in and crush the strike. **Emperor Wilhelm, however, stopped him** and sent an official to negotiate with a delegation from the miners. The strike ended without violence and Bismarck resigned months later. **Wilhelm is reputed to have said, "I do not wish to stain my reign with the blood of my subjects." Yet such measured non-violence obviously did not stay the Emperor's hand in dealing with the Empire's colonies.**

Key terms: Silesia, strike

Contrast: Bismarck wants to use the military to crush a strike but Emperor Wilhelm insisted on negotiating with the workers.

Contrast: despite taking a soft approach on the strikes, apparently the Emperor took a violent approach to foreign affairs and dealing with overseas colonies

Main Idea: The German Empire was marked by contradictions in having amazing success and liberalization in some areas (voting rights, worker supports) while meeting with disastrous failure of authoritarian policies in others (treatment of Catholics, foreign policy) and it should be remembered for more than just starting World War I.

7. B is correct. The author speaks most positively about the Empire's creation of support for workers, expansion of voting rights, and scientific and industrial advances. This is an example of worker support.

    A, C: These limitations on voting rights would get disapproval from the author.

    D: The author strongly disapproved of Germanization and spoke of it as a failure.

8. A is correct. In the final paragraph, we're told that there were contrasting approaches to authoritarianism and that Bismarck wished to take a violent, authoritarian approach to dealing with a domestic crisis. That is contrasted with the Emperor who took a non-violent approach, but apparently was violent in foreign policy and "dealing with its colonies."

9. B is correct. The tone of the passage is generally cut-and-dry with a discussion of facts, overlaid with a particular opinion about what was good and bad about the German Empire's policies. It is thus most likely a work by a historian who studies the German Empire. In particular, you can see a tiny bit of frustration in the first paragraph with the fact that most people only know about one part (World War I) of his area of expertise.

    A: The passage speaks positively about social welfare.

    C, D: Suppression of Catholics and discussion about colonialism are only side concerns in the passage and not the overall focus.

10. A is correct. At the end of the passage, we learn that Chancellor Bismarck took a swift, violent, and authoritarian approach to dealing with a domestic crisis. Thus it seems likely that he either actively supported or at least passively approved of other authoritarian strong-arm tactics in domestic policy.

11. D is correct. The discussion about the rail system follows a comment that Germany experienced an unprecedented industrial expansion. Thus moving from almost no rail system to the second largest in the world in the span of forty years emphasizes the swiftness of German industrial expansion.

    A: While the author says that the German industrial expansion was unprecedented, he never argues that it was overall "superior" to other countries.

    B: The author does not make any "what if" predictions.

C: Following the comment about the rail system, the author goes on to cite other German successes, not failures.

12. C is correct. The author starts with a very strongly positive tone, telling us many impressive things about the German Empire at the end of the 19th century. The passage then moves into a discussion of its failures, both domestic and foreign. Thus his respect is balanced by an appreciation of negative aspects.

    B: The author discusses negative aspects of the German Empire.

    A, D: These are concepts not discussed in the passage.

Passage 3 (Questions 13-18)

Olav **Hammer's** scathing **critique of anthroposophy** centers primarily on his assertion that anthroposophy is not science, but **scientism** – the **inappropriate application of the methods of empirical science to all areas of life** and the assertion that the only true knowledge or facts that can be discovered are those revealed through typical scientific methods. Both in subsuming the natural sciences under the umbrella of spiritual "science" and in its **unjustifiable defense of fringe sciences such as biodynamic agriculture**, anthroposophy places itself firmly in the realm of the delusional, holds Hammer.

Key terms: scientism

Opinion: Hammer criticizes anthroposophy as "fringe"; Hammer also seems to think that scientism is a bad thing

Anthroposophy is a philosophy founded at the start of the 20th century by Austrian philosopher and social reformer Rudolf **Steiner**. The core mission of anthroposophy is to **help individuals develop imagination and intuition**, and to **study the spiritual world with the same objective rigor as the natural sciences**. People were expected to develop a supersensory consciousness which could then be used to study the spiritual realm and report back in a way intelligible to those who had not yet developed such consciousness. **Steiner believed that the spiritual realm was real, and had the same objective existence as our material one.**

Key terms: Steiner

Opinion: Steiner thought the spiritual world was objectively real like the physical world; anthroposophy aimed to develop imagination and to study the spiritual world

Steiner defined human nature as existing of four different components – a physical body that is created from and returns to the inorganic world; an etheric body (similar to all living things); an astral body (similar to all sentient beings); and a unique self-aware component called the ego. Humans reincarnate as part of a karmic cycle and are a higher life-form because they are less specialized. This last point reflects anthroposophy's odd view of evolution: a single unspecialized archetype was the progenitor of all animal life and organisms are devolved from this state, rather than evolved towards increasing complexity as in Darwinism.

Key terms: human nature, components

Opinion: author thinks that the anthroposophic view of evolution is "odd"

It was in this discussion of anthroposophical evolution that Steiner's work drew the attention and ire from so many in both philosophical and scientific circles. Steiner's defenders in the middle and later parts of the 20th century emphasized that such criticism ultimately missed the point. While any number of esoteric traditions flourished at the end of the 19th century (most prominently the Theosophy from which anthroposophy derived., none of them come in for

the same criticism as anthroposophy. Defenders such as Herbert Hahn counter that we ought to look at the practical application of anthroposophic ideas and judge the philosophy not on its rarefied esoteric principles, but on its effect in the real world. "Christianity is not to be judged through a meditation on the paradox of how a being, Jesus, could be both fully man and fully God, but rather on the great works and good charity actually demonstrated by Christians," held Hahn. "We only ask the same."

Opinion: Hahn and other defenders of anthroposophy say to look at practical effect, not esoteric principles

Hahn points out the **Waldorf** schools around the world which focus on holistic, developmentally-appropriate education for students at all levels. Waldorf schools typically produce young adults that are far more well-rounded, creative, and who excel at lateral thinking and problem solving, they assert. **Biodynamic agriculture**, developed in the early 1920's laid the foundations for both modern **organic farming** and what would eventually become **Integrated Pest Management**, the gold standard in sustainable agriculture. Finally, Steiner's ideas about **socially responsible financial associations** set the framework for Social Finance that began with the *Gemeinschaftsbank* in Germany in the 1970's.

Key terms: Waldorf, biodynamic agriculture, organic farming, integrated pest management, Gemeinschaftsbank

Opinion: those who defend anthroposophy think that the various things it led to (organic farming, socially responsible banking, etc.) show that it is good

Both critics and defenders of Steiner's work have valid points, so far as they go, but ultimately **end up speaking past one another**.

Opinion: author thinks that the critics and defenders of anthroposophy are simply addressing different points and so not having a real conversation

Main Idea: Steiner's philosophy of anthroposophy tried to apply scientific principles to the spiritual world; this philosophy contained a number of odd views that drew criticism, but defenders point out that work inspired by anthroposophic principles has done good in the world.

13. B is correct. At the beginning of the fourth paragraph, the author tells us that Steiner's odd views about evolution drew attention and criticism. Without those writings, anthroposophy would have been less likely to get such strong criticism.

    A, C, D: Anthroposophy's views on evolution are not tied into either the components of human nature nor agriculture.

14. D is correct. The passage defines scientism as taking empirical science too far – thinking that all aspects of human life should be analyzed through science.

    A, C: These are examples of applying valid empirical science to scientific questions and thus wouldn't qualify as scientism.

    B: There is no application of empirical science here, since it is simply a psychic making a claim about a supernatural ability.

15. D is correct. The passage tells us that Hammer calls anthroposophy delusional based on its nature as scientism – inappropriately using the methods of empirical science in non-scientific ways. Hahn counters that one should evaluate anthroposophy on the basis of its practical effects in the real world.

    A: Hahn would certainly believe this, but we don't know what Hammer has to say about education and Waldorf schools.

    B: Although Hammer says biodynamic agriculture itself is a pseudoscience, we're never told that he would dispute the fact that biodynamic agriculture led to the development of organic farming.

    C: We don't know what Hahn would have to say about this, and Hammer disputes scientism but we're never told he goes so far as to assert that empirical science can't reach out to things like psychology or other social sciences.

16. B is correct. In the passage, the author describes critics and supports of anthroposophy as talking past one another because they address totally different issues and don't even seem to agree on how to judge the issues. Two candidates who approach a topic from radically different views and don't even address each others' points would be an analogous example.

    A, C, D: In each of these cases the people disputing are addressing the same topic using roughly the same framework and so are not talking "past one another".

17. A is correct. The reference to Christianity is made in the fourth paragraph in which we read about Hahn's efforts to defend anthroposophy against critics.

    B, D: The quote does not reference scientism in any way, and scientism is only mentioned in the first paragraph.

    C: While defenders of anthroposophy do point to Waldorf schools and organic farming as positive outcomes, the reference to Christianity is more general, in which defenders are trying to point out that one should judge a worldview through its effects.

18. C is correct. In the fourth and fifth paragraphs we read about the defenders of anthroposophy and Steiner's works. In those paragraphs, they point to all of the good outcomes of people who were working based on anthroposophical ideas (choice D). Hahn also makes an explicit reference to Christianity and he wants anthroposophy to be judged the same way Christianity should be judged (choice A). Finally, defenders point out that lots of esoteric philosophies were present around the same time (choice B) and yet critics don't attack them the same way they do anthroposophy. At no point do anthroposophy's defenders address the idea of scientism at all (choice C).

Passage 4 (Questions 19 – 23)

Political ideals must be based upon ideals for the **individual life**. The aim of politics should be to make the lives of individuals as **good as possible**. There is nothing for the politician to consider outside or above the various men, women, and children who compose the world. The problem of politics is to adjust the relations of human beings in such a way that each severally may have as much of good in his existence as possible. And this problem requires that we should first consider what it is that we think good in the individual life.

Key terms: political ideals, individuals

Opinion: the author thinks that the aim of politics should be to provide the greatest good to everyone

Cause and effect: in order to provide the greatest good, we must understand what is good for an individual

We may distinguish **two sorts of goods**, and two corresponding sorts of impulses. There are goods in regard to which **individual possession** is possible, and there are goods in which **all can share alike**. The food and clothing of one man is not the food and clothing of another; if the supply is insufficient, what one man has obtained is at the expense of some other man. This applies to material goods generally, and therefore to the greater part of the present economic life of the world. On the other hand, **mental and spiritual goods do not belong to one man to the exclusion of another.** If one man knows a science, that does not prevent others from knowing it; on the contrary, it helps them to acquire the knowledge. If one man is a great artist or poet, that does not prevent others from painting pictures or writing poems, but helps to create the atmosphere in which such things are possible. If one man is full of good-will toward others, that does not mean that there is less good-will to be shared among the rest; the more good-will one man has, the more he is likely to create among others. In such matters there is no possession, because there is not a definite amount to be shared; **any increase anywhere tends to produce an increase everywhere**.

Opinion: the authors believes that there are material goods, which are limited, and spiritual goods, which can be shared and increase without limit

Cause and effect: if a person shares a spiritual good, its increase produces an increase in others

There are two kinds of **impulses**, corresponding to the two kinds of goods. There are **possessive impulses**, which aim at acquiring or retaining private goods that cannot be shared; these center in the impulse of property. And there are **creative or constructive impulses**, which aim at bringing into the world or making available for use the kind of goods in which there is no privacy and no possession.

Key terms: impulses, possessive impulses, creative or constructive impulses

Contrast: the author contrasts the impulse associated with the gain of material goods vs creative impulses, aimed at bringing spiritual goods into the world

The **best life is the one in which the creative impulses play the largest part** and the possessive impulses the smallest. This is no new discovery. The Gospel says: "Take no thought, saying, What shall we eat? or What shall we drink? or, Wherewithal shall we be clothed?" The thought we give to these things is taken away from matters of more importance. And what is worse, the habit of mind engendered by thinking of these things is a bad one; it **leads to competition, envy, domination, cruelty**, and almost all the moral evils that infest the world. In particular, it leads to the predatory use of **force**. **Material possessions can be taken by force** and enjoyed by the robber. Spiritual possessions cannot be taken in this way. You may kill an artist or a thinker, but you cannot acquire his art or his thought. You may put a man to death because he loves his fellow-men, but you will not by so doing acquire the love which made his happiness. Force is impotent in such matters; it is only as regards material goods that it is effective. For this reason the **men who believe in force are the men whose thoughts and desires are preoccupied with material goods**.

Contrast: throughout the passage there is a contrast between material and spiritual goods, possessive and creative impulses; in this paragraph the evils of the former are outlined

Cause and effect: possessive impulses drive a person to the gain of material goods, which can cause them to develop all the moral evils of the world; it is better for men to give in to creative impulses

What we shall desire for individuals is now clear: strong creative impulses, overpowering and absorbing the instinct of possession; **reverence for others**; **respect** for the fundamental creative impulse in ourselves. A certain kind of **self-respect** or native pride is necessary to a good life; a man must not have a sense of utter inward defeat if he is to remain whole, but must feel the **courage** and the **hope** and the will to live by the best that is in him, whatever outward or inward obstacles it may encounter. So far as it lies in a man's own power, his life will realize its best possibilities if it has three things: **creative rather than possessive** impulses, **reverence** for others, and **respect** for the fundamental impulse in himself. Political and social institutions are to be judged by the good or harm that they do to individuals. Do they encourage creativeness rather than possessiveness? Do they embody or promote a spirit of reverence between human beings? Do they preserve self-respect?

Cause and effect: individuals should have reverence for others, respect for themselves, and creative impulses; political institutions have the charge to develop this in the people they govern

Main Idea: The author seeks to define what is meant by good to show how a political institution should harbor good for the greatest number of people; the author discusses how possessive and creative impulses cause evil and good respectively.

19. B is correct. The author uses the example of good-will as a spiritual good. It must be something that is intangible and cannot be exhausted.

A: Time, in a certain sense, is a limited resource so this is not as good an option as B.

C, D: These are material goods

20. B is correct. The author states that "the problem of politics is to adjust the relations of human beings in such a way that each severally may have as much of good in his existence as possible." Since the author thinks that each person severally should have as much good as possible, choice B is correct. The author would argue that a separate ideal for each separate man is preferable to one ideal for all men.

A, C: These are all themes or ideas that can be directly inferred from passage information.

D: A world that is completely dominated by competition would be a world in which a focus on possession and material goods would be paramount. In such a world, few would be able to stay focused on spiritual goods.

21. A is correct. The end of the passage reverts to the question of whether political institutions are doing good in stimulating good creative impulses in society over possessive impulses. Thus the author will likely make a statement in answer to the questions he or she asks at the end of the passage.

B, C, D: These are all topics the author could discuss but earlier in the passage.

22. C is correct. The author believes that everyone has the capacity to do good and choose creative impulses over possessive. There is no reason to think that the author would advocate a theory that everyone is morally corrupt at their core or anything similar to this.

A, B: The passage deals with politics and philosophy.

D: The author probably believes this because without said capacity, creative impulses could not be indulged.

23. B is correct. The author states that creative impulses are a large part of the best life and then cites the Bible reference as evidence that it is accepted that the best life places emphasis on creative impulses rather than possessive.

A: This is not the express purpose of the statement.

C: This is true but choice B is better because the statement is evidence of a previously made claim.

D: While it is true that these cannot be stolen, this is not related to the discussion in question.

Passage 5 (Questions 24 – 29)

During most of the **post-World War II era**, **Japan's economy** experienced a remarkable and, to many, enviable period of rapid economic **growth**. Between 1965 and 1980, nominal gross domestic product grew from $91 billion to $1.065 trillion. In the 1980s, Japan had the **highest productivity** of any country in the world. Many Westerners of the time were not only envious but curious. **What had produced** such a dramatic Japanese expansion and economic boom? Attempts were made to study the factors which had turned the "Land of the Rising Sun" into such a brightly shining economic star. Many of these observers had the specific, ideal end **goal** of determining whether this **good fortune could be replicated** in the United States and other Western countries.

Opinion: author thinks Westerners studied the huge success of Japan's economy after WWII with the intention of trying to replicate its success in the U.S. and Europe

One attempt to discern the reasons for Japan's economic success focused on **attitudes** in the workplace. One such approach focused on the differences between the so-called Theory X and Theory Z. **Theory X**, created by management professor Douglas Murray **McGregor**, refers to the viewpoint that **workers are inherently lazy**, dislike their jobs and their careers, and aren't likely to apply themselves to their jobs without the use of constant supervision and prodding. Many observers believed that American workplaces of the era contained a high percentage of people who subscribed to this theory about their workers. But in 1981, a book by Dr. William **Ouchi** described an alternative viewpoint called "**Theory Z**". The book stated that the attitudes in Japanese workplaces **promoted employee satisfaction** and morale by focusing on the employee's well-being, on and off the job, which was **conducive to productivity** and other positive economic benchmarks. For many, this provided an explanation of why Japan had become the world's most productive country.

Contrast: Theory X (workers are lazy; believed by many Americans) vs Theory Z (if workers have high morale, they will be productive)

Other theories, more based in **macroeconomics** than in management theory, saw Japan's success as less a consequence of the employer-employee dynamic and more a consequence of **serendipitous** and not particularly complex **economic trends** which, in the era studied, overlapped with one another. One of these factors was **low worldwide oil prices**, translating into lower prices for gasoline and other essentials of a growing economy such as energy. Another factor related to the speed of **technological advancement**. In economic supply-and-demand theory, newly introduced technological developments can shift the curve of aggregate supply. When this occurs, production increases, causing economic growth, and there is downward pressure on prices, keeping inflation in check. Postwar Japan could advance very rapidly simply by **importing advanced technologies** from other countries **without** having to invest in **costly**

research and development. After a few decades, though, Japan had essentially caught up to the rest of the world in terms of technology. Once Japan reached technological parity with the world's other advanced countries, the playing field was level again – Japan could no longer simply import technological advancement, and was now able to advance technologically only by **creating its own advances** through expensive investment in research and development.

Opinion: other economists think Japan's economic success was due to low oil prices and an ability to quickly import technological advancements, rather than how workers were managed

By the **late 1990s**, **trouble** in the Japanese economy had started to reach a tipping point. **Consumer** spending and **investor** spending were simultaneously **dropping**, and Japan's traditionally low **unemployment** rate was on the **rise**. Concern about weak aggregate demand led to both domestic and international pressure to fix the issue, as Japan's economy was the world's second-largest at the time and there was fear that Japan's economic troubles could affect business cycles in other countries. Facing this, the government decided to apply the **dual fiscal stimuli** of cutting taxes and increasing government spending. Other measures over the next several years followed, **none fully effective**. **Deflation**, which was re-aggravated in some ways by the government's attempts at structural reform, dampened both production and consumer demand, and led to **legitimate fears of a disastrous deflationary spiral**. After experiencing what many call a "**lost decade**" in economic growth, Japan might now be entering a second one.

Contrast: after decades of large success and economic growth, Japan had a lost decade marked by deflation, reduced demand, and increasing unemployment

Main Idea: The main focuses of this passage are first, Japanese attempts to fix the economy in response to pressure, second, lack of success, and third, the causes and effects of deflation.

24. B is correct. The author describes the potential of a deflationary spiral as "disastrous" and the fears of one occurring as "legitimate." He therefore would be more likely than not to support a policy which could block that from happening, even if other risks exist.

A: The author does not indicate that alleviating deflation will prevent a second "lost decade", let alone that Japan will never re-emerge if a second lost decade occurs.

C: No part of the passage indicates that the author believes a successful economy always requires low inflation.

D: No part of the passage indicates the author believes that this is the only factor preventing Japan from developing a strong economy.

25. D is correct. The passage describes how observers attempted to find out why Japan's postwar economy was as successful as it was. Management theories such as Theory X and Theory Z are discussed in the passage to illustrate this, because some observers used them to try to provide an explanation.

A: This may be accurate, but is not why the author discusses the two theories.

B, C: The author is not interested in whether it is true; he's only concerned with how some used management theories to explain Japan's economic success.

26. A is correct. The third paragraph says that "In economic supply-and-demand theory, newly introduced technological developments can shift the curve of aggregate supply." It goes on to describe the positive economic advantages that this aggregate supply curve-shifting is responsible for (economic growth, keeping inflation in check). Thus, once Japan caught up technologically with the rest of the world, it lost these advantages.

B: The passage indicates that expensive research and development is a necessity for technological advancement after parity is reached with other countries. It does not say that there is no longer an impetus to focus on it.

C: Low prices for oil, gasoline and energy are described, but they are described as existing circumstances at the time, not as the effects of any particular cause.

D: According to the passage, an economic situation which kept inflation in check is described, but it existed before Japan achieved technological parity with other countries, not after.

27. A is correct. Here, the last paragraph describes a weak economy, in addition to foreign and domestic pressure to fix it. This indicates that there was sufficient motivation to fix economic problems. The last paragraph also indicates that the measures undertaken by the government were not fully effective.

B: International economic cooperation is not mentioned in the last paragraph – just international economic pressure.

C: The passage says that structural reform worsened deflation; it does not follow that structural reform can limit inflation.

D: The passage indicates that Japan's weak aggregate demand in the 1990s might have affected other countries' business cycles. However, it also says that Japan had the world's second-largest economy. This answer choice says that weak aggregate demand will "significantly" affect the rest of the world – this might not be true of weak aggregate demand in small countries with small economies.

28. D is correct. Based on the last paragraph, the author is discussing facts that indicate that Japan's government has tried several techniques to solve the country's problems, and all failed. The author does not include data suggesting that this will change and tends to suggest the opposite of answer choice D.

A: The author would probably agree with this, because the last paragraph does not say that structural reform solved any problems and it may have actually caused new ones.

B: The author would probably agree with this, because the last paragraph references domestic and international pressure on Japan to fix its economic issues, based on worry that Japanese economic troubles could affect the business cycles of other countries.

C: The author would probably agree with this. The first few paragraphs describe different explanations of Japan's postwar economic success, without indicating that the issue has ever achieved a consensus. The last paragraph describes how attempts to fix Japan's present economic situation have been tried, and have fallen short. There is no indication that a solution has been found that everyone would agree with.

29. C is correct. I: The fact that they wanted to replicate this success in their own countries meant they had a self-interested purpose, which rules out I.

II: This is accurate because the paragraph indicates that they had a purpose, and explains what that purpose was. III: This is correct because of the characterization of them as "curious".

Passage 6 (Questions 30 – 35)

Titian, Velasquez, and Rembrandt are generally acknowledged to be the **greatest masters of painting** the world has known, and to each of them, we happily and fittingly apply the word **genius**. Of all the definitions of that abused word, there is one that states that genius comes not from seeing more than other people, but from **seeing differently**. In this way, we acknowledge a painter as genius when he is able to, beyond his masterly technical skills, **present to us a view** of life or nature that **we have never seen**, but that we are deeply and immediately convinced is a product of deeper vision than our own. The painter has seen it: only because of our shortcomings, and the dimness or narrowness of our outlooks, is it that we do not see it also.

Key terms: Titian, Velasquez, Rembrandt, genius

Opinion: most consider Titian, Velasquez, and Rembrandt to be the greatest masters of painting

Cause and effect: a painter is a genius if he presents us with a view of life or nature that we have never seen

A **great painter** writes us a letter, filled with details of the things he has seen and heard and felt, **giving us a look into the world in which he lives**. A great painter bares his **personality** to us, and personality in art is of inestimable value. We love **Corot's** *Arcadia* landscape because it is the vision, heart, and character of the personality of the artist, distilled and presented directly to us. A **Rembrandt** may express personality **abundantly**. A **Velasquez**, on the other hand, may express personality **negatively**.

Key terms: Corot's *Arcadia*

Contrast: the ways in which Corot, Rembrandt, and Velasquez each present personality are contrasted

Cause and effect: a great painter bears his personality through his work; we love Corot's *Arcadia* because it possess the heart and character of the artist

In judging a painter, we must be vigilant to carefully distinguish between his own personality and the personality of those who interpret him. The more that we give of ourselves to a painter, or any other kind of artist, the more his work returns our giving with appeal and interest. Cleave the wood of your brain and you find the artist reaching out with communications. Raise the stone of your imagination and the artist is revealed.

Contrast: the personality of the artist vs the personality of the person interpreting the artist's work

Cause and effect: the more we give ourselves to a painter, the more their work gives back

There was a certain **critic** who had **devoted his life** to the study of **Reynolds**. Once, while lecturing upon the great achievements of his subject, the critic put a large subject-picture upon the screen: this was not one of Reynolds's happier

efforts, but rather, an **unattractive and obviously labored design** which we know gave Reynolds a sea of troubles. This critic's **analysis** of the picture was so scientific, so interesting, **so absorbing**, that many of the audience were persuaded that they were looking upon a masterpiece. In reality, they had been **hypnotized by** the subtleties of this **critic's** personal approach to Reynolds.

Contrast: the critic's analysis of the painting vs its actual quality

Cause and effect: because the critic's analysis was so interesting, many thought it was a masterpiece

On the other hand, **some criticism** has tended towards **depreciation**, **due to** the predilection of some critics for **objective** as opposed to subjective criticism. As P.G. **Hamerton** once wrote of Rembrandt, "The **chiaroscuro** (treatment of light in a drawing or painting) of Rembrandt is often **false and inconsistent**, and in fact he relied largely on public ignorance. But though arbitrary, it is always conducive to his purpose."

Opinion: P.G. Hamerton believes that Rembrandt's use of lighting is false and inconsistent

Contrast: criticism that tends to over appreciation vs criticism that tends towards depreciation because it is objective

"**Conducive to his purpose!**" Those four words contain **much virtue**. Perhaps more than anybody, Rembrandt knew that his style of lighting was **not** a **facsimile** of nature, that it did not represent the chiaroscuro seen by the average eye. He had an aim, **a vision before him**, and he never hesitated to interpret that particular vision in **his own particular way**. So, who dares to say Rembrandt was disloyal to nature?

Opinion: Hamerton is wrong

Cause and effect: because he had a vision before him, Rembrandt never hesitated to interpret his particular vision in a particular way

Our concern ought to be not what he should have done, but **what he did**, seeing with his own eyes. These are the questions we should ask ourselves: **Is his interpretation of the world beautiful**, profound, stimulating, and suggestive? Does the imprint of his personality in paint add to our own knowledge and hone our aesthetic perception? Does his work **extend our horizons** by showing us visions that our imperfect eyes and minds cannot see except through him?

Opinion: we should be more concerned with what Rembrandt did than with what he should have done; the value in art is how it shows us one artist's vision, not a pure facsimile of nature

Main Idea: The author makes the case that the greatest painters are able to show us a view of life that we have never seen before and bare their personalities to us; Rembrandt is described in detail; in the end, we ought to judge artists not for what we think they should have done, but for what they actually did.

30.   B is correct. As the author writes in the second paragraph, "We love Corot's Arcadia landscape because it is the vision, heart, and character of the personality of the artist, distilled and presented directly to us. A Rembrandt may express personality abundantly."

A: Titian is never spoken of in depth.

C: Velasquez may express personality negatively, which seems at odds with personality as presented by Corot and Rembrandt.

D: This quality is not attributed to Reynolds' work.

31.   C is correct. In the third paragraph, the author writes, "In judging a painter, we must be vigilant to carefully distinguish between his own personality and the personality of those who interpret him." Now, jump ahead to the fourth paragraph and the Reynolds-critic anecdote: an overzealous critic can color a work in a certain way such that the voice of the artist is muted. The critic had audience members believing the work was a masterpiece when it wasn't.

A: This quality is never attributed to Reynolds.

B: This critic seems to have a penchant for subjectivity.

D: The Hamerton anecdote fulfills this choice more accurately.

32.   C is correct. Though the author does mention technical mastery as almost an afterthought, he does make it clear that it is necessary. As he writes in the first paragraph, ". . . We acknowledge a painter as a genius when he is able to, beyond his masterly technical skills, present to us a view of life . . ."

A: This was just proven false.

B: This is never said to be true.

D: Rather, a masterly painter's personality is "distilled and presented directly" to the viewer.

33.   A is correct. In the first paragraph, the author writes that a masterly painter "present[s] to us a view of life or nature that we have never seen, but that we are deeply and immediately convinced is a product of deeper vision than our own." Now, jump to the sixth paragraph, where the author writes his rebuttal to Hamerton's opinion that Rembrandt's treatment of life was unrealistic. The author has already expressed that the great artist shows us a new vision of the world. As he writes, "He had an aim, a vision before him, and he never hesitated to interpret that particular vision in his own particular way." So, the author would say that Rembrandt's unconventional use of lighting, also known as chiaroscuro, is an example of how he shows us a new view of the world that we wouldn't see other-

wise.

B: The author thinks great artists open up their personality to us, but not that we appropriate the artist's personality for ourselves.

C: Well, if two elements make a genius painter, showing us a new vision of the world and expressing one's personality through art, this only does one of those, at least within the context of the passage.

D: This is never said. The author seems to be able to do this without any help from Rembrandt.

34.   C is correct. First of all, as the passage will have us know, we should be wary of anything a critic says, but as all of the answers come from critics, they can cancel each other out (so to speak). Choice C is correct because it is the only statement that expresses something negative about the painter himself and his abilities.

A: Critics depreciated Rembrandt too. This choice has nothing in it about the artist's own abilities and as the author maintains, an artist's genius rests in his ability to relate to viewers.

B: Same.

D: This is representative of how Hamerton viewed Rembrandt, as too unrealistic. As the author points out, a work needs to be realistic, but it must communicate a sense of the artist's personality. So, Choice D describes something that can be lacking from the work of a genius while Choice C describes something that cannot be lacking.

35.   B is correct. It is never said in the passage that the work of great artists is underappreciated. In fact, the passage is quite celebratory of at least a few great artists. Moreover, the Reynolds critic anecdote demonstrates that some critics over appreciate great artists.

Passage 7 (Questions 36 – 40)

The **codes of ethics** of all health care professionals include a **duty to provide care** to patients even at some risk to themselves. In the **Veteran's Health Administration (VHA)**, staff who are not clinicians also have a duty as **Veteran's Administration (VA)** employees to contribute to the mission of VHA in supporting the delivery of health care services. The duty to provide or support the provision of care is strong, but is not absolute and **has certain justifiable exceptions**. Those exceptions become relevant in circumstances when caring for patients imposes a **disproportionate risk** on the health care providers and staff providing that care.

Opinion: the author presents the idea that health care professionals don't always have to provide care in situations that put themselves at a disproportionately large risk

Cause and effect: if the care of a patient imposes a risk for the caregiver, one must consider the circumstances before providing care

The experience in West Africa and elsewhere indicates that caring for patients with **Ebola (EVD)** may involve personal risk to health care providers and others, including the **risk of infection or death**, burden to their families, and possible quarantine or isolation, if exposed. Caring for patients with EVD may also involve a **risk to an entire health care system** if first-line providers become ill or die, leaving the health care system without vital resources to treat EVD as well as other illnesses. Caring for patients with EVD may also involve a **risk to other patients** if providers become infected and then serve as vectors for transmission. To date, the experience in the U.S. has demonstrated that health care providers' exposure can be mitigated by the proper use of **personal protective equipment (PPE)**, that actions can be taken to ensure that an exposed or infected health care provider will not transmit the virus to others, and that an infected health care provider has a good chance of clearing the virus.

Key terms: West Africa, EVD

Contrast: author outlines the risks involved with treating EVD patients and also the ways to prevent its spread

Cause and effect: treating patients with EVD includes a risk of death; if physicians die, other patients and the health care system will suffer; PPE can prevent spread of EVD

In its **Framework for Ebola Preparedness and Response**, VA leadership is initially asking health care providers and staff to indicate their **willingness to volunteer** for Ebola Response Teams at Tier 1 VAMCs. VA has also issued guidance on the Use of Telework or **Authorized Absence** in Cases of Suspected Exposure to Ebola, and is committed to providing PPE and training for its proper use. Those health care professionals and staff who volunteer out of a sense of altruism, compassion, or duty **personify the highest values** of the VA and their professions. In deciding whether to volunteer to care for patients with Ebola, clinicians and staff should consider their professional role-based obligations as well as other obligations to their own health, to colleagues, friends, and family. As a health care organization, **VA has ethical obligations toward its employees, known as the duty of reciprocity**. VA is committed to supporting employees who would bear a larger burden of risk in caring for patients with EVD by reducing the risk of exposure as much as possible through PPE and training in its proper use, maintaining as physically safe and secure a work environment as possible, organizing and delivering care consistent with the best evidence available, and **allowing flexibilities** such as telework and authorized absence for any employee who is asked to be isolated or quarantined.

Key Terms: Ebola Response Teams, Telework

Opinion: author is asking for volunteers for the Ebola Response Teams and outlines the commitments of the volunteers and of VA towards their employees and volunteers

Cause and effect: the duty of reciprocity entails that the VA holds a great obligation toward their own employees

Should the public health situation evolve to a point where there are **not adequate volunteers** to care for patients with EVD, VA is committed to ensuring that principles of solidarity and a **transparent, fair process will be utilized to assign appropriately trained and qualified employees** to work with patients with EVD. Excluding any group of health care providers from reasonable duties in support of EVD response should be made on the basis of a fair and consistent decision-making process to specify the limits or exceptions to employees' duty to provide care.

Cause and effect: in the event that there are not enough volunteers to handle the Ebola crisis, measures will be taken to assign health care workers to the duties of caring for EVD patients

Main Idea: The main idea of the passage is to present some aspects of the VA's Ebola Preparedness and Response procedures; the author outlines how health care workers are chosen to treat EVD patients and talks about the ethics behind the treatment of infectious diseases.

36.   B is correct. The passage seems to be informing people about the workings of an organization and how they will respond to an Ebola outbreak. This is most consistent with a government publication.

   A: This is a work about a government entity, the Veteran's Health Administration, not a private institution.

   C: This is not information you would find in a textbook.

   D: This could be but is not as likely as choice B, as a radio program would be aimed at a much wider audience than those who have an interest in the VA healthcare procedures.

37.   C is correct. The author is trying to inform the audience on the policies of VHA.

   A: This is not the author's purpose, as the passage does not focus on the dangers of Ebola.

   B: There is no mention of a change.

   D: The use of PPE is only briefly mentioned.

38.   D is correct. The passage states that VA has ethical obligations toward its employees, known as the duty of reciprocity.

   A, B, C: These relationships are explored in the passage but are not the specific "duty of reciprocity".

39.   A is correct. Every paragraph of the passage addresses an ethical issue, how to decide whether it is justifiable to treat a patient, how to decide who treats the patient, and so on.

   B: This is outlined somewhat in the passage but the ethical issues are more important to the content of the passage.

   C: This is only a small part of the passage discussion.

   D: This is not at all the main idea of the passage as the notion of a large scale outbreak that the general public needs to worry about is much too broad for the passage.

40.   C is correct. I: It would be foolish not to take the same precautions with EVD patients, since even a 10% risk of death is a high one.

   II: The passage states that health care workers must balance risk to themselves with their obligation to their patients. If there were less risk to themselves, they would be expected to be more involved in the treatment of EVD patients.

   III: The major risk associated with Ebola is that those who contract it have an exceptionally high mortality rate. If the mortality rate were brought down to 10%, the risks of the disease would be much less serious.

Passage 8 (Questions 41 – 47)

Specialists in **non-epidemiological public health** will tend to **advocate** for carrying out **medical testing** that can, if performed correctly, **lead to early detection** of conditions that have substantially lower morbidity and mortality rates when early treatment is indicated as opposed to treating the patient after the condition has progressed further. A medical test known as a **Pap smear** is one such example. Many experts recommend that **women of age 21 and above** should begin to have this **test conducted on a regular basis** as a method of checking for a few different types of developing medical conditions. Dysplasia and cervical cancer, as well as related conditions such as the presence of human papilloma virus (HPV), are conditions which fall into this category. Often, if a Pap smear is conducted and leads to a positive test result – carcinoma in situ and ASCUS/AGUS are two such examples – further testing will be recommended in order to determine whether a hazardous medical condition is or is not present in the patient.

Key terms: Pap smear

Opinion: some public health specialists advocate medical tests to lead to early diagnosis; one example is regular Pap smears for women over 21

However, there are certain demographic groups for whom **Pap testing is not recommended** due to the potential for elevating the patient's anxiety level, extra expense, and the risk that a **false positive** will lead to **unnecessary and invasive follow-up** procedures such as colposcopies or biopsies of the patient's cervix. This is particularly the case for women **under age 21**, for whom **cells** detected by a Pap smear and/or a cytology exam can be expected to **disappear on their own** rather than develop further. In general, **false negative** test results of a Pap test are **not cause for concern** if testing is done regularly, because the cells missed by this initial Pap test will divide and grow over time, reaching the point where a follow-up Pap test will detect them. Another reason why certain demographic groups are being dissuaded from Pap testing under current guidelines is that a false positive would probably lead to the patient's treatment provider recommending additional Pap smears, and these could likely lead to consequences analogous to those of the initial test.

Opinion: author thinks women under 21 shouldn't get Pap smears to avoid false positives leading to unnecessary and invasive follow-up procedures

Contrast: false positives can lead to unnecessary follow up vs false negatives aren't a concern

Cause and effect: for women under 21, abnormalities in a Pap smear may just clear up

Interestingly, a combination of a **"better-safe-than-sorry"** attitude in the medical community, as well as **inadequate data** regarding effectiveness of Pap testing, affected Pap testing guidelines in ways that, in all likelihood, led to **excessive** testing of most demographic groups in past years. **More recent guidelines**, based on new data taken from organized population-based studies conducted in a number of different countries, indicate that little to no benefit accrues when Pap testing is done every year as opposed to **every three years**. The guidelines in the United States, promulgated by the **American Cancer Society** and others, have been updated to reflect this. Additionally, the guidelines now reflect that testing **every five years** is adequate if a Pap test is **combined** with a separate **test for HPV**, as this virus is one of the most frequent causes of cervical cancer.

Key terms: American Cancer Society, test for HPV

Opinion: author and ACS both believe Pap smears can be done every three years

Contrast: old practice (Pap every year) vs new practice (Pap every three or five years)

Cause and effect: excessive concern and a lack of good data led to over-testing with Pap smears

In examining these guidelines, it is worth noting the **harmful effects** of conducting **excessively frequent Pap smears**, not only for **patients** but for the wider **health care system**. The medical literature has indicated that, due largely to follow-up testing, the cost of **Pap test-related visits can cost over $1,000**, despite the fact that a Pap test itself will typically cost only $25 or so. As a result, the new guidelines not only can **prevent** invasive and **possibly damaging** medical procedures or **follow-up** procedures, but they can **prevent the unnecessary use of scarce resources** that our health care system can ill afford to waste. In this way, more **harmful solutions**, such as the **rationing of care**, can be avoided through the intelligent use of evidence-based medicine to determine the true effectiveness of testing, and allowing for the revision of previous assumptions.

Key terms: Pap test-related visits can cost over $1,000

Opinion: author believes that excessive Pap testing is harmful and expensive for the patient and the larger system; author thinks that rationing of care is a bad solution to dealing with limited healthcare resources

Main Idea: Medical tests such as the Pap smear can be very beneficial by allowing earlier detection and treatment of disease but such tests should only be done when the data suggest that there is a net benefit, because excessive testing can be expensive and harmful for both the patient and the wider healthcare system.

41. A is correct. The fourth paragraph describes how the recently revised guidelines are based on recent population-based studies. The fifth paragraph indicates that evidence-based medicine forms the basis for these aforementioned guidelines.

   B: Pap tests, used for screening, are mentioned in the passage, but the author never connects these to evidence-based medicine.

   C: Lower morbidity and mortality rates due to Pap smear testing are mentioned in the passage. However, the author's discussion of evidence-based medicine is limited to its ability to revise previous assumptions, not its ability to lower morbidity or mortality rates.

   D: The author never connects evidence-based medicine to the overlap between HPV and cervical cancer.

42. B is correct. It is discussed in the fifth paragraph. The author makes it clear that it is a critically important way to prevent harm, both to patients and to the wider health care system. The word "ethical" does not appear, but harm is discussed, and this answer is a better response than the other three available answer choices.

   A: Informed consent is not discussed in the passage.

   C: Information sharing is not discussed in the passage.

   D: Preventing mortality is mentioned in the first paragraph, but the author never indicates that it is a factor that should be prioritized over other factors.

43. D is correct. The view that preventing certain categories of disease, as opposed to other categories of disease, is not discussed in the passage. Since this is an EXCEPT question, D is the right answer.

   A: The third paragraph discusses the viewpoint in this answer choice.

   B: The second and fourth paragraphs discuss the viewpoint in this answer choice.

   C: The second paragraph discusses this viewpoint, specifically as it relates to the under-21 demographic.

44. C is correct. III is a correct response because it does NOT change the analysis of whether Pap testing should be conducted – it is independent of how much testing currently is or isn't done for other conditions.

   I: This is incorrect because if carcinoma grows more quickly than previously thought, it actually would lead to a conclusion that Pap testing should be done more often to catch developing cancerous conditions.

   II: This is also not an appropriate response because the fact that potentially dangerous cells will disappear on their own in the under-21 demographic group is an important reason why a false negative test result is not cause for concern in that group.

45. D is correct. The passage is primarily concerned with describing how recent studies comprise evidence-based medicine that has led to improved guidelines about Pap testing. These new guidelines reduce harm and provide benefits. The passage also provides background information to support this thesis.

   A: The connection between HPV and cervical cancer is mentioned twice, but only in discrete ways that the author does not attempt to connect to the rest of the passage.

   B: The author uses the first paragraph to highlight the connection between positive test results and lower morbidity and mortality rates; however, the rest of the passage tends to focus on the benefits of limiting the frequency of Pap testing, not the benefits of conducting it.

   C: The collection of evidence is somewhat taken for granted in this passage; issues surrounding how the evidence was collected are not discussed.

46. C is correct. The last sentence of paragraph 2 mentions "consequences analogous to those of the initial test." This refers to consequences of an initial Pap smear which has a false positive test result; these consequences are discussed in the first sentence of paragraph 2. They include elevating the patient's anxiety level (making I correct) and the risk that a false positive will lead to biopsies of the patient's cervix (making II correct). However, III is incorrect because false negative test results are mentioned in another part of the paragraph which discusses why a false negative result is not a cause for concern.

47. A is correct. The author states in the last paragraph that the new guidelines save money, conserve resources and prevent rationing from being necessary to save resources in the health care system. However, he does not take into account the viewpoint that a reduction in Pap testing qualifies as rationing of health care – he assumes that there is no overlap between the two.

   B: The author cites evidence that these studies have been conducted. He does not assume, without evidence, that they have been conducted.

   C: The author discusses examples of how early-stage screening can detect such conditions as dysplasia and cervical cancer and explains what comprises a positive test result. He does not make any assumptions to fill the gaps.

   D: This answer choice is an extreme statement. The author does not assume that anxiety will be elevated whenever there is a positive test result; instead, he merely says that there is a "potential" for this to happen.

Passage 9 (Questions 48 – 53)

In the late 1960s, following the success of the civil rights movement for African Americans, **Mexican-Americans** began to form and develop the **Chicano movement**. The origin of the word Chicano is debated: it may be from a transcription of the Nahuatal word "**Meshico**," (**Nahuatal** was the language primary of the Aztecs) which denoted one from the Meshica Pueblo (eventually a shift in the Spanish language led to using an "he" for previous "sh" sounds, denoted by an "x": thus some proponents prefer the spelling "Xicano" to reflect the etymology), or it may be a bastardization of the Spanish word "Mexicano." While it served as a **derogatory** term for Mexican-Americans in the first part of the 20th century, suggesting that their **identity was lost by living in the U.S.** rather than Mexico, it was **reclaimed by activists** in the latter half, much as "Black" was in the African-American movement. The term was meant to **reclaim both ethnic and political identity** (another term, "la raza," or "the race," also serves a similar function). As actor and activist **Cheech Marin** writes: "**Hispanic** is a census term that some [governmental worker] made up to include all Spanish-speaking brown people. It is especially annoying to Chicanos because it is a catch-all term that includes the Spanish conqueror. By definition, it favors European cultural invasion, not indigenous roots." Thus **Chicano was meant to evoke a particular identity: a Spanish-speaking person with indigenous roots** (such as the Aztec heritage evoked by "Meshico"), rather than a person of European descent who came to Mexico after Columbus's European discovery of the New World. People with indigenous blood had lower social, and thus economic, status in colonial Mexico; politically, then, the Chicano movement addressed these **inequalities** as well as questions of ethnic identity. **Today** some Mexican-Americans steer away from the term because of its politicized element: Nahuatal; **Latino** identifies all Spanish speaking inhabitants of the New World, stressing their indigenous heritage in a way that "Hispanic" does not.

Key terms: Chicano, Cheech Marin, Hispanic, Latino

Opinion: Cheech Marin argues that the term Hispanic favors the European roots of Mexican-Americans rather than their indigenous roots

Contrast: Mexican-American vs Chicano vs Hispanic vs Latino; European vs Indigenous roots

Cause and effect: new terms came into vogue for Mexican-American identity based on the political, ethnic, and generic affiliations of the time

The **Chicano movement's** political origin was spurred on by labor activists such as Cesar **Chavez** and Delores **Huerta**; its roots, therefore, gave models of both male and female participation. The **academic**, side, however, arose from more solely **masculine** models. Mexican writers such as Octavio **Paz** and José **Vasconcelos**, both of whom had lived in America for part of their careers and wrote of a cosmic race made up of people of Mexican descent, were the primary influences in academic Chicano studies. It was this tradition that shaped much of early academic Chicano studies, and indeed the masculine ending of the word reflects this focus.

Key terms: Cesar Chavez, Delores Huerta, Octavio Paz, José Vasconcelos

Contrast: gender distribution of the political vs academic roots of the Chicano movement

Cause and effect: the masculine based tradition of writers such as Paz and Vasconcelos shaped the focus of early academic Chicano studies

In 1987, **Gloria Anzaldúa's Borderlands/La Frontera: The New Mestiza** addressed the issue of **gender** in Chicano studies particularly by ushering in an era of Chicana studies. In 1981, she and **Cherrie Moraga** had edited This Bridge Called my Back: Writings by Radical Women of Color, but Borderlands/ La Frontera more specifically addressed the heritage of Mexican American women. Anzaldúa begins the work with an "**autohistoria**," or personal history. She draws upon the experiences of her family, who had lived for many years in the Rio Grande Valley, first a part of Mexico, then ceded to Texas and the United States. **Originally landowners**, the Anzaldúa family were displaced and had to work as laborers on their own land. Anzaldúa extends her analysis by tracing the history of the Native Americans who migrated from the Bering Straits down to Mexico, passing through the American Southwest on their way. Anzaldúa writes that "our Spanish, Indian, and mestizo ancestors" returned to "the U.S. Southwest as early as the sixteenth century … thus making Chicanos originally and secondarily indigenous to the Southwest. Indians and mestizos from central Mexico intermarried with North American Indians. The **continual intermarriage between Mexican and American Indians** and Spaniards formed an even greater mestizaje." Anzaldúa's terms her work "the new Mestiza." The translation of mestiza is "a woman of mixed parentage" (particularly Spanish and Native American), but for Anzaldúa the term mixed extends to the many "border crossings" she encountered in her daily life, reaching out to disenfranchised women of all races and sexualities. While Mestiza has not caught on as a descriptive term, Anzaldúa's work raised attention to gender disparities in academic studies of Mexican-American identity, so that practitioners commonly refer to **Chicano and Chicana studies** or, typographically, as **Chican@** studies.

Key terms: 1987, Gloria Anzaldúa's *Borderlands/La Frontera: The New Mestiza*; Cherrie Moraga; Rio Grande Valley; the new Mestiza; Chican@

Opinion: Anzaldúa argues that the mestiza identity of Chican@s allows for more border crossings and mixed identities

Main Idea: The passage discusses various terms that have been used to define the Mexican-American movement, analyzing the various political, linguistic, ethnic, and gender-based connotations.

48. C is correct. In the second paragraph, the author discusses the word Chicano and argues that "the masculine ending of the word reflects this focus." This implies that masculine Spanish words end in "O," and Anzaldúa advocates the term "mestiza" in discussing women of Mexican-American descent, so a male would be a mestizo.

    A: Anzaldúa advocates the term "mestiza" in discussing women of Mexican-American descent, not Chicano, as in choice A.

    B: It is suggested that the "a" ending is feminine, eliminating choice B

    D: Anzaldúa uses the term "mestizaje," but there is no indication that "aje" is a valid ending grammatically.

49. A is correct. Both "Hispanic" and "Latino" are described as referring to all Spanish-speaking people in the Americas, so the preference for "Latino" must relate to a part of a person's identity beyond just language.

    B: The passage suggests that language is not the only factor in identity.

    C: The passage does not make the extreme claim that no Mexican-American identifies with this term.

    D: Gender identity is not linked with either of these terms.

50. A is correct. The passage focuses on the different terms for the Mexican-American movement discussing issues of language, politics, ethnicity, and gender.

    B: The passage discusses migration through the Rio Grande Valley, but does make claims as to first inhabitants as in choice

    C: Anzaldúa employed the term mestiza, not Chican@.

    D: The passage suggest that Paz and Vasconcelos did not address the concerns of female Mexican-Americans, but not that they were not useful to the Mexican-American movement as a whole.

51. B is correct. The passage discusses the changes in pronunciation in words over time, focusing on the change in the "x" sound.

    A, C: there is no discussion of why certain terms are chosen by people, as in choices A and C.

    D: The passage does not focus on where any particular food stuffs are grown.

52. A is correct. The passage discusses the various political and identity based reasons terms such as Latino, La Raza, and Mestiza are employed. Hispanic, however, is, according to one source cited in the passage, "a census term that some [governmental worker] made up to in-

clude all Spanish-speaking brown people. It is especially annoying to Chicanos because it is a catch-all term that includes the Spanish conqueror. By definition, it favors European cultural invasion, not indigenous roots." Thus Hispanic is the LEAST like the others, making choice A the credited answer.

    B, C, D: These are all mentioned in the passage as terms about political and ethnic identity.

53. D is correct. The passage discusses Anzaldúa's parsing of the history of Rio Grande valley, suggesting that the indigenous people passed through it on their way to Mexico, and then returned by the 16th century, after the early 1500s.

    A: The migration back to Mexico took place after the migration from the Bering Strait.

    B: Anzaldúa argues that the long history of mestizaje in the Rio Grande Valley is part of the ancestral claim of Mexican-Americans in the Rio Grande, not a detriment to it.

    C: The passage argues that "continual intermarriage between Mexican and American Indians and Spaniards formed an even greater mestizaje," not that it is impossible.

SECTION 3
53 Questions, 90 Minutes
Use an answer grid from the back of the book to record your answers

Passage 1 (Questions 1-5)

Over the 40 years from 1973 to 2013, John Shelby Spong, the Episcopalian bishop for the Diocese of Newark, published 24 books in which he detailed the evolution of his thinking about Biblical scripture, the nature of God, and the very foundation of Christianity itself – the divinity of Jesus. As a student and mentee of Bishop John Robinson, a man considered one of the major forces shaping liberal Christian theology through the middle of the 20th century, Spong found himself moving away from the conservative literalism of his childhood and grappling with how to understand Christian faith and teachings in a post-Copernican, post-Darwinian world.

Liberal Christian theology itself does not proscribe any particular dogmas – one may find theologians working in the liberal tradition in Catholicism, Protestant churches, Orthodox seminaries, and even fundamentalist evangelical Christian study groups. Rather, the "liberal" in liberal Christian theology focuses on a method for studying the Bible. It seeks an attempt at objectivity and rational study in line with Enlightenment ideals.

In Spong's case, his approach to his faith and Bible study culminated in 2002 with the publication of *A New Christianity for a New World*. Seeing himself as akin to Martin Luther, who began the reformation that created numerous Protestant churches, Spong centered his work around twelve areas that needed reform.

Spong begins by challenging the literal truth of many basic elements of Christian mythology – the virgin birth, the fall from Paradise, the physical resurrection of Christ's body, the ability of prayer to change outcomes in the physical world, and the connection of life after death to notions of reward and punishment.

In line with progressive political views common in the Western world, Spong asserts that all people are made in God's image and deserve respect. As such, Christian churches should not reject or discriminate against any person on the basis of some external description, whether related to race, gender, sexual orientation, or disability.

Spong saved his most radical challenge to Christianity for his final point: theism is dead. Any understanding we are to create of God cannot depend on the classic notion of a theistic deity (that is, a god who is a supernatural all-powerful being that intervenes in the world). We no longer believe in miracles, Spong holds, and so we should no longer believe in God as a being who works miracles in the world. Spong never clearly takes a stance on deism – the belief that an all-powerful god was the creator of the universe, but that after the act of creation does not in any way act to change the operation of the universe.

Somewhat ironically, his rejection of most Christian myths and even his rejection of theism as a philosophy is not what has led to strongest public response. Rather, one of the minor points buried in the middle of Spong's list of reforms has generated an outcry from seemingly all quarters of the Christian world: his assertion that the cross as a symbol of love and sacrifice is a barbaric idea based on primitive concepts of God and should be dismissed. Perhaps the rest of Christendom is not yet ready to surrender its barbarism, for by Spong's own account, his suggestion that we should not give the cross and crucifix the pride of place as Christianity's central symbols has been met with everything from fiery condemnations from other pulpits and even hate mail and death threats.

1. The passage implies that Spong believes that:

   A. theology does not present eternal, unchanging truths, but rather must change based on contemporary ideas.

   B. Jesus was not a divine being.

   C. God is an all-powerful creator but he no longer acts to affect events in the world.

   D. liberal Christian theology encourages a worthwhile but ultimately impossible standard since no person can ever be truly objective.

2. The author seems to think that the reaction of some other Christians to Spong's points for reform:

   A. is odd because Spong's biggest challenge relates to theism but the strongest reaction has been against Spong's dismissal of the cross.

   B. is barbaric.

   C. will only intensify as Spong's views become more widely known.

   D. is founded on academic disagreement about Spong's philosophical positions rather than emotion.

3. A fundamentalist Christian who believes in the literal truth of the Bible would likely disagree with Spong:

   A. that Jesus is an example of God's divinity.

   B. on minor technical points of Christology but not on the major issues.

   C. on nearly every point Spong raises in A New Christianity for a New World.

   D. when Spong asserts that prayer is capable of creating a change in the physical world through God's intercession.

4. Which of the following would the author classify as an example of a liberal Christian theological dogma?

   A. The virgin birth of Jesus

   B. The perfection of paradise in the Garden of Eden and man's fall from that perfection

   C. The efficacy of prayer

   D. None of the above

5. The author implies that the core belief of Christianity is:

   A. a God that is an all-powerful creator but who does not interfere in the operations of creation.

   B. the nature of Jesus as an incarnation of God.

   C. the truth of the written word in the Bible.

   D. the sacrifice and redemption symbolized by the cross.

Passage 2 (Questions 6-11)

The Federal Reserve ("the Fed") is a collection of twelve regional banks across the US that function as a quasi-governmental agency designed to help manage the banking system and money supply of the United States. The Fed is run by a board of governors appointed by the President and the Fed's area of authority is controlled by Congressional statute. Nonetheless, it is not a governmental agency, as the Fed can set monetary policy without requiring approval from any governmental body, and the Fed does not rely on appropriations from the government to pay its operating budget.

The process by which the Federal Reserve was founded in 1913 and ended up in its current form is, as is ever the case in politics, a matter of compromise in which the "winner" is only evident much after the fact.

The first two central banking system in the US were, at best, moderate successes. Each was given a limited 20 year charter and both the First Bank of the United States (1791-1811) and the Second Bank of the United States (1817-1836) failed to win enough support to have their charters renewed. The period from 1836-1913 was known as "free banking" during which banks operated with little coordination and less oversight. During this time, the financial system saw a number of enormous financial crises culminating in the Panic of 1907, during which the stock market lost over half its value – a feat never replicated in history.

Seeking to prevent future crashes and bank runs, a group lead by Republican Senate leader Nelson Aldrich began meetings in secret. Joined by representatives from JP Morgan Bank, Rockefeller Bank, and other financial industry insiders, the group eventually developed a framework for a central bank called the Aldrich plan. The plan called for a single, privately-controlled, centralized bank called the National Reserve Association which would have the power to control the money supply and would issue currency as a liability of the bank, not the U.S. government. The Association would be controlled by a board of electors voted in by member banks around the country.

Opposition, spearheaded by Democratic presidential candidate William Jennings Bryan, expressed distrust of a system that would put so much power in the hands of the New York City-based banking elite, with little government control. A Congressional subcommittee, the Pujo Committee, found that the financial system consisted of a "vast and growing concentration of control and credit in the hands of a comparatively few men" and that "the peril is manifest when we find the same man can be a director in a dozen different banks . . . representing the same class of interests" and that this close relationship among banking elites created a "pretense of competition" among different financial institutions.

After months of debate and amendments, the Federal Reserve Act was passed in December, 1913. Getting the bill through Congress cost President Woodrow Wilson nearly all of his political capital among his fellow Democrats.

The Democrats had wanted a plan in which the reserve system and currency supply would be directly owned by the federal government. A more right-leaning wing of the Democratic party (primarily representing southern and western states) advocated for a privately-controlled but decentralized system of reserve banks spread around the country. While not government owned or controlled, this decentralized system would be free of control by New York elites.

In the end, the compromise created a decentralized system of reserve banks run by a board of directors appointed by the president, representing an amalgamation of private and government control. The currency would be created by the U.S. Treasury department and would be a liability of (owned by) the government, but the money supply would be regulated by the Fed. The key point of contention – who would control interest rates (and thus manage inflation) – went to backers of the Aldrich plan, as the presidentially-appointed directors would not be able to control interest rates, thus cutting out government control.

In time, it became obvious that the compromise consisted very largely of the ideas behind the Aldrich plan. The New York Federal Reserve Bank, although nominally of the same power as the other reserve banks around the country, soon became a "first among equals" with the other banks simply following the New York Fed's lead on all policy issues.

6. The author's attitude towards the Federal Reserve can best be described as:

A. populist opposition.

B. academic interest.

C. self-interested support.

D. apathy and vague disgust.

7. William Jennings Bryan would most likely approve of which of the following policies regarding a country's central bank?

A. A rule requiring that each bank have a board of directors to provide oversight and that members of the board may not sit on the boards of directors for multiple banks

B. A system in which control over monetary policy is entrusted to a few individuals working in private banks who have the most expertise and knowledge, allowing them to make the best decisions

C. A rule in which banks are allowed to actively collaborate with one another to help reduce redundancy and waste in the financial system

D. A system in which several central banks are allowed to manage their own affairs, permitting one of the central banks to take the lead and set policy for the whole country

8. Which of the following represents a key difference between the National Reserve Association and the Federal Reserve Act?

A. The National Reserve Association did not include any mechanism for oversight and management of the central bank.

B. The Federal Reserve Act permitted oversight by a single central bank in New York that would manage policy for the other regional banks.

C. Whether the interest rates that banks were allowed to charge when issuing loans would be controlled by government dictate

D. Whether currency in use around the country was a liability of a private bank or the US government

9. The passage suggests that had the Second Bank of the United States had its charter extended indefinitely, which one of the following would have occurred?

A. The Panic of 1907 would have been less likely to occur or would likely have been less severe.

B. Senators like Nelson Aldrich would not have wanted a central banking system that was independent of government control.

C. Less power would have been gathered into the hands of a small number of people who were members of the New York banking elite.

D. William Jennings Bryan would have been able to secure the presidency instead of running and losing three times.

10. The author suggests that during the negotiations that lead up to the passage of the Federal Reserve Act, which of the following was true?

A. Members of the Pujo committee all voted against the final form of the Federal Reserve Act.

B. Those who pushed for more private control of the currency won out in debates.

C. Conservative members of the Democratic party in Congress were pleased with the final form of the bill.

D. Members of the various factions in Congress did not understand which faction's view was most closely represented by the final bill.

11. The passage implies that if a Congressman disagrees with a Fed policy, he can:

A. withhold approval for that policy during a formal vote in Congress.

B. encourage his fellow Representatives to reduce the Fed's budget.

C. lobby his fellow Representatives to alter the Fed's mandate, removing that policy from the Fed's control.

D. move to impeach individual members of the Federal reserve board that advocated for that policy.

Passage 3 (Questions 12-18)

The heavy toll exacted by the co-occurrence of multiple chronic conditions is demonstrated by its effect on death, quality of life, hospitalizations, outpatient visits, health care costs, and other health care metrics. We found that the largest relative increase in the percentage of adults with two or more chronic conditions occurred in the youngest group, albeit over a small baseline. If sustained, this increase would have implications for the health of the nation in future decades. Not only does the number of chronic conditions have serious implications for disease, death, and health care costs, but specific combinations of chronic conditions may also negatively or positively influence health and economic outcomes. Specific combinations of chronic conditions may affect quality of life, functional recovery, disability, health care use, health care costs, and polypharmacy (the use of multiple medications by a patient). Furthermore, combinations of comorbidity may also affect survival after serious conditions such as heart failure. For example, the combination of chronic kidney disease and dementia was associated with greatly reduced survival among hospitalized patients with heart failure.

Our study has limitations. First, the self-reported nature of the data likely led to an underestimate of the true prevalence of the chronic conditions. For example, the prevalence of self-reported diabetes underestimates the gold standard prevalence estimated from self-reported data and blood measurements of glucose by about a third to a half. Recent national data about the trends of cardiovascular disease, cancer, chronic obstructive pulmonary disease, and arthritis based on information other than self-report are not available. Therefore, our results require confirmation with other data based on more rigorous assessments of chronic conditions. Second, we were not able to measure undiagnosed disease; therefore, an alternative explanation of the increase in the percentage of adults having one or more chronic conditions is that awareness of these conditions may have improved in the face of a stable prevalence of conditions, thus contributing to the apparent trend. However, the increase in the prevalence of diabetes noted in our study is consistent with data from the National Health and Nutrition Examination Survey in which questionnaires were complemented with measurements of plasma glucose.

Another possible limitation is that the decrease in response rates during the study period raises the possibility that the results may have been subject to a bias. If participants who increasingly refused to participate were healthier than participants who opted to participate, a trend showing an increase in multiple chronic conditions may have represented an artifact. However, the lack of information about the health of adults who refused to participate precludes a thorough exploration of this possibility.

The reports of other investigators continue to shape and strengthen our knowledge base characterizing the prevalence and heterogeneity of multiple chronic conditions. Various studies provide estimates of the prevalence of multiple chronic conditions. A recent NHIS analysis of data on 9 chronic conditions showed that 21.0% of adults aged 45 to 64 years and 45.3% of adults aged 65 years or older had 2 or more chronic conditions. That study examined only adults aged 45 or older. In comparison, we found that 14.7% of adults had 2 or more lifestyle-related chronic conditions in 2009, and 4.5% had 3 or more. Many of these analyses used different sets of chronic conditions in establishing their indices. Prevalence estimates of multiple chronic conditions are clearly influenced by the number of conditions that are considered: the more conditions that are included in a study, the higher the estimates will be. Thus, because we restricted our analyses to 5 chronic conditions that are leading sources of disease and death and that are strongly related to lifestyle factors, the estimates of the noninstitutionalized US population generated in our study are lower than those found elsewhere. Consequently, our analyses yield a complementary perspective on a subset of multiple chronic conditions that had not been previously considered.

12. Based on the passage, bias in the study might occur due to the fact that

   A. many people are unwilling to admit that they have life-threatening conditions.

   B. participants with more health problems were more likely to participate.

   C. participants with fewer health problems were more likely to opt out.

   D. many researchers are apt to over-diagnose chronic conditions due to their training.

13. Based on the passage it can be assumed that the study's authors sought other data in order to:

   A. accurately identify specific co-occurrences of comorbidity.

   B. identify studies with better response rates.

   C. confirm their results and further develop their pool of information.

   D. reshape their initial research questions.

14. The authors mention the combination of kidney disease and dementia in order to:

   A. urge that heart patients be screened for signs of dementia.

   B. identify the most common type of comorbidity currently seen in the USA.

   C. demonstrate one of the groupings that may affect mortality.

   D. suggest the limitations of increased knowledge about co-occurrences.

15. According to the authors, the study's limitations:

   A. are minor and do not affect the outcomes.

   B. prove the inaccuracy of participant response.

   C. do not prevent the accumulation of valuable perspectives on concurrent chronic conditions.

   D. could be avoided through better participant education as to the clinical levels of common lifestyle diseases.

16. Suppose previously undiagnosed genetic disease X was discovered to be the most common chronic condition in the nation. The study authors would most likely:

   A. exclude it in fear of a bias against genetic diseases.

   B. exclude it because it does not reflect lifestyle choices.

   C. include it to more accurately reflect the exact number of endemic multiple conditions.

   D. include it to correct the study's propensity to generate lower co-occurrence estimates than others.

17. Which of the following would most weaken the author's claims about the increase in co-occurrence of diseases in younger adults?

   A. Decreased response rates to health surveys in the younger age groups.

   B. Data that shows no change in health care costs and outcomes over the next 30 years.

   C. An increase in negative outcomes during hospitalizations and health incidents.

   D. Data that demonstrates co-occurrence most frequently happens between three diseases.

18. Based on the passage, all of the following are limitations in the study EXCEPT:

   A. the reluctance of healthier subjects to participate.

   B. the self-reported nature of the data collected.

   C. the inability to measure undiagnosed diseases.

   D. decreased response rates in the latter part of the study.

Passage 4 (Questions 19 – 23)

Every regional "cooking culture," so to speak, contains within it a blend of influences ranging from history to geography. The modern and historical cuisine from Eastern Europe provides a particularly good case study of the various factors which can shape the culinary history of specific cultures. One of the main reasons for this is due to the fact that the countries of Eastern Europe have, historically, existed in proximity to the former Ottoman Empire, to Russia, to the Balkans, to the nations of Central Europe, and – of course – to each other. The influences in question are therefore both internal and external.

Eastern Europeans began their excursions into food culture the way most societies did – using what they had on hand at the time. The earliest examples of regional cooking stemmed from a combination of available ingredients with the needs of local populations. The Baltic and Black Seas are home to a wide variety of fish and seafood, and further inland, the fertile farmlands and woodlands provided wild game and a very favorable environment for grain farming. Grain provided not only the means for making bread and noodles, but also feed for ducks, pigs, lambs, and dairy cows. This abundance lent itself to the widespread use of cream cheese, sour cream, ham, sausage, and, of course, dishes such as dumplings which used both animal meat and dough products from grain. Wild mushrooms added to the diversity of ingredients to choose from, and additional diversity occurred due to exchanges between the culture of each Eastern European country and those of its neighbors.

Indigenous influence on Eastern European cooking was supplemented in other ways which affected the cuisine of today as well as that of earlier historical periods; one such category of influence involves countries which are not, themselves, bordering the region or within it. The question of how this might have been can be answered by looking to an unexpected corner of history; specifically, the history of marriage. For centuries, European marriages among the upper classes were largely political in nature. It was thought to be – and, in many cases, it proved to be – a useful way to build alliances and outmaneuver adversaries. Of course, such events have consequences both intended and unintended; scholars have determined that one of the latter was to have brought the Eastern European food into contact with the contemporary cuisine of Russia, Italy, Germany, and – despite the geographical distance – Turkey and France. This cross-cultural contact allowed for a significant degree of overlap and borrowing from one culture to another. Last but not least, European contact with the Americas meant that food products from the New World such as maize and potatoes eventually became available, and this allowed for Eastern Europeans to experiment with, and create, still more dishes with ever more diversity than would have been possible using only Old World ingredients.

Another phenomenon is the spread of Eastern European cooking to other countries. To name one example, Ukrainian refugees from earlier time periods brought much of their cooking culture to North America, Canada in particular. Interestingly, one reason why this type of cuisine has taken root in North America is the exact same reason why it originally took root in Eastern Europe – because of the ready availability of local ingredients. Products such as beets, potatoes, and cucumbers are just a few examples. In 1957, a cookbook by Savella Stechishin called "Traditional Ukrainian Cookery," was published covering a wide range of cooking topics inspired by Ukrainian recipes, but also building on them. In doing so, it synthesized original Eastern European traditions with local innovations.

19. What best summarizes the main idea of the passage?

    A. It surveys the features that separate Eastern European cooking from those of other regions.

    B. It identifies the ways in which marriages between upper classes assisted in achieving political goals.

    C. It explains the impact that the discovery of the New World had on Eastern Europe.

    D. It highlights how a subcategory of Eastern European culture and other cultures experienced mutual influence.

20. The phrase "indigenous influence on Eastern European cooking" is a reference to:

    I. The local availability of flora and fauna

    II. Political marriages importing culinary traditions of other countries

    III. The influence of the Ottoman Empire, Russia, the Balkans and Central Europe

    A. I only

    B. I and II only

    C. I and III only

    D. I, II and III

21. The author discusses North America for each of the following reasons EXCEPT:

    A. highlighting the diversity caused by the combination of Canadian products and Eastern European cooking practices.

    B. highlighting the overlap between indigenous food products of two distinct regions.

    C. highlighting changes and adjustments made by locals to an aspect of an imported foreign culture.

    D. highlighting the spread of influence traceable to immigration.

22. The author's attitude towards the mixing of North American and Eastern European influences can best be described as:

    A. tentative approval.

    D. reluctant acceptance.

    C. qualified admiration.

    D. measured appreciation.

23. One staple of many Eastern European dishes not mentioned in the passage is kohlrabi, a vegetable related to cabbage. A new recipe with dumplings containing kohlrabi rather than meat would be:

    A. more likely to be tried in Eastern Europe, where there is a strong history of using kohlrabi in cooking.

    B. more likely to be tried in North America, where there is a pre-existing pattern of building on imported cuisine.

    C. more likely to be tried in the past, before New World ingredients were introduced.

    D. None of the above

Passage 5 (Questions 24 – 29)

Take, for instance, the Australian movie *The Babadook*, released to limited audiences internationally in 2014. It certainly contains many stereotypical horror components, including the supernatural title character, the child who appears to see things others do not, and the young, imperiled woman haunted by both her past and fears of the future. Yet the film stands out amongst the slew of horror movies that are released each year: film director William Friedkin, responsible for *The Exorcist*, ranked it with horror classics such as *Psycho*, *Alien*, and *Diabolique*, adding "I've never seen a more terrifying film…It will scare the hell out of you as it did me."

In part, director Jennifer Kent developed such a strong response through her canny use of many of the features of the genre. Myth is frequently at the heart of good horror, as the attempt to explain the unknown merges into the horror posed by such forces. Kent cannily creates her own mythology, the Babadook, a mysterious, shadowed figure that comes to the house when one is asleep. Centering around childhood fears of sleep and dreams, the Babadook is explicated, naturally, through a picture book that Samuel, the child in the film, finds and asks his mother, Amelia, to read. As Amelia comes to believe in, and fear, the Babadook, she attempts multiple times to throw away or burn the book, only to have it reappear each time. This speaks to the power of myth and legend even in our modern society: although modernity would seem to sweep away such fears, they continue to persist.

One set of myths Kent exploits particularly well is those that center on motherhood. Of course, bad mothers have been a persistent trope of terror from the earliest days of story-telling, as evidenced by the plethora of fairy-tales which feature evil stepmothers. *The Babadook* references such horrors as it asks the viewer to question Amelia's own role in the horror taking place: she is frequently angry at her son and can become violent. Is she the monster that he fears? The answer remains creepily ambiguous at the end of the movie. At the same time, horror can also deal with the fears of being a mother: a long line of tales in which mothering is equated with fear, from Victor Frankenstein through Mia Farrow in *Rosemary's Baby*, manifest qualms about how mothering can overtake a woman's life and mind. The scenes in which Samuel attempts to hunt the Babadook with a homemade weapon, causing considerable damage, speaks to the literal and metaphorical violence inherent within children.

This ability to play with both sides of a trope is one of the most remarkable elements of Kent's technique. Her use of the supernatural is another prime example. The scenes in which the Babadook appears are wonderfully creepy and invest the supernatural with a palpable reality. It is quite possible, the viewer believes, that the Babadook does exist and is terrorizing Amelia and Samuel. Yet the growing awareness of the stress that Amelia lives under as a single parent struggling with her grief from the death of her husband and an imaginative, overly active child, paired with the last minute appearance of the ghost of her late husband, also make it quite possible that she is imagining all these events. Thus a more realistic reading, in which the supernatural only exists as a manifestation of psychological trauma, is also available to the viewer. Kent again masterfully inhabits the ambiguity between possible readings, finding horror in the lack of certainty.

24. Based on the passage, how can we know that bad mothers have been a staple of terror for a long time?

   A. Tales such as *Frankenstein*

   B. The enduring persistence of myth

   C. Evil stepmothers in fairy tales

   D. Images in picture books

25. The first paragraph of the passage seems aimed at:

   A. placing *The Babadook* within a larger context.

   B. explaining why *The Babadook* is the best horror movie in recent years.

   C. comparing *The Babadook* to horror movies from other nations.

   D. deciding which components of a movie make it most scary.

26. With which of the following statements about *The Babadook* would the author be most likely to agree?

   A. It is most significant for its complex depiction of the fears surrounding motherhood.

   B. Like many other horror movies, it relies on myth as the primary means of introducing fear.

   C. It is particularly effective in its ambiguity as to interpretation.

   D. By depicting psychological trauma, it avoids predictability.

27. Suppose that a director's cut was released in which the main events of the movie were depicted as flashbacks for Amelia, discussing her former psychosis with a psychiatrist. The author of the passage would most likely react with:

   A. disapproval, because doing so creates more reason as to the causes of the horror.

   B. dislike, because it seems to imply that women can be reduced to violence by motherhood.

   C. enjoyment, because there was more certainty as to why events in the movie took place.

   D. approval, because it plumbed the depths of psychological manifestation in the film.

28. Which of the following, if true, would most strengthen the author's argument about myth in horror movies?

   A. Explaining its close relation to legend

   B. A study that demonstrates that any attempt to explain the unknown results in increased feelings of control and security

   C. Divorcing myth from modernity

   D. Demonstrating that not only horror movies, but soap operas too, depend upon symbols drawn from myths

29. Based on the passage, the best definition of a trope is:

   A. something that induces terror.

   B. a growth towards a certain element.

   C. a theme or idea in a story.

   D. an element of a fairy-tale or myth.

Passage 6 (Questions 30 – 36)

In the pantheon of corrupt politicians, William Magear Tweed – or "Boss" Tweed – is arguably one of the most corrupt. It has been estimated that during his political reign in New York City (roughly from 1852 until 1873) Tweed engineered a political machine that controlled city government and defrauded the city of millions of dollars – perhaps as much as $200 million in the currency of the time – routing public and private funds into his own pockets and those of his friends.

Tweed began his public career as a founding member of a volunteer fire company; at the time, such companies competed against each other, were often tied to street gangs, and drew the allegiance of neighboring ethnic communities. More importantly, the volunteer fire companies often were seen as recruiting grounds for political parties. Tweed caught the attention of local Democratic politicians, who noticed his particular mixture of conviviality and ruthlessness, and they backed his run for city alderman – Tweed's first political position.

Although he was elected to the United States House of Representatives in 1852, and to the New York State Senate in 1867, Tweed's greatest influence came from his appointment to numerous city boards and commissions: he was School Commissioner, Deputy Street Commissioner, and President of the Board of Supervisors, among other things. Perhaps his most powerful position, though, was "boss" of Tammany Hall, the Democratic Party political machine that was hugely influential in 19th century New York City and State politics. Through Tammany, Tweed was able to spread his influence, by appointing friends to office and controlling contracts and public projects.

Perhaps Tweed's boldest and most corrupt project was the New York County Courthouse on Chambers Street, described at the time as "The House that Tweed Built." In 1858, the New York State Legislature approved "a sum not exceeding $250,000" (close to $6 million today) for the construction and furnishing of New York City's courthouse. At the time, this was considered substantial; however, the project ultimately cost $12 million, which is equivalent to about $200 million in today's dollars. (In contrast, the land for New York's Central Park cost New York $5 million; the Alaska purchase amounted to less than half the amount paid for the courthouse.) The New York County Courthouse was the costliest public building that had yet been built in the United States.

How Tweed operated is no mystery: he had placed many of his cronies in key positions – including the city's mayor and comptroller – which allowed him to enact legislation in his favor, control the courts, and operate virtually unchecked. Tradesmen's bills were outrageously inflated, with "gratuities" of up to 65% added for politicians. For example, plasterwork charges amounted to $3 million; not coincidentally, the plasterer was the Tammany Hall "grand marshal." $250,000 – the amount originally allotted for the entire building – was billed for purchase of brooms. The amount of carpeting ordered (at a cost of $5 million) exceeded by many times the building's floor space.

The depth and breadth of the ring of corruption were formidable. There was little attempt at subtlety; it was widely known that vast swaths of the city's government were under the ring's control. Although The New York Times had been mounting a largely unsuccessful campaign to investigate the Tweed Ring's corruption, it was the widely distributed weekly political cartoons of Thomas Nast that finally turned the populace against the corrupt government and brought about Tweed's downfall. Tweed was arrested for his crimes in 1871, and the Tweed Ring was finally forced from power. Ironically, Tweed's trial was held in the still-incomplete courthouse. He was convicted of 204 counts, but he escaped from custody and fled to Spain, only to be recaptured by Spanish officials who recognized him from one of Nast's cartoons. Tweed was brought back to New York City, where he died in prison in 1878.

30. Why does the author describe Tweed's beginnings as a volunteer firefighter?

    A. To suggest that Tweed had political ambitions at an early age

    B. To contrast his early life with the corruption of his later years

    C. To trace Tweed's corruption prior to his earliest political position

    D. To highlight the workings of the Democratic party political machine

31. Which of the following might be another way of describing Tweed's "conviviality and ruthlessness" (paragraph 2)?

    A. Although Tweed seemed civic-minded, he was actually phenomenally corrupt.

    B. Tweed was helpful to his friends, but brutal to his enemies.

    C. Tweed was able to get along with others but did what was necessary to pursue his own ends.

    D. Although Tweed was a public servant, he was widely feared.

32. Of the following, which provides the most appropriate title for the passage?

    A. Corruption in New York City: 1852-1873

    B. Tammany Hall: The Rise and Fall of the Democratic Party Political Machine

    C. Boss Tweed and Thomas Nast: A Cartoonist Takes on Corruption and Wins

    D. Boss Tweed and Tammany Hall: Corruption on a Grand Scale

33. What purpose do the specific amounts mentioned in paragraph 4 serve in advancing the main point of the passage?

    A. They highlight the difference between currency values in Tweed's time with those of today.

    B. They underscore the scale of Tweed's corruption.

    C. They illustrate the lavishness of the New York County Courthouse.

    D. They criticize the public for its failure to recognize corruption.

34. In the 1870s, much of the immigrant population of New York was not literate. How might this fact have influenced the mechanism by which Tweed was ousted from office?

    A. Illiterate people could not read newspaper accusations against Tweed, but they responded to Thomas Nast's political cartoons.

    B. Illiterate immigrants had little knowledge of the politics of 19th century New York.

    C. Because Thomas Nast was a cartoonist, he was ignored by political insiders but appreciated by immigrants.

    D. If The New York Times had been more concerned with the issue of illiteracy, they would have been more successful in rallying the immigrant population.

35. Which of the following is NOT mentioned as a means by which William Tweed influenced New York City politics?

    A. Positioning his friends in places of power

    B. Diverting public monies towards friends and cronies

    C. Promoting public projects according to his personal wishes

    D. Preventing the media from reporting on his corruption

36. The irony that the author mentions in paragraph 6 can best be described as which of the following?

    A. It was a humble cartoonist who brought about Tweed's downfall.

    B. Despite Tweeds riches, he died in prison.

    C. Tweed's trial was held in the New York County Courthouse.

    D. Spanish police recognized Tweed through one of Nast's cartoons

Passage 7 (Questions 37 – 42)

Nancy Armstrong has recently suggested that we view nineteenth century literature as grappling with "a conceptual divide between the biological body providing the envelope of a unique consciousness— and one's membership, by virtue of that same body, in a heterogeneous continuum of living flesh—what Foucault calls 'a multiplicity of man' or 'man-as-species'" (531). Novels that do this, she contends, "joined Victorian intellectuals—Darwin among them—who grappled with the relationship between man as conscious being and man as a biological species, a problem they bequeathed to future theorists of liberal society" (532). Armstrong's formulation makes differing definitions of identity the root of "problems" in both political and evolutionary theory. While traditional depictions of both nineteenth century evolution and liberalism suggest a binary between individual and group identities in which individuality "wins out" over community, neither discourse can operate in this dialectical capacity: instead, each stance is interimplicated, simultaneous, rather than in a struggle for existence.

Charles Dickens makes it clear in *Our Mutual Friend* that clearly defining the boundaries between an individual and its larger community proves more difficult than might appear at first glance. When the villainous Silas Wegg first visits Venus's shop, Venus boasts that:

I've gone on improving myself in my knowledge of Anatomy, till both by sight and by name I'm perfect. Mr. Wegg, if you was brought here loose in a bag to be articulated, I'd name your smallest bones blindfold equally with your largest, as fast as I could pick 'em out, and I'd sort 'em all, and sort your vertebra, in a manner that would equally surprise and charm you.

Evolutionary images—the articulated skeletons and differing species in Venus's shop—become a means to think through how the individual can be defined. Venus anatomizes the human body itself into a discrete set of parts with independent existences that nevertheless take on meaning in their conglomerate, Weggian, form.

Wegg poses a particular problem because his amputated leg bone will not fit into one of the model skeletons by which Venus makes a living. "I can't work you into a miscellaneous one, no how," he tells Wegg: "Do what I will, you can't be got to fit." This moment of exception emphasizes the general permeability between individual and community: not only can the human body be figured as a collection of smaller parts, but those parts can, generally, be assembled and re-assembled regardless of origin. Venus's troubled attempt to unite an increasingly atomized body can be compared to Michel Foucault's formulation, almost a century later, of citizenship with a liberal society. In "trying to discover how multiple bodies, forces, energies, matters, desires, thoughts, and so on, are gradually, progressively, actually and materially constituted as subjects, or as the subject," Foucault posits citizenship as a balancing act between individuality and community that is invested in "discover[ing] how a multiplicity of individuals and wills can be shaped into a single will or even a single body that is supposedly animated by a soul known as sovereignty."

Dickens' graphic representation of the shifting relations between body parts and bodies does not just echo some of the key problems of liberalism; it also metaphorizes the simultaneity of individuality and community presented by Darwin's formulation of evolution. Take, for example, one of Darwin's most famous metaphors, which appears at the end of The Origin: the "tangled bank clothed with many plants of many kinds …birds singing on the bushes …various insects flitting about, and… worms crawling through the damp earth" (489). The bank, which at first glance seems both monolithic and uniform, becomes, through exploration, a complex collation of multiple individuals. It is an object complete in itself, but composed of many different individuals, each with different, and competing, agendas. As with Wegg's leg, the bank reveals the essential instability, or rather, interimplication, of identities.

37. Based on the passage, a dialectical relation is one in which:

    A. one idea is shown to have clear superiority over another.

    B. two ideologies interact with and reshape each other.

    C. multiplicity and simultaneity is encouraged.

    D. conceptual divides are common and accepted.

38. The author suggests all of the following pairs share ideas in common EXCEPT:

    A. Foucault and Dickens.

    B. Dickens and Darwin.

    C. Foucault and Armstrong

    D. Armstrong and Darwin.

39. Based on the passage, the author would be most likely to say which of the following about the relations between literature and other cultural forces?

    A. When it focuses on man-as-species, it is able to illuminate pressing issues of government and sovereignty.

    B. Because of its reliance on characterization and plot, literature tends not to comment on science or politics.

    C. Literature reflects the concerns that were circulating in the larger society through its use of images and metaphors.

    D. They highlight the importance of the individual in contradistinction to a growing emphasis on communal concerns.

40. Suppose that in discussing Mr. Wegg's leg, Venus praised how well it would fit into almost any skeleton he was constructing of miscellaneous parts. The author of the passage would most likely state that such a moment:

    A. troubled the division between individual and community it wished to establish.

    B. reinforced how clearly individuals could be reassembled into a community.

    C. reinforced the evolutionary connection by showing how one element might transform to another.

    D. belied the permeability between structures necessary to reinforce the evolutionary elements referenced.

41. In the passage, the example of Mr. Wegg's leg serves to:

    I. demonstrate connections between liberal and evolutionary images.

    II. emphasize the movement between individual and community.

    III. bring the classification of the individual into question.

    A. I only

    B. III only

    C. II and III only

    D. I, II and III

42. The author most likely includes the details of birds, insects, and worms from Darwin's description in The Origin in order to:

    A. demonstrate his commitment to deconstructing seeming solidity into multiple needs and wants.

    B. suggest that his metaphors are identical to Dickens', although with different subject matter.

    C. highlight the emphasis on different species evident in early evolutionary texts.

    D. stress the need for complexity in dealing with both scientific and political issues.

Passage 8 (Questions 43 – 47)

In what we may term "prescientific days", people were in no uncertainty about the interpretation of dreams. When they were recalled after awakening they were regarded as either the friendly or hostile manifestation of some higher powers, demoniacal and Divine. With the rise of scientific thought the whole of this expressive mythology was transferred to psychology; today there is but a small minority among educated persons who doubt that the dream is the dreamer's own psychical act.

But since the downfall of the mythological hypothesis, an interpretation of the dream has been wanting. The conditions of its origin; its relationship to our psychical life when we are awake; its independence of disturbances which, during the state of sleep, seem to compel notice; its many peculiarities repugnant to our waking thought; the incongruence between its images and the feelings they engender; then the dream's evanescence, the way in which, on awakening, our thoughts thrust it aside as something bizarre, and our reminiscences mutilate or reject it—all these and many other problems have for many hundred years demanded answers which up till now could never have been satisfactory. Before all there is the question as to the meaning of the dream, a question which is in itself double-sided. There is, firstly, the psychical significance of the dream, its position with regard to the psychical processes, as to a possible biological function; secondly, has the dream a meaning—can sense be made of each single dream as of other mental syntheses?

Three tendencies can be observed in the estimation of dreams. Many philosophers have given currency to one of these tendencies, one which at the same time preserves something of the dream's former over-valuation. The foundation of dream life is for them a peculiar state of psychical activity, which they even celebrate as elevation to some higher state. Schubert, for instance, claims: "The dream is the liberation of the spirit from the pressure of external nature, a detachment of the soul from the fetters of matter." Not all go so far as this, but many maintain that dreams have their origin in real spiritual excitations, and are the outward manifestations of spiritual powers whose free movements have been hampered during the day.

In striking contradiction with this the majority of medical writers hardly admit that the dream is a psychical phenomenon at all. According to them dreams are provoked and initiated exclusively by stimuli proceeding from the senses or the body, which either reach the sleeper from without or are accidental disturbances of his internal organs. The dream has no greater claim to meaning and importance than the sound called forth by the ten fingers of a person quite unacquainted with music running his fingers over the keys of an instrument. The dream is to be regarded, says Binz, "as a physical process always useless, frequently morbid." All the peculiarities of dream life are explicable as the incoherent effort, due to some physiological stimulus, of certain organs, or of the cortical elements of a brain otherwise asleep.

But slightly affected by scientific opinion and untroubled as to the origin of dreams, the popular view holds firmly to the belief that dreams really have got a meaning, in some way they do foretell the future, whilst the meaning can be unraveled in some way or other from its oft bizarre and enigmatical content. The reading of dreams consists in replacing the events of the dream, so far as remembered, by other events. This is done either scene by scene, *according to some rigid key*, or the dream as a whole is replaced by something else of which it was a *symbol*. Serious-minded persons laugh at these efforts—"Dreams are but sea-foam!" To my amazement, the popular view grounded in superstition, and not the medical one, comes nearer to the truth about dreams.

43. Which of the following best describes the author's portrayal of the widely accepted view of dreams in what he terms "prescientific days"?

    A. In prescientific days, dreams were usually understood to be spiritual rather than psychological in origin.

    B. In prescientific days, educated persons understood that dreams were psychological rather than physiological in origin.

    C. People in prescientific days were much more aware of the meaning of dreams than are people today.

    D. Only people with knowledge of mythology could accurately interpret dreams in prescientific days.

44. Which of the following statements best captures the conclusion that the author puts forth at the passage's end?

    A. The popular view of dreams is grounded in superstition, while the medical view is not.

    B. Because the popular view of dreams is unconcerned with the origin of dreams, it is of little interest to serious-minded people.

    C. The popular view of dreams, which looks to unraveling the meaning of dreams, provides the best framework for interpreting dreams.

    D. Interpreting dreams by use of a rigid key is not serious minded, and thus not useful to medical writers.

45. The author describes all of the following theories regarding the interpretation of dreams EXCEPT:

    A. dreams can be interpreted by the same method by which we interpret music.

    B. dreams may reflect a higher state or spiritual elevation.

    C. the source of dreams lies in physiological processes.

    D. whatever their source, dreams have meanings that we can unravel and interpret.

46. Suppose that a contemporary study of dreams firmly established that sounds in the immediate environment influenced and shaped a dreaming person's dream. If that were the case, which of the following assertions would be most strongly supported by such evidence?

    A. "Dreams are but sea-foam." (paragraph 5)

    B. The dream is a "physical process, always useless, frequently morbid." (paragraph 4)

    C. The dream is "the liberation of the spirit from the pressure of external nature." (paragraph 3)

    D. "Dreams are provoked and initiated exclusively by stimuli proceeding from the senses or the body." (paragraph 4)

47. The analogy that the author draws in paragraph 4 between dreams and nonmusical striking of a keyboard is best summarized by which of the following statements?

    A. The accidental disturbance of internal organs can cause a person unacquainted with music to create meaningful sound on a keyboard.

    B. Looking for meaning in dreams is akin to looking for music in the random striking of keys.

    C. Dreams rarely have any musical content.

    D. A person unacquainted with music is not likely to attempt to seek the meaning of a dream.

Passage 9 (Questions 48 – 53)

In the 1960s, artists such as Walter De Maria, Nancy Holt, and Michael Heizer began to question the traditional placement of art in museums, galleries, and other indoor spaces, and explored the possibility of creating art made for natural landscapes. The works they created, often in remote and inhospitable regions, are often referred to as "earthworks," or "land art." One of the most famous of these constructions is Robert Smithson's Spiral Jetty. Built on the northeastern shore of the Great Salt Lake in Utah, Spiral Jetty is a jutting, counterclockwise spiral composed of over 6,000 tons of mud, basalt rocks, salt crystals, and water hauled from the lake. Smithson chose to build Spiral Jetty in this location in part because of the lake's unusual physical qualities, such as the reddish hue of the water caused by microbes, and the effect that the lake's extreme salinity had on the black basalt rocks, which had been formed from molten lava from extinct volcanoes.

Smithson was particularly interested in the interaction between art and place; more specifically, much of his artwork focused on the idea of entropy, and how the natural world's chance operations create change. When Smithson created Spiral Jetty in 1970, he knew that the lake's fluctuating water levels would influence how much of his earthwork would protrude from the lake's surface. However, it is likely that he miscalculated the degree to which the water level would rise: for 30 years, beginning in 1972, Spiral Jetty was submerged, barely visible from an aerial view, and then only as a ghostly shadow.

In 2002, the jetty reappeared, though much changed; the once-black rocks were now encrusted in glittering white salt crystals. Changes in the composition of the water have altered the hue of the lake to a muted pink. Decades of silt deposits have fleshed out the jetty; it's now easier to walk on it, and low water levels resulting from a prolonged drought in Utah means that the many visitors who flock to the earthwork can do just that, changing the jetty's topography with their steps. The Spiral Jetty of 2015 looks quite different than Smithson's creation of 1970.

Robert Smithson died in a plane crash in 1973, while exploring sites for a new earthwork. At the time he was building Spiral Jetty, he spoke often about his dedication to process art; that the work changed over time was an essential element of his constructions. That said, however, it is not clear about whether Smithson would have wanted to take steps to preserve his work; in an interview with an art historian given just before his death, Smithson said that he thought that the jetty could "take care of itself," but also intimated that he planned for his work to be permanent.

Smithson's widow, the artist Nancy Holt, believed that her husband did indeed want his work preserved, and advocated that Spiral Jetty be augmented with more rocks to bring it closer to its original state. The Dia Foundation in New York City, which has owned the jetty since Holt bequeathed it to them in 1999, has considered adding more rocks in order to preserve the iconic artwork. Yet some fans of Spiral Jetty find this solution appalling, and insist that it runs counter to Smithson's intent that his work change with the fluctuations of the natural world. As one curator put it, "When refurbishing earthworks, you don't want to create a Tussaud's wax sculpture. Earthworks," he said, "were not made to last forever. There is a danger when restoring them to make a more perfect thing than was originally done."

48. According to the passage, which of the following would be most likely to be described by the term "earth-work"?

   A. An exhibit in which an artist created a realistic cave, complete with flora and fauna, within a large art gallery

   B. A series of photographs taken over a decade, documenting the melting of an iceberg in the far northern Atlantic Ocean

   C. A massive metal arc, placed in a public plaza

   D. A series of large-scale rings carved into an ice field in a remote Canadian location

49. Which of the following is NOT mentioned as a factor in the changing appearance of Spiral Jetty?

   A. The effect of salt crystals coating the basalt rocks

   B. The addition of basalt rocks to elevate the jetty

   C. Variation in the composition of the surrounding water

   D. Foot traffic from visitors traversing the jetty

50. Suppose the text of an interview were discovered in which Robert Smithson described how he envisioned Spiral Jetty in 50 years' time. How would such information influence the Dia Foundation's decisions regarding the maintenance of the artwork?

   A. It would shed light on whether a possible restoration reflected Smithson's original intent.

   B. It would support the foundation's desire to restore Spiral Jetty to its original state.

   C. It would prevent opponents of the restoration from interfering in the rebuilding of the jetty.

   D. It would underscore the importance of letting natural processes continue unimpeded.

51. Why does the author suggest in paragraph 2 that Smithson miscalculated in building Spiral Jetty?

   A. The author assumes that Smithson would want the jetty restored to its original state.

   B. The author thinks Smithson didn't realize the jetty would be almost continuously under water.

   C. The author implies that Smithson did not truly accept the forces of entropy.

   D. The author suggests that Smithson chose the wrong materials to build the jetty.

52. What did the curator mentioned in paragraph 5 most likely mean by cautioning "when refurbishing earthworks, you don't want to create a Tussaud's wax sculpture"?

   A. Restoring the earthwork to a too-perfect state will make it artificial and inauthentic.

   B. Refurbishing the jetty will make it look like a wax sculpture.

   C. By definition, earthworks should never be restored.

   D. Restoration is appropriate for museum works but not for earthworks.

53. According to the passage, which of the following is the most likely cause of the recent decrease in the level of the water surrounding Spiral Jetty?

   A. Foot traffic on top of the jetty

   B. Change in composition of the surrounding water

   C. Lengthy drought in Utah

   D. It is impossible to know.

This page intentionally left blank.

SECTION 3

Answer Key

1	A	12	C	23	B	34	A	45	A
2	A	13	C	24	C	35	D	46	D
3	C	14	C	25	A	36	C	47	B
4	D	15	C	26	C	37	A	48	D
5	B	16	B	27	A	38	D	49	B
6	B	17	B	28	D	39	C	50	A
7	A	18	A	29	C	40	B	51	B
8	D	19	D	30	A	41	D	52	A
9	A	20	A	31	C	42	A	53	C
10	D	21	A	32	D	43	A		
11	C	22	D	33	B	44	C		

Passage 1 (Questions 1-5)

Over the 40 years from 1973 to 2013, John Shelby **Spong**, the Episcopalian bishop for the Diocese of Newark, published 24 books in which he **detailed the evolution of his thinking** about Biblical scripture, the nature of God, and **the very foundation of Christianity itself – the divinity of Jesus**. As a student and mentee of Bishop John **Robinson**, a man considered one of the major forces shaping **liberal Christian theology** through the middle of the 20th century, Spong found himself **moving away from the conservative literalism of his childhood** and grappling with how to understand Christian faith and teachings in a post-Copernican, post-Darwinian world.

Key terms: Robinson, liberal Christian theology

Opinion: Spong moved away from literalism into liberal Christian theology and wrote about his thinking through his books

Liberal Christian theology itself does not proscribe any particular dogmas – one may find theologians working in the liberal tradition in Catholicism, Protestant churches, Orthodox seminaries, and even fundamentalist evangelical Christian study groups. Rather, the "liberal" in liberal Christian theology focuses on a **method for studying the Bible**. It seeks an attempt at **objectivity and rational study** in line with Enlightenment ideals.

Opinion: liberal Christian theology is not a set of beliefs or dogmas, but an attempt to study the Bible through objectivity and rational study

In Spong's case, his approach to his faith and Bible study culminated in 2002 with the publication of *A New Christianity for a New World*. Seeing himself as akin to Martin **Luther**, who began the reformation that created numerous Protestant churches, Spong centered his work around twelve areas that needed **reform**.

Key terms: A New Christianity for a New World, Luther

Opinion: Spong thought that Christianity needed reform

Spong begins by **challenging the literal truth of many basic elements of Christian mythology** – the virgin birth, the fall from Paradise, the physical resurrection of Christ's body, the ability of prayer to change outcomes in the physical world, and the connection of life after death to notions of reward and punishment.

Opinion: Spong thinks that many elements of Christian mythology are not literally true

In line with **progressive political views common in the Western world**, Spong asserts that all people are made in God's image and deserve respect. As such, **Christian churches should not reject or discriminate against any person on the basis of some external description**, whether related to race, gender, sexual orientation, or disability.

Opinion: Spong thinks Christianity should be able to embrace people regardless of things like gender, race, or sexual orientation

Spong saved his **most radical challenge** to Christianity for his final point: **theism is dead**. Any understanding we are to create of God cannot depend on the classic notion of a theistic deity (that is, a god who is a supernatural all-powerful being that intervenes in the world). **We no longer believe in miracles, Spong holds, and so we should no longer believe in God as a being who works miracles in the world**. Spong never clearly takes a stance on **deism** – the belief that an all-powerful god was the creator of the universe, but that after the act of creation does not in any way act to change the operation of the universe.

Key terms: deism

Opinion: author thinks that Spong's stance against theism is his most radical challenge; Spong thinks that since we no longer believe in miracles we have to update our theology as well

Somewhat ironically, his rejection of most Christian myths and even his rejection of theism as a philosophy is not what has led to the strongest public response. Rather, one of the **minor points** buried in the middle of Spong's list of reforms has generated an outcry from seemingly all quarters of the Christian world: **his assertion that the cross as a symbol of love and sacrifice is a barbaric idea based on primitive concepts of God and should be dismissed**. Perhaps the rest of Christendom is not yet ready to surrender its barbarism, for by Spong's own account, his suggestion that we should not give the cross and crucifix the pride of place as Christianity's central symbols has been met with everything from **fiery condemnations from other pulpits and even hate mail and death threats**.

Opinion: author thinks that Spong's rejection of the cross as a symbol is a relatively minor reform; Spong believes that the cross represents a barbaric idea

Cause and effect: Spong speaking out against the cross as a Christian symbol lead to condemnation and even death threats

Main Idea: Episcopalian bishop John Shelby Spong advocates for a number of reforms that cut to the core of Christian theology and identity, and in particular his rejection of the cross as a symbol has earned a strong, negative reaction from others.

1. A is correct. The passage tells us: "We no longer believe in miracles, Spong holds, and so we should no longer believe in God as a being who works miracles in the world." Here, Spong is saying our theology – our ideas about God – must change based on contemporary notions about how the world works (or in the case of miracles, how the world doesn't work).

   B: While Spong detailed "the evolution of his thinking" about the divinity of Jesus, nowhere in the passage do we read that Spong thinks Jesus was not divine.

   C: This is deism and Spong never expresses an opinion about it.

   D: Spong works within the liberal Christian theological tradition and so would be unlikely to think of it as giving us "impossible" standards.

2. A is correct. Near the end of the passage, the author asserts that the most radical thing Spong proposes is that God can no longer be understood as a theistic deity, but that what really riled up people in other parts of the Christian community was the issue of the cross as a symbol.

   B: Spong thinks the cross is barbaric, but the author never says that Christians who oppose Spong are giving a barbaric reaction.

   C: The passage never speaks to what will happen in the future.

   D: Rather, Spong seems to have gotten a very emotional reaction with "fiery condemnations" and death threats.

3. C is correct. Spong's various reforms represent a massive break with traditional Christian views and run counter to the literal truth of the Bible in every case. Thus a person who takes a conservative, literalist stance would disagree with Spong right down the line.

   A: Neither Spong nor any other viewpoint detailed in the passage argues that Jesus is not divine.

   B: The disagreement would be more than minor.

   D: Spong does not believe that prayer can cause changes in the physical world.

4. D is correct. In the second paragraph, the passage tells us that liberal Christian theology is a method of studying the Bible and trying to be objective, and is not a dogma or set of dogmas.

5. B is correct. In the first paragraph, the author says "the very foundation of Christianity itself – the divinity of Jesus", implying that the core belief of Christianity is that Jesus is a divine being – God himself.

   A: This is deism, not necessarily Christianity.

C: The author never says whether he believes in the literal truth of the Bible, or how the Bible should be interpreted.

D: The author mentions that Spong thinks Christians need to move past the cross as their main holy symbol.

Passage 2 (Questions 6-11)

The **Federal Reserve ("the Fed")** is a collection of **twelve regional banks** across the US that function as a quasi-governmental agency designed to help **manage the banking system and money supply** of the United States. The Fed is run by a board of governors appointed by the President and the Fed's area of authority is controlled by Congressional statute. Nonetheless, it is not a governmental agency, as the Fed can **set monetary policy without requiring approval from any governmental body**, and the Fed does **not rely on appropriations from the government to pay its operating budget.**

Key terms: Federal Reserve ("the Fed")

Cause and effect: because it does not require government approval for its actions and does not require the government to pay for its budget, the Fed is not a government agency

The process by which the **Federal Reserve was founded in 1913** and ended up in its current form is, as is ever the case in politics, a matter of **compromise** in which the **"winner" is only evident much after the fact.**

Opinion: author thinks that in politics, everything is compromise with no clear winner until much later

The **first two central banks** in the US were, at best, **moderate successes.** Each was given a limited 20 year charter and both the First Bank of the United States (1791-1811) and the Second Bank of the United States (1817-1836) failed to win enough support to have their charters renewed. The period from 1836-1913 was known as **"free banking"** during which banks operated with **little coordination and less oversight.** During this time, the financial system saw a number of enormous financial **crises** culminating in the **Panic of 1907**, during which the stock market lost over half its value – a feat never replicated in history.

Key terms: Panic of 1907

Opinion: author thinks the first two central banks set up in the US were moderately successful

Cause and effect: free banking with its lack of oversight led to panics and crises

Seeking to **prevent future crashes and bank runs**, a group lead by Republican Senate leader Nelson **Aldrich** began meetings in secret. Joined by representatives from **JP Morgan Bank, Rockefeller Bank, and other financial industry insiders**, the group eventually developed a framework for a central bank called the Aldrich plan. The plan called for a **single, privately-controlled, centralized bank called the National Reserve Association** which would have the power to control the money supply and would issue currency as a liability of the bank, not the U.S. government. The Association would be **overseen** by a **board of electors voted in by member banks** around the country.

Opinion: Aldrich and other banking representatives wanted to create a single private central bank overseen by a board voted in by the banks themselves

Cause and effect: Aldrich believed that a single central bank could stop crashes and bank runs

Opposition, spearheaded by Democratic presidential candidate **William Jennings Bryan** expressed **distrust** of a system that would put so much power in the hands of the **New York City-based banking elite**, with little government control. A Congressional subcommittee, the **Pujo Committee**, found that the financial system consisted of a "**vast and growing concentration of control** and credit in the hands of a comparatively **few men**" and that "the **peril** is manifest when we find the same man can be a director in a dozen different banks . . . representing the same class of interests" and that this close relationship among banking elites created a "**pretense of competition**" among different financial institutions.

Key terms: Pujo committee

Opinion: William Jennings Bryan and others who opposed the Aldrich plan worried about too much power in the hands of a small number of elites

After months of debate and amendments, the Federal Reserve Act was passed in December, 1913. Getting the bill through Congress cost President Woodrow Wilson nearly all of his political capital among his fellow Democrats.

Key terms: Federal Reserve Act

Opinion: author suggests that the Act was not popular among Democrats and President Wilson had to work very hard to get it passed

The **Democrats** had wanted a plan in which the reserve system and currency supply would be **directly owned by the federal government**. A more right-leaning wing of the Democratic party (primarily representing **southern and western states**) advocated for a **privately-controlled but decentralized system** of reserve banks spread around the country. While not government owned or controlled, this decentralized system would be **free of control by New York elites.**

Opinion: Democrats favored direct government control over the central bank

Cause and effect: Democrats from southern and western states believed that a decentralized system would take power away from New York elites

In the end, **the compromise created a decentralized system** of reserve banks run by a board of directors appointed by the president, representing an **amalgamation of private and government control**. The currency would be created by the U.S. Treasury department and would be a liability of (owned by) the government, but the money supply would be regulated by the Fed. The **key point of contention** – who would control **interest rates** (and thus manage inflation) – **went to backers of the Aldrich plan**, as the presidentially-appointed directors would not be able to control interest rates, thus cutting out government control.

Cause and effect: compromise created a decentralized system that was a mix of private and public control; compromise removed the ability of government appointees to set interest rates

In time, it became obvious that the **compromise consisted very largely of the ideas behind the Aldritch plan**. The New York Federal Reserve Bank, although nominally of the same power as the other reserve banks around the country, soon became a "first among equals" with **the other banks simply following the New York Fed's lead on all policy issues**.

Opinion: author thinks that the Aldrich plan basically won; author thinks we ended up with a de facto single central bank since all the other Fed branches just follow the lead of the New York Fed.

Main Idea: The creation of the Federal Reserve in 1913 was aimed at stabilizing the financial system and ended up with a system that has a mix of private and public control and a de facto single central bank in the New York Federal Reserve bank.

6.   B is correct. The author seems to a be a historian describing the Fed and the process that lead to its creation. At no point in the passage does the author state his own view about whether the Fed or its structure is a good or bad thing.

7.   A is correct. Bryan expressed concerns about power being too concentrated and the Pujo committee supported this by finding that the same people sit on the board of directors for many banks. Bryan and his supporters would likely agree that to help avoid this concentration of power, a rule should prevent a single person from sitting on multiple boards.

    B, C, D: A concentration of power (in one bank or in a few people) and collaboration between banks are mentioned in the fifth paragraph as things that Bryan would oppose.

8.   D is correct. The fourth paragraph tells us that the Aldrich plan called for a National Reserve Association and that it, a private entity, would issue currency as a liability of the bank. In the next to last paragraph we read that the Federal Reserve Act created a currency that would be a liability of the US government.

    A: The National Reserve Association called for management by a board of electors.

    B: Although this is what happened in practice, it was not designed by the Act itself.

    C: Neither the National Reserve Association nor the Federal Reserve Act gave power to the government to set interest rates for loans.

9.   A is correct. The passage tells us that after the charter for the Second Bank of the United States lapsed, the country was left with "free banking" during which there were a number of crises as a result of a lack of oversight and coordination between banks. Had the Central Bank still remained in operation, they could likely have managed to avoid or reduce the severity of various panics.

    B, C: The views of Aldrich and the private bankers he met with represented a desire for less government control, and the continued existence of a governmentally-owned Central Bank would not necessarily have changed their views or the evolution of the New York banking elite.

10.   D is correct. In the second paragraph, the author mentions that "as is ever the case in politics, a matter of compromise in which the 'winner' is only evident much after the fact." This suggests that after passing the bill, nobody could tell you exactly who "won" the negotiations over the form the bill would take.

    A, C: The passage tells us that the final bill was a compromise but does say how individual people or factions would have felt about the compromise. B: The passage says there was a compromise, with the currency being issued by the US government (Treasure department) but controlled by the Fed, not that one side won the debate.

11.   C is correct. In the first paragraph, the passage says that the Fed's area of authority is controlled by Congressional statute. Thus, it is possible for Congress to pass a law that limits the Fed's authority.

    A, B: These are mentioned in the first paragraph as things the government does NOT control.

    D: Nowhere in the passage is impeachment mentioned.

Passage 3 (Questions 12-18)

The **heavy toll** exacted by the **co-occurrence of multiple chronic conditions** is demonstrated by its effect on death, quality of life, hospitalizations, outpatient visits, health care costs, and other health care metrics. We found that the **largest relative increase in the percentage of adults with two or more chronic conditions occurred in the youngest group**, albeit over a small baseline. If sustained, this increase would have implications for the health of the nation in future decades. Not only does the number of chronic conditions have serious implications for disease, death, and health care costs, but **specific combinations** of chronic conditions may also negatively or positively **influence health and economic outcomes**. Specific combinations of chronic conditions may affect quality of life, functional recovery, disability, health care use, health care costs, and polypharmacy (the use of multiple medications by a patient). Furthermore, combinations of comorbidity may also affect **survival after serious conditions such as heart failure**. For example, the combination of chronic kidney disease and dementia was associated with greatly reduced survival among hospitalized patients with heart failure.

Cause and effect: chronic conditions, especially in combination, can have a big impact on outcomes and affect recovery from things like heart failure

Contrast: the biggest increase in people with two or more chronic conditions was among the young

Our study has limitations. First, the **self-reported nature of the data likely led to an underestimate** of the true prevalence of the chronic conditions. For example, the prevalence of self-reported diabetes underestimates the gold standard prevalence estimated from self-reported data and blood measurements of glucose by about a third to a half. Recent national data about the trends of cardiovascular disease, cancer, chronic obstructive pulmonary disease, and arthritis based on information other than self-report are not available. Therefore, **our results require confirmation with other data based on more rigorous assessments of chronic conditions**. Second, we were not able to measure undiagnosed disease; therefore, an alternative explanation of the increase in the percentage of adults having one or more chronic conditions is that **awareness of these conditions may have improved** in the face of a stable prevalence of conditions, thus contributing to the apparent trend. However, the increase in the prevalence of diabetes noted in our study is consistent with data from the **National Health and Nutrition Examination Survey** in which questionnaires were complemented with **measurements of plasma glucose**.

Key terms: National Health and Nutrition Examination Survey

Opinion: author thinks study has limitations due to reliance on self-reporting

Cause and effect: trend may be due to increased awareness, not increased disease prevalence

Another possible limitation is that the **decrease in response rates** during the study period raises the possibility that the **results may have been subject to a bias**. If **participants who increasingly refused to participate were healthier** than participants who opted to participate, a trend showing an increase in multiple chronic conditions may have represented an **artifact**. However, the lack of information about the health of adults who refused to participate precludes a thorough exploration of this possibility.

Opinion: author thinks there may be bias

Cause and effect: if healthy people dropped out, it would look like more chronic conditions over time

The **reports of other investigators** continue to shape and strengthen our knowledge base characterizing the prevalence and heterogeneity of multiple chronic conditions. Various studies provide estimates of the prevalence of multiple chronic conditions. A recent **NHIS** analysis of data on 9 chronic conditions showed that 21.0% of adults aged 45 to 64 years and 45.3% of adults aged 65 years or older had 2 or more chronic conditions. That study examined only adults aged 45 or older. In comparison, we found that 14.7% of adults had 2 or more lifestyle-related chronic conditions in 2009, and 4.5% had 3 or more. Many of these analyses used different sets of chronic conditions in establishing their indices. Prevalence estimates of multiple chronic conditions are clearly influenced by the number of conditions that are considered: **the more conditions that are included in a study, the higher the estimates will be**. Thus, because **we restricted our analyses to 5 chronic conditions** that are leading sources of disease and death and that are strongly related to lifestyle factors, the estimates of the noninstitutionalized US population generated in our study are **lower** than those found elsewhere. Consequently, our analyses yield **a complementary perspective** on a subset of multiple chronic conditions that **had not been previously considered**.

Key terms: other investigators, NHIS

Cause and effect: the more conditions in your survey, the more co-morbidity you'll find

Opinion: author thinks this study adds a new perspective by only looking at chronic conditions that are lifestyle-related

Main Idea: The authors did a study of people with multiple chronic conditions and looked at health outcomes, but note that their work is limited by the self-reporting nature of the data, possible bias in who chose to respond, and the fact that they limited their study to only five conditions.

12. C is correct. In the third paragraph, the study authors suggest that the decrease in response rates "may have been subject to a bias," adding that "if participants who increasingly refused to participate were healthier than participants who opted to participate, a trend showing an increase in multiple chronic conditions may have represented an artifact." Thus they suggest that a bias may come from healthier patients not responding to the study.

   A, D: There is no discussion of people's willingness to admit their illnesses or researchers' diagnoses.

   B: This is the opposite of what is stated.

13. C is correct. Starting with the second paragraph, the passage evaluates some of the weaknesses of the study and suggests that gathering data from other sources would "confirm" results through "other data based on more rigorous assessments of chronic conditions" and that using "the reports of other investigators" would "continue to shape and strengthen our knowledge base characterizing the prevalence and heterogeneity of multiple chronic conditions." Thus they seek other data to verify their results and the develop their data pool.

   A: While the first paragraph does discuss some pairings of diseases, the need for more data is not based on identifying particular diseases.

   B: The authors target response rates as one of the limitations of their study, but do not identify other studies as having better rates.

   D: There is no discussion of research questions.

14. C is correct. The first paragraph states that "combinations of comorbidity may also affect survival after serious conditions such as heart failure" and then discusses the combination of chronic kidney disease and dementia as an example of one such pairing.

   A: The passage does not focus on particular policy.

   B: The passage doesn't state how frequently they occur.

   D: The second paragraph discusses limitations of the study, but there is no mention in the passage of the limitations of the knowledge gained.

15. C is correct. The passage discusses limitations of the study, but ends by declaring that it still provides valuable insight as to the co-occurrence of a subset of certain lifestyle related diseases.

   A: The authors admit that the study's limitations do affect the results.

   B: The study is not designed to prove whether participant responses are accurate or not.

   D: The authors do not discuss how to avoid the study's limitations.

16. B is correct. They have chosen to include fewer diseases, and thus generate lower occurrences, to focus on the subset of diseases related to lifestyle choices. If a genetic disease were discovered, the study authors would not include it as it was not connected to lifestyle.

   A: The passage doesn't discuss bias against particular diseases.

   C,D: The authors would not include a genetic, rather than lifestyle based, disease.

17. B is correct. The first paragraph discusses the trend in increased co-occurrence of chronic conditions in the youngest group, and states that "specific combinations of chronic conditions may also negatively or positively influence health and economic outcomes." Thus if data from the next 30 years were to show no change in either health or economic outcomes, as in choice B, this would weaken the authors' claims.

   A: the passage discusses decreased response rates in studies, suggesting that healthier people may be declining to respond; this does not affect measured co-occurrence of diseases, since those people are not part of the healthy subset.

   C: This agrees with the author's claims about the effects of increased co-occurrence in younger adults.

   D: The passage says co-occurrence can occur between two or more diseases, so having it happen between three diseases would not affect the authors' claims.

18. A is correct. The second and third paragraphs discuss the limitations of the study, including the self-reported nature of the study, the fact that undiagnosed diseases are not reported, and the decreased respondent rates. While the possibility of a bias in the study due to healthier people not responding is discussed, it is not given as a definite limitation in the study.

Passage 4 (Questions 19 – 23)

Every regional "**cooking culture**," so to speak, contains within it a **blend of influences** ranging from **history** to **geography**. The modern and historical cuisines from **Eastern Europe** provide a particularly good case study of the various factors which can shape the culinary history of specific cultures. One of the main reasons for this is due to the fact that the countries of Eastern Europe have, historically, **existed in proximity** to the former Ottoman Empire, to Russia, to the Balkans, to the nations of Central Europe, and – of course – to each other. The influences in question are therefore both internal and external.

Key terms: cooking culture

Cause and effect: history and geography are two influences that shape the cooking culture in a region

Opinion: author thinks that Eastern Europe's countries, by being placed between several different other cultures, demonstrate the mix of influences on cooking culture

Eastern Europeans **began** their excursions into food culture the way most societies did – using what they **had on hand** at the time. The earliest examples of **regional cooking** stemmed from a combination of available ingredients with the needs of local populations. The **Baltic** and **Black Seas** are home to a wide variety of fish and **seafood**, and further inland, the **fertile farmlands** and woodlands provided wild game and a very favorable environment for grain farming. Grain provided not only the means for making bread and noodles, but also feed for ducks, pigs, lambs, and dairy cows. This abundance lent itself to the **widespread use of** cream cheese, sour cream, ham, sausage, and, of course, dishes such as **dumplings** which used both animal meat and dough products from grain. Wild mushrooms added to the diversity of ingredients to choose from, and **additional diversity** occurred due to **exchanges** between the culture of each Eastern European country and those of its **neighbors**.

Key terms: Baltic, Black Seas, seafood, dumplings

Cause and effect: regional food culture defined first by local resources and by exchange with local neighbors, seas and farmland provided the basis for the available foods

Indigenous influence on Eastern European cooking was **supplemented** in other ways which affected the cuisine of today as well as that of earlier historical periods; one such category of influence involves countries which are not, themselves, bordering the region or within it. The question of how this might have been can be answered by looking to an unexpected corner of history; specifically, the **history of marriage**. For centuries, European **marriages** among the upper classes were **largely political** in nature. It was thought to be – and, in many cases, it proved to be – a useful way to build alliances and outmaneuver adversaries. Of course, such events have consequences both intended and unintended; scholars have determined that one of the latter was to have brought the **Eastern European food into**

contact with the contemporary cuisine of **Russia, Italy, Germany**, and – despite the geographical distance – **Turkey and France**. This cross-cultural contact allowed for a significant degree of overlap and borrowing from one culture to another. Last but not least, European contact with the Americas meant that **food products from the New World** such as maize and potatoes eventually became available, and this allowed for Eastern Europeans to experiment with, and create, still more dishes with ever more diversity than would have been possible using only Old World ingredients.

Key terms: Russia, Italy, German, Turkey, France, New World

Cause and effect: food culture was expanded as political marriages brought Eastern European culture into contact with cultures from across Europe, and was expanded by inclusion of food products like corn and potatoes from the New World

Another phenomenon is the **spread of Eastern European cooking to other countries**. To name one example, **Ukrainian** refugees from earlier time periods **brought much of their cooking culture to North America**, Canada in particular. Interestingly, one reason why this type of **cuisine has taken root** in North America is the exact same reason why it originally took root in Eastern Europe – because of the **ready availability of local ingredients**. Products such as beets, potatoes, and cucumbers are just a few examples. In 1957, a cookbook by Savella **Stechishin** called "Traditional Ukrainian Cookery," was published covering a wide range of cooking topics inspired by Ukrainian recipes, but also building on them. In doing so, it **synthesized** original **Eastern European** traditions with **local innovations**.

Key terms: Stechishin

Cause and effect: Eastern European cuisine spread to the New World due to immigration and the local availability of ingredients

Opinion: author thinks Stechishin was able to synthesize both traditional Ukrainian cuisine and local innovations in her cookbook

Main Idea: This author sought to discuss the various influences on Eastern European cooking culture, its importation to North America, the overlap between cooking ingredients which are native to both regions, and the addition of new innovations to existing Eastern European cooking practices.

19. D is correct. The passage discusses a subcategory of Eastern European culture (specifically, cooking and culinary arts). It also explains the impact that it had on North American cooking (in the last paragraph), and vice versa, as well as mentioning mutual influence between Eastern European cooking culture and that of other countries in Europe (in the third paragraph).

    A: Differences in Eastern European cooking from those of other regions are not discussed.

    B: Political goals are mentioned, but the passage does not go into any detail about how they were accomplished.

    C: The passage only touches briefly on the impact that products from the New World had on Eastern European cuisine.

20. A is correct. Here, I is correct because local plant and animal life (flora and fauna, respectively) qualify as indigenous.

    II: However, because political marriages imported influence from outside the region, they do not qualify as indigenous; therefore II is incorrect.

    III: Likewise, the Ottoman Empire, Russia, the Balkans, and Central Europe do not count as local influences, so III is incorrect.

21. A is correct. Even though the word "diversity" appears throughout the passage, the author does not say anything about greater diversity being formed by combining Canadian food products with Eastern European cooking. In fact, the only discussion of Canadian and North American food products has to do with the local food products that North America and Eastern Europe have in common. This is not something that would result in greater diversity.

    B, C, D: These are all discussed in the last paragraph.

22. D is correct. The author clearly appreciates the mutual influence of North American and Eastern Europe on cuisine – this is conveyed with language such as "building on" and "local innovations", which suggests that the author may see these changes as progress.

    A: The author does not indicate that he only tentatively approves of what he describes.

    B: There is no suggestion of reluctance to accept the cross-cultural exchange in Eastern European traditions.

    C: The author does not indicate that he has any reservations about admiring the crossover in food and cooking practices.

23. B is correct. In the paragraph where the passage discusses North America, it uses language such as "building on" Ukrainian recipes and cooking topics, and "synthesized original Eastern European traditions with local innovations." This is strongly suggestive that new innovations are more likely to be tried in North America. By contrast, there is no language in the passage suggesting that Eastern Europe is especially likely to experiment with cuisine, compared with other regions.

    A: A strong history of using an ingredient does not necessarily mean that new dishes containing that ingredient will appear.

    C: The passage states that introduction of New World ingredients allowed for the creation of new and varied recipes, but there is no suggestion that this made the use of older ingredients less likely.

Passage 5 (Questions 24 – 29)

Take, for instance, the Australian movie *The Babadook*, released to limited audiences internationally in 2014. It certainly **contains many stereotypical horror components**, including the supernatural title character, the child who appears to see things others do not, and the young, imperiled woman haunted by both her past and fears of the future. Yet **the film stands out** amongst the slew of horror movies that are released each year: film director **William Friedkin**, responsible for *The Exorcist*, ranked it with horror classics such as *Psycho*, *Alien*, and *Diabolique*, adding "I've never seen a more terrifying film . . . It will scare the hell out of you as it did me."

Key terms: Australian, *The Babadook*, William Friedkin, *The Exorcist, Psycho, Alien, Diabolique*

Opinion: Friedkin suggested *The Babadook* was one of the most frightening horror movies released

Contrast: contains many stereotypical elements vs being one of the scariest movies around

In part, director **Jennifer Kent** developed such a strong response through her **canny use** of many of the **features of the genre**. **Myth** is frequently at the heart of good horror, as the attempt to explain the unknown merges into the horror posed by such forces. Kent cannily **creates her own mythology**, the Babadook, a mysterious, shadowed figure that comes to the house when one is asleep. Centering around childhood fears of sleep and dreams, the Babadook is explicated, naturally, through a picture **book** that **Samuel**, the child in the film, finds and asks his mother, **Amelia**, to read. As Amelia comes to believe in, and fear, the Babadook, she attempts multiple times to **throw away** or burn the book, only to have it **reappear** each time. This speaks to the power of myth and legend even in our modern society: although modernity would seem to sweep away such fears, they continue to persist.

Key terms: Jennifer Kent, myth, Samuel, Amelia

Cause and effect: because myth attempts to explain the unknown, it aligns well with horror; when Amelia believes in the Babadook she attempts to get rid of the book about it, but fails, which suggests the power myth holds over people

One set of myths Kent exploits particularly well is those that center on **motherhood**. Of course, **bad mothers** have been a persistent trope of terror from the earliest days of story-telling, as evidenced by the plethora of fairy-tales which feature evil stepmothers. *The Babadook* references such horrors as it asks the viewer to **question Amelia's own role** in the horror taking place: she is frequently angry at her son and can become violent. Is she the monster that he fears? The answer remains creepily **ambiguous** at the end of the movie. At the same time, horror can also deal with the fears of being a mother: a long line of tales in which mothering is equated with fear, from **Victor Frankenstein** through **Mia Farrow** in *Rosemary's Baby*, manifest qualms about how mothering

can overtake a woman's life and mind. The scenes in which Samuel attempts to hunt the Babadook with a homemade weapon, causing considerable damage, speaks to the literal and metaphorical **violence inherent within children**.

Key terms: motherhood, Victor Frankenstein, Mia Farrow, *Rosemary's Baby*

Contrast: the fear of evil mothers vs the fear of being a mother

Cause and effect: because the movie shows the possibility of both an evil mother and a mother with an evil offspring, it exploits multiple fears about motherhood

This ability to play with **both sides of a trope** is one of the most remarkable elements of Kent's technique. Her use of the **supernatural** is another prime example. The scenes in which the Babadook appears are **wonderfully creepy** and invest the supernatural with a **palpable reality**. It is quite possible, the viewer believes, that the Babadook does exist and is terrorizing Amelia and Samuel. Yet the growing awareness of the stress that Amelia lives under as a single parent struggling with her grief from the death of her husband and an imaginative, overly active child, paired with the last minute appearance of the ghost of her late husband, also make it quite **possible that she is imagining** all these events. Thus a more realistic reading, in which the supernatural only exists as a manifestation of psychological trauma, is also available to the viewer. Kent again **masterfully** inhabits the **ambiguity between possible readings**, finding horror in the lack of certainty.

Key terms: supernatural

Contrast: the possibility of an actual supernatural character vs the possibility that the supernatural represents psychological turmoil

Cause and effect: because the movie shows the possibility of both an actual supernatural being and a psychological reading of the same, it creates horror through a lack of certainty, as it does in multiple ways

Main Idea: The passage focuses on the film *The Babadook* and why it is so successfully scary; it discusses the use of legend and the multiple readings of both motherhood and the role of the supernatural in the film that are possible, and praises the director's skill in setting up this ambiguity.

24. C is correct. According to the second paragraph, "bad mothers have been a persistent trope of terror from the earliest days of story-telling, as evidenced by the plethora of fairy-tales which feature evil stepmothers."

    A: *Frankenstein* is given as evidence of fears of being a mother, not bad mothers, as in choice A

    B, D: Myth and picture books are discussed earlier and not in reference to mothering.

25. A is correct. The passage begins "Take, for instance, the Australian movie *The Babadook*," suggesting it is giving it as an example, and discusses common elements of the horror genre.

    B, D: The passage does not make definitive judgments as to best or most scary.

    C: No comparisons are made to other nations.

26. C is correct. The passage discusses how multiple readings of both motherhood and the role of the supernatural in the film are possible, and praises the director's skill in setting this up.

    A, B: These are specific claims the author makes, but do not speak to the film as a whole, with terms such as "most significant" in choice A and "primary," as in choice B.

    D: The passage does not discuss predictability.

27. A is correct. The author states that "Kent...masterfully inhabits the ambiguity between possible readings, finding horror in the lack of certainty." Thus a version that made it clear why the events were happening would not be seen favorably.

    B: The new information does not specifically indict motherhood, nor does the author judge depictions of motherhood.

    C: This is the opposite of the main point of the passage.

    D: The author does not state that understanding psychological manifestation is a goal of the movie.

28. D is correct. In the second paragraph, the author argues for "the power of myth and legend even in our modern society: although modernity would seem to sweep away such fears, they continue to persist." Thus an example that showed myth surfacing in another modern form, such as the soap opera, would strengthen the argument.

    A: Myth and legend are already linked in the passage, so showing their relation would not add anything to the argument.

    B: The passage states that myth is related to horror because "the attempt to explain the unknown merges into the horror posed by such forces." Thus showing that explaining the unknown actually results in a decrease in fear would weaken the author's argument.

    C: The passage argues that myth still functions in modern times; stating the opposite would weaken the argument.

29. C is correct. The term trope is used twice in the passage: we are told "bad mothers have been a persistent trope of terror from the earliest days of story-telling," and, in the discussion of the supernatural, "this ability to play with both sides of a trope is one of the most remarkable elements of Kent's technique." Thus we can deduce that a trope has to do with images, themes, or ideas, such as maternity or the ghostly.

    A: There is no indication that tropes cause terror.

    B: While tropism is growth towards something in scientific terms, there is no indication of growth in this context.

    C: Tropes are not linked solely to fairy-tales and myths in the passage.

Passage 6 (Questions 30 – 36)

In the pantheon of **corrupt politicians**, William Magear Tweed – or **"Boss" Tweed** – is arguably one of the most corrupt. It has been estimated that during his political reign in New York City (roughly from 1852 until 1873) Tweed engineered a political machine that controlled city government and **defrauded** the city of **millions of dollars** – perhaps as much as $200 million in the currency of the time – routing public and private funds into his own pockets and those of his friends.

Key terms: corrupt politicians, Boss Tweed

Opinion: Boss Tweed was one of the most corrupt politicians in history

Tweed began his public career as a founding member of a **volunteer fire company**; at the time, such companies competed against each other, were often tied to street gangs, and drew the allegiance of neighboring ethnic communities. More importantly, the volunteer fire companies often were seen as **recruiting grounds for political parties**. Tweed caught the **attention of local Democratic politicians**, who noticed his particular mixture of conviviality and ruthlessness, and they backed his run for city alderman – Tweed's first political position.

Key terms: volunteer fire company

Cause and effect: Tweed founded a volunteer fire company, a common way of entering politics

Opinion: local Democratic politicians admired Tweed's "conviviality and ruthlessness"

Although he was elected to the United States House of Representatives in 1852, and to the New York State Senate in 1867, **Tweed's greatest influence** came from his appointment to numerous **city boards and commissions**: he was School Commissioner, Deputy Street Commissioner, and President of the Board of Supervisors, among other things. Perhaps his most powerful position, though, was **"boss" of Tammany Hall**, the Democratic Party political machine that was hugely influential in 19th century New York City and State politics. Through Tammany, Tweed was able to **spread his influence**, by appointing friends to office and controlling contracts and public projects.

Key terms: Tweed's greatest influence, boss of Tammany Hall

Cause and effect: as boss of Tammany Hall, Tweed was able to gain control of city politics

Perhaps Tweed's boldest and **most corrupt project** was the **New York County Courthouse** on Chambers Street, described at the time as "The House that Tweed Built." In 1858, the New York State Legislature approved "a sum not exceeding $250,000" (close to $6 million today) for the construction and furnishing of New York City's courthouse. At the time, this was considered substantial; however, the

project ultimately cost $12 million, which is equivalent to about $200 million in today's dollars. (In contrast, the land for New York's Central Park cost New York $5 million; the Alaska purchase amounted to less than half the amount paid for the courthouse.) The New York County Courthouse was the **costliest public building** that had yet been built in the United States.

Key terms: New York County Courthouse, costliest public building

Contrast: Central Park and the Alaska purchase each cost less than the courthouse

Opinion: the New York County Courthouse represented Tweed's most corrupt project

How Tweed operated is no mystery: he had placed many of his **cronies** in key positions – including the city's mayor and comptroller – which allowed him to enact legislation in his favor, control the courts, and operate virtually unchecked. Tradesmen's bills were outrageously inflated, with **"gratuities"** of up to 65% added for politicians. For example, plasterwork charges amounted to $3 million; not coincidentally, the plasterer was the Tammany Hall "grand marshal." $250,000 – the amount originally allotted for the entire building – was billed for purchase of brooms. The amount of carpeting ordered (at a cost of $5 million) exceeded by many times the building's floor space.

Key terms: cronies, gratuities

Cause and effect: Tweed gained control by placing his cronies in key positions and made a fortune through kickbacks

The depth and breadth of the **ring of corruption** were formidable. There was little attempt at subtlety; it was **widely known** that vast swaths of the city's government were under the ring's control. Although *The New York Times* had been mounting a largely unsuccessful campaign to investigate the Tweed Ring's corruption, it was the widely distributed weekly **political cartoons of Thomas Nast** that finally turned the populace against the corrupt government and brought about Tweed's downfall. Tweed was arrested for his crimes in 1871, and the Tweed Ring was finally forced from power. Ironically, Tweed's trial was held in the still-incomplete courthouse. He was convicted of 204 counts, but he escaped from custody and fled to Spain, only to be recaptured by Spanish officials who recognized him from one of Nast's cartoons. Tweed was brought back to New York City, where he **died in prison in 1878**.

Key terms: ring of corruption, political cartoons of Thomas Nast

Cause and effect: Nast's cartoons helped expose Tweed's corruption and turn opinion against him

Main idea: In late 19th century New York City, Boss Tweed and his Tammany cronies ran a ring of corruption of staggering proportions which was brought down, in part, by cartoons.

30. A is correct. In paragraph 2, the sentence that begins with "More importantly" points us towards the significance of Tweed's founding a volunteer fire company: politics. The author tells us that political parties often drew members from the volunteer firefighters.

   B, C: The author doesn't portray his early life as particularly pure, but neither does she make the point in this paragraph that Tweed was corrupt from the get-go. The point is that Tweed was politically savvy.

   D: The paragraph focuses more on Tweed's life than on the more general workings of Democratic party politics.

31. C is correct. A person who is convivial is sociable and able to get along with others; contrast this with ruthlessness, a trait which connotes single-minded pursuit of one's goals.

   A: Civic-minded is a misinterpretation of convivial, which, as mentioned above, means sociable.

   B: Remember that paragraph 2 is about Tweed's early days as a firefighter. There's not enough information in that paragraph to support choice B.

   D: Nothing suggests that Tweed was feared.

32. D is correct. This passage focuses on Boss Tweed's corruption: how he manipulated the city, and what he achieved in doing so.

   A: This is too broad, focusing on corruption in general rather than on Tweed and his gang.

   B: This neglects to mention Tweed.

   C: Thomas Nast was instrumental in bringing down Tweed – we get that in the last paragraph of the passage – but since that's a detail rather than a main point, it would make a poor title for this passage.

33. B is correct. Those amounts serve to show just how much money (taxpayers' money, that is) Tweed was spending.

   A: We do get a little helpful comparison between dollar values of then and now, but that's not the point of comparing costs of the vast Alaska purchase vs a single building, for example.

   C: We're told the courthouse was expensive, but not that it was lavish.

   D: Tweed and his cronies are criticized, not the public.

34. A is correct. A significant number of New Yorkers at the time were illiterate, which means they could not read newspaper articles detailing Tweed's excesses. But they could appreciate Nast's biting political cartoons, which fanned the outrage of those who'd missed the newspaper stories.

35. D is correct. Boss Tweed put his friends in positions of authority (paragraphs 3 and 5); he diverted taxpayers' money to his friends (paragraphs 1 and 5); and he pushed through his own pet projects (paragraphs 3 and 4). The only thing the passage does NOT attribute to Tweed is preventing the media from reporting on him, and in fact the passage states that Tweed's corruption was well-known.

36. C is correct. The author mentions the "irony" outright in paragraph 6: Tweed stood trial on hundreds of corruption charges in the very courthouse that represented his most corrupt undertaking. The other choices all represent ironies, but not the one so clearly discussed in the passage in paragraph 6.

Passage 7 (Questions 37 – 42)

Nancy Armstrong has recently suggested that we view nineteenth century literature as grappling with "a conceptual divide between the biological **body** providing the envelope of a **unique consciousness**— and one's membership, by virtue of that same body, in a heterogeneous **continuum of living flesh**—what **Foucault** calls 'a multiplicity of man' or 'man-as-species'" (531). Novels that do this, she contends, "joined Victorian intellectuals—**Darwin** among them—who grappled with the relationship between man as conscious being and man as a biological species, a problem they bequeathed to future theorists of liberal society" (532). Armstrong's formulation makes differing definitions of identity the root of "problems" in both political and evolutionary theory. While traditional depictions of both nineteenth century **evolution** and **liberalism** suggest a binary between **individual** and **group identities** in which individuality "wins out" over community, neither discourse can operate in this dialectical capacity: instead, **each stance** is interimplicated, **simultaneous**, rather than in a struggle for existence.

Key terms: Nancy Armstrong, Foucault, Darwin, evolution, liberalism

Opinion: Armstrong believes that nineteenth century literature grapples with a division between uniqueness and a larger continuum that Foucault defines as "man as species"; she argues that this was like scientists such as Darwin who dealt with the same issues

Contrast: individual vs group identity

Cause and effect: re-assessing the relation between liberalism and evolution allows a new, dialectical, understanding of the relation between individual and community

Charles Dickens makes it clear in *Our Mutual Friend* that clearly defining the boundaries between an individual and its larger community proves more difficult than might appear at first glance. When the villainous **Silas Wegg** first visits Venus's shop, **Venus** boasts that:

I've gone on improving myself in my **knowledge of Anatomy**, till both by sight and by name I'm perfect. Mr. Wegg, if you was brought here **loose** in a bag to be **articulated**, I'd name your smallest bones blindfold equally with your largest, as fast as I could pick 'em out, and I'd sort 'em all, and sort your vertebra, in a manner that would equally surprise and charm you.

Evolutionary images—the articulated skeletons and differing species in Venus's shop—become a means to think through **how the individual can be defined**. Venus anatomizes the human body itself into a **discrete** set of **parts** with independent existences that nevertheless take on **meaning in their conglomerate**, Weggian, form.

Key terms: Charles Dickens, *Our Mutual Friend*, Silas Wegg, Venus

Contrast: human body as discreet parts vs having meaning as a whole

Cause and effect: the ability to sort bones both demonstrates evolutionary ties and shows that bodies are seen as constructed of independent parts that only have meaning as a whole

Wegg poses a particular problem because his amputated leg bone will not fit into one of the model skeletons by which Venus makes a living. "I can't work you into a miscellaneous one, no how," he tells Wegg: "Do what I will, you can't be got to fit." This moment of exception emphasizes the **general permeability between individual and community**: not only can the human body be figured as a collection of smaller parts, but those parts can, generally, be assembled and re-assembled regardless of origin. Venus's troubled attempt to **unite** an increasingly atomized **body** can be compared to Michel **Foucault's formulation**, almost a century later, of **citizenship** with a liberal society. In "trying to discover how multiple bodies, forces, energies, matters, desires, thoughts, and so on, are gradually, progressively, actually and materially constituted as subjects, or as the subject," Foucault posits citizenship as a balancing act between individuality and community that is invested in "discover[ing] how a **multiplicity of individuals** and wills can be shaped into a **single will** or even a single body that is supposedly animated by a soul known as **sovereignty**."

Key terms: citizenship, sovereignty

Opinions: Foucault argues that the central issue of citizenship is figuring out how multiple wills/bodies can be seen as the will of sovereignty, or the state as a whole

Cause and effect: because Wegg's leg does not fit into just any skeleton, he draws attention to how, generally, individual parts can be assembled into a larger collection

Dickens' graphic representation of the shifting relations between body parts and bodies does not just echo some of the key problems of liberalism; it also **metaphorizes** the **simultaneity of individuality and community** presented by Darwin's formulation of evolution. Take, for example, one of **Darwin's** most famous metaphors, which appears at the end of The Origin: the "**tangled bank** clothed with many plants of many kinds …birds singing on the bushes …various insects flitting about, and… worms crawling through the damp earth" (489). The bank, which at first glance **seems** both **monolithic** and uniform, becomes, through exploration, a **complex collation of multiple individuals**. It is an object complete in itself, but composed of many different individuals, each with different, and competing, agendas. As with Wegg's leg, the bank reveals the essential instability, or rather, interimplication, of identities.

Contrast: appearance of one uniform community vs emphasis on all the parts that make it

Cause and effect: because Darwin shows both the whole and its parts, he reveals the way in which identity is neither fully individual nor fully communal

Main Idea: The passage draws connections between literature, science and politics, particularly in terms of how images of individuality and community are handled. It argues that all three discourses point to an interconnection between individuals and community, rather than a struggle between them.

37. A is correct. The first paragraph, in which the term "dialectical" is introduced, likens it to "a binary between individual and group identities in which individuality 'wins out' over community;" one idea having superiority of the other fits this.

    B, C: The dialectical is contrasted to a relationship in which "each stance is interimplicated, simultaneous, rather than in a struggle for existence." Thus interaction and simultaneity are the opposite of dialectical relations.

    D: Since one idea "wins out" over the other, it does not seem that conceptual divides are accepted, as in choice D.

38. D is correct. The author compares Dickens's depiction of Wegg's leg to Foucault's of citizenship in paragraph three, supporting choice A. In the final paragraph, Darwin's depiction of community and individual is linked to Dickens, as in choice B. In the first paragraph, Armstrong uses Foucault's ideas to develop her own, supporting choice C. Choice D is the one that is not supported, making it the credited answer.

39. C is correct. The passage as a whole focuses on the images and language used to describe the relations between the individual and the community, drawing connections between literature and science and connecting them to political issues.

    A: Foucault's idea of "man-as-species" is part of what Armstrong sets up as a conceptual divide in nineteenth century literature, but there is no indication in the passage that literature that focuses specifically on it is particularly illuminating.

    B: The passage links literature with science and politics.

    D: The passage focuses on the way the needs of the individual and the community are balanced with each other.

40. B is correct. The passage states that Mr. Wegg's leg, which won't fit with any other skeletons that Venus makes, is a "moment of exception" that "emphasizes the general permeability between individual and community." Thus if it did fit with other skeletons, it would emphasize that connection.

A: Because it doesn't fit, it demonstrates division; fitting would not trouble that division.

C, D: There is no discussion of the evolutionary imagery in terms of how well Wegg's leg fits with other skeletons.

41. D is correct. The passage states that the skeletons in the shop, of which Mr. Wegg's leg is a part, serve as "evolutionary images" and as a means, ultimately, of imagining "citizenship with[in] a liberal society," supporting choice I. His leg, because it does not fit with other skeletons, "emphasizes the general permeability between individual and community," as in choice II. Because it does not fit with others, though, it "poses a particular problem" and represents a "troubled attempt to unite an increasingly atomized body," supporting choice III.

42. A is correct. In discussing the images in the tangled bank, the author writes that "the bank, which at first glance seems both monolithic and uniform, becomes, through exploration, a complex collation of multiple individuals. It is an object complete in itself, but composed of many different individuals, each with different, and competing, agendas." Thus choice A is the credited answer because it emphasizes the difference that can be seen in the bank.

B: There is no direct comparison with Dickens' metaphors.

C: Species and difference in early evolutionary texts are not the focus of this passage.

D: Political issues are not discussed in this paragraph.

Passage 8 (Questions 43 – 47)

In what we may term "**prescientific days**" people were in **no uncertainty** about the interpretation of **dreams**. When they were recalled after awakening they were regarded as either the friendly or hostile manifestation of some **higher powers**, demoniacal and Divine. With the rise of **scientific thought** the whole of this **expressive mythology** was **transferred to psychology**; today there is but a small minority among educated persons who doubt that the dream is the dreamer's own psychical act.

Opinion: early people thought dreams were from a higher power; educated people today believe dreams come from the dreamer

Cause and effect: scientific thought caused dream interpretation to shift to psychology

But since the downfall of the mythological hypothesis an **interpretation of the dream has been wanting**. The conditions of its origin; its relationship to our psychical life when we are awake; its independence of disturbances which, during the state of sleep, seem to compel notice; its many peculiarities repugnant to our waking thought; the incongruence between its images and the feelings they engender; then the dream's evanescence, the way in which, on awakening, our thoughts thrust it aside as **something bizarre**, and our reminiscences mutilate or reject it—all these and many other **problems have for many hundred years demanded answers** which up till now could never have been satisfactory. **Before all** there is the question as to the **meaning of the dream**, a question which is in itself double-sided. There is, firstly, the psychical significance of the dream, its position with regard to the psychical processes, as to a possible biological function; secondly, has the dream a meaning—can sense be made of each single dream as of other mental syntheses?

Opinion: author thinks there are questions about dreams that have no good answers yet but the most important is the meaning **Contrast:** two possible meanings to dreams – biological function of dreaming vs actual meaning of the dream itself

Three tendencies can be observed in the estimation of dreams. Many **philosophers** have given currency to one of these tendencies, one which at the same time preserves something of the **dream's former over-valuation**. The foundation of dream life is for them a peculiar state of **psychical activity**, which they even celebrate as **elevation** to some higher state. **Schubert**, for instance, claims: "The dream is the liberation of the spirit from the pressure of external nature, a detachment of the soul from the fetters of matter." Not all go so far as this, but many maintain that dreams have their origin in real spiritual excitations, and are the **outward manifestations of spiritual powers** whose free movements have been hampered during the day.

Key terms: Schubert, spiritual excitations

Opinion: some thinkers give dreams high value as spiritual experiences; the author thinks this is over-valuing dreams

In striking contradiction with this the majority of **medical writers** hardly admit that the dream is a psychical phenomenon at all. According to them **dreams** are provoked and initiated exclusively by **stimuli proceeding from the senses or the body**, which either reach the sleeper from without or are accidental disturbances of his internal organs. The dream has **no greater claim to meaning** and importance than the sound called forth by the ten fingers of a person quite unacquainted with music running his fingers over the keys of an instrument. The dream is to be regarded, says **Binz**, "as a physical process **always useless, frequently morbid**." All the peculiarities of dream life are explicable as the incoherent effort, due to some physiological stimulus, of certain organs, or of the cortical elements of a brain otherwise asleep.

Key terms: Binz, incoherent effort

Opinion: doctors see dreams as meaningless things arising from actions of the body

But slightly affected by scientific opinion and untroubled as to the origin of dreams, the **popular view** holds firmly to the belief that dreams **really have got a meaning**, in some way they do foretell the future, whilst the meaning can be unraveled in some way or other from its oft bizarre and enigmatical content. The reading of dreams consists in replacing the events of the dream, so far as remembered, by other events. This is done either scene by scene, *according to some rigid key*, or the dream as a whole is replaced by something else of which it was a *symbol*. Serious-minded persons laugh at these efforts—"Dreams are but sea-foam!" To **my amazement, the popular view grounded in superstition**, and not the medical one, **comes nearer to the truth** about dreams.

Key terms: popular view

Opinion: the popular view says dreams can be interpreted through symbols because there is meaning to dreams; the author agrees

Main Idea: Dreams have been interpreted in four broad ways: the prescientific view of dreams as visitations from a higher power; the philosopher view that dreaming is spiritual; the medical view that dreams are meaningless; and the popular view that the author agrees with, that dreams have meaning that can be interpreted through symbols.

43. A is correct. This question asks about how the author portrays the understanding of dreams in prescientific days. In prescientific days people understood dreams as an the expression of higher powers.

    B: This choice distorts paragraph 1's reference to educated persons – it's educated persons *today* who think of dreams as psychological.

    C: No evidence is present of whether prescientific people were more (or less) aware of the meaning of dreams.

    D: This choice plays on the mention of "expressive mythology" in paragraph 1; knowledge of mythology is not tied to ability to interpret dreams.

44. C is correct. This brunt of this passage is descriptive; we get three different points of view. The author only states his opinion at the end of the passage: the popular view is the right one. Note that in the other paragraphs, we get other points of view.

45. A is correct. Choice A confuses the musical analogy in paragraph 4. So it represents the only theory not mentioned – and is our answer.

    B: Dreams as a higher spiritual state is the thrust of the psychical view described in paragraph 3.

    C: Dreams as the result of physiological processes is a theory elaborated in paragraph 4.

    D: This choice describes the popular view of dreams.

46. D is correct. This question basically says, suppose there were clear evidence that some bodily or sensory event caused or influenced a dreamer's dream. That's the point of view of the medical writers, described in paragraph 4.

    A: This quote minimizes the importance of dreams, but doesn't actually support the medical writers' view.

    B: This is close but goes too far. Yes, the hypothetical study would seem to support the physiological cause of dreams theory – but it would not support the idea that dreams are useless or morbid.

    C: Actually, our hypothetical study would be more likely to discredit this point of view, not support it.

47. B is correct. This question asks about a tricky analogy: from the point of view of the medical writers, to say that there is meaning in dreams (which to them are caused by random biological processes) is like looking for musicality in the random banging on a keyboard (like a piano) by a person who hasn't a clue how to play it.

    A, C: Whether or not dreams have musical content or the dreamer creates musical sounds is irrelevant. Again, the issue of music serves as an analogy, it's not literally about music.

D: The author suggests that a person unacquainted with music is unlikely to randomly create music, but there's no information on whether he or she seeks the meaning of a dream.

Passage 9 (Questions 48 – 53)

In the **1960s**, artists such as Walter De Maria, Nancy Holt, and Michael Heizer began to question the **traditional placement** of art in museums, galleries, and other indoor spaces, and explored the possibility of creating art made for natural landscapes. The works they created, often in remote and inhospitable regions, are often referred to as "**earthworks**," or "land art." One of the most famous of these constructions is **Robert Smithson's Spiral Jetty**. Built on the northeastern shore of the **Great Salt Lake** in Utah, Spiral Jetty is a jutting, counterclockwise spiral composed of over **6,000 tons** of mud, basalt rocks, salt crystals, and water hauled from the lake. Smithson chose to build Spiral Jetty in this location in part because of the lake's unusual physical qualities, such as the **reddish hue** of the water caused by microbes and the effect that the lake's extreme salinity had on the black basalt rocks, which had been formed from molten lava from extinct volcanoes.

Key words: earthworks, Robert Smithson, Spiral Jetty

Contrast: unlike traditional artworks, earthworks are created for natural landscapes

Cause and effect: the Great Salt Lake's physical qualities, color led to Smithson choosing that site

Smithson was particularly interested in the **interaction between art and place**; more specifically, much of his artwork focused on the idea of **entropy**, and how the natural world's chance operations create change. When Smithson created Spiral Jetty in 1970, he knew that the lake's **fluctuating water levels** would influence how much of his earthwork would protrude from the lake's surface. However, it is **likely** that he **miscalculated** the degree to which the water level would rise: for 30 years, beginning in 1972, Spiral Jetty was **submerged**, barely visible from an aerial view, and then only as a ghostly shadow.

Key words: entropy, fluctuating water levels, submerged

Cause and effect: Smithson's artwork is changed by the effects of the environment

Opinion: the author suggests that Smithson didn't realize that the jetty would be submerged for decades

In 2002, the jetty reappeared, though much changed; the once-black rocks were now encrusted in glittering white salt crystals. Changes in the composition of the water have altered the hue of the lake to a muted pink. Decades of silt deposits have fleshed out the jetty; it's now easier to walk on it, and low water levels resulting from a prolonged drought in Utah means that the many visitors who flock to the earthwork can do just that, changing the jetty's topography with their steps. The Spiral Jetty of 2015 looks quite different than Smithson's creation of 1970.

Contrast: the jetty, once comprised of black rocks in red water, now appears as white rocks in muted pink water

Cause and effect: salt encrustation, changes in water composition, and changing water levels have altered Spiral Jetty's appearance

Robert Smithson died in a plane crash in 1973, while exploring sites for a new earthwork. At the time he was building Spiral Jetty, he spoke often about his dedication to **process art**; that the work changed over time was an essential element of his constructions. That said, however, it is not clear about whether Smithson would have wanted to take steps to **preserve his work**; in an interview with an art historian given just before his death, Smithson said that he thought that the jetty could "take care of itself," but also intimated that he planned for his work to be permanent.

Key words: process art, preserve his work

Opinion: the author says it is not clear whether Smithson would have wanted Spiral Jetty preserved

Smithson's **widow**, the artist **Nancy Holt**, believed that her husband **did indeed want his work preserved**, and advocated that Spiral Jetty be augmented with more rocks to bring it closer to its original state. The **Dia Foundation** in New York City, which has owned the jetty since Holt bequeathed it to them in 1999, has considered adding more rocks in order to preserve the iconic artwork. Yet some fans of Spiral Jetty find this solution appalling, and insist that it runs counter to Smithson's intent that his work change with the **fluctuations** of the natural world. As one curator put it, "When refurbishing earthworks, you don't want to create a Tussaud's wax sculpture. **Earthworks**," he said, "**were not made to last forever**. There is a danger when restoring them to make a more perfect thing than was originally done."

Key words: Nancy Holt, Dia Foundation, fluctuations

Opinion: opponents of restoration of the jetty say that restoration would run counter to Smithson's believe in process art; furthermore, restoration might make the piece inauthentic and too perfect and changeless

Main idea: Spiral Jetty, an iconic earthwork, is changing because of environmental effects, but there exists controversy about whether it should be restored.

48. D is correct. The author describes earthworks in the first paragraph. The main point here is that they are artworks that exist outside of a gallery or museum, set in natural landscapes and made to interact with the environment.

    A, B: These can both be eliminated because they are works exhibited in traditional gallery space – they're not earthworks even though their subject is the natural world.

    C: Even though this is an outdoor exhibit, it is not in the remote, natural environment typical of earthworks.

49. B is correct. In paragraph 3, we learn that the salinity of the water, its changing composition, and foot traffic over the jetty all have contributed to its changing appearance. The only element not mentioned is the addition of basalt rocks, choice B. This hasn't been done yet – it is still under consideration.

50. A is correct. A big question regarding whether to restore Spiral Jetty to its original state is what Smithson would have wanted; the artist died before his wishes were made clear. If such a document were found, it might clarify his original intent. Correct choice A says this. The other choices all jump to a conclusion as to what that document would say – and we aren't told that.

51. B is correct. The author implies that while Smithson probably figured that the water levels would fluctuate, he probably didn't think that his artwork would become invisible for decades.

52. A is correct. Think about a figure in a wax museum (like Madame Tussaud's). It is too perfect – unreal, inauthentic, not actually lifelike. The thing about earthworks is that they are changed by the environment in which they exist; they are not as static as works that exist within a museum or gallery. So the curator is concerned that refurbishing an earthwork might make it too perfect.

    B: This is too literal; the curator's comment is meant as a metaphor.

    C, D: The curator doesn't say they should never be restored or that it's inappropriate, but that one must be very careful not to create something too perfect in the restoration process.

53. C is correct. You can find the answer to this question in paragraph 3: "low water levels resulting from a prolonged drought in Utah…"

    A, B: Foot traffic on the jetty, and change in water composition, have both influenced the appearance of Spiral Jetty – but neither is the cause of the decrease in the water level.

SECTION 4

53 Questions, 90 Minutes

Use an answer grid from the back of the book to record your answers

Passage 1 (Questions 1 – 5)

In 1961, Yale University psychologist Stanley Milgram initiated a study that has become perhaps the most notorious psychology experiment to date. Milgram placed an ad in the *New Haven Register* seeking subjects to participate in "a scientific study of memory and learning." Hundreds of subjects – each paid $4 – responded. When participants arrived at Milgram's research lab for the learning and memory study, they were faced with something entirely unexpected. Under the supervision of a lab-coated scientist, each volunteer – known as the "teacher" -- would read a series of words to another person – the "learner," who was hidden behind a partition and hooked up to an electric-shock device. The learner would repeat the words to the best of his ability. Each time the learner made a mistake, the teacher administered an electric shock. Shocks started out mild in intensity (15 volts: labeled "slight shock" on the teacher's control panel) and continued up to 450 volts (labeled "danger: severe shock"). As the shocks increased in severity, the learner would cry out in pain, sometimes citing a heart condition, and pleading with the teacher to stop. If the teacher hesitated or questioned the safety of the learner, the supervising scientist would urge him to continue. The results of the experiment were horrifying: approximately two-thirds of subjects continued to shock the learners to the maximum level, following the urging of the supervisor, even when the learner pled for mercy.

What the subjects did not know until they left the research lab was that the shocks weren't real. The agonized cries were delivered by actors; the learners and supervisor were in on the ruse too. In fact, the study was not about learning and memory at all: it was about obedience to authority. Milgram used the results of his study to support his now-famous claim that ordinary people will obey virtually any order – even to harm and even torture others – given by an authority figure. The findings of Milgram's study have been used to explain some of the darkest episodes of recent history, from the Holocaust to the abuse of prisoners in Abu Ghraib.

Fifty years after Milgram first published his study, however, psychologists and sociologists have started to question Milgram's findings. It's not his data that is at issue. Milgram repeated his study numerous times, and found that the number of people who followed the orders to shock all the way to the end remained at around 65%. In the decades since Milgram's study, few other researchers have attempted to reproduce his experiment because of clear ethical issues. Subjects in Milgram's study were deeply distressed by their experience, some with lasting trauma. In 2007, though, psychologist Jerry Burger performed a slight variation on Milgram's study, limiting the maximum shock value to 150 volts, and found obedience rates virtually equal to Milgram's.

Contrary to Milgram's explanation – that ordinary people will obediently and unthinkingly follow even malevolent authorities – some social scientists today explain the phenomenon as one of social identification. One such psychologist, Alexander Haslam, notes that the supervising "scientist" in Milgram's experiment reminded subjects that their compliance was key to the success of the experiment, and to the more general benefit of science. Subjects identified with these worthy goals. Social identification, says Haslam, is what motivates people to act as followers, and such identification is not thoughtless; rather, it is "the endeavor of committed subjects." The benefit of Haslam's interpretation is twofold. First, it provides a more nuanced explanation for historical atrocities – that functionaries in brutal regimes do more than simply follow orders; and second, it explains why people tend to obey orders more in some situations than in others. In Milgram's experiment, subjects were encouraged to identify with the scientist, and arguably, enlightened society, rather than with the learner behind the partition. Were the experiment designed so that subjects had greater identification with learners, it is likely that Milgram would have seen different results.

1. Of the following, which best describes the "teachers'" understanding of the experiment, as described in the passage?

    A. The "teachers" believed the experiment was testing learning and memory function in the "learners," and that learners were actually receiving shocks.

    B. The "teachers" realized that the experiment was not about learning and memory, but believed that "learners" were receiving shocks.

    C. The "teachers" believed the experiment was testing learning and memory function, but probably knew that the "learners" were not actually receiving shocks.

    D. Both "teachers" and "learners" probably realized that the experiment was not about learning and memory, but felt obligated to complete their portion of the study.

2. According to the author, what was "horrifying" about the results of Milgram's experiment?

    A. Innocent people were subjected to physical pain.

    B. The experiment's subjects experienced emotional distress and trauma.

    C. The experiment was undertaken without regard to the well-being of participants.

    D. A large majority of participants were willing to harm innocent people.

3. Which of the following best describes the ethical concern expressed in paragraph 3?

    A. The maximum voltage in Burger's experiment was still high enough to deliver significant pain.

    B. Burger's study might not be regarded as legitimate because of the limitations he placed on voltage.

    C. It would be wrong to repeat Milgram's experiment, since his subjects had suffered emotional pain from participating.

    D. Milgram's study valued the abstract scientific progress more than individual human lives.

4. The author cites which of the following as the primary difference between Milgram's explanation of the behavior he observed, and Haslam's explanation of Milgram's findings?

    A. Haslam believed that subjects followed orders because they identified with the scientist and his goals, whereas Milgram believed that his subjects obeyed authority figures without much examination.

    B. Haslam believed that fewer of Milgram's subjects would have followed orders if they had identified more fully with the supervising scientist.

    C. Haslam believed that Milgram's experiment does not provide an adequate explanation for historic atrocities such as the Holocaust and Abu Ghraib.

    D. Haslam believed that Milgram's subjects obeyed without thinking, whereas Milgram saw the subjects as deliberately choosing to inflict pain.

5. In the last paragraph, the author suggests that a certain change in Milgram's experiment's design would have yielded different results. Which of the following expresses the most likely difference?

    A. Fewer subjects would have agreed to participate in Milgram's study.

    B. Fewer subjects would have continued to shock the learners to the maximum level.

    C. The study would have attracted a different demographic of participants.

    D. Milgram's study would have been accorded greater legitimacy.

Passage 2 (Questions 6 – 11)

The names go together as do those of Shelley and Keats or Fortnum and Mason. Even to people who seldom or never look seriously at a picture they have stood, these ten years, as symbols of modernity. They are preeminent: and for this there is reason. Matisse and Picasso are the two immediate heirs to Cezanne. They are in the direct line: and through one of them a great part of the younger generation comes at its share of the patrimony. To their contemporaries they owe nothing: they came into the legacy and had to make what they could of it. They are the elder brothers of the movement, a fact which the movement occasionally resents by treating them as though they were its elder sisters.

Even to each other they owe nothing. Matisse, to be sure, swept for one moment out of his course by the overwhelming significance of Picasso's abstract work, himself made a move in that direction. But this adventure he quickly, and wisely, abandoned; the problems of cubism could have helped him nothing to materialize his peculiar sensibility. And this sensibility—this peculiar reaction to what he sees— is his great gift. No one ever felt for the visible universe just what Matisse feels; or, if one did, he could not create an equivalent. Because, in addition to this magic power of creation, Matisse has been blessed with extraordinary sensibility both of reaction and touch, he is a great artist; because he trusts to it entirely he is not what for a moment apparently he wished to be—a chef d'ecole.

Picasso, on the other hand, who never tried to be anything of the sort, is the paramount influence in modern painting— subject, of course, to the supreme influence of Cezanne. All the world over are students and young painters to whom his mere name is thrilling; to whom Picasso is the liberator. His influence is ubiquitous: even in England it is immense. Not only those who for all their denials— denials that spring rather from ignorance than bad faith— are mere apes of the inventor of cubism, but artists who float so far out of the mainstream as the Spensers and the Nashes, Mr. Lamb and Mr. John, would all have painted differently had Picasso never existed.

Picasso is a born chef d'ecole. His is one of the most inventive minds in Europe. Invention is as clearly his supreme gift as sensibility is that of Matisse. His career has been a series of discoveries, each of which he has rapidly developed. A highly original and extremely happy conception enters his head, suggested, probably, by some odd thing he has seen. Forthwith he sets himself to analyze it and disentangle those principles that account for its peculiar happiness. He proceeds by experiment, applying his hypotheses in the most unlikely places. Before long he has established what looks like an infallible method for producing an effect of which, a few months earlier, no one had so much as dreamed. This is one reason why Picasso is a born chef d'ecole. And this is why of each new phase in his art the earlier examples are apt to be the more vital and well nourished. At the end he is approaching that formula towards which his intellectual effort tends inevitably. It is time for a new discovery.

6.   Based on the passage, Matisse:

   A. considered Cezanne a more important influence in his art than Picasso.

   B. was overly sensitive about his work and its influence.

   C. highlighted the problems of cubism by stressing its relation to materiality.

   D. briefly dabbled in abstract art before dismissing it.

7.   The author assumes which of the following in comparing Matisse and Picasso?

   A. Artists' achievements can be measured not just in the quality of their works, but in their effect on the larger field.

   B. Picasso's cubism raised stronger emotions than Matisse's innovations.

   C. There can only be one chef d'ecole per artistic generation.

   D. In order to assess an artist, one must understand both who they are heirs to and the heirs to their own aesthetics.

8.   Based on the passage, a chef d'ecole has all of the following qualities EXCEPT:

   A. great influence on other artists.

   B. complete faith in one's natural talents and ways of viewing the world.

   C. a keen interest in experimenting and creating new techniques.

   D. the ability to make innovations seem inevitable.

9.   Suppose that a painter in the time period in which this review was written insisted that his work was so innovative as to be totally unlike Picasso's. The author of the review would most likely state that:

   A. Picasso's influence was so widespread that even painters outside the conventional path were affected by his work.

   B. such a claim arises from a misreading of who invented cubism, thus cementing Picasso's influence.

   C. Picasso's desire to be a chef d'ecole was the most likely reason for the painter's disavowal of his influence.

   D. this denial of Picasso's influence most probably emerged from ignorance of Picasso's religious conviction.

10.   Based on the passage, when Picasso had fully developed a phase of his art, his works were apt to be:

   A. aiming towards a new discovery.

   B. formulaic and less full of life.

   C. frequently copied by others.

   D. sold for higher prices though less vital.

11.   The author suggests that "the movement occasionally" treats Matisse and Picasso "as though they were its elder sisters" in order to:

   A. belie the frequently formulaic approach of these artists in modern innovation.

   B. highlight their frequently feminine styles and innovations.

   C. demonstrate the lack of relevance these artists have in more modern works.

   D. employ dismissive treatment to assert its dislike of their power.

Passage 3 (Questions 12 – 18)

We all know something about time: we know it as past, present, and future, we know it as being divisible into successive parts, and we know that all that happens, happens in time. Those who have pondered it a great deal are likely to tell us that time is a necessity of thought, that time is and must be infinite, and that it is infinitely divisible. You will notice that these are the same statements that were made regarding space, and as they have just been critiqued, we won't dwell on them long. However, we must not pass over them altogether.

As far as time being necessary, we must admit that we cannot annihilate or think away time, and that it means nothing to attempt such a task. Whatever time is, it does not seem to be of a nature that we can demolish it. But is it necessarily absurd to speak of a system of things – albeit, not a system of things in which there is change and succession, an earlier and later, but still, a system of things of some sort – in which there are no time relations? Of course, this problem is merely theoretical, for no such system exists in the world.

As for the infinity of time, may we not ask on what grounds anyone could venture to assert this? No one can say that infinite time is a given in his experience. If we cannot directly perceive this infinity, must we not then seek some proof of it? The only proof appears to be contained in this statement: we cannot conceive of a time before which there was no time, nor of a time after which there will be no time. This is a proof that is no proof, for here it is written out: we cannot conceive of a time in the time before which there was no time, nor of a time in the time after which there will be no time. We might as well say: we cannot conceive of a number the number before which was no number, nor of a number the number after which will be no number. Whatever may be said of the conclusion, the argument is weak.

Turning to the consideration of time as infinitely divisible, we find ourselves facing the same difficulties that showed themselves when we considered space as infinitely divisible. Certainly no one is ever conscious of the infinite number of parts of the minute that just passed. Nevertheless, shall he claim it did contain an infinite number of parts? How did it succeed in passing? How did this minute even begin to pass? If the minute is infinitely divisible, there is no end to the number of parts into which it can be divided, those parts are all successive, no two parts can pass at once, and they must all proceed in a certain order.

Something must pass first. What could it be? If that something has parts and is divisible, the whole of it cannot pass first. Rather, it must pass bit by bit, as does the whole minute. If it is infinitely divisible, we find ourselves with the same problem we faced at the outset. Therefore, whatever passes first cannot have parts. So, let us assume it has no parts and bid it Godspeed! Has the minute begun? By hypothesis, our minute is infinitely divisible, composed of parts, and those parts of other parts, and so on without end. We cannot, through division, come to any part which itself is not composed of smaller parts. Therefore, the partless thing that passed is not part of the minute. Rather, it is still waiting at the gate, and no member of its platoon can prove it has the right to lead the rest.

12. According to the passage, when we are studying some-thing that is typically regarded as given, but we cannot directly perceive it, what ought we to do?

    A. Deny claims made by those who professionally study the topic

    B. Deny claims popularly believed to be true

    C. Reflect deeply upon it

    D. Seek proof of it

13. Which of the following most closely identifies the prob-lem underlying the fourth paragraph?

    A. How can human beings even begin to attempt to con-ceive of infinity?

    B. How can a provably finite amount of time be proven to be infinitely divisible?

    C. How can something that is infinite be composed of individual finite moments?

    D. How can we actually prove something whose only proof is rhetorical, not physical?

14. Which of the following most likely describes the au-thor's intent in including the question in the second paragraph?

    A. To suggest that time is merely an invention of the hu-man mind that we attach to instances of change

    B. To address the fact that time is completely unavoid-able, from both a practical and theoretical perspective

    C. To question whether the statements he makes in the first two sentences of the paragraph are 100% true

    D. To challenge the authority of "those who have pon-dered it a great deal" and empower laypeople

15. Based upon the passage, which of the following state-ments is someone who has pondered time a great deal most likely to believe?

    A. Thought could not exist without time.

    B. That which passes before a minute has no parts.

    C. Time could not exist without thought.

    D. That which passes before a minute has infinite parts.

16. Suppose the author is in the process of hiring an ap-prentice to help him in his work on time. He is looking for someone who already has somewhat of a working knowledge of the subject matter. Assuming all the ap-plicants are equally intelligent, which of the following will the author most likely hire?

    A. The applicant who studies rhetoric

    B. The applicant who studies geometry

    C. The applicant who studies space

    D. The applicant who studies clock- and watch-making

17. All of the following statements about time are true EXCEPT:

    A. it is necessarily infinite.

    B. it is divisible into infinite, concurrent parts.

    C. it is a necessity of thought.

    D. it is present in all systems of things.

18. According to the passage, which of the following state-ments about space is true?

    I. It is a necessity of thought.

    II. It is infinitely divisible.

    III. Space is the partless thing that leads to time.

    A. II only

    B. II and III

    C. I and II

    D. I, II, and III

Passage 4 (Questions 19 – 23)

A blind man once said, when asked if he would not be glad to have his eyesight, "to improve the organs I have, would be as good as to give me that which is wanting in me." This sentence sums up the whole aim of blind education. Dr. Eichholtz, a noted educator of the blind, says: "Education of the blind absolutely fails in its object, in so far as it fails to develop the remaining faculties to compensate for the want of sight. Touch and sight must be developed by means which practically in all respects are dissimilar. A blind man discerns the sensation from the real presence of an object at his fingers' end, only by the force or weakness of that very sensation." So, then, let us consider that, to the blind, fingers are eyes, and remember that they have ten instead of two. As I have been blind since early infancy, my own case offers an illustration in point.

Blindness does not lead to any refinement of the senses of touch, hearing or smell, but to a greater keenness in the interpretation of the information furnished by these senses. Diderot says, "the help which our senses reciprocally afford to each other, hinders their improvement," and so the person in possession of all the senses regards the blind man as a marvel of intelligence and skill, just because, on losing his eyesight, his remaining senses come to the rescue, and he continues to live and move and have his being without the most precious of all physical senses. In the world of the blind child eyesight plays no part, and so the other senses are made to do double duty, and the extent to which these may be cultivated is limited only by the mentality of the child, its early training and environment.

I think hearing is the first sense to be cultivated, both in the infant and the adult suddenly deprived of eyesight. Through its ears, the child recognizes voices, detects different footfalls, is enabled to measure distance with a fair degree of accuracy, and can form a very clear idea as to the shape and dimensions of a room. All this information is conveyed to the normal child through the eyes. One writer has said, "but a distinction should be made between sensitiveness and an ability to use the sense, between native sensory capacity of the sense organ, and the acquired ability to use that capacity."

The second sense to be developed in the blind child is that of touch, and this development begins at a very early date, supplementing the sense of hearing. Long before the child is old enough to read, its fingers have become its eyes, and each of the ten fingers carries its quota of information to the active brain, the amount and quality of this information increasing with the mental development. In addition to the fingers, the nerves of the face and those of the feet contribute their share of information. The child learns to detect differences in climatic condition by the feel of the air on its face. I have often heard very young blind children exclaim, "It feels like rain! It feels like a nice day! The air feels heavy! The wind feels soft! The wind is rough today !" The nerves of the feet contribute their share of helpful knowledge, calling attention to differences in the ground often unnoticed by the eye, telling whether the path is smooth or rough, grassgrown or rock-strewn. The auditory and pedal nerves are mutually helpful, the ear recording and classifying the sounds made by the feet, often guiding them aright by recalling certain peculiarities of sound— whether the ground is hollow", whether the sidewalk is of board or cement, and whether there is a depression here or a raised place there. I often wonder how deaf-blind people walk as well as they do, when they can not hear their footfalls. I find walking much more difficult when on a crowded thoroughfare, or when passing a planing mill or boiler factory.

19. Which of the following visual abilities cannot be taken up by other well-trained senses?

    A. The ability to judge the dimensions of a room

    B. The ability to distinguish color

    C. The ability to determine shape and texture of an object

    D. The ability to recognize different individuals

20. Which of the following does the passage author NOT cite as a factor in the degree of sensitivity in a blind person's other senses?

    A. The reciprocal help of other senses

    B. Their learning environment

    C. Their mental ability

    D. Their quality of training

21. According to Diderot:

    A. blind education cannot cause other senses to fully compensate for the loss of sight.

    B. a blind person's way of sensing the world is entirely dissimilar from the sighted; he has ten eyes instead of two.

    C. the average person does not properly develop their individual sense faculties as they use others as crutches.

    D. one must distinguish native sensory capacity and the trained ability to make use of that capacity.

22. Based on the passage, it's reasonable to expect that in an indoor space suddenly losing all light, the individual best able to navigate would be

    A. a recently blinded child with acute hearing.

    B. an older man with average hearing who has been without sight since childhood.

    C. a very young child with all her senses.

    D. an adult with perfect eyesight and hearing.

23. Which of the following titles most accurately describes the passage?

    A. The Philosophy of Education for the Blind

    B. Survey of the Senses

    C. Several Methods for Coping with Blindness

    D. The Methodology of Education for the Blind

Passage 5 (Questions 24 – 29)

Pottery sherds found archeologically in colonial sites serve multiple purposes. They help to date the sites, they reflect cultural and economic levels in the areas of their use, and they throw light on manufacture, trade, and distribution.

Satisfying instances of these uses were revealed with the discovery in 1935 of two distinct but unidentified pottery types in the excavations conducted by the National Park Service at Jamestown, Virginia, and later elsewhere along the eastern seaboard. One type was an elaborate and striking yellow sgraffito ware, the other a coarse utilitarian kitchen ware whose red paste was heavily tempered with a gross water-worn gravel or "grit." Included in the latter class were the components of large earthen baking ovens.

The sgraffito pottery is a red earthenware, coated with a white slip through which designs have been incised. An amber lead glaze imparts a golden yellow to the slip-covered portions and a brownish amber to the exposed red paste. The gravel-tempered ware is made of a similar red-burning clay and is remarkable for its lack of refinement, for the pebbly texture caused by protruding bits of gravel, and for the crude and careless manner in which the heavy amber glaze was applied to interior surfaces. Once seen, it is instantly recognizable and entirely distinct from other known types of English or continental pottery. A complete oven, now restored at Jamestown, is of similar paste and quality of temper. It has a roughly oval beehive shape with a trapezoidal framed opening in which a pottery door fits snugly.

Following the initial discoveries at Jamestown there was considerable speculation about these two types. Worth Bailey, then museum technician at Jamestown, was the first to recognize the source of the sgraffito ware as "Devonshire." Bailey also noted that the oven and the gravel-tempered utensils were made of identical clay and temper. However, in an attempt to prove that earthenware was produced locally, he assumed, perhaps because of their crudeness, that the utensils were made at Jamestown. This led him to conjecture that the oven, having similar ceramic qualities, was also a local product. He felt in support of this that it was doubtful "so fragile an object could have survived a perilous sea voyage."

Since these opinions were expressed, much further archeological work in colonial sites has revealed widespread distribution of the two types. Bailey himself noted that a pottery oven is intact and in place in the John Bowne House in Flushing, Long Island. A fragment of another pottery oven recently has been identified among the artifacts excavated by Sidney Strickland from the site of the John Howland House, near Plymouth, Massachusetts; and gravel-tempered utensil sherds have occurred in many sites. The sgraffito ware has been unearthed in Virginia, Maryland, and Massachusetts.

Such a wide distribution of either type implies a productive European source for each, rather than a local American kiln in a struggling colonial settlement like Jamestown. Bailey's attribution of the sgraffito ware to Devonshire was confirmed in 1950 when J. C. Harrington, archeologist of the National Park Service, came upon certain evidence at Barnstaple in North Devon, England. This evidence was found in the form of sherds exhibited in a display window of C. H. Brannam's Barnstaple Pottery that were uncovered during excavation work on the premises. These are unmistakably related in technique and design to the American examples. A label under a fragment of a large deep dish in the display is inscribed: "Piece of dish found in site of pottery. In sgraffiato. About 1670." This clue opened the way to further investigations, the results of which relate the sgraffito ware, the gravel-tempered ware, and the ovens to the North Devon towns and to a busy commerce in earthenware between Barnstaple, Bideford, and the New World.

24. In the third paragraph, the author uses the phrase "instantly recognizable and entirely distinct" in order to:

    A. bolster a viewpoint about the links between pottery products found in areas distant from each other.

    B. highlight the superior nature of particular types of pottery as compared with more average pottery.

    C. show how people of both historical and modern time periods appreciated the pottery discussed in the passage.

    D. explain why Worth Bailey was able to connect the pottery's origin with "Devonshire" before his contemporaries were able to do so.

25. What, if true, would bolster the conclusion that some of the pottery described in the passage had a European origin?

    I. Sgraffito artifacts being excavated in England with styles similar to colonial sgraffito pieces

    II. Discovering similarities between colonial pottery from archeological sites and contemporary English pottery in private collections

    III. A letter dating from colonial times stating that the pottery manufactured in the colonies was similar in appearance to the pottery available for purchase in England

    A. I and II only

    B. I and III only

    C. II and III only

    D. I, II and III

26. Of the following categories referenced in the first paragraph, which is the passage primarily concerned with?

    A. Helping to date archaeological sites

    B. Revealing insights into the contemporary culture and economy

    C. Providing information relating to manufacturing, trading and distributing pottery

    D. None of the above

27. The author's purpose in citing the discovery of pottery ovens in Maryland, Massachusetts, Virginia, and Long Island is to:

    A. provide support for a thesis regarding historical manufacturing and distribution centers.

    B. highlight the sophistication of colonial manufacturing and distribution.

    C. demonstrate that Bailey was correct in determining that earthenware was produced locally.

    D. show how pottery-related products which were too fragile to survive a sea voyage could nonetheless find their way to a large percentage of the English colonies.

28. The author's purpose in referencing an assumption made by Bailey is to:

    A. indicate that he may not have correctly determined the source of pottery as Devonshire.

    B. indicate that he may have reached a conclusion in advance of sufficient evidence collection.

    C. show that Bailey was incorrectly promoted to his position as Jamestown's museum technician.

    D. show that assumptions made by researchers sometimes reflect available evidence.

29. What would it imply if archeological evidence were unearthed in London showing examples of sgraffito which matched the American examples more closely than was the case with the examples from Barnstaple and Bideford?

    A. That Barnstaple and Bideford can be ruled out as the original earthenware sources

    B. That sgraffito only originated in London and the gravel-tempered ware originated in the other two locations

    C. That the source of sgraffito was evenly distributed between the three locations in question

    D. That the "European source" referenced in the passage may have been London rather than the other two locations

Passage 6 (Questions 30 – 34)

Concerning the origin of the American game of baseball there exists considerable uncertainty. A correspondent of Porter's Spirit of the Times, as far back as 1856, begins a series of letters on the game by acknowledging his utter inability to arrive at any satisfactory conclusion upon this point; and a writer of recent date introduces a research into the history of the game with the frank avowal that he has only succeeded in finding "a remarkable lack of literature on the subject."

In view of its extraordinary growth and popularity as "Our National Game," the author deems it important that its true origin should, if possible, be ascertained, and he has, therefore, devoted to this inquiry more space than might at first seem necessary.

In 1856, within a dozen years from the time of the systematization of the game, the number of clubs in the metropolitan district and the enthusiasm attending their matches began to attract particular attention. The fact became apparent that it was surely superseding the English game of cricket, and the adherents of the latter game looked with ill-concealed jealousy on the rising upstart. There were then, as now, persons who believed that everything good and beautiful in the world must be of English origin, and these at once felt the need of a pedigree for the new game. Some one of them discovered that in certain features it resembled an English game called "rounders," and immediately it was announced to the American public that baseball was only the English game transposed. This theory was not admitted by the followers of the new game, but, unfortunately, they were not in a position to emphasize the denial. One of the strongest advocates of the rounder theory, an Englishman himself, was the writer for out-door sports on the principal metropolitan publications. In this capacity and as the author of a number of independent works of his own, and the writer of the "baseball" articles in several encyclopedias and books of sport, he has lost no opportunity to advance his pet theory. Subsequent writers have, blindly, it would seem, followed this lead, until now we find it asserted on every hand as a fact established by some indisputable evidence; and yet there has never been adduced a particle of proof to support this conclusion.

While the author of this work entertains the greatest respect for that gentleman, both as a journalist and man, and believes that baseball owes to him a monument of gratitude for the brave fight he has always made against the enemies and abuses of the game, he yet considers this point as to the game's origin worthy of further investigation, and he still regards it as an open question.

When was baseball first played in America? The first contribution which in any way refers to the antiquity of the game is the first official report of the "National Association" in 1858. This declares "The game of baseball has long been a favorite and popular recreation in this country, but it is only within the last fifteen years that any attempt has been made to systematize and regulate the game." The italics are inserted to call attention to the fact that in the memory of the men of that day baseball had been played a long time prior to 1845, so long that the fifteen years of systematized play was referred to by an "only."

Colonel Jas. Lee, elected an honorary member of the Knickerbocker Club in 1846, said that he had often played the same game when a boy, and at that time he was a man of sixty or more years. Mr. Wm. F. Ladd, my informant, one of the original members of the Knickerbockers, says that he never in any way doubted Colonel Lee's declaration, because he was a gentleman eminently worthy of belief.

30. Which of the following best describes the author's feeling toward the theory that baseball was transposed from the English game of "rounders"? The author thinks that:

    A. certain English-born men made up the theory out of a sense of English pride.

    B. the theory is plausible but lacks any evidence.

    C. certain English-born men propagated the theory out of a misunderstanding of facts.

    D. the theory is probably true, but desires to find concrete evidence.

31. Suppose it were discovered that the first mention of rounders as a game in England was in 1804, which of the following expresses how the author would most likely be affected by this news? The author would:

    A. be forced to recognize that rounders gave way to baseball.

    B. maintain the convictions he or she already held.

    C. be glad that more research was being done into the origin of rounders.

    D. feel more justified in believing that baseball is of uniquely American origin.

32. Which of the following would provide the strongest evidence that baseball originated prior to 1845?

    A. The testimony of Oliver Wendell Holmes that he played baseball at Harvard in 1828.

    B. A 1860 newspaper report that several Harvard graduates remember playing baseball at Harvard in 1828.

    C. The finding of a labeled diagram of a baseball diamond in Harvard's archives, dated to 1828.

    D. The finding of a bat created in 1828 similar to those used for baseball.

33. Which of the following is most likely the subject of the next paragraph after the end of the passage?

    A. The futility in trying to ascertain the exact date that baseball came about

    B. The futility in trying to ascertain the exact manner that baseball was invented

    C. The incompatibility of the timeline of baseball's origin and the claim it descended from cricket

    D. The incompatibility of the timeline of baseball's origin and the claims in the third paragraph

34. What is the purpose of the last sentence of the first paragraph?

    A. To provide evidence in favor of the author's ideas concerning baseball's origin

    B. To provide additional evidence that there is much uncertainty surrounding baseball's origin

    C. To provide additional evidence that there has been little thought or research put into the question of baseball's origin

    D. To give the reason that the author will take whatever space necessary to bring the question of baseball's origin into light

Passage 7 (Questions 35 – 39)

It should be observed that each kind of rhetoric has its own appropriate style. The style of written prose is not that of spoken oratory, nor are those of political and forensic speaking the same. Both written and spoken have to be known. To know the latter is to know how to speak good Greek. To know the former means that you are not obliged, as otherwise you are, to hold your tongue when you wish to communicate something to the general public.

The written style is the more finished: the spoken better admits of dramatic delivery – like the kind of oratory that reflects character and the kind that reflects emotion. Hence actors look out for plays written in the latter style, and poets for actors competent to act in such plays. Yet poets whose plays are meant to be read are read and circulated: Chaeremon, for instance, who is as finished as a professional speech-writer; and Licymnius among the dithyrambic poets. Compared with those of others, the speeches of professional writers sound thin in actual contests. Those of the orators, on the other hand, are good to hear spoken, but look amateurish enough when they pass into the hands of a reader. This is just because they are so well suited for an actual tussle, and therefore contain many dramatic touches, which, being robbed of all dramatic rendering, fail to do their own proper work, and consequently look silly.

Thus strings of unconnected words, and constant repetitions of words and phrases, are very properly condemned in written speeches: but not in spoken speeches -- speakers use them freely, for they have a dramatic effect. In this repetition there must be variety of tone, paving the way, as it were, to dramatic effect; e.g. "This is the villain among you who deceived you, who cheated you, who meant to betray you completely." This is the sort of thing that Philemon the actor used to do in the Old Men's Madness of Anaxandrides whenever he spoke the words "Rhadamanthus and Palamedes," and also in the prologue to the Saints whenever he pronounced the pronoun "I." If one does not deliver such things cleverly, it becomes a case of "the man who swallowed a poker." So too with strings of unconnected words, e.g. "I came to him; I met him; I besought him." Such passages must be acted, not delivered with the same quality and pitch of voice, as though they had only one idea in them. They have the further peculiarity of suggesting that a number of separate statements have been made in the time usually occupied by one. Just as the use of conjunctions makes many statements into a single one, so the omission of conjunctions acts in the reverse way and makes a single one into many. It thus makes everything more important: e.g. "I came to him; I talked to him; I entreated him" -- what a lot of facts! the hearer thinks -- "he paid no attention to anything I said." This is the effect which Homer seeks when he writes,

Nireus likewise from Syme (three well-fashioned ships did bring),

Nireus, the son of Aglaia (and Charopus, bright-faced king),

Nireus, the comeliest man (of all that to Ilium's strand).

If many things are said about a man, his name must be mentioned many times; and therefore people think that, if his name is mentioned many times, many things have been said about him. So that Homer, by means of this illusion, has made a great deal of Nireus though he has mentioned him only in this one passage, and has preserved his memory, though he nowhere says a word about him afterwards.

35. Based on the passage, omitting conjunctions leads to:

    A. combining multiple ideas into one statement.

    B. confusion as to who is being addressed.

    C. making the subject seem more important.

    D. reversing the previously stated idea.

36. The author's pairing of written and spoken rhetoric is similar to his pairing of which of the following?

    A. Poetic and dramatic

    B. Chaeremon and Licymnius

    C. Political and forensic

    D. Greek and Latin

37. According to the author, reading a text meant to be spoken can make it seem silly because:

    A. the skillful use of conjunctions and pronouns is only revealed orally.

    B. prose is a higher art and its power is revealed through reading it carefully.

    C. without dramatic effects and tone, such orations do not fully communicate their meaning.

    D. focusing on the political and forensic content of speeches draws attention to the proper work of rhetoric.

38. Suppose a follower of the writer of this passage advertised a class focused on written rhetoric. Which would be the most likely campaign slogan?

    A. Impress your friends with your control of tone and voice!

    B. Share your ideas fluently with the larger community!

    C. Learn to write in a wide variety of genres and styles!

    D. Stop hindering your communication with unconnected ideas!

39. Which of the following, if written by a writer that focused on works meant to be read, would most weaken the author's claims?

    A. A speech that was highly polished and sophisticated

    B. A speech that contested a recent political decision through the use of theatrical techniques

    C. A speech that seemed to favor content over device

    D. A speech that was rendered insignificant when read aloud by an accomplished orator

Passage 8 (Questions 40 – 46)

Ought the State to support the arts? There is certainly much to be said on both sides of this question. It may be said, in favor of the system of voting supplies for this purpose, that the arts enlarge, elevate, and harmonize the soul of a nation; that they divert it from too great an absorption in material occupations; encourage in it a love for the beautiful; and thus act favorably on its manners, customs, morals, and even on its industry. It may be asked, what would become of music in France without her Italian theatre and her Conservatoire; of the dramatic art, without her Théâtre-Français; of painting and sculpture, without our collections, galleries, and museums? It might even be asked, whether, without centralization, and consequently the support of the fine arts, that exquisite taste would be developed which is the noble appendage of French labor, and which introduces its productions to the whole world? In the face of such results, would it not be the height of imprudence to renounce this moderate contribution from all her citizens, which, in fact, in the eyes of Europe, realizes their superiority and their glory?

To these and many other reasons, whose force I do not dispute, arguments no less forcible may be opposed. It might first of all be said, that there is a question of distributive justice in it. Does the right of the legislator extend to abridging the wages of the artisan, for the sake of, adding to the profits of the artist? M. Lamartine said, "If you cease to support the theatre, where will you stop? Will you not necessarily be led to withdraw your support from your colleges, your museums, your institutes, and your libraries? It might be answered, if you desire to support everything which is good and useful, where will you stop? Will you not necessarily be led to form a civil list for agriculture, industry, commerce, benevolence, education? Then, is it certain that Government aid favours the progress of art?" This question is far from being settled, and we see very well that the theatres which prosper are those which depend upon their own resources.

I am, I confess, one of those who think that choice and impulse ought to come from below and not from above, from the citizen and not from the legislator; and the opposite doctrine appears to me to tend to the destruction of liberty and of human dignity.

But, by a deduction as false as it is unjust, do you know what economists are accused of? It is, that when we disapprove of government support, we are supposed to disapprove of the thing itself whose support is discussed; and to be the enemies of every kind of activity, because we desire to see those activities, on the one hand free, and on the other seeking their own reward in themselves. Thus, if we think that the State should not interfere by taxation in religious affairs, we are atheists. If we think the State ought not to interfere by taxation in education, we are hostile to knowledge. If we say that the State ought not by taxation to give a fictitious value to land, or to any particular branch of industry, we are enemies to property and labor. If we think that the State ought not to support artists, we are barbarians, who look upon the arts as useless.

Against such conclusions as these I protest with all my strength. Far from entertaining the absurd idea of doing away with religion, education, property, labor, and the arts, when we say that the State ought to protect the free development of all these kinds of human activity, without helping some of them at the expense of others--we think, on the contrary, that all these living powers of society would develop themselves more harmoniously under the influence of liberty; and that, under such an influence no one of them would, as is now the case, be a source of trouble, of abuses, of tyranny, and disorder.

40. As quoted in the second paragraph, Lamartine favors an argument strategy in which:

    A. the opposing position is shown to contradict well-established principles.

    B. his own position is shown to be supported by empirical evidence.

    C. the opposing position leads to a slippery slope problem in which logic gives no clear end to the position.

    D. his own position is supported by logical consistency and rational thought.

41. Which of the following is most likely a statement made by the author of the passage?

    A. My faith is in mankind, not in the legislator.

    B. My faith is in the legislator, not in mankind.

    C. An activity which is neither aided by supplies, nor regulated by government, is an activity destroyed.

    D. An activity which is aided by supplies, or regulated by government, is destined to fail.

42. Which of the following are arguments from the passage given for government funding of the arts?

    I. Ceasing funding of the arts gives reason to cease funding of other essential institutions.

    II. Economists do not approve of the arts.

    III. Government funding keeps the arts alive.

    A. II only

    B. III only

    C. I and II only

    D. I and III only

43. Which of the following best describes the author's attitude towards government?

    A. He or she is cynical toward government and thinks it wasteful.

    B. He or she is respectful of government as a force for advancement of society.

    C. He or she is cautiously fearful of government's power being overextended.

    D. He or she is tolerant of government's evils.

44. Which of the following will the author most likely agree with or support?

    A. Legislation increasing the cap on government funding for the arts

    B. Legislation allowing for the creation of a state-funded religion

    C. Legislation imposing restrictions on government funding of museums

    D. Legislation imposing a cap on artists' wages

45. What is the main purpose of the first paragraph of the passage?

    A. Present the main argument against the author's opinion

    B. Present the main argument in favor of the author's opinion

    C. Outline the benefits that the arts provide to European society

    D. Outline the form of the arts that are currently funded by the government

46. What is the purpose of the statement "if we think that the State should not interfere by taxation in religious affairs, we are atheists"?

    A. To draw attention to the discrimination against economists

    B. To show that religious affairs should be separate from government affairs

    C. To explain that economists are illogical or barbaric

    D. To ridicule that the author's ideas should draw accusations of disapproving of the arts

Passage 9 (Questions 47 – 53)

The scientific enterprise is built, in the ideal sense, upon the notion of free, full sharing of information made in the course of scientific discovery. While such a system of information-sharing can allow more rapid progress as various scientists build upon each others' work, it provides no particular inherent safeguards against inaccuracy in reported findings nor in full reporting of findings that may be quite important, if the researcher making such findings doesn't recognize their importance. Imagine, for a moment, that Alexander Fleming took no particular note of the fact that bacteria did not seem to grow in the area of the Penicillium fungi . . .

The full sharing of information would entail explanation, in painstaking detail, of the methods used to uncover certain results. But such a lengthy, exhaustive description would quickly generate a sheer volume of information that would be impossible to manage. One may argue that lab techniques could be referenced in shorthand (e.g. "a standard H&E stain revealed that . . .") but even there two significant problems arise.

First is the incorrect assumption that the exact physical materials used are largely fungible. For example, when conducting a titration, chemists would assume that the acid purchased from one scientific supply company is functionally identical to that same acid when purchased from a different company. While this may have been a workable assumption in the early- or mid-twentieth century, the increasing complexity and hyper-sensitivity of modern experiment, along with findings from chaos theory demonstrating the vast impact of tiny fluctuations in starting conditions, the basic inter-exchangeability of different experimental apparatuses and reagents is no longer valid.

Even more problematic is the issue of variations in the individual skill of the researchers involved. A study that requires surgical ablation of a portion of the test animal's brain will generate vastly different outcomes if the ablation procedure is carried out by a well-meaning and skilled researcher who simply lacks the masterful level of skill required. As it is practically impossible to address the first issue, and literally impossible to address the second issue when communicating scientific results, the foundation of the scientific enterprise begins to appear much shakier than initially supposed.

These problems only compound when we look beyond the full sharing of information itself. If the goal of science is to produce theories which make replicable predictions about how the world "really is" we see how damning the problems of full-information sharing become. After all, science is supposed to be the general, not the specific. It is the enterprise of "we" as opposed the artist's enterprise of "I". Thus it becomes no science at all to assert, "when this gifted surgeon carries out this procedure on a lab animal's brain, this is the result." If there is no other surgeon in the world who can replicate this feat, then the whole notion of replicability shows itself invalid ab initio.

The solution that suggests itself (to the extent that there even is one) is either a sharp delimiting of science to a far smaller ambit, or a fundamental shift away from the basic logical positivism that provides the philosophical undergirding that supports all of science back to the Enlightenment. The former is the more palatable, perhaps, but it is actually the second that is more feasible. Territory hard-acquired is never willingly surrendered and asking the scientific community to give up the realms of the very small, very large, and very complicated is a fool's errand. Instead, we must seek the shift in perspective that is harder to achieve but that pains less.

47. Which paragraph of the text most strongly suggests that the passage author is a philosopher?

    A. Paragraph 1

    B. Paragraph 2

    C. Paragraph 3

    D. Paragraph 6

48. For which of the following assertions does the author provide support by a concrete example?

    A. Science is founded on making predictions.

    B. An alternative philosophy to logical positivism must be found.

    C. Researchers assume experimental materials are fungible.

    D. Curtailing the areas that science investigates would solve many problems.

49. Suppose the passage author is tasked with developing the first-year science curriculum at a new university. He would most likely include which of the following in the course of study?

    A. Math courses that address chaos theory

    B. Courses on lab techniques that emphasize developing manual dexterity and technical skill

    C. Writing courses that emphasize how to concisely convey full information about an experiment

    D. Courses on the philosophical foundations of science that emphasize views other than logical positivism

50. If several of the most prominent scientific journals switch to a publishing format that permits online links to exhaustive details about the exact procedures used, including video footage of procedures being carried out, this would most *challenge* which of the following passage claims?

    A. A gifted surgeon could generate experimental results that would be difficult or impossible to replicate.

    B. It would be impossible to manage the volume of information entailed in full information sharing.

    C. Narrowing science to a smaller set of fields is the best path forward when fixing several problems inherent in science.

    D. Certain lab techniques can be referenced in shorthand.

51. In the final paragraph, the author's use of the phrase, "sharp delimiting of science to a far smaller ambit," most nearly means:

    A. shifting away from the arrogance of science that implies that science is the solution to every problem.

    B. limiting science departments to using certain types of experimental materials to aid in reproducibility.

    C. reducing the areas of inquiry that are investigated by science.

    D. eliminating science's reliance on the philosophy of logical positivism.

52. Which of the following claims, if made by the author in another publication, would most contradict the main argument here?

    A. "In the case of aerospace engineering, especially, exacting standards have ensured that the 'replaceable parts' notion that began centuries ago is now indispensible."

    B. "Several artists' communes have created works that require collective effort both in their creation and appreciation."

    C. "The skill of an individual researcher may certainly turn up results that are valuable."

    D. "The stunning successes of empiricism and positivism demonstrate that repeatable, scientific predictions are not just one way forward but the only way forward."

53. The author's overall tone can best be described as:

    A. abstract but engaged.

    B. concerned and exasperated.

    C. dismissive and uninterested.

    D. academic but emotional.

This page intentionally left blank.

SECTION 4

Answer Key

1	A	12	D	23	A	34	B	45	A
2	D	13	B	24	A	35	C	46	D
3	C	14	C	25	D	36	C	47	D
4	A	15	A	26	C	37	C	48	C
5	B	16	C	27	A	38	B	49	D
6	D	17	B	28	B	39	B	50	B
7	A	18	C	29	D	40	C	51	C
8	B	19	B	30	A	41	A	52	D
9	A	20	A	31	B	42	D	53	A
10	B	21	C	32	C	43	C		
11	D	22	B	33	D	44	C		

Passage 1 (Questions 1 – 5)

In 1961, Yale University psychologist Stanley **Milgram** initiated a study that has become perhaps the most notorious **psychology experiment** to date. Milgram placed an ad in the *New Haven Register* seeking subjects to participate in "a scientific **study of memory and learning**." Hundreds of subjects – each paid $4 – responded. When participants arrived at Milgram's research lab for the learning and memory study, they were faced with something entirely unexpected. Under the supervision of a lab-coated scientist, each volunteer – known as the "teacher" -- would read a series of words to another person – the "learner," who was hidden behind a partition and hooked up to an electric-shock device. The learner would repeat the words to the best of his ability. Each time the learner made a mistake, the teacher administered an electric shock. **Shocks** started out mild in intensity (15 volts: labeled "slight shock" on the teacher's control panel) and continued up to 450 volts (labeled "danger: severe shock"). As the shocks increased in severity, the learner would cry out in pain, sometimes citing a heart condition, and pleading with the teacher to stop. If the teacher hesitated or questioned the safety of the learner, the **supervising scientist would urge him to continue**. The results of the experiment were horrifying: approximately **two-thirds of subjects continued to shock the learners** to the maximum level, following the urging of the supervisor, even when the learner pled for mercy.

Key terms: Milgram, psychology experiment, study of memory and learning, shocks

Cause and effect: experiment subjects ("teachers") gave "learners" increasingly severe shocks as part of a supposed experiment in learning and memory; two-thirds of the subjects kept shocking to the maximum and most dangerous level

What the subjects did not know until they left the research lab was that the **shocks weren't real**. The agonized cries were delivered by actors; the learners and supervisor were in on the ruse too. In fact, the study was not about learning and memory at all: it was about **obedience to authority**. Milgram used the results of his study to support his now-famous claim that **ordinary people will obey virtually any order** – even to harm and even to torture others – given by an **authority figure**. The findings of Milgram's study have been used to explain some of the darkest episodes of recent history, from the Holocaust to the abuse of prisoners in Abu Ghraib.

Key term: obedience to authority

Contrast: the experiment was not actually about learning and memory – it was testing subjects obedience to authority

Opinion: psychologist Stanley Milgram asserted that ordinary people will follow orders, even when it means harming others

Fifty years after Milgram first published his study, however, psychologists and sociologists have started to **question Milgram's findings**. It's not his data that is at issue. Milgram repeated his study numerous times, and found that the number of people who followed the orders to shock all the way to the end remained at around 65%. In the decades since Milgram's study, **few** other researchers have attempted to **reproduce** his experiment because of clear **ethical issues**. (Subjects in Milgram's study were deeply distressed by their experience, some with lasting trauma.) In 2007, though, psychologist Jerry **Burger** performed a slight variation on Milgram's study, limiting the maximum shock value to 150 volts, and found **obedience rates virtually equal** to Milgram's.

Key terms: ethical issues, Burger

Cause and effect: no one repeated Milgram's experiment for nearly 50 years, because it seemed unethical to inflict emotional pain knowingly on the subjects; however, Burger performed a variation in 2007, in which subjects thought they were inflicting much milder shocks

Contrary to Milgram's explanation – that ordinary people will obediently and unthinkingly follow even malevolent authorities – some social scientists today explain the phenomenon as one of **social identification**. One such psychologist, Alexander **Haslam**, notes that the supervising "scientist" in Milgram's experiment reminded subjects that their compliance was key to the success of the experiment, and to the more **general benefit of science**. Subjects identified with these **worthy goals**. Social identification, says Haslam, is what motivates people to act as followers, and such identification is not thoughtless; rather, it is "the endeavor of committed subjects." The benefit of Haslam's interpretation is twofold. First, it provides a more nuanced explanation for historical atrocities – that functionaries in brutal regimes **do more than simply follow orders**; and second, it explains why people tend to obey orders more in some situations than in others. In Milgram's experiment, subjects were encouraged to **identify with the scientist**, and arguably, **enlightened society**, rather than with the learner behind the partition. Were the experiment designed so that subjects had **greater identification with learners**, it is likely that Milgram would have seen different results.

Key terms: social identification, Haslam

Contrast: psychologist Haslam believes that subjects were obedient not because they simply followed authority (as Milgram said) but because they identified with the supervising scientist and science in general; he calls this phenomenon "social identification"

Opinion: the author suggests that if Milgram encouraged subjects to identify with learners, rather than with scientist and science, fewer subjects would have gone all the way with shocks

Main idea: Milgram's experiment tested the degree to which people would follow orders even when it meant harming others. He believed that his experiment showed that ordinary people are blindly obedient to authority, but recent psychologists say Milgram's results illustrate social identification.

1. A is correct. The subjects of Milgram's experiment (the "teachers") believed they were participating in a study of learning and memory, and that the shocks were real. As we're told in paragraph 2, it wasn't until the subjects left the lab that they learned that they were not actually shocking the "learners."

2. D is correct. There's a lot that could be called horrifying in Milgram's experiment – but this question is asking for the author's viewpoint. You can find the answer at the end of paragraph 1. There, the author says that the results of Milgram's experiment that are horrifying – that the majority of participants were willing to shock innocent people to death.

3. C is correct. Take a look at paragraph 3. The ethical issue mentioned here is that the subjects in Milgram's experiment were traumatized by their experience. You probably can think of many other ethical issues around this study – but remember, your answer needs to be based on information in the passage.

4. A is correct. To summarize: Milgram believed that the reason his subjects were so compliant was because they were unthinkingly following authority, and theorized that such obedience was behind many instances of inhumane behavior in history. Haslam, however, believed that the subjects were compliant because they were identifying with the supervising scientist and all he represented – it was social identification and not obedience to authority at work.

    B: Haslam probably would say that fewer subjects would have followed orders if they'd identified more with the learner, not the scientist.

    C: We don't really have enough information to support or reject this choice.

    D: Haslam thought the subjects were making a somewhat conscious choice to inflict shocks, but Milgram seemed to think they were following blindly.

5. B is correct. The passage ends with the suggestion that if the subjects in Milgram's study were prompted to identify with the learner, not the scientist, fewer people would have conceded to shock the learners so severely.

Passage 2 (Questions 6 – 11)

The names go together as do those of **Shelley** and **Keats** or **Fortnum** and **Mason**. Even to people who seldom or never look seriously at a picture they have stood, these ten years, as symbols of modernity. They are preeminent: and for this there is reason. **Matisse** and **Picasso** are the two immediate heirs to **Cezanne**. They are in the direct line: and through one of them a great part of the younger generation comes at its share of the patrimony. To their contemporaries they owe nothing: they came into the legacy and had to make what they could of it. **They are the elder brothers of the movement**, a fact which the movement occasionally resents by treating them as though they were its elder sisters.

Key terms: Shelley, Keats, Fortnum, Mason, Matisse, Picasso, Cezanne

Contrast: Matisse and Picasso in contrast to their contemporaries and followers

Cause and effect: Cezanne's work influenced Matisse and Picasso who have influenced a new generation of artists

Even to each other they owe nothing. Matisse, to be sure, swept for one moment out of his course by the overwhelming significance of Picasso's abstract work, himself made a move in that direction. But this adventure he quickly, and wisely, abandoned; the problems of cubism could have helped him nothing to materialize his peculiar sensibility. And this **sensibility**—this peculiar reaction to what he sees—is his **great gift**. No one ever felt for the visible universe just what Matisse feels; or, if one did, he could not create an equivalent. Because, in addition to this magic power of creation, Matisse has been blest with extraordinary sensibility both of reaction and touch, he is a great artist; because he trusts to it entirely he is not what for a moment apparently he wished to be—a **chef d'ecole**.

Key terms: sensibility, chef d'ecole

Contrast: styles and sensibilities of Matisse and Picasso

Cause and effect: Matisse was briefly influenced by Picasso, but realized Picasso's style did not suit his sensibilities; because Matisse trusts entirely to his sensibility, he is a great artist, but not a chef d'ecole

Picasso, on the other hand, who never tried to be anything of the sort, is **the paramount influence in modern painting**—subject, of course, to the supreme influence of Cezanne. All the world over are students and young painters to whom his mere name is thrilling; to whom Picasso is the liberator. His influence is ubiquitous: even in England it is immense. Not only those who for all their denials— denials that spring rather from ignorance than bad faith— are mere apes of the inventor of cubism, but **artists who float so far out of the mainstream** as the Spensers and the Nashes, Mr. Lamb and Mr. John, **would all have painted differently had Picasso never existed**.

Opinion: students and young painters think of Picasso as a liberator

Contrast: those who admire Picasso vs those who deny his importance vs those outside the mainstream

Cause and effect: Picasso's style and influence has changed how a wide variety of artists paint

Picasso is a born **chef d'ecole**. His is one of the **most inventive minds in Europe**. Invention is as clearly his supreme gift as sensibility is that of Matisse. His career has been a series of **discoveries**, each of which he has rapidly developed. A highly original and extremely **happy conception** enters his head, suggested, probably, by some odd thing he has seen. Forthwith he sets himself to **analyze** it and disentangle those principles that account for its peculiar happiness. He proceeds by **experiment**, applying his hypotheses in the most unlikely places. Before long he has established what looks like an infallible **method** for producing an effect of which, a few months earlier, no one had so much as dreamed. This is one reason why Picasso is a born chef d'ecole. And this is why of **each new phase** in his art the **earlier examples** are apt to be the **more vital** and well nourished. At the end he is approaching that formula towards which his intellectual effort tends inevitably. It is time for a new discovery.

Key terms: chef d'ecole

Contrast: Picasso's ability to establish a method for an effect vs no one else even realizing the need for that effect

Cause and effect: Picasso operates through discovery: he sees something, it inspires a new idea, he analyzes what is exciting about that idea and then figures out how to do it well; this makes him a chef d'ecole; it also means that once he has mastered the new technique, his works are less vital than when he is developing the technique

Main Idea: The passage suggests that Matisse and Picasso are the two greatest modern artists, but because Picasso is always analyzing his reactions and creating new techniques, he is more of a chef d'ecole than Matisse, who trusts his instincts wholly.

6. D is correct. The second paragraph states that "Matisse, to be sure, swept for one moment out of his course by the overwhelming significance of Picasso's abstract work, himself made a move in that direction. But this adventure he quickly, and wisely, abandoned." Thus he did briefly explore abstract art.

   A: The passage never addresses Matisse's attitudes about his artistic forbearers.

   B: While the passage highlights Matisse's sensibility, it does not suggest he is overly sensitive.

   C: The passage does not connect cubism and materiality.

7. A is correct. The passage describes the specific artistic achievements of Matisse and Picasso, and also assesses whether each is a chef d'ecole, or one who affects others in the field.

   B, C: The passage does not directly discuss the emotions raised by cubism, or the number of chef d'ecoles per generation.

   D: While the passage does mention who Matisse and Picasso were heirs to and their effect on others, it does not suggest this is of prime importance in assessing their work or that it "must" be understood.

8. B is correct. In discussing Matisse, the author writes that he "has been blest with extraordinary sensibility both of reaction and touch, he is a great artist; because he trusts to it entirely he is not what for a moment apparently he wished to be—a chef d'ecole." Thus the passage suggests that faith in one's work is NOT a quality of a chef d'ecole.

   A, C, D: In the discussion of Picasso, who the author terms a chef d'ecole, we are told he is a "paramount influence in modern art," that "his career has been a series of discoveries," and that when he creates a new technique he has "established what looks like an infallible method for producing an effect of which, a few months earlier, no one had so much as dreamed."

9. A is correct. The author states that both those who deny his influence and those who are far from the mainstream "would…have painted differently had Picasso never existed." Thus a claim that an artist's work was completely unrelated to Picasso's would have been met with skepticism.

   B, C: The passage does not discuss either controversy over who invented cubism or Picasso's desire to be a chef d'ecole.

   D: While the passage suggests that some dismiss Picasso from "ignorance rather than bad faith," it does not address religious faith.

10. B is correct. The author states that in "each new phase in his art the earlier examples are apt to be the more vital and well nourished. At the end he is approaching that formula towards which his intellectual effort tends inevitably. It is time for a new discovery." Thus when his art is fully developed, we can assume it is less vital and exciting.

    A: This suggests his late work is more, rather than less, vital.

    C, D: The degree to which his work is copied or costs is not mentioned in the passage.

11. D is correct. In the first paragraph, the author suggests that other artists display some jealousy and their "resent[ment]" by treating Matisse and Picasso as "elder sisters."

    A, C: Choices A and C both suggest that other artists look down on Matisse and Picasso's work, which is not stated in the passage.

    B: The suggestion is that the other artists felt jealousy about Matisse and Picasso and thus treated them as "elder sisters"; there is no suggestion that they found their work to be feminine as in choice B.

Passage 3 (Questions 12 – 18)

We all know something about **time**: we know it as **past, present**, and **future**, we know it as being **divisible** into **successive parts**, and we know that all that happens happens in time. **Those who have pondered it a great deal** are likely to tell us that time is a **necessity of thought**, that time is and must be **infinite**, and that it is infinitely divisible. You will notice that these are the same statements that were made regarding **space**, and as they have just been critiqued, we won't dwell on them long. However, we must not pass over them altogether.

Contrast: that which we know vs that which those who have pondered it more know

As far as time being necessary, we must admit that we cannot **annihilate** or **think away** time, and that it means nothing to attempt such a task. Whatever time is, it does not seem to be of a nature that we can demolish it. But is it **necessarily absurd** to speak of a **system of things** – albeit, not a system of things in which there is **change** and **succession**, an **earlier** and **later**, but still, a system of things of some sort – in which there are no **time relations**? Of course, this problem is **merely theoretical**, for no such system exists in the world.

Opinion: even though it's crazy to "think away time" we should ponder what it would mean to have a theory that has no time

As for the infinity of time, may we not ask on what **grounds** anyone could venture to assert this? No one can say that infinite time is a given in his **experience**. If we cannot **directly perceive** this infinity, must we not then seek some **proof** of it? The only proof appears to be contained in this statement: we cannot conceive of **a time before which there was no time**, nor of **a time after which there will be no time**. This is a proof that is no proof, for here it is written out: we cannot conceive of **a time in the time before which there was no time**, nor of **a time in the time after which there will be no time**. We might as well say: we cannot conceive of a **number** the number before which was no number, nor of a number the number after which will be no number. Whatever may be said of the **conclusion**, the **argument** is weak.

Contrast: knowing time is infinite vs experiencing it, experiencing vs proof

Opinion: we can't directly experience the infinity of time, so we go for a proof; but author thinks that "the argument is weak".

Turning to the consideration of time as infinitely divisible, we find ourselves facing the **same difficulties** that showed themselves when we considered space as infinitely divisible. Certainly no one is ever **conscious** of the infinite number of parts of the **minute** that just **passed**. Nevertheless, shall he claim it did contain an infinite number of parts? How did it succeed in passing? How did this minute even **begin to pass**? If the minute is infinitely divisible, there is **no end** to the number of parts into which it can be divided, those parts

are all successive, no two parts can pass at once, and they must all proceed in a **certain order**.

Contrast: time as infinitely divisible vs space; not being conscious of the infinite parts of a minute vs claiming it has infinite parts

Cause and effect: because time seems infinitely divisible, it creates a paradox about how a minute can actually pass

Something must **pass first**. What could it be? If that something has parts and is divisible, **the whole** of it cannot pass first. Rather, it must pass **bit by bit**, as does the whole minute. If it is infinitely divisible, we find ourselves with the same problem we faced at the outset. Therefore, whatever passes first cannot have parts. So, let us assume it has no parts and bid it Godspeed! Has the minute begun? By **hypothesis**, our minute is infinitely divisible, composed of parts, and those parts of other parts, and so on without end. We cannot, through **division**, come to any part which itself is not composed of smaller parts. Therefore, the **partless thing** that passed is not part of the minute. Rather, it is still waiting at the gate, and no member of its platoon can prove it has the right to lead the rest.

Contrast: the whole of it passing first vs it passing bit by bit; partless thing vs the minute; partless thing vs member of its platoon

Cause and effect: since time is infinitely divisible, it seems impossible for time to pass since the first to pass must be a single "chunk" of time that itself cannot be divided further

Main Idea: The author discusses time, contrasting what laymen and philosophers know about; we run into problems we cannot prove, like the infinite divisibility of time. We have these assumptions that seem to make sense, and yet, we do not really have means to truly and fully address the nature of "time".

12. D is correct. In the third paragraph we read, "As for the infinity of time, may we not ask on what grounds anyone could venture to assert this? No one can say that infinite time is a given in his experience. If we cannot directly perceive this infinity, must we not then seek some proof of it?" It seems the infinity of time is taken as a given, yet the author questions how any person can directly experience this.

A, B: He's not calling on us to deny claims, but to find proof for them.

C: Yes, we need to reflect deeply, but the author, when asking about proof, seems to be seeking something tangible.

13. B is correct. There are two problems that arise: how can a finite minute be infinitely divisible, and how can such a minute succeed in passing, let alone begin to pass. Choice B satisfies the first question, and the second question is not reflected in any of the choices.

A: That question is not addressed here.

C: Rather, how can something that is finite (a minute) be composed of individual, infinite moments?

D: This is more in the third paragraph.

14. C is correct. Here is that question without the bit in the middle: "But is it necessarily absurd to speak of a system of things in where there are no time relations?" He's asking, are we positive that it is always absurd to speak of a system with no time? Or, are we positive that time cannot be done away with? Of course, he says the problem is only theoretical, for no such system exists in the world. But, he still questions those first two sentences.

A: This suggestion is not being made.

B: Rather, he's challenging this notion.

D: This doesn't seem to be an "us vs them" thing. Lay people would likely agree that time is unavoidable.

15. A is correct. The author writes, "Those who have pondered it a great deal are likely to tell us that time is a necessity of thought..."

B: The author brings this up, not "those who have pondered much".

C: This is the reverse of the correct answer.

D: Rather, it must be partless. We know from the last sentence that this doesn't work either.

16. C is correct. As the author writes in the first paragraph, "You will notice that these are the same statements that were made regarding space, and as they have just been critiqued, we won't dwell on them long." This statement implies that an understanding of space will be helpful in understanding time.

A: Though rhetoric is used here, there is never a case made that an understanding of it is helpful in understanding time.

B: Geometry is not mentioned.

D: This answer may be a bit tempting, but no point is made about watch making being helpful here. Time is being studied as an abstract, philosophical problem – not as a practical, engineering issue that a watchmaker would focus on.

17. B is correct. Rather, it is divisible into infinite, successive parts.

A, C, D: These are all stated as true in the passage.

18. C is correct. Items I and II are stated as true in the passage. Item III is never stated. We never know what this "partless thing" actually is. Moreover, space, like time, can be divided into infinite parts, as we know from the first paragraph.

Passage 4 (Questions 19 – 23)

A blind man once said, when asked if he would not be glad to have his eyesight, "to **improve the organs I have**, would be as good as to give me that which is wanting in me." This sentence sums up the **whole aim of blind education. Dr. Eichholtz**, a noted educator of the blind, says: "Education of the blind absolutely fails in its object, in so far as it fails to develop the remaining faculties to compensate for the want of sight. **Touch** and **sight** must be developed by means which practically in all respects are dissimilar. A blind man discerns the sensation from the real presence of an object at his fingers' end, only by the force or weakness of that very sensation." So, then, let us consider that, **to the blind, fingers are eyes**, and remember that they have ten instead of two. As I have been blind since early infancy, my own case offers an illustration in point.

Key terms: blind education, Dr. Eichholtz

Contrast: sight vs touch, in all respects dissimilar

Cause and effect: blind education develops different senses as alternatives, not replacements, for sight

Blindness does **not** lead to any **refinement** of the senses of touch, hearing or smell, but to a **greater keenness** in the interpretation of the information furnished by these senses. **Diderot** says, "the help which our senses reciprocally afford to each other, hinders their improvement," and so the person in possession of all the senses regards the blind man as a marvel of intelligence and skill, just because, on losing his eyesight, his **remaining senses come to the rescue**, and he continues to live and move and have his being without the most precious of all physical senses. In the world of the blind child eyesight plays no part, and so **the other senses are made to do double duty**, and the extent to which these may be cultivated is limited only by the mentality of the child, its early training and environment.

Key terms: Diderot

Contrast: lack of sight coupled with improved development of other senses

Cause and effect: other senses are not more sensitive, but mind's interpretation is improved

I think **hearing** is the **first** sense to be **cultivated**, both in the infant and the adult suddenly deprived of eyesight. Through its ears, the child recognizes voices, detects different footfalls, is enabled to measure distance with a fair degree of accuracy, and can form a very clear idea as to the shape and dimensions of a room. All this information is conveyed to the normal child through the eyes. One writer has said, "but a **distinction** should be made between **sensitiveness** and an **ability to use the sense**, between native sensory capacity of the sense organ, and the acquired ability to use that capacity."

Contrast: sound-based determination of surroundings vs instant visual awareness

Cause and effect: blind child's developed hearing allows for judgment of room dimensions, distances, and recognition of individuals by step or speech

The **second** sense to be developed in the blind child is that of **touch**, and this development **begins at a very early date**, supplementing the sense of hearing. Long before the child is old enough to read, its **fingers have become its eyes**, and each of the ten fingers carries its quota of information to the active brain, the amount and quality of this information increasing with the mental development. In addition to the fingers, the nerves of the **face and those of the feet** contribute their share of information. The child learns to detect differences in climatic condition by the feel of the air on its face. I have often heard very young blind children exclaim, "It feels like rain! It feels like a nice day! The air feels heavy! The wind feels soft! The wind is rough today !" The nerves of the feet contribute their share of helpful knowledge, calling attention to differences in the ground often unnoticed by the eye. telling whether the path is smooth or rough, grassgrown or rock-strewn. The **auditory and pedal nerves are mutually helpful**, the ear recording and classifying the sounds made by the feet, often guiding them aright by recalling certain peculiarities of sound— whether the ground is "hollow", whether the sidewalk is of board or cement, and whether there is a depression here or a raised place there. I often wonder how deaf-blind people walk as well as they do, when they can not hear their footfalls. I find walking much more difficult when on a crowded thoroughfare, or when passing a planing mill or boiler factory.

Cause and effect: the blind use their sense of touch to enhance the information they get from hearing, especially when it comes to the sense of touch in their feet to help in walking

Main Idea: Education of the blind is predicated on training of other senses to meet the same information-gathering needs by different means.

19. B is correct. No mention of color is made in the passage, and indeed, recognizing color by touch is very far-fetched. The other abilities can be taken over by other senses: sound (choice A and D) and touch (choice C).

20. A is correct. Answer choice A comes from a quote of Diderot's, not the passage author.

21. C is correct. Each of these answer choices pulls from the passage, but only one is attributable to Diderot. A simple search of Diderot's quotation in paragraph two reveals answer choice C as a match.

22. B is correct. Since the passage repeatedly makes the point that the other senses don't actually become more sensitive in the absence of sight, but the information is more exactly interpreted, a recently-blind, untrained child will be little better off than a sighted individual suddenly in the dark. The older adult who has been blind for some time should be best able to navigate the room, even if his hearing is not the most acute, since he has the experience to interpret sound information to understand his surroundings.

23. A is correct. The overall goal of the passage is to give an overview of the underlying theory of education for the visually-impaired. The titles in answer choices B and C are out of scope, and C, additionally, is inaccurate. There aren't several methods: a single general idea of education for the blind is presented. Now, choosing between answer choices A and D is not so easy, but recall again the main idea of the passage. The main underlying idea of blind education is elucidated throughout, while no specific, practical steps are given. So, Philosophy of Education is a superior match to the topic of the passage rather than Methodology of Education.

Passage 5 (Questions 24 – 29)

Pottery sherds found archeologically in **colonial** sites serve multiple purposes. They help to **date** the sites, they reflect cultural and economic **levels** in the areas of their use, and they **throw light on manufacture, trade, and distribution.**

Cause and effect: the bits of pottery at colonial sites give lots of information

Satisfying instances of these uses were revealed with the discovery in **1935** of **two distinct** but unidentified pottery types in the excavations conducted by the National Park Service at **Jamestown, Virginia**, and later elsewhere along the eastern seaboard. One type was an **elaborate** and striking yellow **sgraffito** ware, the other a **coarse utilitarian kitchen** ware whose red paste was heavily tempered with a gross water-worn gravel or "**grit.**" Included in the **latter** class were the components of **large earthen baking ovens**.

Contrast: elaborate sgraffito vs coarse grit-filled kitchen ware including baking ovens

Opinion: author thinks discovering these two types of pottery was "satisfying"

The **sgraffito** pottery is a **red** earthenware, coated with a white slip through which designs have been incised. An **amber** lead **glaze** imparts a **golden yellow** to the slip-covered portions and a brownish amber to the exposed red paste. The **gravel-tempered ware** is made of a similar red-burning clay and is **remarkable** for its **lack of refinement**, for the **pebbly texture** caused by protruding bits of gravel, and for the **crude and careless manner** in which the heavy amber glaze was applied to **interior** surfaces. once seen, it is instantly recognizable and **entirely distinct** from other known types of **English or continental pottery**. A **complete oven**, now restored at Jamestown, is of **similar** paste and quality of temper. It has a roughly oval beehive shape with a trapezoidal framed opening in which a pottery door fits snugly.

Contrast: sgraffito pottery is covered in designs vs the crude earthenware

Following the initial discoveries at Jamestown, there was considerable speculation about these two types. Worth **Bailey**, then museum technician at Jamestown, was the **first to recognize** the source of the sgraffito ware as "**Devonshire**." Bailey also noted that the oven and the gravel-tempered utensils were made of identical clay and temper. However, in an attempt to prove that earthenware was produced locally, he assumed, perhaps because of their crudeness, that the **utensils** were made at Jamestown. This led him to conjecture that the **oven**, having similar ceramic qualities, was also a **local** product. He felt in support of this that it was **doubtful** "so fragile an object could have **survived a perilous sea voyage.**"

Key terms: Bailey, Devonshire

Opinion: Bailey believes the sgraffito is from Devonshire, and the gravel ones were made locally

Since these opinions were expressed, much further archeological work in colonial sites has revealed **widespread distribution** of the two types. Bailey himself noted that a pottery **oven is intact** and in place in the **John Bowne House** in Flushing, **Long Island**. A fragment of another pottery oven recently has been identified among the artifacts excavated by Sidney **Strickland** from the site of the John Howland House, near Plymouth, **Massachusetts**; and gravel-tempered utensil sherds have occurred in many sites. The **sgraffito** ware has been unearthed in **Virginia**, Maryland, and **Massachusetts**.

Key terms: John Browne House, Long Island, Strickland, Massachusetts, Virginia

Cause and effect: discoveries have shown both the gravel and sgraffito were in different states

Such a **wide distribution** of either type implies a **productive European source** for each, rather than a local American kiln in a struggling colonial settlement like Jamestown. Bailey's attribution of the sgraffito ware to **Devonshire** was **confirmed** in 1950 when J. C. **Harrington**, archeologist of the National Park Service, came upon certain **evidence** at Barnstaple in **North Devon, England**. This evidence was found in the form of sherds exhibited in a display window of C. H. Brannam's Barnstaple Pottery that were uncovered during excavation work on the premises. These are **unmistakably related** in technique and design to the **American examples**. A label under a fragment of a large deep dish in the display is inscribed: "Piece of dish found in site of pottery. In sgraffiato. About 1670." This clue opened the way to further investigations, the results of which relate the sgraffito ware, the gravel-tempered ware, and the ovens to the North Devon towns and to a busy commerce in earthenware between Barnstaple, Bideford, and the New World.

Key terms: Harrington, North Devon, England

Cause and effect: wide presence of pottery suggests they were made in England, not locally and this was confirmed by evidence in Devonshire

Main Idea: Two types of pottery that were different (fine sgraffito vs crude gravelware) were found throughout the eastern US and were traced to an origin in Devonshire, England.

24. A is correct. The passage is focused on the geographical source of pottery. The main view is that such products seem to have been from England. One piece of evidence is the style of the colonial pottery is similar to pottery from England, as distinct from other styles. This bolsters the connection between the pottery in these locations.

    B: This is incorrect – there is nothing in the tone of the passage which indicates the author views some types of pottery as superior to "average" pottery.

    C: There is nothing in the passage relating to how people appreciate the pottery.

    D: The passage doesn't indicate that the evidence allowed Bailey to develop his theory before others.

25. D is correct. I is correct because a common design can be evidence of a common origin. II is also correct because English pottery that is contemporary with colonial pottery can also be evidence of a shared origin. Finally, in III, a contemporary letter would provide evidence even though it's not direct archeological proof.

26. C is correct. The passage describes two types of colonial pottery (2nd and 3rd paragraphs), the possible sources (4th paragraph), details about where the pottery has been found (fifth), and evidence relating to the pottery's origin (last paragraph). These relate to the manufacture, trade and distribution of the pottery.

    A: This is mentioned in the first paragraph, and in passing in the last paragraph. It isn't the main point of the passage.

    B: The passage only sporadically mentions culture and there is next to no mention of the contemporary economy.

27. A is correct. The thesis in question is that, historically, manufacturing and distribution of pottery (and probably related products such as ovens) originated in England. This is supported by the list of colonies where pottery ovens were found, and the implication such a wide distribution was unlikely to come from Jamestown.

    B: The passage indicates the manufacturing appears to have been in England, not the colonies.

    C: The passage undercuts Bailey's theory about local production. It does so in the fourth paragraph and the first sentence of the last paragraph.

    D: The idea that pottery-related products were too fragile to survive a sea voyage is an assumption made by Bailey.

28. B is correct. Bailey assumed fragile earthenware could not have survived a sea voyage, and that they must have been made locally. However, the next two paragraphs say that archeological work which took place later discovered similar pottery in a wide variety of colonial locations, and that "such a wide distribution of either type implies a productive European source for each".

    A: The passage says that Bailey "was the first to recognize the source of the sgraffito ware as Devonshire." The word "recognize" means that this determination was accurate, not a mistake.

    C: The discussion of Bailey's assumption is limited to a particular part of his analysis, not whether he should have his position as museum technician.

    D: The discussion of Bailey's assumption is followed by evidence that it was most likely incorrect, not that it lined up.

29. D is correct. The passage indicates that the evidence that Barnstaple and Bideford could have originated the earthenware found in the American colonies comprises similarities between samples found in each place. If earthenware found in London is more similar, then this provides stronger evidence of a London origin.

    A, B: Even though the similarities between American pottery and London-sourced pottery are stronger than the similarities between American pottery and that from Barnstaple and Bideford, this still constitutes evidence that the original source was London. It is also possible that pottery originated from Barnstaple and Bideford which was even more similar to American pottery, but these examples have yet to be excavated.

    C: There is no evidence that sgraffito pottery came from the three locations in equal quantities.

Passage 6 (Questions 30 – 34)

Concerning the **origin** of the **American** game of **baseball** there exists considerable **uncertainty**. A correspondent of Porter's Spirit of the Times, as far back as **1856**, begins a series of letters on the game by acknowledging his utter **inability** to arrive at any **satisfactory conclusion** upon this point; and a writer of recent date introduces a research into the history of the game with the frank avowal that he has only succeeded in finding "a remarkable lack of literature on the subject."

Key terms: American, baseball, 1856

Opinions: the author believes there is uncertainty about baseball's history

In view of its extraordinary growth and popularity as "**Our National Game**," the author deems it **important that its true origin** should, if possible, be ascertained, and he has, therefore, devoted to this inquiry more space than might at first seem necessary.

Key terms: Our National Game

Cause and effect: the author devoted much space to the inquiry of baseball's origin because he or she deems it important

In **1856, within a dozen years** from the time of the **systematization** of the game, the number of clubs in the metropolitan district and the enthusiasm attending their matches began to attract particular attention. The fact became apparent that it was surely **superseding** the English game of **cricket**, and the adherents of the latter game looked with ill-concealed jealousy on the rising upstart. There were then, as now, **persons** who believed that **everything good** and beautiful in the world must be of **English** origin, and these at once felt the need of a pedigree for the new game. Some one of them discovered that in **certain features it resembled** an English game called "**rounders**," and immediately it was announced to the American public that baseball was only the English game transposed. This theory was not admitted by the followers of the new game, but, unfortunately, they were not in a position to emphasize the denial. One of the strongest advocates of the rounder theory, an Englishman-born himself, was the writer for out-door sports on the principal metropolitan publications. In this capacity and as the author of a number of independent works of his own, and the writer of the "baseball" articles in several encyclopedias and books of sport, he has lost no opportunity to **advance his pet theory**. Subsequent writers have, **blindly**, it would seem, followed this lead, until now we find it asserted on every hand as a fact established by some indisputable evidence; and yet there has never been adduced a **particle of proof** to support this conclusion.

Key terms: cricket, English, rounders

Opinions: the author does not agree that baseball descended from rounders; the author believes that the propagation of this rumor is the work of proud Englishmen

Cause and effect: the propagation of rumors led to the masses believing that baseball descended from rounders

While the author of this work entertains the **greatest respect for that gentleman**, both as a journalist and man, and believes that baseball owes to him a monument of gratitude for the brave fight he has always made against the enemies and abuses of the game, he yet considers this point as to **the game's origin worthy of further investigation**, and he still regards it as an **open question**.

Opinions: the author respects the man that said baseball came from rounders, but does not believe his idea is true

When was baseball first played in America? The first contribution which in any way refers to the antiquity of the game is the first official report of the "National Association" in 1858. This declares "The game of baseball has long been a favorite and popular recreation in this country, but it is only within the last fifteen years that any attempt has been made to systematize and regulate the game." The italics are inserted to call attention to the fact that in the memory of the men of that day baseball had been played a long time prior to 1845, so long that the fifteen years of systematized play was referred to by an "only."

Key terms: National Association, 1858, fifteen years, systematize, prior to 1845

Opinion: the author concludes that baseball must have been around prior to 1845

Colonel Jas. Lee, elected an honorary member of the **Knickerbocker Club** in **1846**, said that he had often played the same game when a boy, and at that time he was a man of **sixty** or more years. Mr. Wm. F. **Ladd**, my informant, one of the original members of the Knickerbockers, says that he never in any way doubted Colonel Lee's declaration, because he was a gentleman eminently worthy of belief.

Opinions: the author thinks Lee's testimony is evidence that baseball was played years ago

Cause and effect: if Colonel Jas. Lee is to be believed, then baseball would have been around for decades prior to 1846

Main Idea: The author seeks to provide an account of the origin of baseball; the author apparently believes it to be of American origin and tries to debunk the theory that it descended from an English game and offers evidence that the game is quite a bit older than the mid-nineteenth century.

30. A is correct. The author states that concerning the theory, "there has never been adduced a particle of proof to support this conclusion." The author also states that those who prescribe to the theory do so "blindly" and that those who first supported the theory were persons "who believed that everything good and beautiful in the world must be of English origin."

   B: The author seems to be hostile toward the idea.

   C: The author never mentions that the English faithful might have some misunderstanding.

   D: The author does not believe the theory to be true.

31. B is correct. The author seems to care very little for whatever arguments are given in favor of the theory that rounders gave way to baseball. Since the statement in the question is not conclusive evidence that rounders gave way to baseball, there is no reason to think the author would change his or her views.

   A: There is not sufficient evidence for the author to be so swayed.

   C: There is no reason to thinking the author cares about research being done into rounders.

   D: The statement in the stem does not support this conclusion.

32. C is correct. The testimony of a person is never as good as a concrete piece of evidence that can be carefully scrutinized. Of choices C and D, choice C is better because it is obviously specific to the game of baseball.

   A, B, D: These are all certainly evidence in favor of the proposition but are not as strong as C.

33. D is correct. The paragraphs at the end of the passage attempt to lay out a timeline for the age of baseball in America. One gets the feeling that the author is laying out the timeline in an attempt to debunk the theory posited in the third paragraph about rounders. It is expected that the author use the information developed at the end of the passage to provide evidence against the theory about rounders.

   A: There is mention of the uncertainty surrounding baseball but the author does not seem to think it a futile effort to find the truth.

   B: There is more discussion of dates at the end of the passage than the manner of baseball's invention.

   C: There was no claim that baseball descended from cricket.

34. B is correct. The main idea of the first paragraph is that there is much uncertainty surrounding baseball's origin, not that there hasn't been much effort to ascertain the truth.

   A: The author does not present his or her ideas until later in the passage.

   C: This is not the argument of the first paragraph.

   D: There is no reason to think that this is the author's intention with the last sentence of the first paragraph. He or she mentions the space taken only in the second paragraph.

Passage 7 (Questions 35 – 39)

It should be observed that **each kind of rhetoric** has its own **appropriate style**. The style of written prose is not that of spoken oratory, nor are those of political and forensic speaking the same. **Both written and spoken have to be known.** To know the latter is to know how to **speak good Greek**. To know the former means that you are not obliged, as otherwise you are, to hold your tongue when you wish to communicate something to the **general public**.

Contrast: written vs oratory

Opinion: author thinks each form of rhetoric has a style unique to its own form

Cause and effect: to know written rhetoric is to be able to communicate to the general public; to know oral rhetoric is to speak good Greek

The **written** style is the **more finished**: the **spoken** better admits of **dramatic delivery** – like the kind of oratory that reflects character and the kind that reflects emotion. Hence **actors** look out for **plays** written in the latter style, and poets for actors competent to act in such plays. Yet poets whose plays are meant to be read are read and circulated: **Chaeremon**, for instance, who is as finished as a **professional speech-writer**; and **Licymnius** among the dithyrambic poets. Compared with those of others, the **speeches of professional writers sound thin** in actual contests. Those of the orators, on the other hand, are good to hear spoken, but **look amateurish** enough when they pass into the hands of a **reader**. This is just because they are so well suited for an actual tussle, and therefore contain many dramatic touches, which, being robbed of all dramatic rendering, fail to do their own proper work, and consequently look silly.

Key terms: Chaeremon, Licymnius

Contrast: writing for dramatic delivery vs for reading

Cause and effect: things written for oratory contain dramatic touches to be used when delivering a speech and may look silly when simply read; those who create rhetoric that is meant to be read end up sounding thin when read aloud

Thus **strings** of unconnected words, and constant **repetitions** of words and phrases, are very properly condemned in written speeches: but not in **spoken** speeches -- speakers use them freely, for they have a **dramatic effect**. In this repetition there must be variety of tone, paving the way, as it were, to dramatic effect; e.g. "This is the villain among you who deceived you, who cheated you, who meant to betray you completely." This is the sort of thing that **Philemon** the actor used to do in the Old Men's Madness of **Anaxandrides** whenever he spoke the words "**Rhadamanthus and Palamedes**," and also in the prologue to the Saints whenever he pronounced the pronoun "I." If one does not deliver such things cleverly, it becomes a case of "the man who swallowed a poker." So too with strings of **unconnected words**, e.g. "I came to him; I met him; I besought him."

Such passages **must be acted**, not delivered with the same quality and pitch of voice, as though they had only one idea in them. They have the further peculiarity of suggesting that a number of separate statements have been made in the time usually occupied by one. Just as the use of **conjunctions** makes **many** statements **into** a single **one**, so the **omission of conjunctions** acts in the reverse way and **makes a single one into many**. It thus makes everything more important: e.g. "I came to him; I talked to him; I entreated him" -- what a lot of facts! the hearer thinks -- "he paid no attention to anything I said." This is the effect which Homer seeks when he writes,

Nireus likewise from Syme (three well-fashioned ships did bring),

Nireus, the son of Aglaia (and Charopus, bright-faced king),

Nireus, the comeliest man (of all that to Ilium's strand).

If many things are said about a man, his name must be mentioned many times; and therefore people think that, if his name is mentioned many times, many things have been said about him. So that **Homer**, by means of this **illusion**, has made a great deal of though he has **mentioned him only in this one passage**, and has **preserved his memory**, though he nowhere says a word about him afterwards.

Contrast: use of unconnected and/or repeated phrases in written vs spoken speeches

Cause and effect: using tone allows unconnected phrases to have dramatic effect; using conjunctions makes many statements one; omitting them makes a single statement seem like many

Main Idea: The passage differentiates between written and spoken rhetoric, stressing that the use of tone and other dramatic touches allows for meaning in spoken orations that would seem silly when written.

35. C is correct. In the third paragraph, the author states that "just as the use of conjunctions makes many statements into a single one, so the omission of conjunctions acts in the reverse way and makes a single one into many. It thus makes everything more important".

    A: Using, not omitting, conjunctions makes many statements into one.

    B: Confusion as to the addressee is not discussed in the passage.

    D: Omitting conjunctions "acts in a reverse way" to combining statements by using conjunctions; it does not reverse ideas.

36. C is correct. The first paragraph states that "The style of written prose is not that of spoken oratory, nor are those of political and forensic speaking the same," thus suggesting that written and spoken are in a similar relationship of opposition as are political and forensic.

    A, B: These pairings are portrayed as similar rather than in opposition.

    D: Latin is never mentioned in the passage.

37. C is correct. The passage focuses on the differences between written and oral rhetoric, arguing that spoken rhetoric allows for dramatic touches and delivery that do not come across in the written form.

    A: The discussion of conjunctions and pronouns discusses both oral and written examples.

    B: There is no comparison of prose to other art forms in the passage.

    D: The political and forensic are presented as contrasting types of communication, like spoken and written, not as what makes a certain kind of communication effective, eliminating choice D.

38. B is correct. The passage states that mastering written rhetoric "means that you are not obliged, as otherwise you are, to hold your tongue when you wish to communicate something to the general public." Thus a focus on speaking well to a larger community would be in agreement with the ideas of the passage.

    A, C: Tone and variety of genres are not discussed in the passage.

    D: The passage discusses how unconnected words can be a problem in written communication, but it is not a major focus of the power of written communication.

39. B is correct. Speeches written by professional writers, we learn in the second paragraph, can "sound thin in actual contests" as opposed to those of orators which "are so well suited for an actual tussle, and therefore contain many dramatic touches, which, being robbed of all dramatic rendering, fail to do their own proper work, and consequently look silly." Thus professional writers do not use the dramatic effects of professional orators, so a speech written by one that used theatrical techniques would oppose the claims in the passage.

    A: The passage states that professional writing is "more finished," or polished, as in choice A.

    C: Content is never discussed in the passage, and thus would not strengthen or weaken the author's argument.

    D: This agrees with the author's claims about written speeches.

Passage 8 (Questions 40 – 46)

Ought the State to support the arts? There is certainly **much to be said on both sides** of this question. It may be said, in favours of the system of voting supplies for this purpose, that the **arts enlarge**, elevate, and harmonize the **soul of a nation**; that they divert it from too great an absorption in material occupations; encourage in it a love for the beautiful; and thus act favorably on its manners, customs, morals, and even on its industry. It may be asked, what would become of music in France without her **Italian theatre** and her **Conservatoire**; of the dramatic art, without her **Théâtre-Français**; of painting and sculpture, without our collections, galleries, and museums? It might even be asked, whether, without centralization, and consequently the support of the fine arts, that **exquisite taste** would be developed which is the **noble appendage of French labor**, and which introduces its productions to the whole world? In the face of such results, would it not be the height of imprudence to renounce this moderate contribution from all her citizens, which, in fact, in the eyes of Europe, realizes their superiority and their glory?

Key terms: arts, Italian theatre, Conservatoire, Theatre-Francais

Opinion: the opinions of those who believe the state ought to support the arts are presented in this paragraph

Cause and effect: it is asked what would become of the arts in Europe without state funding; some suspect that they would flounder

To these and many other reasons, whose force I do not dispute, arguments no less forcible may be **opposed**. It might first of all be said, that there is a question of **distributive justice** in it. Does the right of the **legislator** extend to **abridging the wages of the artisan, for the sake of, adding to the profits of the artist**? M. **Lamartine** said, "If you cease to support the theatre, where will you stop? Will you not necessarily be led to withdraw your support from your colleges, your museums, your institutes, and your libraries?" It might be answered, if you desire to support everything which is good and useful, where will you stop? Will you not necessarily be led to form a civil list for agriculture, industry, commerce, benevolence, education? Then, is it certain that Government aid favours the progress of art? This question is far from being settled, and we see very well that the **theatres which prosper** are those which **depend upon** their **own resources**.

Key terms: distributive justice, legislator, own resources

Opinion: the author believes that the arts will flourish on their own without government aid; the author believes that the government must choose carefully what to support

Contrast: this paragraph presents views in contrast to those presented in the first paragraph

Cause and effect: if you desire to support everything good, you will be led to try supporting more than is prudent; the theaters which prosper are those which depend upon their own resources

I am, I confess, one of those who think that choice and **impulse ought to come from below and not from above**, from the **citizen** and not from the **legislator**; and the opposite doctrine appears to me to tend to the **destruction of liberty** and of human dignity.

Opinion: author states his opinion that the state should not support the arts so that the artistic impulse comes from citizens rather than the government

But, by a deduction as false as it is unjust, do you know what **economists** are accused of? It is, that **when we disapprove of government support, we are supposed to disapprove of the thing itself** whose support is discussed; and to be the enemies of every kind of activity, because we desire to see those activities, on the one hand **free**, and on the other **seeking their own reward** in themselves. Thus, if we think that the State should not interfere by taxation in religious affairs, we are atheists. If we think the State ought not to interfere by taxation in education, we are hostile to knowledge. If we say that the State ought not by taxation to give a fictitious value to land, or to any particular branch of industry, we are enemies to property and labor. If we think that the State ought not to support artists, we are barbarians, who look upon the arts as useless.

Contrast: economists are accused of disapproving of things which they think ought not to have government support

Cause and effect: if the accusation discussed is true, then economists are accused of being atheists or barbarian

Against such conclusions as these I **protest with all my strength**. Far from entertaining the absurd idea of doing away with religion, education, property, labor, and the arts, when we say that the State ought to **protect** the **free development** of all these kinds of human activity, without helping some of them at the expense of others--we think, on the contrary, that all these living powers of society would **develop themselves more harmoniously** under the influence of **liberty**; and that, under such an influence no one of them would, as is now the case, be a source of trouble, of abuses, of tyranny, and disorder.

Key terms: protect, develop themselves

Opinion: the author's main opinion is expressed; he or she believes that the arts will develop themselves and will do so better without government involvement

Cause and effect: liberty will promote the development of the arts

Main Idea: The author believes that the state should not support the arts because the arts will flourish under the influence of the people in the society alone, and in making this argument the author presents both sides.

40. C is correct. In the second paragraph, Lamartine asks us "Where will you stop?" essentially saying if you want government to stop supporting the arts, you'd also have to ask it to remove support from many other good things since there's no clear line between the arts and other good things we would absolutely want the government to support.

41. A is correct. The author believes that human society will promote the arts better than government intervention.

    B: This is the opposite of what the author thinks.

    C, D: The author does not believe that government involvement will necessarily result in failure (nor its converse) but rather that things flourish more with "liberty" – that is, freedom from government meddling.

42. D is correct. Choice I is mentioned in the second paragraph. Choice III is the main argument presented in the first paragraph. II: Even if this is true, it is not an argument for government funding of the arts.

43. C is correct. The author believes that government has a place in society but that it should not be involved to too great a degree in the affairs of the people.

    A, D: The author is not altogether against government thinking it must be evil or wasteful.

    B: The author is not completely for government as a force for good.

44. C is correct. The author believes that institutions will flourish on their own without government aid. Specifically, the passage talks about art. Since museums are mainly artistic in nature, the author would agree with restrictions on government funding of museums.

    A: The author would disagree with this.

    B: The author probably would not agree with government support for religion.

    D: The author believes that the less imposition by government on the affairs of the arts, the better.

45. A is correct. The first paragraph expresses the opinions of those who are for government funding of the arts.

    B: The opposite is true.

    C: The benefits that the arts provide are mentioned, but only in service of the overall argument that the government should fund them. Plus, the focus is on France, not all of Europe.

    D: This never occurs in the passage

46. D is correct. The author uses the example in question in order to emphasize the absurdity of the accusation leveled against economists. Just because an economist will disagree with taxation in religious affairs, as most would, does not mean he or she is an atheist.

    A: The purpose is not to draw attention to the discrimination itself, but to its falsehood.

    B: This is not the point of the statement – although we may guess that the author would support separation of church and state, the main idea of this passage speaks only to the arts.

    C: The author would not argue that economists are illogical or barbaric.

Passage 9 (Questions 47 – 53)

The **scientific** enterprise is built, in the ideal sense, upon the notion of **free, full sharing** of information made in the course of scientific discovery. While such a system of information-sharing can **allow more rapid progress** as various scientists build upon each others' work, it provides no particular inherent safeguards against **inaccuracy** in reported findings nor in full reporting of findings that may be quite important, if the researcher making such findings **doesn't recognize their importance**. Imagine, for a moment, that Alexander **Fleming** took no particular note of the fact that bacteria did not seem to grow in the area of the *Penicillium* fungi . . .

Key terms: Fleming, *Penicillium*

Cause and effect: science relies on sharing info for rapid progress

Contrast: info sharing doesn't protect against inaccuracies or failure to recognize important discoveries

The **full sharing** of information would entail **explanation**, in painstaking detail, of the **methods** used to uncover certain results. But such a lengthy, exhaustive description would quickly generate a **sheer volume of information that would be impossible to manage**. One may argue that lab techniques could be referenced in **shorthand** (e.g. "a standard H&E stain revealed that . . .") but even there two significant **problems** arise.

Cause and effect: full info sharing would generate unmanageable amounts of information

Opinion: author thinks there are problems with using shorthand

First is the **incorrect assumption** that the exact physical **materials** used are largely **fungible**. For example, when conducting a titration, chemists would assume that the **acid purchased from one scientific supply company is functionally identical to that same acid when purchased from a different company**. While this may have been a workable assumption in the early- or mid-twentieth century, the increasing complexity and hyper-sensitivity of modern experiment, along with findings from **chaos theory** demonstrating the vast impact of tiny fluctuations in starting conditions, the basic **inter-exchangeability** of different experimental apparatuses and reagents is **no longer valid**.

Opinion: a scientist would assume a certain chemical is the same regardless of who sold it; author thinks this is an invalid assumption.

Even more **problematic** is the issue of **variations** in the individual **skill** of the researchers involved. A study that requires surgical ablation of a portion of the test animal's brain will generate vastly different outcomes if the ablation procedure is carried out by a well-meaning and skilled researcher who simply lacks the masterful level of skill required. As it is practically impossible to address the first issue, and literally

impossible to address the second issue when **communicating** scientific results, the **foundation of the scientific enterprise begins to appear much shakier** than initially supposed.

Opinion: author thinks variation in researcher skill is a big problem

Cause and effect: it is impossible to communicate researcher skill, so foundation of science based on communication is shaky

These problems only compound when we look beyond the full sharing of information itself. If the goal of science is to produce theories which make **replicable predictions** about how the world "really is" we see how damning the **problems of full-information sharing** become. After all, science is supposed to be the general, not the specific. It is the enterprise of "we" as opposed the artist's enterprise of "I". Thus it becomes no science at all to assert, "when this gifted surgeon carries out this procedure on a lab animal's brain, this is the result." If there is no other surgeon in the world who can replicate this feat, then **the whole notion of replicability shows itself invalid** *ab initio*.

Cause and effect: problems with communication get worse when that communication is extended to predictions

Opinion: author thinks predictions based on work by unusually skilled researchers makes repeatability invalid

The **solution** that suggests itself (to the extent that there even is one) is either a sharp **delimiting of science** to a far smaller ambit, or a fundamental **shift away from the basic logical positivism** that provides the **philosophical** undergirding that supports all of science back to the Enlightenment. The former is the more palatable, perhaps, but it is actually the **second that is more feasible**. Territory hard-acquired is never willingly surrendered and asking the scientific community to give up the realms of the very small, very large, and very complicated is a fool's errand. Instead, we must seek the **shift in perspective** that is harder to achieve but that pains less.

Opinion: author thinks solution to these problems is limiting the areas of science ("giving up the very small, very large...") or changing the philosophy of science

Main Idea: Science has a serious problem with the communication of information that it is based on, and the repeatable predictions that come out of this communication; these problems can be solved by limiting science's areas or by changing its philosophy.

47. D is correct. Throughout the text, the author takes an abstract, philosophical view of science but in the final paragraph he reveals that his solution to the problem is based on a change in philosophy. Thus in paragraph 6 he most clearly reveals that he is likely a philosopher himself.

48. C is correct. In the third paragraph, the author explains what he means by "fungible" by giving a concrete example relating to an acid purchased from one company or another.

49. D is correct. At the end of the passage, we get the author's solutions to the problems in the passage: a change in philosophy. Thus, given a chance to develop his own curriculum, he would likely emphasize this change in philosophy early on.

50. B is correct. In the second paragraph, the author tells us that a truly full amount of information sharing would generate a huge amount of information and it would be impossible to manage. If modern information technology and the internet would, instead, make it reasonable to have full information available to those who want or need it, while still maintaining most journal articles at a manageable length, then the claim of unmanageability would then be false.

51. C is correct. In the final paragraph, the author uses a very academic phrase but then later clarifies it by bringing up the idea of "giving up" the realms of the very small, very large, or very complicated. So reducing the "ambit" of something seems to refer to reducing the areas that it studies or works on.

52. D is correct. The author's main argument is that problems of information-sharing and prediction making mean that science has serious flaws and that the only solutions are to limit science or change its philosophy. If the author had written elsewhere about the success of science and logical positivism, that would contradict his main thesis.

53. A is correct. The author is certainly engaged with the material and has some clear notions about how science should be fixed, while addressing the topics in a very philosophical, abstract way.

SECTION 5

53 Questions, 90 Minutes

Use an answer grid from the back of the book to record your answers

Passage 1 (Questions 1 – 6)

It would be easy to peg Eudora Welty as a "southern writer." Born in Jackson, Mississippi in 1909, she wrote prolifically about life in both actual and fictional southern towns. While nearly all her works are set in the American South, the themes that she addresses are broad and universal, and often explore her characters' sense of place. One of Welty's finest novels, *Optimist's Daughter,* is such a work. In a distinctly southern voice, Welty tackles issues of class, morality, memory, and the meaning of "home."

The novel centers on Laurel Hand, a Mississippian living in Chicago, who is summoned to a New Orleans hospital where her father, well-loved small-town Mississippi Judge Clint McKelva, is about to undergo a serious eye operation. In the hospital, Laurel, a reserved, introspective middle-aged widow, meets the Judge's new wife: Fay, a brash, petulant, and uncultured Texan, younger than Laurel, eager to hold on to the safety and security that her unlikely marriage to the aging judge provides. Something goes awry with the Judge's surgery, and after weeks of convalescence he dies, to Laurel's deep sorrow and Fay's profound annoyance.

Welty is too skillful a writer to partition her novel into broad, cartoonish dualities, and it is with grace and subtlety that she draws distinctions between Laurel's soft-focus past and Fay's hard-eyed present; between genteel Mississippians and roughshod Texans; between unabashed materialism and well-bred restraint. Still, *Optimist's Daughter* is a novel of contrasts, and we are riveted as we watch Laurel wrestle with them as she seeks to find greater understanding of her family's life and acceptance of her father's choice of Fay.

Welty is particularly skilled at capturing the particulars of regional speech. Fay's redneck family, the Chisoms – Bubba, Wendell, and Mama – show up unannounced at Judge McKelva's funeral, and their rough and raucous speech contrasts with that of Laurel's childhood Mississippi friends – soft-spoken but gossipy spinsters with names like Miss Adele and Miss Tennyson Bullock. Yet despite Welty's gentle parodying, none of the characters fall into caricature. Never does Welty hit a false note: each character feels true, not just as a representation, but as a real being. In the hands of a lesser writer, Laurel would be too much the gentlewoman, representing the gracious past, and Fay the outsider, the shallow materialist who brings unwanted change to the small sleepy town. Instead, our utter sympathy with Laurel is mitigated by her slight priggishness, and by our knowledge that she abandoned the comfortable confines of Mount Salus, Mississippi, for life in a Chicago apartment. Similarly, our disgust with Fay is softened by her childishness and vulnerability, as well as her enduring but perhaps misguided effort to build herself a life better than the squalor she left in East Texas.

Optimist's Daughter looks squarely at a particular (yet fictitious) place, and lovingly yet humorously populates it for readers, using fine and well-picked detail. As Laurel prepares to say a permanent farewell to her childhood home, Fay coolly assesses her future there, finding fault with items that swell with significance to Laurel. Different ideas about place clash: Laurel's urge to hold on to her past bumps up against Fay's unambiguous desire to determine her future. In a final and poignant scene, Laurel and Fay clash over an old breadboard, dear to Laurel but meaningless to Fay, but for the fact that it is now hers. Laurel's relinquishing the breadboard to Fay – after coming close to striking her with it – dovetails with her recognition that she can release her grip on the past, and leave Fay to keep, or abandon, the house and all within it. Though both have called Mount Salus, Mississippi, home, for each it was a distinctly different place, one changed for each by the other.

1. According to the passage, why is it inaccurate to refer to Welty as a southern writer?

   A. Not all of her novels are set in the American South.

   B. Welty does not particularly identify as a Southerner.

   C. Welty's works address universal themes that are relevant to many.

   D. The themes of *Optimist's Daughter* are dependent on the characters' identity as Southerners.

2. What does the author achieve by including the names of Fay's family and Laurel's friends?

   A. It helps to illustrate the distinctions of class and culture that divide the two women.

   B. It prevents the reader from making generalizations regarding the cultures that define Laurel and Fay.

   C. It allows the author to criticize Laurel's social snobbishness.

   D. It illustrates the poverty and ignorance of Fay's family.

3. What does the author mean when she says that Welty is "too skillful to partition her novel into broad, cartoonish dualities"?

   A. Welty is successful in addressing solemn issues rather than more superficial topics.

   B. Welty creates contrasts, but does so with care and subtlety.

   C. Welty avoids comparisons between past and future.

   D. Welty uses regional speech to illustrate cultural differences.

4. Of the following, which captures the author's opinion of *Optimist's Daughter*?

   A. *Optimist's Daughter* is extremely effective at portraying the "soul" of the South.

   B. Its one flaw is Welty's unwillingness to root the novel in a truly realistic place.

   C. Its excellence lies in its use of detail to address universal issues.

   D. Despite Welty's protests, she should be categorized as a southern writer.

5. Of the following, which is NOT described as a fundamental difference between Laurel and Fay?

   A. Laurel has lived her adult life alone, but Fay has always relied on others.

   B. Laurel is from a higher socioeconomic class than Fay.

   C. Laurel tends to look towards the past, while Fay leans towards the future.

   D. Laurel is restrained in her speech, but Fay speaks her mind.

6. Based on information in the last paragraph of the passage, which of the following might describe an action Laurel might take if the novel were to continue?

   A. Laurel attempts to gain a better understanding of Fay's background.

   B. Laurel leaves Mount Salus, but with a greater sense of peace with her past.

   C. Laurel finally accepts Fay, and suggests that she and Fay share the Mount Salus home.

   D. Laurel sees Mount Salus more clearly, recognizing its flaws.

Passage 2 (Questions 7 – 11)

Maimonides is well known amongst Jewish scholars for his contributions to medicine and for his extensive writings on ethical and legal issues. During the Middle Ages, Maimonides wrote a comprehensive commentary on Jewish oral law and oral tradition. While modern scientific rigor has since proven Maimonides' medical writings obsolete, his philosophical work in the field of rabbinic law still holds authority in the Jewish religion.

In Judaism there exists a religious duty to give called "*tzedaka*". *Tzedaka* is loosely translated into English as "charity", although the classical Hebrew roots of the word more correctly correspond with the English word "justice". Maimonides writes that the proper execution of *tzedaka* is more important than any other Jewish duty. In order to illustrate his view of ideal *tzedaka*, Maimonides identified eight levels of *tzedaka* and arranged these levels in order of merit.

The highest level of *tzedaka* on this list describes an act that fosters self-sufficiency, such as the endowment of an interest-free loan or an offer of business partnership. If a poor person is given a loan to start a business, this person will then be able to create his or her own funds. This person will no longer require charity and will be able to partake in the act of *tzedaka* as a benefactor. Vitally, offering a poor person a business partnership requires that we do not look down on him and treat him with the same dignity as a rich man.

The seven following levels of *tzedaka* are all variations on a similar theme. The second-best level entails giving anonymously to an anonymous recipient. This is done to minimize any embarrassment or shame that the recipient may feel, and prevents the benefactor from boastfulness. This act necessitates the involvement of an organizing force such as a synagogue. The third level entails giving anonymously to a recipient whose identity is known (to the benefactor), and the fourth level giving publicly to an unknown recipient, as if announcing one's donation.

The final and least meritorious mode of *tzedaka* according to Maimonides is giving "with sadness". A reluctant donation is ranked lower than a willing but inadequate donation (level 7). Maimonides interprets *tzedaka* as a method for ensuring economic stability as well as respecting the poor. A system that jeopardizes the dignity of the poor is not justified by any potential financial benefits. Maimonides writes that a benefactor who publicly chastises the poor is not completing an act of *tzedaka*, even if, as he puts it, he gives a poor man "1000 gold coins".

In 2014, a charity campaign called "the ice bucket challenge" gained popularity via social media. In order to raise money for amyotrophic lateral sclerosis research, participants would publicly post videos of themselves being doused with a bucket of ice cold water and donating to the cause before nominating three other people to do the same.

The ice bucket challenge most closely resembles level four of Maimonides's eight levels, "giving publicly to an un-known recipient". This act of charity would not be ideal for Maimonides, who would prefer anonymous and private donations. While *tzedaka* originally intends to help those in need quietly but effectively, ubiquitous social media campaigns have turned philanthropy into a public spectacle. The Internet has effectively eliminated the need for face-to-face contact while making a donation. It would be far more virtuous to use this facet of the World Wide Web to preserve anonymity while performing *tzedaka*.

7. Which of the following would be the most exemplary according to Maimonides' view of *tzedaka*?

    A. Starting a public fundraiser for a specific local homeless person

    B. Donating a large sum of money privately to an unknown recipient

    C. Donating a goat to a needy family in Uganda so that it will produce cheese and generate income

    D. Lending a friend 1,000 dollars without interest

8. Which of the following are necessary conditions for *tzedaka* according to Maimonides?

    I. For the recipient to become self-sustaining

    II. For the dignity of the recipient to be respected

    III. A financial contribution from a benefactor

    A. I only

    B. III only

    C. II and III only

    D. I, II and III

9. Which of the following is an assumption that the author makes in the first paragraph of the passage?

    A. Jews hold Rabbinic law to a higher authority than scientific evidence.

    B. Old ethical and legal theories hold more validity than outdated scientific theories.

    C. Maimonides' philosophical work has always been more important that his contributions to medicine.

    D. Maimonides' scientific findings were never useful.

10. Which of the following assertions would most *weaken* the author's argument?

    A. Foundations that collect money for medical research are not comparable to poor individuals.

    B. Receiving donations publically is demeaning.

    C. The general public was eager to participate in the ice bucket challenge.

    D. The ALS ice bucket challenge raised 5 million dollars.

11. What is the most likely meaning of the phrase "with sadness" in the passage?

    A. While crying

    B. Unwillingly

    C. Mournfully

    D. While feeling pain

Passage 3 (Questions 12 – 16)

The mushroom is a highly prized article of food that can be as easily grown as many other vegetable products of the soil, with as much pleasure and profit. Below it is shown, in particular, that this peculiar plant is singularly well-adapted to the needs of all manner of people, and for whom the mushroom has become a standard crop for home use, the city market, or both. It is directly in their line of business; is a winter crop, requiring their care when outdoor operations are at a standstill, and they can most conveniently attend to growing mushrooms. Using manure on a mushroom crop before using it on other crops provides a wealth of advantages. After having borne a crop of mushrooms it is thoroughly rotted and in good condition for early spring crops; and for seed beds of tomatoes, lettuces, cabbages, cauliflowers, and other vegetables; in other words, it is the best kind of manure.

In most large gardens, one can find a mushroom house, where the growing of mushrooms is an easy matter; in more modest gardens where there is no such convenience, the gardener has to trust to his own ingenuity as to where and how she is to grow the mushrooms. But so long as she has an abundance of fresh manure, she can usually find a place to make the beds. In the toolshed, the potting-shed, the wood-shed, the stoke-hole, the fruit-room, the vegetable-cellar, the cow-house or horse-stable, the carriage-house, barn-cellar, woodshed, or house-cellar, she can surely find a corner; or, handier still, a convenient room under the green-house benches, where she can make some beds. But the best place is, perhaps, the cellar. An empty stall in a horse-stable is a capital place, and not only affords room for a full bed on the floor, but for rack-beds as well. Failing all of these she can start in August or September and make beds outside, as the London market gardeners do.

Those who keep horses should, at least, grow mushrooms for their own family use and perhaps for market as well. They are so easily raised, and they take up so little space that they commend themselves particularly to those who have only a village or suburban lot, and, in fact, only a barn. And they are not a crop for which we have to make a great preparation and need a large quantity of manure. No matter how small the bed may be, it will bear mushrooms; and if we desire we can add to the bed week after week, as our store of manure increases, thereby keeping up a continuous succession of mushrooms.

No one can grow mushrooms better or more economically than the farmer. She has already the cellar-room, the fresh manure and the loam at home, and all she needs is some spawn with which to plant the beds. Nothing is lost. The manure, after having been used in mushroom beds, is not exhausted of its fertility, but, instead, is well rotted and in a better condition to apply to the land than it was before being prepared for the mushroom crop. The farmer will not feel the little labor that it takes. There is no secret whatever connected with it, and skilled labor is unnecessary to make it successful. The commonest farm hand can do the work,

which consists of turning the manure once every day or two for about three weeks, then building it into a bed and spawning and molding it. Nearly all the labor for the next ten or twelve weeks consists in maintaining an even temperature and gathering and marketing the crop.

12. If the excerpt were the first chapter of a book, which of the following would most likely be the title of the book?

A. Edible Mushrooms and How to Distinguish Them

B. Mushrooms: How to Grow Them

C. Mushroom Culture: its Extension and Improvement

D. Mushrooms of America, Edible and Poisonous

13. Which of the following is the LEAST reasonable inference to be made from the passage?

A. Mushrooms enhance the fertility of manure.

B. Mushrooms grow best in the winter.

C. Mushrooms grow best at higher elevations.

D. Mushrooms grow best in dark places.

14. Which of the following can most reasonably be inferred from the passage?

A. The author's intention is to sell a product.

B. The author's intention is to offer instructions on how to grow mushrooms.

C. The author's intention is to develop an economic theory surrounding the selling of mushrooms.

D. The author's intention is to present his or her research into the biology of mushroom germination.

15. Suppose it were found that mushrooms can be grown just as easily in the summer as in the winter, how would this affect the author's argument that mushroom growing is an economically smart choice?

A. It would undermine one of the author's main points, that mushrooms are unique in that they can be grown in the winter.

B. It would not affect the author's arguments that mushrooms are unique in that they can be grown in the winter.

C. It would undermine the author's suggestion that mushrooms should be grown in the winter.

D. It would support the author's contention that mushrooms require minimal labor to grow.

16. Which of the following is a sentence the author would most likely NOT use in continuing his or her discourse on mushrooms?

A. An underground cellar is the best of all structures in which to grow mushrooms.

B. Fresh mushrooms, like good fruit and handsome flowers, are a product of the garden that is always acceptable.

C. The raising of mushrooms is within the reach of nearly every one.

D. The industry is one to which men are better suited than women and children.

Passage 4 (Questions 17 – 23)

The study of ethics is perhaps most commonly conceived as being concerned with the questions "What sort of actions ought men perform?" and "What sort of actions ought men avoid?" It is conceived as dealing with human conduct and as deciding what is virtuous and what is vicious among the kinds of conduct among which, in practice, people are called upon to choose. Owing to this view of the province of ethics, it is sometimes regarded as the practical study to which all others may be opposed as theoretical. The good and the true are sometimes spoken of as independent kingdoms: the former belonging to ethics, while the latter belongs to the sciences.

This view, however, is doubly defective. In the first place, it overlooks the fact that the object of ethics, by its own account, is to discover true propositions about virtuous and vicious conduct, and that these are just as much a part of truth as true propositions about oxygen or the multiplication table. The aim is not practice, but propositions about practice; and propositions about practice are not themselves practical, any more than propositions about gases are gaseous. One might as well maintain that botany is vegetable or zoology animal. Thus the study of ethics is not something outside science and co-ordinate with it: it is merely one among sciences.

The first step in ethics, therefore, is to be quite clear as to what we mean by good and bad. Only then can we return to conduct, and ask how right conduct is related to the production of goods and the avoidance of evils.

Good and Bad, in the sense in which the words are here intended (which is, I believe, their usual sense), are ideas which everybody, or almost everybody, possesses. These ideas are apparently among those which form the simplest constituents of our more complex ideas, and are therefore incapable of being analyzed or built up out of other simpler ideas. When people ask "What do you mean by good?" the answer must consist, not in a verbal definition such as could be given if one were asked "What do you mean by pentagon?" but in such a characterization as shall call up the appropriate idea to the mind of the questioner. This characterization may, and probably will, itself contain the idea of good, which would be a fault in a definition, but is harmless when our purpose is merely to stimulate the imagination to the production of the idea which is intended. It is in this way that children are taught the names of colors; they are shown (say) a red book, and told that that is red; and for fear they should think red means book, they are shown also a red flower, a red ball, and so on, and told that these are all red. Thus the idea of redness is conveyed to their minds, although it is quite impossible to analyze redness or to find constituents which compose it.

In the case of good, the process is more difficult, both because goodness is not perceived by the senses, like redness, and because there is less agreement as to the things that are good than as to the things that are red. This is perhaps one reason that has led people to think that the notion of good could be analyzed into some other notion, such as pleasure or object of desire. A second reason, probably more potent, is the common confusion that makes people think they cannot understand an idea unless they can define it—forgetting that ideas are defined by other ideas, which must be already understood if the definition is to convey any meaning. When people begin to philosophize, they seem to make a point of forgetting everything familiar and ordinary; otherwise their acquaintance with redness or any other color might show them how an idea can be intelligible where definition, in the sense of analysis, is impossible.

17. Which of the following would be the most *surprising* statement by the author given the passage information?

    A. We ought to act in the way we believe most likely to create as much good as possible.

    B. When you are studying any matter, ask yourself only what are the facts.

    C. Ethical statements are relative and cannot be said to be true or false.

    D. Ethics is a department of philosophy and psychology.

18. The author uses the first paragraph in order to do which of the following?

    A. Present the argument that the author will expound upon throughout the passage

    B. Present an argument that the author will discredit

    C. Present the main theme of the passage by use of an analogy

    D. Present the author's purpose in writing the passage

19. What is the purpose of the statement that "botany is vegetable"? To illustrate the absurdity of saying that:

    A. science is practical

    B. propositions about practice are theoretical

    C. ethics is purely practical

    D. a science is purely theoretical

20. Which of the following is NOT a problem in defining "good" discussed in the passage?

    A. It is feared that some might think good means the act of doing good.

    B. It is impossible to understand good unless by experience.

    C. Good is not easily perceived.

    D. In trying to define good, one must use the notion of good in the definition.

21. Which of the following would the author argue is LEAST similar to the word good in terms of one's ability to define it?

    A. Salty

    B. Yellow

    C. Warmth

    D. Sun

22. With which of the following statements would the author most likely agree?

    A. Most ideas or notions are not made up of indefinable constituent ideas.

    B. Characterizations of good and bad rarely presuppose the notions of good and bad.

    C. Characterizations of good and bad are a means of calling up the right ideas.

    D. We may say that a thing is good when on its own account it ought to exist.

23. Which of the following would the author most likely treat later on in continuation of this work?

    A. An analysis of "right" and "wrong"

    B. The history of ethics

    C. The philosophy of religion

    D. A discussion of war and its characterization as bad

Passage 5 (Questions 24 – 28)

A classic, according to the usual definition, is an old author canonized by admiration, and an authority in his particular style. The word classic was first used in this sense by the Romans. With them not all the citizens of the different classes were properly called *classici*, but only those of the chief class, those who possessed an income of a certain fixed sum. Those who possessed a smaller income were described by the term *infra classem*, below the preeminent class. The word *classicus* was used in a figurative sense by Aulus Gellius, and applied to writers: a writer of worth and distinction, *classicus assidu-usque* scriptor, a writer who is of account, has real property, and is not lost in the proletariat crowd. Such an expression implies an age sufficiently advanced to have already made some sort of valuation and classification of literature.

At first the only true classics for the moderns were the ancients. The Greeks, by peculiar good fortune and natural enlightenment of mind, had no classics but themselves. They were at first the only classical authors for the Romans, who strove and contrived to imitate them. After the great periods of Roman literature, after Cicero and Virgil, the Romans in their turn had their classics, who became almost exclusively the classical authors of the centuries which followed. The middle ages, which were less ignorant of Latin antiquity than is believed, but which lacked proportion and taste, confused the ranks and orders. Ovid was placed above Homer, and Boetius seemed a classic equal to Plato. The revival of learning in the fifteenth and sixteenth centuries helped to bring this long chaos to order, and then only was admiration rightly proportioned. Thenceforth the true classical authors of Greek and Latin antiquity stood out in a luminous background, and were harmoniously grouped on their two heights.

Meanwhile modern literatures were born, and some of the more precocious, like the Italian, already possessed the style of antiquity. Dante appeared, and, from the very first, posterity greeted him as a classic. Italian poetry has since shrunk into far narrower bounds; but, whenever it desired to do so, it always found again and preserved the impulse and echo of its lofty origin. It is no indifferent matter for a poetry to derive its point of departure and classical source in high places; for example, to spring from Dante rather than to issue laboriously from Malherbe.

If it is desired, names may be applied to this definition which I wish to make purposely majestic and fluctuating, or in a word, all- embracing. I should first put there Corneille of the Polyeucte, Cinna, and Horaces. I should put Moliere there, the fullest and most complete poetic genius we have ever had in France. Goethe, the king of critics, said:—

"Moliere is so great that he astonishes us afresh every time we read him. He is a man apart; his plays border on the tragic, and no one has the courage to try and imitate him. His Avare, where vice destroys all affection between father and son, is one of the most sublime works, and dramatic in the highest degree. In a drama every action ought to be im-portant in itself, and to lead to an action greater still. In this respect Tartuffe is a model. What a piece of exposition the first scene is! From the beginning everything has an important meaning, and causes something much more important to be foreseen. The exposition in a certain play of Lessing that might be mentioned is very fine, but the world only sees that of Tartuffe once. It is the finest of the kind we possess. Every year I read a play of Moliere, just as from time to time I contemplate some engraving after the great Italian masters."

24. Which of the following is an assertion that is supported by evidence in the passage?

    A. The Romans are the fathers of classic literary works.

    B. The Greeks were the first artistically enlightened civilization in Europe.

    C. The Italians are the fathers of classical poetry.

    D. Moliere was the greatest poetic genius in history.

25. What is the author's overall attitude toward the classification of works of art as classics?

    A. He attempts to develop a concrete set of rules that determine whether a work is a classic.

    B. He attempts to develop a set of rules but incorporates some amount of subjective personal taste.

    C. He determines in an entirely subjective manner whether a work is a classic.

    D. He allows each person their own interpretation of which works qualify as a classic.

26. Given the information in the passage, one would most reasonably assume that Tartuffe is considered a classic because:

    A. of its classification as a drama.

    B. it was written by Moliere.

    C. each element in the play has its own significance.

    D. the climax of the play is reached near the beginning.

27. Given the passage discussion, which of the following works of art would be most reasonably considered to be a classic?

    A. An epic poem by Ovid

    B. A poem by Malherbe

    C. An Italian poem written during the renaissance

    D. A marble statue produced by the Italian master Michelangelo

28. What purpose does the phrase "natural enlightenment of mind" (paragraph 2) have in the context of the whole passage?

    I. To explain why the Greeks were able to produce classic works of art

    II. To explain why the Greeks had no classic works of art but their own

    III. To explain why the Romans only produced classics after the Greeks

    A. I only

    B. II only

    C. III only

    D. I and II only

Passage 6 (Questions 29 – 35)

But in some branches of economic inquiry and for some purposes, it is more urgent to ascertain new facts, than to trouble ourselves with the mutual relations and explanations of those which we already have. While in other branches there is still so much uncertainty as to whether those causes of any event which lie on the surface and suggest themselves at first are both true causes of it and the only causes of it, that it is even more urgently needed to scrutinize our reasoning about facts which we already know, than to seek for more facts.

For this and other reasons, there always has been and there probably always will be a need for the existence side by side of workers with different aptitudes and different aims, some of whom give their chief attention to the ascertainment of facts, while others give their chief attention to scientific analysis; that is taking to pieces complex facts, and studying the relations of the several parts to one another and to cognate facts. It is to be hoped that these two schools will always exist, each doing its own work thoroughly, and each making use of the work of the other. Thus best may we obtain sound generalizations as to the past and trustworthy guidance from it for the future.

Those physical sciences, which have progressed most beyond the points to which they were brought by the brilliant genius of the Greeks, are not all of them strictly speaking "exact sciences." But they all aim at exactness. That is they all aim at precipitating the result of a multitude of observations into provisional statements, which are sufficiently definite to be brought under test by other observations of nature. These statements, when first put forth, seldom claim a high authority. But after they have been tested by many independent observations, and especially after they have been applied successfully in the prediction of coming events, or of the results of new experiments, they graduate as laws. A science progresses by increasing the number and exactness of its laws; by submitting them to tests of ever increasing severity; and by enlarging their scope till a single broad law contains and supersedes a number of narrower laws, which have been shown to be special instances of it.

Although the subject-matter of some progressive physical sciences is not, at present at least, capable of perfectly exact measurement; their progress depends on the multitudinous co-operation of armies of workers. They measure their facts and define their statements as closely as they can: so that each investigator may start as nearly as possible where those before him left off. Economics aspires to a place in this group of sciences, because its measurements are seldom exact, and are never final; yet it is ever working to make them more exact, and thus to enlarge the range of matters on which the individual student may speak with the authority of his science. Let us then consider more closely the nature of economic laws, and their limitations. Every cause has a tendency to produce some definite result if nothing occurs to hinder it. Thus gravitation tends to make things fall to the ground, but when a balloon is full of gas lighter than

air, the pressure of the air will make it rise in spite of the tendency of gravitation to make it fall. The law of gravitation states how any two things attract one another; how they tend to move towards one another, and will move towards one another if nothing interferes to prevent them. The law of gravitation is therefore a statement of tendencies.

29. The author discusses the law of gravitation in order to:

    A. contrast the predictive powers of physics with those of economics.

    B. better understand exact sciences.

    C. demonstrate statements of tendencies.

    D. explain the causes that may hinder definite results in data collection.

30. Based on the passage, how can scientific analysis best be defined?

    A. Boiling down multiple observations into testable provisional statements

    B. Dissecting issues in order to be able to ascertain which facts are true and which are erroneous

    C. Emphasizing mutual relations rather than obtaining new facts

    D. Dividing a complicated issue into its component parts and defining those parts' relations to each other

31. Based on the passage, it can be inferred that the author values cooperation because:

    A. in war situations with countless armies, only cooperative economies flourish.

    B. unlike the more exact sciences, economics requires accumulation of data.

    C. competition acts as a false interference that hinders the process.

    D. it leads to more complete knowledge achieved more quickly.

32. The speaker assumes which of the following about uncertainty in causes?

    A. Physical sciences are the best way to erase the uncertainty in causes that arises from a reliance on logic.

    B. The reasoning behind proximal causes can shadow the true causes.

    C. It is best to ascertain the reasoning that leads people to think the way they do about data rather than seek the root of that data.

    D. Uncertainty in causes can be ascribed to various tendencies.

33. The author focuses on science in this passage in order to:

    A. assert that economics, too, requires regularity and the accumulation and analysis of data.

    B. contrast it to economics, which focuses more on predicting the future than explaining the past.

    C. explain how laws of tendencies rule economic theory.

    D. enlarge the explanatory scope of economics.

34. Suppose that it was discovered that economists currently focus on scientific analysis, with very few involved in ascertaining facts. Based on the passage, the author would most likely believe:

    A. while they would be able to create accurate predictions as to the future, it would not be based on sound knowledge of the past.

    B. it is unlikely that economists are doing their best work due to a lack of complete information.

    C. that such a move was a positive one because the subject matter of economics should aim for precision, as defined by scientific analysis.

    D. that such a divide was unlikely, since the work of each school depended on the other.

35. Based on the passage, all of the following are signs of a branch of science progressing EXCEPT:

    A. passing stringent observations and experiments and predicting future events.

    B. creating an overarching law that explains multiple previous laws.

    C. increasing the accuracy of laws.

    D. increasing the accuracy of predictions.

Passage 7 (Questions 36 – 42)

What exactly does Wagner mean historically? He represents *the rise of the actor in music*, an event of great moment that leads me not only to think, but also, to fear. Never before have the uprightness and genuineness of musicians been put to such a dangerous test. It is obvious now that great success is no longer the achievement of the genuine, for in order to get it, you must be an actor! The mob success of Victor Hugo and, of course, Richard Wagner, prove that in declining civilizations, wherever and whenever the mob is given the choice, genuineness becomes superfluous and unfavorable. The actor alone still kindles great enthusiasm, and therefore, it is his golden age that is now dawning.

With drums and fifes, Wagner marches at the vanguard of all artists in declamation, display, and virtuosity. He began by winning over the conductors, the scene-shifters, the stage-singers, and of course, the orchestra; he delivered them from monotony. Wagner's movement has spread even to the land of knowledge: entire sciences pertaining to music are beginning to slowly rise out of centuries of scholasticism. The people of this movement have a perfect right to honor Wagner: in him, they recognize their highest type, and because his work managed to inflame them with his own ardor, they feel themselves made powerful. It is in this sphere that Wagner's influence has actually been beneficent, for never before has there been so much thinking, willing, and pure industry in it. Wagner endowed these artists with a new conscience: what they now expect and actually attain for themselves, they never even began to seek out before Wagner's time, for they were too modest then.

Another spirit prevails on the stage, for Wagner rules there that the most difficult things are to be expected, blame is always severe, praise is very scarce, and that the good and the excellent have become the rule. Taste is no longer necessary, and truly, neither is a good voice, for Wagner's work is sung only with ruined voices, making for a more dramatic effect. Even talent is now out of the question: the decadent, Wagnerian ideal, expressiveness at all costs, is hardly compatible with talent. All this is required for the achievement of this ideal is virtue, or, that is to say, training, automatism, and self-denial. Wagner's stage does not require taste, voices, nor gifts, but it does require one thing: Germans!

For Wagner's purposes, this is the definition of a German: an obedient man with long legs. After all, there is deep significance in the fact that the rise of Wagner coincided with the rise of the "Empire," for both phenomena are proof of one and the same thing: obedience and long legs. Never before have people been more obedient and never before have they been so effectively and efficiently ordered about. More particularly, the conductors of Wagnerian orchestra are worthy of an age that will be one day referred to by posterity, with timid awe, as the classical age of war.

Wagner fully understood how to command, and therefore, was in this respect a great teacher. He commanded others as a man who, with a lifelong practice of self-discipline, exercised an unyielding will over himself. In fact, Wagner was perhaps the greatest example of self-violence in the whole history of art.

36. All of the following statements about Wagner are true EXCEPT:

    A. he inspired many people to industriousness.

    B. his work often calls for singers with ruined voices.

    C. his greatest ideal requires reflection, naturalism, and indulgence.

    D. because he knew how to control himself and others, he was a great teacher.

37. Which of the following statements about the passage are true?

    I. Wagner's rise in influence directly brought about the rise of the "Empire."

    II. In a declining civilization, genuineness necessarily becomes superfluous and unfavorable.

    III. Wagner's movement began when he won over musicians by giving them compelling drama to work with.

    A. II only

    B. III only

    C. I and II only

    D. I, II, and III

38. Based upon the passage, which of the following is most likely the author's intended meaning for the word "actor"?

    A. One who works upon the stage

    B. One who is not genuine

    C. One who makes things happen

    D. One who is adored by the people

39. According to the passage, which of the following is the most accurate reason why Wagner's stage requires Germans?

    A. Because it requires actors with great strength

    B. Because it is extremely nationalistic in tone

    C. Because it runs like an efficient, well-oiled machine

    D. Because it is, beyond else, about building community

40. Based upon the passage, which of the following statements most accurately captures the difference between Wagner's effect on the land of knowledge and the spirit of the stage?

    A. Wagner's effect on academia ended up being more influential than his effect on the stage.

    B. Wagner empowered academics but forced severe restrictions on the stage.

    C. Wagner secretly preferred the world of academia to the world of the stage.

    D. Wagner did not care for academics and therefore did not challenge them as he did theatre artists.

41. Based upon the passage, which of the following statements is the author most likely to believe?

    A. Civilization is in a downward spiral.

    B. Wagner is the greatest musician of all time.

    C. Wagner was less interested in nationalism than he was in great voices.

    D. Wagner's extreme self-discipline was matched only by Hugo's.

42. Suppose a modern composer were seeking to fully emulate the life and work of Wagner, in order to create a grander, more traditional body of work than rest of his contemporaries. If he had to emulate one essential quality of Wagner's, based upon the passage, what would it be?

    A. Imbuing his work with the sensations of war

    B. Throwing taste out the window

    C. Nationalism beyond all else

    D. Expressiveness at all costs

Passage 8 (Questions 43 – 46)

Considering how difficult it is for men to hold a newly acquired state, some may justly wonder how Alexander the Great became the master of Asia in only a few years, and how his successors maintained their rule of empire. Because Alexander died before the empire's full settlement, it would have been reasonable for the people of the empire to rebel. Yet, Alexander's successors maintained it, and in truth, they met no harsher difficulties than those which arose from their own ambitions.

Of the principalities for which records are available, there are two different ways of governance: either by a prince and his servants, the latter of whom help manage the kingdom by the prince's favor and permission, or else by a prince and his barons, the latter of whom hold their offices not by princely assignation, but by the antiquity of their blood. These barons rule their own states with their own subjects who recognize and follow their rule with sincere affection. Meanwhile, in those states ruled by a prince and his servants, the prince himself is held with the highest consideration, for in all of the principality there is no one considered superior to him. If the subjects of this state do yield their obedience to another, it is to a minister or an official, and in so doing they show no sincere affection. In our time, the prime examples of these two governments are the Turk and the King of France.

The monarchy of the Turk is ruled solely by one lord, the Turk himself, and the rest are his servants. His kingdom is divided into sanjaks and to each of these he sends ministers and officials that he may shift and change as he pleases. On the other hand, the King of France is seated in the midst of the ancient body of lords, all of whom have their own loyal subjects. These lords have their own prerogatives for rule: the King alters them only at his own risk.

It is evident that it would be of great difficulty to seize the kingdom of the Turk, and yet it is also evident that it would be of great ease to hold the kingdom once conquered. This is because a potential usurper will clearly not be called into the kingdom by the Turk, nor will he be assisted in his revolt by the minsters and officials. As these ministers are all essentially slaves and bondmen, they can only be corrupted from their allegiance to the Turk with great difficulty. Even if they are corrupted, these ministers hold little esteem in the eyes of the people and thus cannot motivate them to raise arms against their beloved Turk. Therefore, whosoever attacks the Turk must note this and must know that his success will depend more on his own army's strength than on the revolt of others.

However, if the Turk is conquered, and if he is defeated in such a way that he cannot replace his armies, the only thing left the usurper has to fear is the family of the Turk. If the royal family is killed, there is nothing left to fear, as the ministers and officials have little credit with the people. As the conqueror did not rely upon these people for his usurpation, he need not fear them after it.

On the contrary, a usurper can easily enter the Kingdom of France by winning over some malcontented baron, desirous of change. Such men as this can open the way into the Kingdom and make victory easy, but here lies the problem: if you wish to hold the Kingdom, you will meet with innumerable difficulties, both from the barons who have assisted you and from those you have defeated. In this case, it is not sufficient to have exterminated the royal family, for the lords of the Kingdom remain to lead fresh movements against you. If you are unable to satisfy or exterminate them, the state is lost whenever time brings the opportunity.

43. Based upon the passage, the author most likely agrees with which of the following statements?

   A. Alexander's successors could hold the Asian empire because it was comparable to the Turk's kingdom.

   B. Alexander's successors could hold the Asian empire because it was comparable to the kingdom of France.

   C. Alexander's successors could hold the Asian empire thanks in large part to the sovereign lords of Asia.

   D. Alexander's successors could hold the Asian empire because the people were desirous of change.

44. The author's discussion of the two examples of principalities is most likely made in order to:

   A. provide an argument for the truism that governance and conquest are incredibly difficult.

   B. demonstrate the eternal complexity of human governance and society.

   C. demonstrate the duality of the governance of principalities in his own era.

   D. provide insight into how Alexander's successors were able to hold the Asian empire.

45. Based upon the passage, it can be inferred that the author believes the most efficient way for both scholars and rulers to determine proper policy and practices is to:

   A. act in accordance with the opinions of the people, expressed through popular vote.

   B. examine contemporary or historical precedents that are relevant to current questions.

   C. work closely with thought experiments based upon general historical precedence.

   D. conduct polls in which the ministers and officials of the state are asked their opinion.

46. Suppose the enterprising young ruler of State A wants to conquer State B, which is ruled by a prince and a collection of lords whose positions were determined by their birth. According to the passage, what two things are necessary for the young usurper from State A to conquer and hold State B?

   A. The usurper must incite revolts against the ruler of State B by undermining his royal claim, and then he must assassinate the ruler in such a way that the people of State B unanimously support the usurper.

   B. The usurper must choose a disgruntled lord to befriend and then incite widespread revolt against the ruler of State B.

   C. The usurper must befriend a disgruntled lord of State B and then exterminate all other lords, including the one he befriended.

   D. The usurper must incite revolts against the ruler of State B and then exterminate all the uncooperative lords of State B.

Passage 9 (Questions 47 – 53)

It has been well said that the "conquest of fear" is the best indication we have that civilization has really advanced mankind to a higher level. When we speak of the "conquest of fear" we do not mean that fear itself has entirely disappeared; that can never be. We mean only that much unreasonable fear has been dissipated. I believe that the sum-total of fear has greatly diminished with the progress of the world, but as the amount of fear cannot be weighed or measured, we have no criterion of values.

There is now widespread confidence in the orderly succession of natural laws. People no longer live in daily dread of the spirits of darkness, and are not afraid of the unknown; an eclipse of the sun or the coming of a comet does not strike terror into the hearts of the community.

Epidemics, also, follow natural laws. They come, rise, reach their height and virulence, and decline according to known biological rules. The trained epidemiologist can tell at once by looking at the curve of annual prevalence of typhoid fever of a city whether the people are drinking badly infected water or not. A milk outbreak has its own special characteristics that permit speedy recognition. Certain diseases recrudesce annually with the regularity of our crops. I know of one health officer of one of our large cities who each year takes a mean advantage of the seasonal prevalence of typhoid fever by instituting a newspaper sanitary campaign in September. The health department then claims the credit for the inevitable decline in October.

In fact, the natural history of disease has risen almost to the dignity of a science. In many instances, at least, we are able to control and foretell the phenomena of disease prevalence. For this, of course, we have to thank largely the patient researches into the causes of the communicable infections, and especially the scientific and self-sacrificing studies into their modes of transmission. Useful and trustworthy results have been obtained only by exact laboratory methods. The rapid accumulation of this real knowledge has robbed infection of the superstitious dread in which it was formerly held. We are no longer tied helpless in the face of a devastating plague, and in our ignorance blame it on the supernatural wrath of an irresponsible power. Now we fight back, for we have the knowledge that gives courage and conquers fear.

Fear is lessening, but we would not want it to disappear entirely, for while it is a miserable sensation, it has its uses in the same sense that pain may be a marked benefit to the animal economy, and in the same sense that fever is a conservative process. Reasonable fear saves many lives and prevents much sickness. It is one of the greatest forces for good in preventive medicine, and at times it is among the most useful instrument in the hands of the sanitarian.

The indifference to disease can be just as dangerous. I have noticed a nonchalance towards yellow fever in Vera Cruz, Santiago, and other tropical places where "familiarity breeds a species of contempt," and the fatalistic tendency of mankind accepts the inevitable, though a Lazear laid down his life as the result of a mosquito bite to save his fellow-men. It is lack of fear of yellow fever that permits it to smolder in an endemic focus, just as the lack of fear of typhoid fever permits it to smolder in Boston, Philadelphia, Washington, and other American cities. A sharp epidemic of typhoid fever is a good lifesaver. The fear it instills builds filter plants, spends money and awakens energy for other necessary and expensive sanitary improvements.

47. In asserting in the first paragraph that the fear in the world has held back world progress, the author:

  A. supports his view with specific data.

  B. summarizes his main view that fear is bad.

  C. bolsters his position with logic and reasoning.

  D. acknowledges the speculative nature of his opinion.

48. The author implies that without the advance of science, people would:

  A. be more likely to fear natural events like eclipses.

  B. lose their healthy fear of epidemics.

  C. have a roughly equal level of public health because fear would provide protection equal to the advances of science.

  D. be more indifferent to more of life's dangers including sickness.

49. According to the passage, all of the following has contributed to understanding the natural history of a disease EXCEPT:

  A. empirical observations.

  B. patient and physician sacrifice.

  C. fear of the disease.

  D. improved scientific techniques.

50. Based on the passage, it can be inferred that the author would:

  A. encourage a patient who has contracted an infectious disease not to fear its progression.

  B. encourage patients who haven't contracted a disease not to fear infected individuals.

  C. attempt to raise public alarm during the outbreak of a contagious disease.

  D. discourage public education to prevent public over confidence and indifference.

51. The author utilizes the example of typhoid fever in Vera Cruz, Santiago, in order to:

  A. provide evidence for the benefits of unreasonable fear.

  B. caution against an excess of fear.

  C. give an example of the benefits of modern epidemiology.

  D. caution against public indifference to a disease.

52. According to the passage, it can be inferred that the public's best defense against an epidemic is:

  A. adequate levels of reasonable fear.

  B. low levels of unreasonable fear.

  C. public health education and intervention.

  D. prior experience with similar diseases.

53. Which of the following, if true, would most weaken the author's main argument?

  A. A study indicates that countries with the lowest levels of fear regarding a disease have the lowest incidence of infection.

  B. A study indicates that the levels of societal education, not fear, is the most important predictor of response to an epidemic.

  C. A study indicates that public fear of an infectious disease has led to a higher incidence of chronic illness.

  D. A study indicates that the level of societal fear regarding an infectious disease has no impact on its spread.

This page intentionally left blank.

SECTION 5

Answer Key

1	C	12	B	23	A	34	B	45	B
2	A	13	C	24	B	35	D	46	C
3	B	14	B	25	B	36	C	47	D
4	C	15	B	26	C	37	B	48	A
5	A	16	D	27	D	38	B	49	C
6	B	17	C	28	D	39	C	50	A
7	C	18	B	29	C	40	B	51	D
8	C	19	C	30	D	41	A	52	C
9	B	20	A	31	D	42	D	53	D
10	A	21	D	32	C	43	A		
11	B	22	C	33	A	44	D		

Passage 1 (Questions 1 – 6)

It would be easy to peg **Eudora Welty** as a "**southern writer.**" Born in Jackson, Mississippi in 1909, she wrote prolifically about life in both actual and fictional southern towns. While nearly all her **works are set** in the American **South**, the themes that she addresses are broad and **universal**, and often explore her characters' **sense of place**. One of Welty's finest novels, *Optimist's Daughter,* is such a work. In a distinctly southern voice, Welty tackles issues of class, morality, memory, and the meaning of "home."

Key terms: Eudora Welty, Optimist's Daughter

Opinion: although Eudora Welty's works are set in the south, her themes are universal

The novel centers on **Laurel Hand**, a Mississippian living in Chicago, who is summoned to a New Orleans hospital where her father, well-loved small-town Mississippi **Judge Clint McKelva**, is about to undergo a serious eye operation. In the hospital, Laurel, a reserved, introspective middle-aged widow, meets the Judge's new wife: **Fay**, a brash, petulant, and uncultured Texan, younger than Laurel, eager to hold on to the safety and security that her unlikely marriage to the aging judge provides. Something **goes awry with the Judge's surgery**, and after weeks of convalescence he **dies**, to Laurel's deep **sorrow** and Fay's profound **annoyance**.

Key Terms: Laurel Hand, Judge Clint McKelva, Fay

Cause and effect: a mishap during surgery kills the judge

Contrast: Laurel experiences sorrow and Fay experiences annoyance when the judge dies

Welty is **too skillful** a writer to partition her novel into broad, **cartoonish dualities**, and it is with **grace and subtlety** that she draws **distinctions** between **Laurel's** soft-focus past and **Fay's** hard-eyed present; between genteel Mississippians and roughshod Texans; between unabashed materialism and well-bred restraint. Still, *Optimist's Daughter* is a **novel of contrasts**, and we are riveted as we watch Laurel wrestle with them as she seeks to find greater understanding of her family's life and acceptance of her father's choice of Fay.

Contrasts: Welty draws subtle distinctions between Laurel and Fay, past and present, and social classes

Opinion: author thinks that Welty is skillful in keeping the comparisons subtle

Welty is **particularly skilled** at capturing the particulars of **regional speech**. Fay's redneck family, the Chisoms – Bubba, Wendell, and Mama – show up unannounced at Judge McKelva's funeral, and their rough and raucous speech **contrasts** with that of Laurel's childhood Mississippi friends – soft-spoken but gossipy spinsters with names like Miss Adele and Miss Tennyson Bullock. Yet despite Welty's **gentle parodying**, **none** of the characters fall into **caricature**. Never does Welty hit a false note: each character feels true, not just as a representation, but as a real being. In the hands of a lesser writer, Laurel would be too much the gentlewoman, representing the gracious past, and Fay the outsider, the shallow materialist who brings unwanted change to the small sleepy town. Instead, our utter **sympathy** with **Laurel** is mitigated by her slight **priggishness**, and by our knowledge that she abandoned the comfortable confines of Mount Salus, Mississippi, for life in a Chicago apartment. Similarly, our **disgust** with **Fay** is **softened** by her childishness and **vulnerability**, as well as her enduring but perhaps misguided effort to build herself a life better than the squalor she left in East Texas.

Cause and effect: the author uses contrasting details to demonstrate the differences between Laurel's world and Fay's

Contrast: our sympathy for Laurel and disgust with Fay are contrasted by other aspects of their characters

Opinion: author thinks that the characters feel especially genuine and are not caricatures

Optimist's Daughter looks squarely at a particular (yet fictitious) place, and **lovingly** yet **humorously populates** it for readers, using fine and well-picked detail. As **Laurel** prepares to say a **permanent farewell** to her childhood home, **Fay** coolly assesses her future there, **finding fault** with items that swell with significance to Laurel. Different ideas about place **clash**: Laurel's urge to hold on to her past bumps up against Fay's unambiguous desire to determine her future. In a final and poignant scene, Laurel and Fay clash over an old breadboard, dear to Laurel but meaningless to Fay, but for the fact that it is now hers. **Laurel's** relinquishing the breadboard to Fay – after coming close to striking her with it – dovetails with her recognition that she can **release her grip on the past**, and leave Fay to keep, or abandon, the house and all within it. Though both have called Mount Salus, Mississippi, **home**, for each it was a distinctly different place, one changed for each by the other.

Cause and effect: Laurel and Fay clash over an old breadboard, and through this clash Laurel realizes that it is time to let go of her past.

Contrast: Laurel says goodbye to a place full of significance but Fay takes a coldly materialistic view

Main idea: Eudora Welty demonstrates her masterful writing in *Optimist's Daughter*, which uses careful detail to address universal themes of home, identity, and place; its voice is distinctly southern, but its scope is broad.

1. C is correct. The author says at the very beginning that although Eudora Welty is from Mississippi and sets her novels in the south, she explores issues and themes that are universal.

   A: While true, this is irrelevant. Welty's universal themes are what make her more than just a "southern" writer.

   B: Welty was born in Mississippi and thus it is very likely that she does identify as a southerner.

   D: This is the opposite of the author's general thesis about Welty's universal themes.

2. A is correct. What does knowing that Fay's relative is named "Bubba" and Laurel's close friend is "Miss Tennyson Bullock" do for us? It helps us understand the class and cultural divide that separates Fay – poor, from rural Texas – and Laurel – more comfortable, from small town Mississippi.

   B: Actually it helps the reader gain an understanding of each woman's culture.

   C: The author makes it clear in paragraph 4 that Welty is sympathetic to both characters, and writes in a way that helps the reader feel that way too.

   D: Knowing that Fay's people are "Bubba" and "Mama" help us understand who they are, but this choice leaves out the larger point made – that the names help us understand both Fay and Laurel, and appreciate the difference between them.

3. B is correct. The author is saying here that Welty draws the contrasts between the world of Fay and the world of Laurel skillfully, and by doing so makes them more rich and real to us.

   A: The contrast between solemnity and superficiality isn't addressed by the passage.

   C: This is the opposite of what the author states. The contrast between Laurel and Fay hinges in large part on the fact that Laurel is focused on the past and Fay is focused on the future.

   D: The author believes that Welty does have particular skill in capturing the regional dialects of her characters, but dialect is not addressed as a part of the "dualities" asked about in the question.

4. C is correct. The author is clearly praising Welty's skillful writing in *Optimist's Daughter*. She notes Welty's careful use of detail, ability to capture particulars of speech, and skill in creating characters who seem authentic and true – AND her tenaciousness in tackling universal issues, such as the notion of "home."

5. A is correct. We're told in paragraph 2 that Laurel is widowed, so she seems to have lived with a husband. We don't know anything from the passage about Fay's life before she married Judge McKelva – except that she's from Texas, and poor. The other choices are all differences between the two women that are described in the passage.

6. B is correct. At the end of the passage, we learn that in one of the final scenes of the novel, Laurel has the realization that she can ease her grip on the past, and allow Fay make her home in Laurel's childhood house if she so chooses. She has reached some sort of understanding, and is ready to move on, literally and emotionally. Given this, if the author were to write more it would probably be about Laurel leaving town, and her greater sense of ease.

   A: The last paragraph implies that Laurel has as good an understanding as she needs of Fay's background already – there's no suggestion that Laurel will look backwards towards that.

   C: Laurel seems to have made peace in her own mind, but there's no indication that they will share a home.

   D: It's unlikely that were the novel to continue, Laurel would turn to the flaws of Mount Salus.

Passage 2 (Questions 7 – 11)

Maimonides is well known amongst **Jewish scholars** for his contributions to **medicine** and for his extensive writings on **ethical** and legal issues. During the Middle Ages, Maimonides wrote a comprehensive commentary on Jewish oral law or oral tradition. While modern scientific rigor has since proven Maimonides's medical writings obsolete, his **philosophical work** in the field of rabbinic law **still holds authority** in the Jewish religion.

Key terms: Maimonides

Opinion: Maimonides is an important writer on Jewish ethics

Contrast: Maimonides's medical writings are obsolete but his ethical writing still holds

In Judaism there exists a religious duty to give called "*tzedaka*". *Tzedaka* is loosely translated into English as "**charity**", although the classical Hebrew roots of the word more correctly correspond with the English word "**justice**". Maimonides writes that the proper execution of *tzedaka* is **more important than any other Jewish duty**. In order to illustrate his view of ideal *tzedaka*, Maimonides identified **eight levels** of *tzedaka* and arranged these levels in order of merit.

Key terms: tzedaka

Opinion: Maimonides asserts that tzedaka is the most important duty

Contrast: tzedaka is translated as charity but the classical Hebrew word better fits justice

The **highest** level of *tzedaka* on this list describes an **act that fosters self-sufficiency**, such as the endowment of an interest-free loan or an offer of business partnership. If a poor person is given a loan to start a business, this person will then be able to create his or her own funds. This person will no longer require charity and **will be able to partake in the act of** *tzedaka* **as a benefactor**. Vitally, offering a poor person a business partnership requires that we **do not look down** on him and treat him with the same dignity as a rich man.

Opinion: when offering tzedaka as a benefactor, we must not look down on the poor person

Cause and effect: self-sufficient charity is best b/c the recipient will be able to act as a beneficiary

The seven following levels of *tzedaka* are all variations on a similar theme. The **second-best** level entails **giving anonymously** to an **anonymous recipient**. This is done to **minimize** any **embarrassment** or shame that the recipient may feel, and prevents the benefactor from boastfulness. This act necessitates the involvement of an organizing force such as a synagogue. The third level entails giving anonymously to a recipient whose identity is known (to the benefactor), and the fourth level giving publicly to an unknown recipient, as if announcing one's donation.

Contrast: contrasts between the levels: Level 2: anonymous, Level 3: anonymous giving to known recipient, Level 4: announcing donation to an unknown recipient

The final and **least meritorious** mode of *tzedaka* according to Maimonides is **giving "with sadness"**. A **reluctant donation** is ranked **lower** than a willing but inadequate donation (level 7). Maimonides interprets *tzedaka* as a method for ensuring economic stability as well as respecting the poor. A system that jeopardizes the dignity of the poor is not justified by any potential financial benefits. Maimonides writes that a benefactor who **publicly chastises** the poor is **not** completing an act of *tzedaka*, even if, as he puts it, he gives a poor man "1000 gold coins".

Opinion: Maimonides thinks level 7 is willing but inadequate giving and the bottom, level 8 is giving reluctantly

Contrast: chastising someone for being poor is so bad, it's not even level 8 – it is not an act of tzedaka at all, regardless of how much you give

In 2014, a charity campaign called "**the ice bucket challenge**" gained popularity via social media. In order to raise money for amyotrophic lateral sclerosis research, participants would **publicly post videos** of themselves being doused with a bucket of ice cold water and donating to the cause before nominating three other people to do the same.

Key terms: ice bucket challenge, amyotrophic lateral sclerosis, publicly

The ice bucket challenge **most closely resembles level four** of Maimonides's eight levels, "giving publicly to an unknown recipient". This act of charity would **not be ideal** for Maimonides, who would prefer anonymous and private donations. While *tzedaka* originally intends to help those in need quietly but effectively, ubiquitous **social media** campaigns have turned **philanthropy into a public spectacle**. The internet has effectively eliminated the need for face-to-face contact while making a donation. It would be far more virtuous to use this facet of the world wide web to preserve anonymity while performing *tzedaka*.

Opinion: Author thinks social media is too public and could be improved with anonymity

Contrast: internet should be a tool for anonymous charity but it is not being used as such today

Cause and effect: putting the video up publicly on YouTube makes "ice bucket challenge" participants operate on level 4 of tzedaka

Main Idea: Maimonides had ethical writings that still carry weight in the Jewish community, especially as to the religious duty of *tzekaka*, and Maimonides classified the eight levels ranging from gifts that encourage self-sufficiency as the most righteous down to gifts that are given reluctantly as the least meritorious; the author seems to think social media campaigns like the Ice Bucket Challenge, while good acts, qualify as a less than exemplary act of giving.

7. C is correct. This question requires you to understand the "most exemplary" action to be level 1 of *tzedaka* (all of paragraph 3 in the passage is devoted to this concept). Specifically we are looking for an action that fosters self sufficiency. Here, choice C gives a good example of fostering self-sufficiency.

    A, D: Maimonides considers anonymity of both the bene-factor and recipient to be important. These may well be acts of *tzedaka,* but they are not exemplary.

    B: This describes Maimonides' level 2 of *tzedaka*, but not the first.

8. C is correct. The question is asking for *necessary* con-ditions, not what is *exemplary*. All 8 levels of *tzedaka* are still *tzedaka*. II is stated in the passage explicitly. All the levels are expressions of respect to poor people. While III is not explicitly stated in the passage, the definition of *tzedaka* is "a religious duty to give", and all levels deal with some sort of financial contribution.

    I: This looks attractive because it's Maimonides's ideal form of *tzedaka*. Levels 2-8, however, do not cause the recipient to become self-sustaining. Since those levels are still considered *tzedaka*, this cannot be a necessary condition.

9. B is correct. The passage asserts that: "While modern scientific rigor ha[s] since proven Maimonides' medical writings obsolete, his philosophical work [is relevant today]"

    A: This is not an assumption the author makes. He does say that Maimonides' laws are respected today by Jew-ish scholars, but nothing about how Jews see scientific evidence.

    C: The word "always" in this answer choice makes it incorrect. The author doesn't compare Maimonides' contributions to medicine and philosophy in medieval ages. His medical works may well have been more important at the time, we simply do not know. The passage information does not support this answer.

    D: The word "never" makes this option incorrect. See option C.

10. A is correct. The author's argument is that the ALS ice bucket challenge is not an ideal form of charity (as read through Maimonides' levels of *tzedaka*). In order for his argument to be valid, his comparison between a monetary donation to poor people and donations to a research foundation must be valid. Remember that Maimonides was writing specifically about helping poor people through monetary donations. The author assumes that he would feel the same about helping sick people through a research foundation; however such a foundation was not likely to exist in Maimonides' time. This is an assumption that the author makes that can be directly challenged to weaken his argument.

    B: This supports Maimonides' levels of *tzedaka*, which is not explicitly an argument of the author.

    C: This is irrelevant to the author's argument.

    D: This does not weaken the author's argument. More money does not equal better *tzedaka*.

11. B is correct. From the passage: [the lowest level is giving] "with sadness". A reluctant donation is ranked lower than a willing but inadequate donation (level 7); "with sadness" is followed by "reluctant".

    A, C: These options take the word "sadness" literally. Maimonides is not likely to condemn a person for donating while crying.

Passage 3 (Questions 12 – 16)

The **mushroom** is a highly prized article of food that can be as easily grown as many other vegetable products of the soil, with as much **pleasure** and **profit**. Below it is shown, in particular, that this peculiar plant is **singularly well-adapted to the needs of all manner of people**, and for whom the mushroom has become a standard crop for **home use**, the **city market**, or both. It is directly in their line of business; is a winter crop, requiring their care when outdoor operations are at a standstill, and they can most conveniently attend to growing mushrooms. Using manure on a mushroom crop before using it on other crops provides a wealth of advantages. **After** having borne a crop of **mushrooms** it is thoroughly rotted and in good condition for early spring crops; and for seed beds of tomatoes, lettuces, cabbages, cauliflowers, and other vegetables; in other words, it is the **best kind of manure**.

Key Terms: mushroom, home use, city market, winter crop, manure

Opinion: author seems to think highly of mushrooms and mushroom farming; author believes the practice enjoyable and profitable

Cause and effect: using manure on mushrooms first will enhance its utility with other crops

In most large **gardens,** one can find a **mushroom house**, where the growing of mushrooms is an easy matter; in more modest gardens where there is no such convenience, and the gardener has to trust to his own ingenuity as to where and how she is to grow the mushrooms. But so long as she has an abundance of fresh manure, she can usually find a place to make the beds. In the **toolshed**, the potting-shed, the wood-shed, the stoke-hole, the fruit-room, the vegetable-cellar, the cow-house or horse-stable, the carriage-house, barn-cellar, woodshed, or house-cellar, she can **surely find a corner**; or, handier still, a **convenient room under the greenhouse benches**, where she can make some beds. But the **best** place is, perhaps, the **cellar**. An empty stall in a horse-stable is a capital place, and not only affords room for a full bed on the floor, but for rack-beds as well. Failing all of these she can start in August or September and make beds outside, as the London market gardeners do.

Cause and effect: it appears that a shed or underground area are best for growing mushrooms

Those who **keep horses** should, at least, grow mushrooms for their own family use and perhaps for market as well. They are so easily raised, and they take up so little space that they commend themselves particularly to those who have only a **village** or **suburban lot**, and, in fact, only a **barn**. And they are not a crop for which we have to make a great preparation and need a large quantity of manure. **No matter how small the bed** may be, it will bear mushrooms; and if we desire we can add to the bed week after week, as our store of manure increases, thereby keeping up a continuous succession of mushrooms.

Opinion: the author believes that those who keep horses, villagers, and people with barns should grow mushrooms, especially since mushrooms can be grown in a very small area

No one can grow mushrooms better or more economically than the **farmer**. She has already the cellar-room, the fresh manure and the loam at home, and all she needs is **some spawn** with which to plant the beds. Nothing is lost. The manure, after having been used in mushroom beds, is not exhausted of its fertility, but, instead, is well rotted and in a **better condition** to apply to the land than it was before being prepared for the mushroom crop. The farmer will not feel the little labor that it takes. There is no secret whatever connected with it, and **skilled labor** is **unnecessary** to make it successful. The commonest farm hand can do the work, which consists of turning the manure once every day or two for about three weeks, then building it into a bed and spawning and molding it. Nearly all the labor for the next ten or twelve weeks consists in maintaining an even temperature and gathering and marketing the crop.

Opinions: the author believes that farmers are best suited to grow mushrooms and that it is easy to do so

Cause and effect: mushrooms grow best at even temperatures

Main Idea: The main idea of the passage is to inform the reader of the utility and pleasure of growing mushrooms; the author introduces some main points as to who should grow mushrooms, how, and why.

12. B is correct. The passage is all about growing mushrooms, making B the best choice.

    A: There is no discussion of eating the mushrooms or which are edible.

    C: This is beyond the scope of the passage.

    D: The author does not discuss poisonous mushrooms in the passage, nor do we get any reference to American mushrooms.

13. C is correct. There is no mention of elevation in the passage and it is unreasonable to assume that elevation will play much of a role in the productivity of mushroom growing.

    A: The passages states this directly in the first and last paragraphs.

    B: The passage states that mushrooms are a winter crop.

    D: The passage implies that mushrooms grow best when they are kept contained in a box or cellar where no light will reach them.

14. B is correct. The passage explains the profitability of growing mushrooms and offers a brief introduction to the process of growing mushrooms. The author will likely expound further how to best grow mushrooms as his or her intent seems educational.

    A: The passage makes no mention of a product the author is trying to sell.

    C: There's no discussion of economics in the passage.

    D: The passage is not highly rigorous with the science and does not discuss germination at all.

15. B is correct. The fact that mushrooms can also grow in the summer does not mean they are no longer special for being able to grow in the winter.

    A: This is false.

    C: The author would still suggest that they be grown in the winter when other activities come to a stand still.

    D: There is no connection between the information in the question stem and this answer.

16. D is correct. The author believes that any class of person can and should be involved in growing mushrooms. He or she would not likely state that men are better suited for the job than women and children. The author states that very little labor is involved and that it can be done indoors.

    A: The author states that a cellar is probably the best place to grow mushroom.

    B: This statement agrees with the author's attitude toward mushrooms.

    C: This statement agrees with the author's opinions expressed in the passage.

Passage 4 (Questions 17 – 23)

The study of **ethics** is perhaps most commonly conceived as being concerned with the questions "What sort of **actions** ought men **perform**?" and "What sort of actions ought men **avoid**?" It is conceived as dealing with **human conduct** and as deciding what is **virtuous** and what is **vicious** among the kinds of conduct among which, in practice, people are called upon to choose. Owing to this view of the province of ethics, it is sometimes regarded as *the* **practical** study to which all others may be opposed as **theoretical.** The **good** and the **true** are sometimes spoken of as independent kingdoms: the former belonging to ethics, while the latter belongs to the sciences.

Opinion: some people view ethics as dealing with practical issues

Contrast: the study of virtuous and vicious actions is the aim of ethics; the good is thought to be under ethics, while the true is under science

This view, however, is **doubly defective.** In the first place, it overlooks the fact that the object of ethics, by its own account, is to **discover true propositions** about virtuous and vicious conduct, and that these are just as much a part of truth as true propositions about oxygen or the multiplication table. The aim is not practice, but propositions about practice; and **propositions** about practice are **not themselves practical**, any more than propositions about gases are gaseous. One might as well maintain that botany is vegetable or zoology animal. Thus the **study of ethics** is not something outside science and co-ordinate with it: it is **merely one among sciences.**

Opinion: author believes that ethics is "one among sciences" and that the study of virtue and vice is theoretical and that practice is not its aim

Contrast: the author's ideas that ethics aims at truth vs the view that ethics aims at practice/conduct

Cause and effect: if one maintains that ethics is practical, one may assume that the study of anything is that thing itself (e.g. that zoology "is animal")

The **first step** in **ethics**, therefore, is to be quite clear as to what we mean by **good** and **bad.** Only then can we return to **conduct**, and ask how right conduct is related to the production of goods and the avoidance of evils.

Opinion: author thinks first step in ethics is defining good and bad

Good and Bad, in the sense in which the words are here intended (which is, I believe, their usual sense), are **ideas** which everybody, or almost everybody, possesses. These ideas are apparently among those which form the **simplest constituents** of our more complex ideas, and are therefore **incapable** of being **analyzed** or built up out of other simpler ideas. When people ask "What do you mean by good?" the answer must consist, not in a verbal definition such as could

be given if one were asked "What do you mean by pentagon?" but in such a characterization as shall call up the appropriate idea to the mind of the questioner. This characterization may, and probably will, itself contain the idea of good, which would be a fault in a definition, but is harmless when our purpose is merely to **stimulate the imagination** to the production of the idea which is intended. It is in this way that children are taught the names of **colors**; they are shown (say) a red book, and told that that is red; and for fear they should think red means book, they are shown also a red flower, a red ball, and so on, and told that these are all red. Thus the **idea** of **redness** is **conveyed** to their minds, although it is quite **impossible to analyze redness** or to find constituents which compose it.

Opinion: the author believes that good or bad is the simplest of any idea and can not be broken down further or analyzed (uses the analogy of teaching red via example)

Cause and effect: we teach good and bad (or "red") by stimulating the imagination not by giving a definition

In the case of good, the process is more difficult, both because goodness is **not perceived** by the **senses**, like redness, and because there is **less agreement** as to the things that are good than as to the things that are red. This is perhaps one reason that has led **people to think that the notion of good could be analyzed** into some other notion, such as **pleasure** or object of **desire.** A second reason, probably more potent, is the common confusion that makes people think they cannot understand an idea unless they can define it—forgetting that ideas are defined by other ideas, which must be already understood if the definition is to convey any meaning. When people begin to philosophize, they **seem to make a point of forgetting everything familiar and ordinary**; otherwise their acquaintance with redness or any other color might show them how an idea can be **intelligible** where **definition**, in the sense of analysis, **is impossible.**

Contrast: common sense (things can be understood without a formal definition) vs philosophizing

Cause and effect: it is difficult to define good because it is not easily perceived and there is less agreement as to what is good.

Opinion: author thinks that good cannot be analyzed down into another concept like pleasure

Main Idea: Some mistakenly think the aim of ethics is good conduct when, in fact, ethics is a science aiming at making true statements about what is good; the ideas of good and bad themselves are the simplest constituents of ideas and cannot be analyzed further into simpler ideas even though some people wrongly think that "good" or "bad" requires a formal definition reducing it to something like "pleasure".

17. C is correct. The author states that ethics is a science and thus implies that truth can be found in ethical statements. We should expect the author to believe that ethical statements are either true or false.

18. B is correct. The first paragraph presents the ideas about ethics that are commonly believed – that ethics is about conduct. The author presents the ideas only to disagree with them to make his or her point that ethics is about arriving at true statements about conduct.

19. C is correct. The phrase in question was used directly after and in support of the statement that propositions about practice are not themselves practical, implying that the study of ethics has no aim in practicality but in theory.

    A: The author may believe this but the statement was not intended to illustrate it.

    B: The author believes that propositions about practice are theoretical.

    D: The author probably believes that a science is theoretical. Either way the statement is dealing with ethics not another science.

20. A is correct. This "fear" is never discussed by the author and is thus the correct answer.

    B: The passage discusses how it is impossible to understand good by analysis or definition. It is implied that only through experience or example can good be understood.

    C: This is stated in the last paragraph.

    D: This is expounded upon in the fourth and fifth paragraphs.

21. D is correct. The sun is an object with a specific definition.

A, B, C: These words are difficult to define in the sense that good is difficult to define. They are all direct perceptions that one can perceive, or stimulate in the imagination, but telling someone the definition of the word "yellow" or "salty" will not let them understand them. You must show them a yellow object, or let them taste a salty food.

22. C is correct. Choice C gives the answer that much of the passage tries to explain; characterization of good and bad serve to enlighten the mind as to the true nature of good and bad, despite lacking formal definitions. They "stimulate the imagination".

    A: The author states that at the base of most ideas are indefinable constituent ideas.

    B: The author would say that they always do.

    D: There is no indication that the author would attempt a definition of good like this.

23. A is correct. The author appears to be approaching the topic of ethics from as neutral and objective a standpoint as possible. His or her aim is purely academic. Similar to the discussion of good and bad, it is most reasonable to assume the author could analyze right and wrong.

    B: If the author was going to expound further on the history of ethics, he or she would have done so before moving on to a discussion of good and bad.

    C: There has been no discussion of religion or hint that the author would discuss it.

    D: As the author discussed how difficult defining "good" was without giving an example, it would not follow that he or she would discuss "bad" with an example.

Passage 5 (Questions 24 – 28)

A **classic**, according to the usual definition, is an old author **canonized** by admiration, and an authority in his particular style. The word classic was first used in this sense by the **Romans**. With them not all the citizens of the different classes were properly called *classici*, but only those of the chief class, those who possessed an income of a certain fixed sum. Those who possessed a smaller income were described by the term *infra classem*, below the preeminent class. The word *classicus* was used in a figurative sense by **Aulus Gellius**, and applied to writers: a writer of worth and distinction, *classicus assiduusque* scriptor, a writer who is of account, has real property, and is not lost in the proletariat crowd. Such an expression implies an age sufficiently advanced to have already made some sort of valuation and classification of literature.

Key terms: classic, canonized, Romans, classici, infra classem, Aulus Gellius

Cause and effect: the term "classic" has its origin with respect to literature and the arts

At first the only true classics for the moderns were the ancients. The **Greeks**, by peculiar good fortune and natural enlightenment of mind, had no classics but themselves. They were at first the only classical authors for the Romans, who strove and contrived to imitate them. After the great periods of Roman literature, after **Cicero** and **Virgil**, the Romans in their turn had their classics, who became almost exclusively the classical authors of the centuries which followed. The **middle ages**, which were less ignorant of Latin antiquity than is believed, but which **lacked proportion and taste**, confused the ranks and orders. **Ovid** was placed above **Homer**, and **Boetius** seemed a classic equal to **Plato**. The revival of learning in the fifteenth and sixteenth centuries helped to bring this long chaos to order, and then only was **admiration rightly proportioned**. Thenceforth the true classical authors of Greek and Latin antiquity stood out in a luminous background, and were **harmoniously grouped on their two heights**.

Key terms: Greeks, Cicero, Virgil, middle ages, Ovid, Homer, Boetius, Plato

Cause and effect: the people of the middle ages are said to have wrongly ranked some of the ancient poets and artists above others; the revival of learning fixed this

Meanwhile modern literatures were born, and some of the more precocious, like the **Italian**, already possessed the style of antiquity. **Dante** appeared, and, from the very first, posterity greeted him as a classic. Italian poetry has since shrunk into far narrower bounds; but, whenever it desired to do so, it always found again and preserved the impulse and echo of its lofty origin. It is no indifferent matter for a poetry to derive its point of departure and classical source in high places; for example, to **spring from Dante** rather than to **issue laboriously from Malherbe**.

Key terms: the Italian, Dante, Malherbe

Opinion: the author attempts to objectively analyze which works of art are classics but his or her opinion probably plays a large role

Contrast: Dante is contrasted to Malherbe, the former a great poet, the latter supposedly less great

Cause and effect: because of its origins in greatness, Italian poetry is able to revive itself "whenever it desired to do so"

If it is desired, names may be applied to this definition which I wish to make purposely majestic and fluctuating, or in a word, all- embracing. I should first put there **Corneille of the Polyeucte, Cinna**, and **Horaces**. I should put **Moliere** there, the fullest and most complete **poetic genius** we have ever had in France. **Goethe**, the **king of critics**, said: "Moliere is so great that he astonishes us afresh every time we read him. He is a man apart; his plays border on the tragic, and no one has the courage to try and imitate him. His **Avare**, where vice destroys all affection between father and son, is one of the most sublime works, and dramatic in the highest degree. In a **drama every action ought to be important in itself**, and to lead to an action greater still. In this respect **Tartuffe** is a model. What a piece of exposition the first scene is! From the beginning everything has an important meaning, and causes something much more important to be foreseen. The exposition in a certain play of Lessing that might be mentioned is very fine, but the world only sees that of Tartuffe once. It is the finest of the kind we possess. **Every year I read a play of Moliere**, just as from time to time I contemplate some engraving after the great **Italian masters**."

Key terms: Corneille of the Polyeucte, Cinna, Horaces, Moliere, Avare, Tartuffe, Italian masters

Opinion: author believes Moliere to be one of the greatest poetic geniuses ever

Cause and effect: since Goethe is praised as "king of critics" we can assume the author believes and is influenced by Goethe's criticisms

Main Idea: The author attempts to describe what a "classic" work of art is; he gives several examples of the classic authors and artists and provides a framework for how to tell if an individual is able to produce classics.

24. B is correct. The passage states that the Greeks were the first civilization to create classics and that they had natural enlightenment of mind.

   A: There is no evidence to support this. The Greeks probably deserve this distinction.

   C: The Italians are mentioned as great poets but this is too strong a claim.

   D: Moliere is praised as one of the greatest French poets but there is no evidence to support that he was the greatest in all of history.

25. B is correct. The author tries to define a classic with a set of rules. However, whether a work fulfills the rules is somewhat up to interpretation. The author's taste comes in, for example, when he suggests that Homer should be placed above Ovid.

   A: The set of rules is not concrete. The classification of artistic works can have no such set of rules.

   C: The author believes that there are some qualifications that need to be met.

   D: The author has no problem denying others' opinions about which works of art are classics.

26. C is correct. The passage states that Tartuffe is a great drama because "in a drama every action ought to be important in itself, and to lead to an action greater still."

   A: A drama is not necessarily a classic.

   B: This does not necessarily mean it is a classic. Even a genius like Moliere could produce a substandard work.

   D: This is not mentioned in the passage.

27. D is correct. Goethe compares Tartuffe, which he considers a classic, to one of the works of the Italian masters. Michelangelo is one of the most widely revered sculptors of all time, thus a statue produced by him has the greatest chances of being considered a classic by the author.

   A: The author specifically calls out Ovid in a context that puts him below Homer, suggesting the author's low opinion of Ovid.

   B: Malherbe is said to be a lesser poet than Dante.

   C: This could be a classic but is too broad a category to be the correct answer.

28. D is correct. I: The phrase in question was included to explain why the Greeks were able to produce works of art. II: Since they were the first to experience this natural enlightenment of mind, this explains why they were the first to produce classic works of art. III: The phrase has nothing to do with the Romans.

Passage 6 (Questions 29 – 35)

But in some branches of **economic inquiry** and for some purposes, it is more **urgent** to **ascertain new facts**, than to trouble ourselves with the mutual relations and explanations of those which we already have. While in **other branches** there is still so much uncertainty as to whether those causes of any event which lie on the surface and suggest themselves at first are both true causes of it and the only causes of it, that it is even more **urgently** needed to **scrutinize our reasoning** about facts which we already know, than to seek for more facts.

Contrast: some branches of economic theory require new facts while others require scrutinizing the reasoning about those facts

Cause and effect: when it is unclear as to whether a seeming cause is the true or only cause, it is best to focus on the reasoning about the facts

For this and other reasons, there always has been and there probably **always will be a need** for the existence side by side of **workers with different aptitudes and different aims**, some of whom give their chief attention to the ascertainment of **facts**, while others give their chief attention to **scientific analysis**; that is taking to pieces complex facts, and studying the relations of the several parts to one another and to cognate facts. It is to be hoped that these two schools will always exist; each doing its own work thoroughly, and each making use of the work of the other. Thus best may we obtain sound generalizations as to the past and trustworthy guidance from it for the future.

Contrast: workers who focus on ascertaining facts vs those who do scientific analysis

Cause and effect: when the two schools of analysis make use of each other's work, we best obtain sound generalizations about the past and guidance to the future

Those **physical sciences**, which have progressed most beyond the points to which they were brought by the brilliant genius of the **Greeks**, are not all of them strictly speaking "**exact sciences.**" But they all aim at exactness. That is, they all aim at precipitating the result of a multitude of observations into provisional **statements**, which are sufficiently **definite** to be brought under test by other observations of nature. These statements, when first put forth, seldom claim a high authority. But **after they have been tested** by many independent observations, and especially after they have been applied successfully in the prediction of coming events, or of the results of new experiments, they graduate as **laws**. A science **progresses** by **increasing** the number and exactness of its **laws**; by submitting them to tests of ever increasing severity; and by enlarging their scope till a single broad law contains and supersedes a number of narrower laws, which have been shown to be special instances of it.

Contrast: provisional statements vs laws

Cause and effect: multiple observations are shaped into provisional statements, which are tested and applied to experiments and predictions and then become laws; science progresses when there are more laws which are more exact, more tested, and with a broader scope

Although the subject-matter of some **progressive physical sciences** is not, at present at least, capable of perfectly exact measurement; their progress depends on the multitudinous co-operation of armies of workers. They measure their facts and define their statements as closely as they can: so that each investigator may start as nearly as possible where those before him left off. **Economics aspires to** a place in this group of **sciences**: because though its measurements are seldom exact, and are never final; yet it is ever working to make them more exact, and thus to enlarge the range of matters on which the individual student may speak with the authority of his science. Let us then consider more closely the nature of economic laws, and their limitations. Every cause has a tendency to produce some definite result if nothing occurs to hinder it. Thus gravitation tends to make things fall to the ground, but when a balloon is full of gas lighter than air, the pressure of the air will make it rise in spite of the tendency of gravitation to make it fall. **The law of gravitation** states how any two things attract one another; how they tend to move towards one another, and will move towards one another if nothing interferes to prevent them. The law of gravitation is therefore a statement of tendencies.

Contrast: not being capable of exact measurement vs needing workers cooperating to measure facts exactly

Cause and effect: in economic laws, causes produce results if nothing hinders them from doing so, as does the law of gravitation

Main Idea: The passage suggests that economics should be treated like a physical science both in terms of a drive towards greater accuracy and predictive power and in its reliance on statements of tendencies.

29.   C is correct. The final paragraph introduces the idea of the "tendency to produce some definite result if nothing occurs to hinder it," as part of the "nature of economic laws, and their limitations," and then discusses gravity in depth as "a statement of tendencies".

A: The passage seeks to compare physics and economics, not contrast them.

B: The focus is on understanding economics, not exact sciences, as in choice B.

D: There is no focus on what can hinder the definite results, just the general tendencies.

30.   D is correct. The passage states that scientific analysis is "taking to pieces complex facts, and studying the relations of the several parts to one another and to cognate facts".

A: The third paragraph discusses developing the scope of a law and testing it as ways of expanding science, not doing analysis.

B: While scientific analysis is about dissecting issues, the passage does not discuss ascertaining truth value.

C: The passage stresses the acquisition of new facts.

31.   D is correct. The passage discusses cooperation several times, stating that "progress depends on" it and at its best "each investigator may start as nearly as possible where those before him left off." Thus it stresses completeness and not replicating work.

A: While the cooperating scientists are described as "armies," there is no discussion of war.

B: Cooperation in economics is not contrasted with that in other sciences. Presumably, the author would think all sciences require cooperation.

C: Interferences, discussed in the last paragraph, are not contrasted with cooperation.

32.   C is correct. In the second paragraph, the author discusses "uncertainty as to whether those causes of any event which lie on the surface and suggest themselves at first are both true causes of it and the only causes of it," adding that "it is even more urgently needed to scrutinize our reasoning about facts which we already know, than to seek for more facts".

A: Uncertainty is discussed in relation to physical sciences, not in opposition to them.

B: There is no discussion of proximal causes in the passage.

D: Tendencies are discussed as a form of scientific law in the passage, not as causes, as in choice D.

33.   A is correct. The passage asserts that economics is a form of science, and that sciences accumulate and explain facts and develop laws about them.

B: Economics is seen as a form of science, not in contrast to it.

C: The passage states that economic laws are statements of tendencies, but not that these are laws that rule over economics.

D: Advancing economics may entail enlarging the scope of it, but this question is specifically asking about the parallels between economics and the hard sciences.

34.   B is correct. When discussing those who gather data vs those who analyze it, the author states that "it is to be hoped that these two schools will always exist; each doing its own work thoroughly, and each making use of the work of the other. Thus best may we obtain sound generalizations as to the past and trustworthy guidance from it for the future." Thus the credited answer is choice B, which suggests that with only one group working, sound generalizations could not be reached.

A: The passage states that the two schools working together lead to sound generalizations and trustworthy guidance, but does not suggest that simply focusing on analysis would only lead to one result.

C: The passage is against just analysis or just data collection.

D: While the passage suggests economics depends on both "schools," it does not imply the schools depend on each other to function.

35.   D is correct. The passage states that "a science progresses by increasing the number and exactness of its laws" as in choice C, "by submitting them to tests of ever increasing severity" as in choice A, "and by enlarging their scope till a single broad law contains and supersedes a number of narrower laws, which have been shown to be special instances of it," as in choice B. Thus choice D is the one not discussed, and the credited answer. Accuracy of prediction is suggested as part of what makes a statement a law, not science progressing.

Passage 7 (Questions 36 – 42)

What exactly does **Wagner** mean historically? He represents *the rise of the actor in music,* an event of great moment that leads me not only to think, but also to fear. Never before have the **uprightness** and **genuineness** of musicians been put to such a **dangerous test**. It is obvious now that **great success** is no longer the achievement of **the genuine**, for in order to get it, you must be an actor! The **mob success** of Victor **Hugo** and, of course, Richard Wagner, prove that in **declining civilizations**, wherever and whenever the mob is given **the choice**, **genuineness** becomes **superfluous** and unfavorable. The actor alone still kindles great enthusiasm, and therefore, it is his golden age that is now dawning.

Key terms: Wagner, *the rise of the actor in music,* Hugo

Contrast: having genuineness vs being an actor; the mob vs genuineness in a declining civilization

Cause and effect: because of the rise of the actor in music, the genuineness of musicians is put to a dangerous test; we know that in declining civilizations, genuineness is not preferred

With drums and fifes, Wagner marches at **the vanguard** of **all artists** in declamation, display, and virtuosity. He began by winning over the **conductors**, the scene-shifters, the stage-singers, and of course, the **orchestra**; he delivered them from monotony. Wagner's **movement** has spread even to **the land of knowledge**: entire **sciences** pertaining to music are beginning to slowly rise out of **centuries of scholasticism**. The people of this movement have a perfect right to honor Wagner: in him, they recognize their highest type, and because his work managed to inflame them with his own ardor, they feel themselves made powerful. It is in this sphere that **Wagner's influence** has **actually** been **beneficent**, for never before has there been so much **thinking**, **willing**, and **pure industry** in it. Wagner endowed these artists with a new conscience: what they now expect and actually attain for themselves, they never even began to seek out before Wagner's time, for they were too modest then.

Key terms: the vanguard, all artists, centuries of scholasticism

Contrast: monotony vs Wagner's style; the ardor of Wagner vs the empowerment of his followers

Cause and effect: by winning over conductors and the orchestra, Wagner began his movement; because of Wagner's movement, entire sciences pertaining to music are slowly rising out of centuries of scholasticism

Another **spirit** prevails on **the stage**, for Wagner rules there that **the most difficult things** are to be **expected**, blame is always severe, praise is very scarce, and that **the good** and **the excellent** have become the **rule**. Taste is no longer necessary, and truly, **neither is a good voice**, for Wagner's work is sung only with ruined voices, making for a more **dramatic effect**. Even talent is now out of the question: the **decadent**,

Wagnerian ideal, **expressiveness at all costs**, is hardly compatible with talent. All this is required for the achievement of this ideal is virtue, or, that is to say, training, automatism, and self-denial. **Wagner's stage** does **not** require **taste**, **voices**, **nor gifts**, but it does require one thing: **Germans**!

Contrast: good vs ruined, expressiveness vs talent

Cause and effect: because Wagner's work is sung with ruined voices, a good voice is no longer necessary; because the ideal of expressiveness at all costs is not compatible with talent, talent is also out of the question

For **Wagner's purposes**, this is **the definition of a German**: an **obedient** man with **long legs**. After all, there is **deep significance** in the fact that **the rise of Wagner** coincided with **the rise of the "Empire,"** for both phenomena are proof of one and the same thing: obedience and long legs. Never before have people been more obedient and never before have they been so effectively and efficiently **ordered about**. More particularly, the conductors of Wagnerian orchestra are worthy of an age that will be one day referred to by posterity, with timid awe, as **the classical age of war**.

Key terms: the definition of a German, an obedient man with long legs, the classical age of war

Cause and effect: the rise of Wagner's style and of the "Empire" both hinged on the German people having obedience and effectiveness

Wagner fully understood how **to command**, and therefore, was in this respect a **great teacher**. He commanded others as a man who, with a lifelong practice of self-discipline, exercised an **unyielding will over himself**. In fact, Wagner was perhaps the greatest example of **self-violence in the whole history of art**.

Cause and effect: because Wagner understood how to command, he was a great teacher; Wagner understood this because of his lifelong self-discipline

Main Idea: The author seeks to define Wagner's meaning and place in history; he describes how this was beneficial to people in the world of knowledge, but perhaps was more negative in the world of the stage; the author compares the rise of Wagner's influence to the rise of the German empire, associating Wagner with order, imperialism, and war.

36. C is correct. Rather, his greatest ideal, expressiveness at all costs, requires virtue, "or, that is to say, training, automatism, and self-denial." Choice C reflects this opposites of these qualities.

37. B is correct. III is true because Wagner's movement began when he won over the artists involved in playing his music and making it happen on stage by delivering them from monotony. In other words, he made the work more interesting, more compelling.

    I: This is false because the rise of Wagner and the rise of the Empire coincided, being driven by the central motivating impulse of "obedience and long legs."

    II: This is false because it misses a crucial part of the statement that it references: the part that read "wherever and whenever the mob is given the choice." So, a declining civilization does not necessarily lead to genuineness going out of favor, but when the mob gets to decide, it does.

38. B is correct. First of all, the rise of the actor in music puts the "uprightness and genuineness of musicians" to a more dangerous test than ever before. Second of all, "It is obvious now that great success is no longer the achievement of the genuine, for in order to get it, you must be an actor!" Therefore, an actor must be something that is or is least close to the opposite of genuine.

    A: It is never said that Wagner is anything close to a stage actor.

    C: Well, he certainly does make things happen, but in the first paragraph, actor is more used as a foil to genuineness and uprightness.

    D: Certainly he was adored by the people, but this does not necessarily relate to his representing the rise of the actor in music. In fact, in a time when civilization was not declining, a person might have to be more genuine to be admired.

39. C is correct. According to the passage, Germans are obedient and have long legs. Therefore, they can easily and efficiently be told what to do, and can likely carry it out with strength and efficiency as well. "Never before have people been more obedient and never before have they been so effectively and efficiently ordered about." So, the quality that makes Germans so desirable to Wagner in producing his works are these: obedience and long legs.

    A: This is true, but misses the obedient part.

    B: Again, it's not just because Germans are German, but because the author thinks that they have certain innate qualities.

    D: Blame being severe and praise being scarce don't seem like the best way to build a community.

40. B is correct. What Wagner did in the "land of knowledge" was instill a bit of his own ardor, infusing that field with more "thinking, willing, and pure industry" than it had ever had before. On the contrary, "Another spirit prevails on stages," and this spirit is much more stringent and strict.

    A: This is never said and may in fact be the opposite of the truth.

    C: This is also never said. If it had been so, might he have been an academic instead of a composer?

    D: This is never said either.

41. A is correct. "The mob success of Victor Hugo and, of course, Richard Wagner, prove that in declining civilizations, wherever and whenever the mob is given the choice, genuineness becomes superfluous and unfavorable." As Wagner is successful here, we can assume that civilization is declining, that it is in a downward spiral.

    B: This is never said, and we know that the author has some problems with and fears about Wagner.

    C: This is the opposite of what is said in the passage, as the author makes the point that Wagner's music does not require a great voice.

    D: We never get a mention of Hugo's self-discipline, and because Wagner practiced such an unyielding self-discipline over himself, the author writes that he "was perhaps the greatest example of self-violence in the whole history of art."

42. D is correct. As the author writes in the third paragraph, "The decadent, Wagnerian ideal, expressiveness at all costs, is hardly compatible with talent." This is the Wagnerian ideal, expressiveness at all costs: it is the principle that guides the rest of his qualities, characteristics, and approaches to art. Therefore, if a student were to emulate Wagner and had only one attribute to take on, this would be it.

    A: Rather, we get a sense that the Wagnerian *conductors* are the ones that imbue the work with a sense of war.

    B: This is to serve the central principle, expressiveness at all costs.

    C: While the author seems to think Wagner's work required Germans, we're never told that Wagner himself or that Wagner's work was fundamentally nationalistic.

Passage 8 (Questions 43 – 46)

Considering how **difficult** it is for men to **hold** a newly acquired state, some may justly wonder how **Alexander the Great** became the **master of Asia** in only a few years, and how his **successors maintained** their rule of empire. Because Alexander **died before the empire's full settlement**, it would have been reasonable for the people of the empire to **rebel**. **Yet**, Alexander's **successors maintained it**, and in truth, they met no harsher difficulties than those which arose from their own ambitions.

Contrast: the difficulty in acquiring a newly held state vs how Alexander the Great and his successors managed to do it

Cause and effect: because Alexander died before the empire had been fully settled, we would have expected rebellion

Of the **principalities** for which **records** are available, there are two different ways of governance: either by a **prince and his servants**, the latter of whom help manage the kingdom by the prince's favor and permission, or else by a **prince and his barons**, the latter of whom hold their offices not by princely assignation, but by the antiquity of their blood. These barons rule their own states with their own subjects who recognize and **follow their rule with sincere affection**. Meanwhile, in those states ruled by a prince and his servants, the prince himself is held with the highest consideration, for in all of the principality there is no one considered superior to him. If the subjects of this state do yield their obedience to **another**, it is to a **minister** or an **official**, and in so doing they show **no sincere affection**. In our time, the prime examples of these two governments are the **Turk** and the King of **France**.

Contrast: governance by the prince vs governance by the prince and barons, barons vs servants, the Turk vs the King of France

Cause and effect: because the barons hold their offices by the antiquity of their blood, they rule their own subjects; when the subjects of this kind of state yield obedience to another besides the Prince, it is to a servant of the prince's and they show him no real affection

The **monarchy** of the **Turk** is ruled solely by **one lord**, the Turk himself, and the rest are his servants. His kingdom is divided into **sanjaks** and to each of these he sends **ministers and officials** that he may shift and change as he pleases. On the other hand, the King of **France** is seated in the midst of the **ancient body of lords**, all of whom have their own loyal subjects. These **lords have their own prerogatives** for rule: the King alters them only at his own risk.

Key terms: sanjak

Contrast: the sole monarchy of the Turk vs the ancient body of lords in France

Cause and effect: because the monarchy of the Turk is ruled solely by one lord, the Turk can send ministers and officials

to sanjaks as he pleases and may shift and change them as he pleases as well; because the members of the ancient body of lords of France have their own loyal subjects and their own prerogatives for rule, the King alters them only at his own risk

It is evident that it would be of great **difficulty** to **seize** the kingdom of the **Turk**, and yet it is also evident that it would be of **great ease to hold the kingdom** once conquered. This is because a potential usurper will clearly not be called into the kingdom by the Turk, nor will he be assisted in his revolt by the ministers and officials. As these ministers are all essentially slaves and bondmen, they can only be corrupted from their allegiance to the Turk with great difficulty. Even if they are corrupted, these ministers hold little esteem in the eyes of the people and thus cannot motivate them to raise arms against their beloved Turk. Therefore, **whosoever attacks the Turk** must note this and must know that his success will **depend** more on his **own army's strength** than on the revolt of others.

Contrast: the difficulty of seizing the Kingdom of the Turk vs the ease of holding it

Cause and effect: a potential usurper's success will rely upon his own army's strength and not the revolts of others

However, if the **Turk** is **conquered**, and if he is defeated in such a way that he **cannot replace his armies**, the only thing left the usurper has to fear is the **family** of the Turk. If the **royal family is killed**, there is **nothing left to fear**, as the ministers and officials have little credit with the people. As the conqueror did not rely upon these people for his usurpation, he need not fear them after it.

Contrast: the family of the Turk vs the ministers and officials of the Turk

Cause and effect: if the royal family is killed, the usurper has nothing left to fear

On the contrary, a **usurper** can **easily enter the Kingdom of France** by winning over some **malcontented baron**, desirous of change. Such men as this can open the way into the Kingdom and make victory easy, but here lies the problem: if you wish to **hold the Kingdom**, you will meet with **innumerable difficulties**, both from the barons who have assisted you and from those you have defeated. In this case, it is not sufficient to have exterminated the royal family, for the lords of the Kingdom remain to lead fresh movements against you. If you are unable to satisfy or exterminate them, the state is lost whenever time brings the opportunity.

Contrast: the difficulty of entering the Turk's Kingdom vs the ease of entering the Kingdom of France; the ease of victory in taking France vs the innumerable difficulties in holding it

Cause and effect: a malcontented baron who is desirous of change can be easily won over, entrance France and victory, are made easy; because the lords remain to lead fresh movements against you, it is not sufficient to have exterminated the royal family

Main Idea: Holding a conquered state is hard, so how did Alexander the Great make it seem so easy? The author describes two kinds of principalities, one ruled by the prince and barons, one ruled by the prince and servants; he then examines the relative ease or difficulty of conquering and then holding them; in so doing, it implies that Alexander's conquest of Asia was made manageable because the Asian empire consisted mostly of states like that of the Turk, which were easy to hold.

43. A is correct. In response to the question posed in the first paragraph (how did Alexander the Great's successors maintain his empire?), the author presents the two primary examples of principalities. Only one of them, in which a prince has sole rule and employs servants as minister and officials, represents a principality that would be relatively easy to hold after conquering it (though it would be difficult to take initially).

   B: The Asian empire is more comparable to the Turk's kingdom.

   C: In a state with a prince and his servants ruling, the lords of the realm are not sovereign in their power.

   D: This is possible, but within the context of the paragraph, in a state with a prince as sole ruler, the people admire no one more than the ruler. It is in the other type of principality that a baron, desirous of change, may help a usurper.

44. D is correct. The first paragraph poses the central question, and the following paragraphs seek to answer it through examples of the major two types of principalities.

   A: Conquest is seemingly not so difficult in the case of a state in which a ruler is tempered by a class of lords with hereditary claims to power.

   B: This is true, but too general and vague for this context.

   C: There would seem to be duality between the two types of principalities mentioned, but they are mentioned for the purpose of answering the central question.

45. B is correct. The entire passage is essentially an attempt to answer the central question posed in the first paragraph: the passage's primary method is to employ a basic analysis of the two primary types of principalities and to try and answer that question within the framework of that analysis.

   A: This passage does not suggest the author would value a popular vote.

   C: The passage does not employ thought experiments based upon historical precedence as much as analysis of two types of governments that were contemporary to the author.

   D: This idea is also not mentioned in the passage, and in fact, the author may be against it, as the ministers and officials of both types of principalities will have a bias, either in favor of or against the prince.

46. C is correct. The scenario given here is representative of the second type of principality of which the Kingdom of France is an example. Choice C is the only option that includes two true statements about how this kind of principality can be both conquered and held successfully.

   A: The problem here is that in this type of principality, people will still have allegiance to their respective lords.

   B: This will not help hold the kingdom because sovereign lords will still be around to lead "fresh movements."

   D: The problem here is that inciting revolts against the ruler of State B will no guarantee that the state can be conquered, as people will still keep allegiances to their lords. Moreover, the author states that all lords, even those that are trusted, should be exterminated.

Passage 9 (Questions 47 – 53)

It has been well said that the "**conquest of fear**" is the best indication we have that **civilization** has really **advanced** mankind to a higher level. When we speak of the "conquest of fear" we do not mean that fear itself has entirely disappeared; that can never be. We mean only that **much unreasonable fear has been dissipated**. I believe that the sum-total of fear has greatly diminished with the progress of the world, but as the amount of fear cannot be weighed or measured, we have no criterion of values.

Opinion: author argues that the conquest of fear doesn't refer to the disappearance of fear, just that the levels of unreasonable fear has dissipated and that this indicates the advancement of civilization

There is now widespread confidence in the **orderly succession of natural laws**. People no longer live in daily dread of the spirits of darkness, and are **not afraid of the unknown**; an eclipse of the sun or the coming of a comet does not strike terror into the hearts of the community.

Cause and effect: widespread confidence in the order of natural laws and decrease in superstitious beliefs is evidence to the decrease in unreasonable fear

Epidemics, also, **follow natural laws**. They come, rise, reach their height and virulence, and decline according to known biological rules. The trained epidemiologist can tell at once by looking at the curve of annual prevalence of typhoid fever of a city whether the people are drinking badly infected water or not. A **milk** outbreak has its **own special characteristics** that permit speedy recognition. Certain diseases **recrudesce** annually with the **regularity** of our crops. I know of one health officer of one of our large cities who each year takes a mean advantage of the seasonal prevalence of typhoid fever by instituting a newspaper sanitary campaign in September. The health department then claims the credit for the inevitable decline in October.

Cause and effect: epidemics follow patterns dictated by biological rules and natural laws, the confidence in which the author previously associated with the dissipation of unreasonable fear

In fact, the **natural history of disease** has risen **almost** to the **dignity of a science**. In many instances, at least, we are able to **control and foretell the phenomena** of disease prevalence. For this, of course, we have to thank largely the **patient researches** into the causes of the communicable infections, and especially the scientific and **self-sacrificing studies** into their modes of transmission. Useful and trustworthy results have been obtained only by **exact laboratory methods**. The rapid accumulation of this **real knowledge** has **robbed** infection of the **superstitious** dread in which it was formerly held. We are **no longer tied helpless** in the face of a devastating plague, and in our ignorance blame it on the supernatural wrath of an irresponsible power. Now we **fight back**, for we have the knowledge that gives courage and conquers fear.

Opinion: author believes that advancing scientific knowledge has elevated epidemiology to the full dignity of a science, and in doing so has helped to conquer our fear of infectious diseases

Cause and effect: advancing science and the study of infectious diseases has given us a better grasp for the logic and science of disease transmission, lessening our fear of it

Fear is lessening, but we would **not want it to disappear entirely**, for while it is a miserable sensation, it **has its uses** in the same sense that pain may be a marked benefit to the animal economy, and in the same sense that **fever** is a conservative process. **Reasonable fear saves** many lives and prevents much sickness. It is **one of the greatest forces for good in preventive medicine**, and at times it is among the most useful instrument in the hands of the sanitarian.

Opinion: author believes that reasonable fear can at times be the most useful tool for preventing the spread of diseases.

Contrast: reasonable fear hear is contrasted as a positive force for preventing the spread of diseases vs unreasonable fear which has been gladly gotten rid of

The **indifference** to disease can be just as **dangerous**. I have noticed a **nonchalance** towards yellow fever in **Vera Cruz**, Santiago, and other tropical places where "familiarity breeds a species of contempt," and the **fatalistic tendency of mankind** accepts the inevitable, though a **Lazear** laid down his life as the result of a mosquito bite to save his fellow-men. It is **lack of fear** of yellow fever that permits it to **smolder in an endemic focus**, just as the lack of fear of typhoid fever permits it to smolder in Boston, Philadelphia, Washington, and other American cities. A **sharp epidemic** of typhoid fever is a **good lifesaver**. The **fear it instills builds filter plants, spends money** and awakens energy for other necessary and expensive sanitary improvements.

Key terms: Vera Cruz, Lazear

Opinion: author believes that a lack of reasonable fear can be deadly, so much so that he believes that a sharp outbreak of a disease could be a positive force in the long run.

Cause and effect: without reasonable fear a disease is more likely to spread through a community, as a result sharp epidemics that instill fear might be beneficial in the long run

Main idea: The conquest of fear refers to the conquest of unreasonable fear and superstition; however, we do not want to lose the reasonable fear we have in the face of a disease, as that fear saves lives.

47. D is correct. In the first paragraph the author acknowledges "fear cannot be weighed or measured, we have no criterion".

48. A is correct. In the second paragraph, the author implies that due to our confidence in natural laws, we no longer fear things like eclipses or comets.

49. C is correct. In the fourth paragraph the author states that our understanding of diseases can be attributed to "scientific and self-sacrificing studies into the modes of disease transmission", and that specifically those studies were conducted using "exact laboratory techniques". Answer choice A, B, and D are therefore incorrect. Furthermore while the author states that reasonable fear helps prevent the spread of a disease, it does not contribute to our understanding of it.

50. A is correct. The author states that reasonable fear helps to prevent the spread of a disease. However once an individual has contracted it there is no sense in living in fear of its progression because that fear would not help the individual to overcome it.

    B: The author states that a lack of fear of infected individuals, and therefore the disease itself, allows diseases to continue to propagate, which he would not encourage.

    C: While the author believes that reasonable fear of a disease is beneficial, public *alarm* would be too strong and likely fall into the category of unreasonable fear.

    D: Public education regarding the transmission of a disease is critical to preventing its spread, and the author would likely argue that it would help to instill a beneficial amount of reasonable fear, not the opposite.

51. D is correct. The author uses the example of typhoid fever in Vera Cruz to emphasize his point that public indifference to a disease can be dangerous.

    A: The example of Vera Cruz is used to caution against indifference to a disease, and therefore it does not provide specific evidence for the benefits of unreasonable fear. The author generally takes a negative tone towards unreasonable fear at the start of the passage.

    B: The author believes the community in Vera Cruz does not fear typhoid fever enough.

    C: Vera Cruz is used as a cautionary example, not as an example of the benefits of epidemiology.

52. C is correct. The passage states that fear is one of the "greatest forces for good in preventive medicine, and at times it is among the most useful instrument in the hands of the sanitarian", therefore answer choice A is tempting. Public health education and intervention, however, would raise levels of reasonable fear through education while also promoting techniques to prevent disease communication. The author makes a point of saying that a sharp epidemic of typhoid can raise fear enough to get people moving on public health interventions like building filter plants.

    B: The author states that unreasonable fear is good to avoid, however it would not be the best defense against an epidemic.

    D: A population that had previously exposed to a disease, but remained uneducated or indifferent to the methods of its spread (Santa Cruz example), would not be expected to fair any better in the face of an epidemic.

53. D is correct. A study that indicated that the level of public fear had no impact on its spread would directly contradict one of the author's main arguments.

    A: A country may not fear a disease *because* it has a low incidence of infection, not the other way around. The finding therefore wouldn't weaken the author's main argument.

    B: Even if societal education is the *most* important predictor of a response to an epidemic, levels of societal fear may also play a significant role. The findings could therefore still be consistent with the author's main argument.

    C: The author and passage are not concerned with chronic illness.

SECTION 6

53 Questions, 90 Minutes

Use an answer grid from the back of the book to record your answers

Passage 1 (Questions 1 – 6)

In 1947, the French artist Jean Dubuffet coined the term *art brut* to describe works created by artists who resided outside of artistic culture. *Art brut*, or "raw art" was, to Dubuffet "uncooked" – pure and unadulterated, uninfluenced by artistic convention, fashion, or intellectual trends. Writing about *art brut,* Dubuffet said "those works created from solitude and from pure and authentic creative impulses – where the worries of competition, acclaim and social promotion do not interfere – are, because of these very facts, more precious than the productions of professionals."

Dubuffet's interest in *art brut* can be seen in the larger cultural context of the rejection of the art establishment by early to mid 20th century artists. The Dada, Cubist, Futurist, and Surrealist movements all abandoned certain cultural conventions in favor of new and sometimes jarring expressions. Artists like Pablo Picasso and Henri Matisse looked away from "high" culture and towards so-called primitive or naïve art, and incorporated elements in their work. While Dubuffet's description makes the work of those artists sound quite idyllic, the solitude of the artists he was applauding often stemmed from their institutionalization. Dubuffet's initial introduction to this sort of art was probably through a book entitled *Artistry of the Mentally Ill,* published in 1922 by a German psychiatrist. A massive volume illustrating the artwork of thousands of psychiatric patients across Europe, it drew the attention of several avant-garde artists of the time, including Dubuffet. Psychotics, mediums, religious fanatics, eccentrics – these were the artists whose outpourings were labeled "raw."

Several decades after Dubuffet's use of the term *art brut*, English art critic Roger Cardinal coined the term "outsider art" in 1972 to describe the work of artists outside of traditional art culture. To Cardinal, outsider art was a somewhat broader category than that described by Dubuffet; it included not just the works of artists with profound mental illness, but also works of people outside of the mainstream – geographically or socially isolated, living with disabilities, or simply untrained. In the United States, curators and critics began to look at American folk art differently, and the lines between folk art and outsider art began to blur: what critics conceived of as folk art, generally thought to embody traditional forms and social values, began to include more marginal and individualistic expressions.

The parameters of outsider art have continued to expand dramatically. Today, outsider art is seen less as pathological and more as the creative expression of individuals not conditioned by art history or art world trends. Outsider artists come from all walks of life and cultures; the common denominator they share is raw creativity. Visionary art, folk art, naïve art: whatever the label, the common thread is that the artists are not traditionally schooled in art-making. Still, some of these artists have achieved enormous commercial success. Over the past two decades, outsider art has become a highly saleable art category, with several journals covering the subject, a yearly Outsider Art Fair in New York, repre-sentation of artists in respected galleries, and exhibition of works of outsider artists in major museums worldwide. It is ironic that the mainstream art world has embraced the outsiders, widely exhibiting their work, profiting on the efforts of those seemingly unaware of the art world's machinations. The question arises, too, of how artists working in some degree of isolation are influenced by attention and acclaim; does that attention necessarily bring the art world's own pathologies – which Dubuffet sought to defy in celebrating *art brut?*

1. The passage suggests that which of the following might be a critique of the mainstream art world, according to Jean Dubuffet?

    A. It produces work that is technically skillful but lacking in true creativity.

    B. It interferes with authentic creativity.

    C. It values fame more than talent.

    D. It does not acknowledge the avant-garde.

2. According to the passage, which of the following describes a difference between folk art and outsider art?

    A. Outsider art is often more individualistic, while folk art reflects elements and forms of a culture.

    B. Folk art may include formally trained artists, whereas outsider artists are self-taught.

    C. Outsider artists are more likely to have profound mental illness than are folk artists.

    D. Folk artists are more likely than outsider artists to be accepted by the art establishment.

3. Which of the following best describes the lives of early artists creating art brut?

    A. They were artists who had rejected the artistic convention of the day.

    B. They considered themselves to be in the avant-garde.

    C. Their solitude stemmed from profound mental illness or institutionalization.

    D. Their artistic creativity was often mistaken for psychosis.

4. Of the following, which reflects the paradox the author describes at the end of the passage?

    A. The conception of what is defined as outsider art has become unclear.

    B. Commercial success and critical attention may affect the purity of outsider artists.

    C. Outsider art has decreased the importance of traditional folk art forms.

    D. The term outsider art now includes artists who are not self-taught.

5. According to the author, outsider art may be characterized by all of the following EXCEPT:

    A. creation by religious visionaries.

    B. incorporation of some traditional cultural forms.

    C. inclusion of academically trained artists.

    D. critical acclaim and commercial success.

6. Suppose a contemporary artist were to create work that incorporated traditional Native American art forms. According to the passage, would that artist be considered an outsider?

    A. Possibly, if the artist was self-taught and working in some degree of isolation.

    B. Possibly, if the artist had not achieved commercial success.

    C. No, because the artist would be considered a folk, not outsider, artist.

    D. Yes, because traditional art forms are now considered outsider art.

Passage 2 (Questions 7 – 13)

Tularaemia is a bacterial zoonotic disease of the northern hemisphere. The bacterium (*Francisella tularensis*) is highly virulent for humans and a range of animals such as rodents, hares and rabbits. It may cause epidemics and epizootics. Tularaemia is transmitted to humans (i) by arthropod bites, (ii) by direct contact with infected animals, infectious animal tissues or fluids, (iii) by ingestion of contaminated water or food, or (iv) by inhalation of infective aerosols. There is no human-to-human transmission.

Tularaemia is reported from most countries in the northern hemisphere, although its occurrence varies widely from one region to another. In some countries, endemic regions with frequent outbreaks are close to regions that are completely free of tularaemia. There is also a wide variation with time. In an endemic area, tularaemia may occur annually within a 5-year period, but may also be absent for more than a decade. The reasons for this temporal variation in the occurrence of outbreaks are not well understood. When, after a long lapse, the first case of a new outbreak appears, the disease may be more or less forgotten and is therefore not easily diagnosed. *F. tularensis* subspecies *tularensis* (type A) is one of the most infectious pathogens known in human medicine. The infective dose in humans is extremely low: 10 bacteria when injected subcutaneously and 25 when given as an aerosol (McCrumb, 1961; Saslaw et al., 1961; Saslaw et al., 1961). For example, on Martha's Vineyard in the United States of America, two adolescents contracted respiratory tularaemia after mowing a grassed area (Feldman et al., 2001). It is believed that an aerosol of *F. tularensis* subspecies *tularensis* was generated after the carcass of a rabbit which had died of tularaemia was accidentally shredded by the lawnmower.

The risk posed by tularaemia can be properly managed, provided the public health system is well prepared. In order to avoid laboratory-associated infection, safety measures are needed and consequently clinical laboratories do not generally accept specimens for culture. However, since clinical management of cases depends on early recognition, there is an urgent need for diagnostic services. In addition to its natural occurrence, *F. tularensis* causes great concern as a potential bioterrorism agent. The present guidelines on tularaemia (i) provide background information on the disease, (ii) describe the current best practices for its diagnosis and treatment in humans, (iii) suggest measures to be taken in case of epidemics and (iv) provide guidance on how to handle *F. tularensis* in the laboratory. The target groups for these guidelines include clinicians, laboratory personnel, public health workers, veterinarians, and any other person with an interest in zoonoses.

The guidelines are the result of an international collaboration, initiated at a WHO meeting in Bath, United Kingdom of Great Britain and Northern Ireland in 2003, continued in Umeå, Sweden, in 2004 and finalized in Geneva, Switzerland, in 2005. Each chapter of the guidelines was developed by a selected group of scientists with extensive developmental work and general experience relevant to the field

covered. Chairs of each group met regularly throughout the process to ensure consistency and for critical review. The document was also subject to internal and external peer reviews. As with many other areas, understanding of the nature of tularaemia and its causative agent is evolving rapidly across all aspects discussed in the guidelines, including taxonomy, epidemiology, epizootiology, detection, diagnostics, therapy and prophylaxis. It is envisaged therefore that modifications to these guidelines will become necessary every three years.

7. Based on the passage, clinical laboratories are loath to accept suspected tularaemia specimens because:

   A. the extremely low infective dose means detection is frequently difficult.

   B. temporal infrequency means that diagnosis can be difficult.

   C. a lack of protocol results in a high risk of laboratory-associated infection.

   D. clinical management requires rapid and early recognition.

8. Based on the passage it can be assumed that zoonotic means which of the following about the vector?

   A. It can only be transmitted between non-human animals.

   B. It is more readily transmitted between non-human animals.

   C. It can transfer from animal to human, but not vice versa.

   D. It never transmits between humans.

9. The author most likely discusses temporal variation in outbreaks in order to:

   A. argue that diseases that are forgotten can be the most dangerous health risks.

   B. analyze why such variations occur in order to develop safety measures.

   C. hypothesize why some strains of tularaemia are so infective.

   D. suggest a reason why diagnosis of tularaemia is crucial.

10. This passage can best be described as a(n):

    A. assessment of the bioterrorist threat tularaemia may pose at the present time.

    B. justification for the WHO issued guidelines that will follow.

    C. case history of aerosol based spread of infectious vectors.

    D. manifesto for the need for better clinical resources in combatting tularaemia.

11. Suppose that a year after these guidelines were issued, dramatic new findings on the epidemiology of tularaemia came to light. WHO would most likely recommend that:

    A. scientists wait for a period of three years in order to assess the validity of such claims in clinical practice.

    B. a panel of scientists with experience in the field meet to develop modifications to the current recommendations.

    C. issues of epizootiology get renewed attention based on these new findings.

    D. foreign intelligence agencies such as the CIA and MI-5 be apprised of new bioterrorism threats.

12. Based on the passage, the origin of a case of tularaemia in humans could be:

    I. while camping, drinking from a pool at the campsite that infected rabbits had frequented.

    II. while cleaning a barn in the country, uncovering a nest of spiders and receiving several bites on limbs but not the trunk.

    III. on a hunting trip, nicking an infected hare from a 25 foot distance, resulting in a blood spray, though not a kill.

    A. I only

    B. III only

    C. I and II only

    D. II and III only

13. One reason this document was aimed at laboratory personnel, amongst others, was the assumption that if:

    A. clinicians are warned about possible outbreaks in a timely manner, they can prevent them from happening.

    B. the reason for temporal spacing was better understood, then diagnostic services would be more efficacious.

    C. tularaemia was to be used as a bioterrorism agent, the rapidity of diagnosis would be crucial is ending the outbreak.

    D. laboratories were more willing to accept probable tularaemia cases, diagnostic speed would be more rapid.

Passage 3 (Questions 14 – 18)

First, as to the science of numbers. So far as the acquirements of the Phoenicians on this subject are concerned it is impossible to speak with certainty. The magnitude of the commercial transactions of Tyre and Sidon necessitated a considerable development of arithmetic, to which it is probable the name of science might be properly applied. A Babylonian table of the numerical value of the squares of a series of consecutive integers has been found, and this would seem to indicate that properties of numbers were studied. According to Strabo the Tyrians paid particular attention to the sciences of numbers, navigation, and astronomy; they had, we know, considerable commerce with their neighbors and kinsmen the Chaldaeans; and B'ockh says that they regularly supplied the weights and measures used in Babylon. Now the Chaldaeans had certainly paid some attention to arithmetic and geometry, as is shown by their astronomical calculations; and, whatever was the extent of their attainments in arithmetic, it is almost certain that the Phoenicians were equally proficient, while it is likely that the knowledge of the latter, such as it was, was communicated to the Greeks. On the whole it seems probable that the early Greeks were largely indebted to the Phoenicians for their knowledge of practical arithmetic or the art of calculation, and perhaps also learnt from them a few properties of numbers. It may be worthy of note that Pythagoras was a Phoenician; and according to Herodotus, but this is more doubtful, Thales was also of that race.

Geometry is supposed to have had its origin in land-surveying; but while it is difficult to say when the study of numbers and calculation—some knowledge of which is essential in any civilized state—became a science, it is comparatively easy to distinguish between the abstract reasonings of geometry and the practical rules of the land-surveyor. Some methods of land-surveying must have been practiced from very early times, but the universal tradition of antiquity asserted that the origin of geometry was to be sought in Egypt. That it was not indigenous to Greece, and that it arose from the necessity of surveying, is rendered the more probable by the derivation of the word from γη˜, the earth, and μετρέω, I measure. Now the Greek geometricians, as far as we can judge by their extant works, always dealt with the science as an abstract one: they sought for theorems which should be absolutely true, and, at any rate in historical times, would have argued that to measure quantities in terms of a unit which might have been incommensurable with some of the magnitudes considered would have made their results mere approximations to the truth. The name does not therefore refer to their practice. It is not, however, unlikely that it indicates the use which was made of geometry among the Egyptians from whom the Greeks learned it. This also agrees with the Greek traditions, which in themselves appear probable; for Herodotus states that the periodical inundations of the Nile (which swept away the landmarks in the valley of the river, and by altering its course increased or decreased the taxable value of the adjoining lands) rendered a tolerably accurate system of surveying indispensable, and thus led to a systematic study of the subject by the priests.

We have no reason to think that any special attention was paid to geometry by the Phoenicians, or other neighbors of the Egyptians. A small piece of evidence which tends to show that the Jews had not paid much attention to it is to be found in the mistake made in their sacred books, where it is stated that the circumference of a circle is three times its diameter: the Babylonians also reckoned that π was equal to 3.

14. Which of the following is a conclusion that can be reached from the information in the first paragraph?

    A. The Greeks had a base of mathematical knowledge they inherited from the Babylonians.

    B. The Greeks had a base of mathematical knowledge they inherited from the Phoenicians.

    C. The Chaldeans had a base of mathematical knowledge they inherited from the Phoenicians.

    D. The Chaldeans were the first to develop a systematic approach to arithmetic.

15. Which of the following might necessitate a civilization's development of a system of surveying?

    A. Living near the ocean where seasonal typhoons consistently wipe out life near the shore

    B. Living as nomads following herds of bison

    C. Living as farmers and using diverted rainwater for irrigation

    D. Living in seaside caves and fishing for food

16. Which of the following assumptions can be made based on information in the passage?

    A. The Egyptians had a more accurate approximation for π than 3.

    B. The Greeks likely assumed that π was 3 as well.

    C. The Phoenicians inherited their geometry knowledge from the Babylonians.

    D. The Jews inherited their geometry knowledge from the Babylonians.

17. Which of the following is a conclusion that can be reached from the information in the passage?

    A. The Greeks were the first to use geometry.

    B. The Phoenicians were the first to use geometry.

    C. The Egyptians were the first to use geometry.

    D. The Babylonians were the first to use geometry.

18. Suppose a Phoenician record were found that labeled the correct value of π as the ratio of a circle's circumference to its diameter. How would this finding compare with the information in the passage?

    A. It would disagree with the author's claim that no neighbors of the Egyptians were interested in geometry.

    B. It would support the author's claim that Pythagoras was a Phoenician.

    C. It would support the author's claim that Pythagoras was a geometrician.

    D. It would support the author's claim that the Egyptians inherited some knowledge of geometry from the Phoenicians.

Passage 4 (Questions 19 – 25)

At this point you may think that the primary use of logic in the real world is to deduce conclusions from workable premises and to satisfy yourself that conclusions deduced by others are correct. If only it were! Society would be far less disposed to panics and other delusions, and politics especially would be an entirely different thing if even a majority of the arguments that are regularly broadcast across the world were correct. Rather, I fear the inverse is true. For every one workable pair of premises that leads to a logical conclusion you meet in newspapers or magazines or other media, you will find five that lead to no conclusion at all. Even when the premises are workable, for every one instance where the writer draws a correct conclusion, there are ten where they draw an incorrect one.

In the case of the former, you may say, "The premises are fallacious." In the case of the latter, "The conclusion is fallacious." The primary use you will find for your new logical skills will actually be in detecting these two types of fallacies.

You can detect the first kind, fallacious premises, when, after marking them out on the larger diagram, you attempt to move those marks to the smaller diagram. You will take the four compartments, one by one, and ask for each one, "What mark can I place here?" For every one, the answer will be, "Nothing." This of course shows that there is no conclusion at all. For example: "All soldiers are brave. Some Englishmen are brave. Therefore, some Englishmen are soldiers." This statement looks like a syllogism, with a conclusion drawn from two premises, and might easily fool a less experienced logician, but not you. Rather, you would simply set out the premises and then calmly proclaim them to be fallacious: you wouldn't condescend to ask what conclusion the writer professed to find, knowing that no matter what it is, it must be wrong. You would be safe like the wise mother who said, "Mary, go up to the nursery, see what Baby's doing, and tell him not to do it."

You can detect the more difficult to spot second kind, fallacious conclusions, only after marking both diagrams, reading of the correct conclusion, and then comparing it with the conclusion drawn by the writer. Keep in mind, however, you ought not to immediately claim a conclusion to be fallacious simply because it is not identical to the correct one. Rather, it may be a part of the correct conclusion, and be correct as far as it goes. In this case, you would call it a defective conclusion. Take for example this syllogism: "All unselfish people are generous. No misers are generous. Therefore, no misers are unselfish." These premises, expressed in letters, are as follows: "All not-x are m. No y are m."

The correct conclusion would be, "All not-x are not-y," or in other words, "All unselfish people are not misers," while the conclusion by the writer is, "No y are not-x," which is the same as "No not-x are y," and so is part of "All not-x are not-y." In this case, you would simply claim a defective conclusion. The same problem would arise if you were in a bakery and a little boy came in, put down two pence, and marched off with a bun worth a single penny. You would shake your head and say, "Defective conclusion. Poor chap!" Perhaps at this point you would ask the lady behind the counter whether she would let you eat the bun left behind by that poor chap, and perhaps she would reply, "You shall not!"

19. Which of the following most likely preceded this passage in the book the passage was drawn from?

    A. A detailed account of the current state of media

    B. A depiction of how logic ideally functions in the real world

    C. An explanation of how to use the two diagrams

    D. A thorough introduction to inductive reasoning

20. Based upon the passage, the author likely believes which of the following statements?

    A. More people can set up their premises correctly than can draw their conclusions accurately.

    B. More people can draw their conclusions accurately than can set up their premises correctly.

    C. Most people who follow media and politics tend not to be interested in logic and reasoning.

    D. Most people who follow media and politics tend to be intimidated by logic and reasoning.

21. Which of the following is the most likely reason why the author uses letters to express the second logical fallacy, but not the first?

    A. The second syllogism is more complicated than the first.

    B. The first syllogism is obviously false to all people while the second is not.

    C. The second type of fallacy is more egregious than the first.

    D. The first syllogism is entirely incorrect, but the second is partially correct.

22. Say the author presents his readers with a syllogism expressed in letters: "All x are not-m. All y are m. Therefore, all x are not-y and all y are not-x." Which of the following spelled out syllogisms correctly corresponds to this?

    A. All Dragons are not real. All Scotchmen are real. Therefore, all dragons are not Scotchmen and all Scotchmen are not dragons.

    B. No anchovy pizzas are delicious. All rotten eggs are not delicious. Therefore, all anchovy pizzas are rotten eggs and all rotten eggs are anchovy pizzas.

    C. All brown hair is lustrous. All blonde hair is also lustrous. Therefore, all people with brown hair and all people with blonde hair have lustrous hair.

    D. All shoes and hats are smelly. All comets are not smelly. Therefore, all hats and shoes are not comets and all comets are not hats nor shoes.

23. According to the passage all of the following statements about deductive reasoning in the real world are true EXCEPT:

    A. it draws a conclusion from premises.

    B. it is mostly misunderstood.

    C. it is primarily used to reveal fallacies.

    D. it cannot be used to satisfy oneself that the conclusions deduced by others are correct.

24. Based upon the passage, which of the following statements are true?

    I. A less experienced logician is more likely to be fooled by the first logical fallacy than the second.

    II. A more experienced logician is less likely to be fooled by the first logical fallacy than the second.

    III. Both types of fallacies are equally likely to fool an experienced logician.

    A. I only

    B. II only

    C. II and III only

    D. I, II, and III

25. Based upon the passage, how would the author use letters to express the syllogism in the third paragraph with fallacious premises?

    A. All x are m. Some not-y are m. Therefore, some not-y are x.

    B. All x are m. Some y are m. Therefore, some y are x.

    C. All x are m. Some not-y are m. Therefore, some not-y are x.

    D. All x are m. Some y are m. Therefore, some y are not-x.

Passage 5 (Questions 26 – 32)

The jenny, invented in 1765 by the weaver James Hargreaves, was the first invention to bring about a radical change in the state of English workers. Instead of one spindle like the spinning-wheel used before, the jenny carried sixteen or eighteen spindles, manipulated by hand by a single workman, making it possible to deliver more yarn than ever before. Whereas one weaver used to employ three spinners and had to wait for yarn, there was now more yarn than could actually be woven by the available workers. Because of the diminished cost of production, the price of woven goods shot down, driving the already increasing demand for them even higher.

As such, more weavers were needed, and weaver's wages also rose. Now that the weavers could earn more at their looms, they gradually abandoned farming. At that time, a family of four adults and two children (who were often set to spooling) could earn, with eight hour work days, four pounds sterling per week, and oftentimes more if trade was good. In fact, a single weaver could often earn two pounds a week at his loom. Gradually, the class of farming weavers disappeared, reshaping itself into the class of weavers who lived entirely upon wages and had no property at all, not even the pretended property. Thus, they became working-men, proletarians.

The old relationship between spinner and weaver was destroyed. Up until this historical moment, yarn had been spun and woven under one roof. Now that both the jenny and the loom required a strong hand, men began to spin as well as weave, and whole families lived by spinning while others laid their superseded spinning-wheels aside, and if they did not have the means to purchase a jenny, were forced to live entirely upon the wages of the father. This split of spinning and weaving began the division of labor that has since been perfected.

While the industrial proletariat was birthed from this still imperfect machine, the same machine gave rise to the agricultural proletariat. Up to this point, there had been a vast number of small land owners, yeomen, who had vegetated in the same unthinking peace as their neighbors, the farming weavers. These yeomen cultivated their land in the inefficient fashion of their ancestors and, after remaining stationary from generation to generation, opposed every change with the stubbornness characteristic of creatures of habit. Among them were also many small holders, those who had their land handed down from their fathers by hereditary lease of ancient force of custom, and who had held the land as securely as if it had been their own.

When the new industrial workers withdrew from farming, many of these small holdings became idle, and upon them the new class of large tenants established themselves, holding fifty to two hundred or more acres. Though they were liable to be turned out by year's end, they improved tillage and farming practices to increase the land's yield. Therefore, they could sell produce more cheaply than the yeomen, for whom nothing remained when their farms no longer supported them but to sell it, buy a jenny or loom, or become a farm laborer. Their inherited slowness and inefficient methods left them no alternative when forced to compete with those who managed their holdings with sounder principles and with the advantages bestowed by large scale farming and capital investment in the improvement of soil.

26. According to the passage, which of the following things did men have to do before the invention of the jenny?

    A. Spin wool into yarn

    B. Wait for yarn from spinners

    C. Own large tracts of land

    D. Invest in improving the soil

27. Based upon the passage, which of the following is the most likely reason why the author used the word "vegetated" in the fourth paragraph?

    A. To politely hint at the idiocy and inferiority of the yeomen

    B. To demonstrate that the yeomen were near catatonic in their misperception of reality

    C. To suggest that the yeomen's behavior over time was slow and rooted, like vegetables

    D. To show that the yeomen are slightly more intelligent than the farming weavers

28. Based upon the passage, which of the following statements is the author most likely to believe about the disruptive nature of inventions?

    A. Any invention that can increase wages for workers must be considered beneficial to the proletariat.

    B. The jenny, like many other inventions, was ultimately worth the cultural erosion it brought about.

    C. Inventions ought to be somehow moderated so as not to entirely disrupt fragile systems of commerce.

    D. For better or worse, inventions that increase efficiency empower the most efficient and wealthy.

29. Which of the following is the best reason why the large tenants were so successful at farming?

    A. They could afford to spend time to improve the capabilities of the land and their tools.

    B. They were more intelligent than the yeomen and were not stuck into age-old ways of thinking.

    C. They had more money than the yeomen, and so could afford to hire more laborers.

    D. They were able to, with the quality of their goods, drive the price of goods up, increasing profit.

30. Say that Mr. James Hargreaves were to travel in time to the present and read about the history of the industrial revolution, beginning with his invention of the jenny. Given the passage, which of the following consequences of his invention would he most regret?

    A. That the jenny brought about sounder principles in farming and capital investment in soil which eventually led to the exploitation of the soil through chemical fertilizers

    B. That the jenny began the division of labor which has since been perfected creating a society in which almost nobody is capable of being self-sufficient

    C. That the jenny brought about the end of the class of farming weavers turning them into a proletariat that was often exploited

    D. That the jenny required weavers to become more efficient

31. All of the following were effects caused by the invention of the jenny EXCEPT:

    A. the price of produce shot down.

    B. the demand for produce shot up.

    C. the demand for investment shot up.

    D. the cost of production shot up.

32. Which of the following statements about spinning and weaving are true?

    I. Before the invention of the jenny, spinning was mostly the occupation of woman and children.

    II. Before the invention of the jenny, spinning and weaving were paired, often in individual homes.

    III. After the invention of the jenny, there was essentially no longer any relationship between spinning and weaving.

    A. II only

    B. I and II

    C. I and III

    D. I, II, and III

Passage 6 (Questions 33 – 38)

By directing the activities of the young, society determines their future, and therefore, its own future. Because at some later date the young will compose the society of that period, the nature of society will be largely informed by the direction of children's activities in the earlier period. This effect, a cumulative movement of action towards a later result, is known as growth.

The first condition of growth is immaturity. This may seem to be a simple truism, that anything that develops must first be undeveloped. But the prefix "im" actually refers to something positive, not merely a lack. To begin, we will look at the words "capacity" and "potentiality," both having a double meaning, one negative and one positive. Capacity can refer to mere receptivity, as in the capacity of a cup. Potentiality may refer to a dormant state: an ability to become something different with the influence of some external force. But capacity also has a power to it, and potentiality has a force to it. So, when we say that immaturity is the possibility of growth, we are not so much referring to the absence of things or abilities which may exist later, we are referring to a positive force that is present: the very ability to develop.

We tend to view immaturity as a lacking and growth as that which fills the void. This is because we view childhood comparatively and not intrinsically: we treat it as a lack because we compare it to adulthood as a fixed standard, and therefore, our attention is set upon what the child lacks, what he will not have until adulthood. In some cases this comparison is legitimate, but if this is our only way of viewing immaturity, we may perhaps be guilty of overconfident analysis.

If children could express themselves articulately, they would tell a different story. Moreover, there is evidence to suggest that for certain moral or intellectual purposes, adults ought to emulate children. The problem of our assumption that immaturity is a negative quality is most apparent when we consider that that it sets up a static end as a standard. Within this conception, the completion of growing is an accomplished growth, a state in which we no longer grow, an ungrowth. We can clearly observe the futility of this conception in the fact that every adult resents the notion of no longer having an ability to grow, and every adult will mourn this loss instead of falling back on all that has been achieved and considering it adequate. Why should there be an unequal measure for adult and child?

Taken in absolute and not comparative terms, immaturity refers to a positive ability: the power to grow. We do not have to draw out latent positive activities from a child, as some education doctrines would have it, for where there is life, there are already eager, impassioned activities. Growth is not something that is done to children. Rather, it is something they do. This positive aspect of immaturity allows us to understand its two primary traits: dependence and plasticity.

It may seem absurd to claim dependence as something positive, but consider this: if helplessness were all there was

to dependence, no development would ever take place and children would grow into adults that would need caring for throughout their whole lives. Dependence is accompanied by growth in ability and is therefore something constructive.

A child's plasticity is his adaptability for growth, and it is something quite different than the plasticity of putty. It is not so much the ability to change form in accord with external pressure, but rather, the ability to learn from experience, to retain something from one experience that will be useful in another. It is the power to modify actions based upon the results of what has happened before. Without this, the acquisition of habits and growth itself would be impossible.

33. Which of the following is the most likely reason why the author wrote the first two sentences of the fourth paragraph?

    A. In order to prove that children have greater wisdom and intuition than adults

    B. In order to provide another side to the argument that immaturity ought to be viewed comparatively

    C. In order to demonstrate how the common way of looking at childhood and immaturity is flawed

    D. In order to persuade the reader to embrace a particular way of looking at childhood

34. Based upon the passage, it is likely that the author most believes which of the following statements?

    A. Most adults reach a point when they are content to stop developing.

    B. A set educational doctrine is not necessary for children to develop.

    C. Immaturity may actually be something that is desirable for all people.

    D. Besides their inferior communication skills, children are actually quite adult-like.

35. According to the passage, why is a child's plasticity so important to his or her development?

    A. Because it is accompanied by growth in ability

    B. Because it is the means for acquiring habits

    C. Because it makes children physically adaptable

    D. Because it is interconnected with latent, positive activities

36. Say an experimental elementary school is developing a new curriculum. The school hires the author of this passage as a consultant. Based upon the passage, it can be inferred that the author would encourage which of the following methods of educating students?

    A. Developing a curriculum of positive activities based upon what the children already do

    B. Developing a curriculum of positive activities based upon what the children ought to be doing

    C. Developing a curriculum based upon a comparison of the relationship of childhood to adulthood

    D. Developing a curriculum meant to heighten the plasticity and dependence of children

37. According to the passage, all of the following statements about immaturity are true EXCEPT:

    A. people tend to view it comparatively.

    B. people tend to view it as a lack of something.

    C. people tend to compare it to adulthood as a variable standard.

    D. people tend to prove the futility of the normative understanding of it.

38. Which of the following statements accurately explains why the author introduced the words "capacity" and "potentiality" in the second paragraph?

    I. They both have a double meaning.

    II. They both can refer to passive and active states.

    III. Viewed positively, they are both synonymous with the author's understanding of immaturity.

    A. I only

    B. I and II only

    C. I and III only

    D. I, II, and III

Passage 7 (Questions 39 – 45)

But it is otherwise with moral laws. These, in contradistinction to natural laws, are only valid as laws, insofar as they can be rationally established a priori and comprehended as necessary. In fact, conceptions and judgments regarding ourselves and our conduct have no moral significance, if they contain only what may be learned from experience; and when any one is, so to speak, misled into making a moral principle out of anything derived from this latter source, he is already in danger of falling into the coarsest and most fatal errors.

If the philosophy of morals were nothing more than a theory of happiness (eudaemonism), it would be absurd to search after principles a priori as a foundation for it. For however plausible it may sound to say that reason, even prior to experience, can comprehend by what means we may attain to a lasting enjoyment of the real pleasures of life, yet all that is taught on this subject a priori is either tautological, or is assumed wholly without foundation. It is only experience that can show what will bring us enjoyment. The natural impulses directed towards nourishment, the sexual instinct, or the tendency to rest and motion, as well as the higher desires of honour, the acquisition of knowledge, and such like, as developed with our natural capacities, are alone capable of showing in what those enjoyments are to be found. And, further, the knowledge thus acquired is available for each individual merely in his own way; and it is only thus he can learn the means by which he has to seek those enjoyments. All specious rationalizing a priori, in this connection, is nothing at bottom but carrying facts of experience up to generalizations by induction (*secundum principia generalia non universalia*); and the generality thus attained is still so limited that numberless exceptions must be allowed to every individual in order that he may adapt the choice of his mode of life to his own particular inclinations and his capacity for pleasure. And, after all, the individual has really to acquire his prudence at the cost of his own suffering or that of his neighbors.

But it is quite otherwise with the principles of morality. They lay down commands for every one without regard to his particular inclinations, and merely because and so far as he is free, and has a practical reason. Instruction in the laws of morality is not drawn from observation of oneself or of our animal nature, nor from perception of the course of the world in regard to what happens, or how men act. But reason commands how we ought to act, even though no example of such action were to be found; nor does reason give any regard to the advantage which may accrue to us by so acting, and which experience could alone actually show. For, although reason allows us to seek what is for our advantage in every possible way, and although, founding upon the evidence of experience, it may further promise that greater advantages will probably follow on the average from the observance of her commands than from their transgression, especially if prudence guides the conduct, yet the authority of her precepts as commands does not rest on such considerations. They are used by reason only as counsels, and by way of a counterpoise against seductions to an opposite course, when adjusting beforehand the equilibrium of a partial balance in the sphere of practical judgment, in order thereby to secure the decision of this judgment, according to the due weight of the a priori principles of a pure practical reason.

39. Based on the passage, which is true of principles of morality?

    A. They aim at producing the greatest happiness.

    B. They must be based in practical reasons.

    C. They are universal, regardless of individual desire.

    D. They can be derived a priori, like natural laws.

40. The passage implies that natural laws:

    A. are less valid than moral laws.

    B. lead to grave errors in morality.

    C. are derived from experience.

    D. must be rationally established.

41. The author assumes that generalizations are morally valuable only when they:

    A. prevent alterations to meet specific desires.

    B. can be shown to be post facto rather than a priori.

    C. are flexible enough to allow for exceptions.

    D. prevent suffering of either self or neighbor.

42. With which of the following statements would the author of the passage be most likely to agree?

    A. Morals must be founded on neither observation nor will towards pleasure.

    B. Rationality can be dangerous when it is used to justify reasons to avoid moral behavior.

    C. Natural and moral laws must be integrated for better understanding.

    D. Generalizations hold no place in moral principles.

43. Suppose that a visitor to a foreign country observed that inhabitants were careful to never injure any animal, including insects, and began to operate similarly to fit in. The author of the passage would suggest that such a decision was ethically:

    A. weak, because it depended on attention to animal nature.

    B. suspect, because it was not founded on understanding or reason.

    C. commendable, because it was founded on the principle of happiness.

    D. worthy, because it created a command as to how to act.

44. Based on the passage, the theory of eudaemonism takes into account all of the following EXCEPT:

    A. personal advantage.

    B. honor.

    C. sexual instinct.

    D. nourishment.

45. Based on the passage, a statement is tautological when it:

    A. establishes a set of rational principles upon which to act.

    B. is assumed without any basis in experience.

    C. requires experience to reinforce what is claimed.

    D. is based upon natural choices and inclinations.

Passage 8 (Questions 46 – 49)

Dogs, pigs, chickens, and carabao appear to have been long in the possession of the Tinguian tribe. Horses, goats, and cattle are now owned by some of the people, but only the former are of sufficient number to be considered important.

The dogs are surly, ill-kept creatures of mongrel breed. They are seldom treated as pets, but are kept for hunting. Well-fed dogs are considered lazy, and hence they are fed only with a rice gruel, which seems to be neither fattening nor satisfactory. When in the village, the miserable creatures wander about under the houses, there to pick up and fight over morsels which may drop from above, or they lie in the ashes of the bonfires, the better to protect themselves from fleas and other enemies. When used in hunting, they are kept in leash until the game is started. When released, they follow the quarry at full cry, and if the game has been injured, they will seldom give up the chase. It is necessary for the hunters to follow the dogs closely and beat them off a slain animal, otherwise they will quickly devour it. They are always rewarded with a part of the intestines and some other portions, so that they may be keen for the next hunt.

Pigs run at large throughout the villages or in the neighboring underbrush. They are fed at night close to the dwellings, and thus become at least half tame. Many spend the hot hours of mid-day beneath the houses, from which they are occasionally driven by the irate housewives, when their squealing and fighting become unbearable. The domestic pigs are probably all descended from the wild stock with which they still constantly mix. Most of the young pigs are born with yellow stripes like the young of the wild, but they lose these marks in a short time. Castration of the young males is usually accomplished when the animals are about two months old.

Considerable numbers of chickens are raised. Nets or coops are arranged for them beneath the houses, but they run at large during the day time. Eggs are an important part of the food supply, but the fowls themselves are seldom killed or eaten, except in connection with the ceremonies. The domestic birds closely resemble the wild fowl of the neighborhood, and probably are descended from them. Except for a few strongly influenced settlements, cock-fighting has no hold upon this people.

The carabao or water buffalo is the most prized and valuable animal possessed by this tribe. As a rule, it is handled and petted by the children from the time of its birth, and hence its taming and breaking is a matter of little moment. In the mountain region about Lakub, where most of the animals are allowed to run half wild, only the strongest are broken. The animal is driven into an A-shaped pen, and a heavy pole is fastened across its neck just behind the horns. It is thus prevented from using its strength, and is loaded or ridden until it becomes accustomed to the treatment. Carabao are used for drawing the sleds and for plowing and harrowing in the lower fields. Should one be seriously injured, it would be killed and eaten; but strong animals are slaughtered only on very rare occasions. Wild carabao are fairly abundant in the mountains. They closely resemble the tame stock, and are generally considered to be derived from animals which have escaped.

46. Given the information presented in the third paragraph, which of the following statements could most reasonably be inferred?

   A. Adult pigs have yellow stripes

   B. Pigs are brought up as pets

   C. Young wild pigs do not have yellow stripes

   D. Pigs are brought up as a source of food

47. Of the following passage assertions, which one is LEAST supported by evidence or an example in the passage?

   A. The carabao is the most prized and valuable animal possessed by the tribe

   B. Domestic pigs are descended from the wild stock

   C. The squealing and fighting of pigs is annoying to some

   D. Well-fed dogs are lazy

48. Which of the following views is most contrary to the author's opinion regarding the treatment of water buffalo?

   A. Water buffalo are more valuable than horses.

   B. Water buffalo are primarily used for transportation.

   C. Water buffalo themselves are a main source of food for the tribe.

   D. Water buffalo are more important to the tribe than chickens and pigs.

49. Suppose that horses, cows, and goats became more abundant in the tribal community. Which of the following describes how they might be viewed by the tribe?

   A. Similar to how the dogs are viewed

   B. Similar to how the pigs are viewed

   C. Similar to how the chickens are viewed

   D. Similar to how the carabao are viewed

Passage 9 (Questions 50 – 53)

We now pass to Plato's central work, *The Republic*, which combines the humor, the vividly drawn characters, and the energetic dialogue of his earlier works with the more serious, more constructive, and more statesmanlike aims of his later career. The dialogue opens beautifully with Socrates and a companion walking home from a festival at the harbor of Athens when they come across some friends who convince them to come to the house of Cephalus, an old friend. The companions find the old man seated in his court and crowned, such as the custom was, for the celebration of a family sacrifice, and beaming happiness for his life well spent.

They all discuss the happiness of old age that comes for those who have done good and not evil, and who are not overly materialistic. To Cephalus, the good life is a very simple matter, centering around duty to God and duty to neighbors, according to what is prescribed and orderly. To him, this is sufficient, but not, of course, to Socrates.

Socrates raises doubts about one's duty in special circumstances, and the discussion is taken up not by Cephalus, "who goes away to the sacrifice," but by his son, and by the Sophist Thrasymachus, whose point is that the real meaning of justice is interest, and that might is right. With an analogy of the arts, Socrates shows that might devoid of justice is mere weakness, and that there is honor even among thieves. However, he does concede that the case for law working among individuals is weak, for they have many conflicting influences, chances, and difficulties that can obscure the relationship between action and happiness.

Therefore, for the sake of the debate, Socrates proposes a state in which justice is "writ large" for the community as a whole. Here, the relationship between individual and community is that of education and training, and many strange theories partially drawn from Sparta, including the equal training of men and women and the community of wives, are woven in. Then, the dialogue shifts, and Socrates raises the role of education from community training to the preparation of the soul for the heavenly life.

To represent the earthly life, Socrates describes men that have been, from birth, bound by chains in a cave, with their backs to the light, able only to see shadows cast upon the wall, shadows which they take as the only realities. Moreover, they can become skilled in interpreting the shadows. If you turn these men to the true light, says Socrates, they are overwhelmed and feel as though they have lost their reality and will be tempted to grope back to the familiar darkness and shadows.

But if they patiently struggle upwards until the sun itself can be seen, through more pain and more dazzling, they at last reach revelation. Now, if they return to the cave, they will see poorly and their fellows will see them as dreamers who have lost their way. Moreover, if these men who have seen heavenly truth try to enlighten these children of darkness and shadows, they may be persecuted or even killed.

Socrates says the world will never be right until those who have had a glimpse of the sun come back to the things of the earth and order them in accordance with the eternal verities. For this reason, if the perfect life is to be lived on earth, the philosopher must be king, and for the training of these ideal rulers, an ideal education is required, an education which Plato calls dialectic.

50.　Based upon the passage, the author most likely agrees with which of the following statements?

　A. Though seeing the sun brings enlightenment, living in the cave is preferable.

　B. Cephalus, his son, and Thrasymachus have no idea what they are talking about.

　C. Law and order can never work among individuals.

　D. Only a very few people have the capacity to rule the ideal state.

51.　Why does Socrates introduce his allegory of the cave?

　A. To illuminate his point that education is preparation of the soul for heavenly life

　B. To depict the misery of man and our hope of salvation in an easy to understand way

　C. To prove that most people are incapable of ruling a city or community

　D. To illustrate what he actually thinks of Cephalus and his simple idea of the good life

52.　Based upon the passage, which of the following statements is most true of dialectic?

　A. It is a form of education best taught to those who are most likely to end up "stuck in the cave."

　B. It is a difficult lifestyle that few will undertake and even fewer will be successful with.

　C. It is the highest of the human arts and should only be studied by the most intelligent.

　D. It is necessary for the equal training of men and women and the community of wives in Sparta.

53.　Say the parents of a child want her to become the President of the United States and they take the passage as a serious guide for her training. Based upon the passage, which of the following might be a reason that the parents would relent in forcing the child to learn via dialectic?

　A. The path of dialectic, of seeing the sun and then returning to the cave to enlighten those still stuck, is very difficult.

　B. The good life described by Cephalus, in its virtuous simplicity and grace, is far more appealing than the struggle of dialectic.

　C. If she is not subtle enough in lining up earthly things with the heavenly verities, she could be persecuted or killed.

　D. Because Socrates is not a politician and has no experience in actual lawmaking, he should not necessarily be trusted on this subject.

This page intentionally left blank.

SECTION 6

Answer Key

1	B	12	C	23	D	34	C	45	C
2	A	13	D	24	B	35	B	46	D
3	C	14	B	25	B	36	A	47	D
4	B	15	C	26	B	37	C	48	C
5	C	16	A	27	C	38	D	49	D
6	A	17	C	28	D	39	C	50	D
7	C	18	A	29	A	40	C	51	A
8	D	19	C	30	C	41	A	52	B
9	D	20	A	31	D	42	A	53	C
10	B	21	D	32	B	43	B		
11	B	22	A	33	C	44	A		

Passage 1 (Questions 1 – 6)

In 1947, the French artist **Jean Dubuffet** coined the term *art brut* to describe works created by artists who resided outside of artistic culture. *Art brut*, or "raw art" was, to Dubuffet "uncooked" – pure and unadulterated, **uninfluenced by artistic convention**, fashion, or intellectual trends. Writing about *art brut,* Dubuffet said "those works created from solitude and from **pure and authentic creative impulses** – where the worries of competition, acclaim and social promotion do not interfere – are, because of these very facts, **more precious** than the productions of professionals."

Key terms: Jean Dubuffet, *art brut*

Opinion: Dubuffet thought that artists who worked outside of artistic culture had pure and authentic creative impulses which created more precious art

Contrast: those who created outside of artistic culture vs those within it

Dubuffet's interest in *art brut* can be seen in the larger **cultural context** of the **rejection of the art establishment** by early to mid 20th century artists. The **Dada**, **Cubist**, **Futurist**, and **Surrealist** movements all abandoned certain cultural conventions in favor of new and sometimes jarring expressions. Artists like Pablo **Picasso** and Henri **Matisse** looked **away from "high" culture** and towards so-called primitive or naïve art, and incorporated elements in their work. While Dubuffet's description makes the work of those artists sound quite idyllic, the **solitude** of the artists he was applauding often stemmed from their **institutionalization**. Dubuffet's initial introduction to this sort of art was probably through a book entitled *Artistry of the Mentally Ill,* published in 1922 by a German psychiatrist. A massive volume illustrating the artwork of thousands of **psychiatric patients** across Europe, it drew the attention of several avant-garde artists of the time, including Dubuffet. Psychotics, mediums, religious fanatics, eccentrics – these were the artists whose outpourings were labeled "raw."

Key terms: cultural context, Dada, Cubist, Futurist, Surrealist, Picasso, Matisse

Cause and effect: the artists working in isolation were often institutionalized psychiatric patients, or people who lived on the margins of society

Several decades after Dubuffet's use of the term *art brut*, English art critic **Roger Cardinal** coined the term "**outsider art**" in 1972 to describe the work of artists outside of traditional art culture. To Cardinal, outsider art was a somewhat **broader category** than that described by Dubuffet; it included not just the works of artists with profound mental illness, but also works of people **outside of the mainstream** – **geographically** or **socially** isolated, living with **disabilities**, or simply **untrained**. In the United States, curators and critics began to look at American **folk art** differently, and the **lines between folk art and outsider art** began to **blur**: what critics conceived of as folk art, generally thought to embody traditional forms and social values, began to include more marginal and individualistic expressions.

Key terms: Roger Cardinal, outsider art, folk art

Opinion: Cardinal used the term outsider art to describe various artists working outside traditional art culture

Cause and effect: the outsider art movement broadened the definition of folk art

The **parameters** of outsider art have continued to **expand dramatically. Today**, outsider art is seen less as pathological and more as the creative expression of **individuals not conditioned by art history** or art world trends. Outsider artists come from all walks of life and cultures; the common denominator they share is **raw creativity**. Visionary art, folk art, naïve art: whatever the label, the common thread is that the artists are not traditionally schooled in art-making. Still, some of these artists have achieved enormous **commercial success**. Over the past two decades, **outsider art** has become a **highly saleable art category**, with several journals covering the subject, a yearly Outsider Art Fair in New York, representation of artists in respected galleries, and exhibition of works of outsider artists in major museums worldwide. It is ironic that the mainstream art world has embraced the outsiders, widely exhibiting their work, profiting on the efforts of those seemingly unaware of the art world's machinations. The question arises, too, of how artists working in some degree of isolation are influenced by attention and acclaim; does that attention necessarily bring the art world's own pathologies – which Dubuffet sought to defy in celebrating *art brut?*

Contrast: outsider art used to be outside the establishment but now outsider art is popular and valuable in the art community

Opinion: author questions whether the popularity and success of outsider artists will influence their work in the very way that Dubuffet criticized the art establishment

Main idea: Art brut and outsider art have evolved from a limited movement focused on the artistic outpourings of institutionalized individuals to a popular and commercially successful art category that encompasses several genres.

1. B is correct. Dubuffet values art brut because it is untouched by the influence of the art establishment, which he accuses of destroying the purity of the artistic creativity.

    A: We don't know whether he thinks mainstream art is technically skillful or not.

    C: Dubuffet probably believed this, but it's not supported by any evidence in the passage.

    D: We don't know if Dubuffet faulted the mainstream world for not acknowledging the avant-garde.

2. A is correct. Paragraph 3 discusses the relationship between folk art and outsider art: folk art usually reflects traditional cultures and values, but outsider art is more individualistic.

    B: No mention of the training of folk artists is in the passage.

    C: No evidence of this, according to the passage. The connections between mental illness and outside art was only one aspect at the very beginning of outsider art, not an enduring quality of it.

    D: There's no way of knowing whether folk art was more or less acceptable to the art establishment.

3. C is correct. In paragraph 2, we learn that the artists Dubuffet first celebrated were often profoundly mentally ill, and likely institutionalized.

4. B is correct. The paradox that is noted is that the attention to and commercial success of outsider artists may be sullying the very purity that defines the category.

5. C is correct. The passage notes that outsider art may be created by religious visionaries or fanatics, may, like folk art, include some traditional forms, and may be acclaimed and successful. The one thing it cannot be is created by artists who have been influenced by artistic convention.

6. A is correct. Paragraph 3 notes the overlap between outsider art and folk art. Outsider artists may be influenced by some traditional forms – for example, wood carving, beading, etc. – but the most important point is that the artist is self-taught and individualistic. It's possible, as correct choice A says, that such an artist might be considered an outsider.

    B: Commercial success does not preclude an artist from being considered an outsider.

    C: The passage notes that the distinction between folk and outsider art is blurry.

    D: But not all traditional art forms are considered outsider art.

Passage 2 (Questions 7 – 13)

Tularaemia is a **bacterial zoonotic** disease of the northern hemisphere. The bacterium (*Francisella tularensis*) is highly virulent for humans and a range of animals such as rodents, hares and rabbits. It may cause epidemics and epizootics. *F. tularensis* is **transmitted to humans** (i) by arthropod bites, (ii) by direct contact with infected animals, infectious animal tissues or fluids, (iii) by ingestion of contaminated water or food, or (iv) by inhalation of infective aerosols. There is **no human-to-human transmission**.

Key terms: Tularaemia, bacterial zoonotic

Contrast: ways disease can spread vs lack of human to human transmission

Cause and effect: arthropod bites, direct contact with infected animals or their bodies, ingesting contaminated water or food and inhaling aerosols can all result in Tularemia

Tularaemia is reported from most countries in the **northern hemisphere**, although its occurrence **varies widely** from one region to another. In some countries, endemic regions with frequent outbreaks are close to regions that are completely free of tularaemia. There is also a **wide variation with time**. In an endemic area, tularaemia may occur annually within a 5-year period, but may also be absent for more than a decade. The reasons for this temporal variation in the occurrence of outbreaks are **not well understood**. When, after a long lapse, the first case of a new outbreak appears, the disease may be more or less forgotten and is therefore not easily diagnosed. *F. tularensis* subspecies *tularensis* (type A) is one of the **most infectious pathogens known in human medicine**. The infective dose in humans is extremely low: 10 bacteria when injected subcutaneously and 25 when given as an aerosol (McCrumb, 1961; Saslaw et al., 1961; Saslaw et al., 1961). For example, on Martha's Vineyard in the United States of America, two adolescents contracted respiratory tularaemia after mowing a grassed area (Feldman et al., 2001). It is believed that an aerosol of *F. tularensis* subspecies *tularensis* was generated after the carcass of a rabbit which had died of tularaemia was accidentally shredded by the lawnmower.

Key terms: endemic regions, F. tularensis subspecies tularensis (type A)

Contrast: endemic areas and frequency of infection in them, with some areas having outbreaks next to those with none and some with frequent outbreaks and others with rare outbreaks

Cause and effect: not having seen an outbreak can lead to issues in diagnosing; a very small amount of bacteria can cause infection

The risk posed by tularaemia can be properly managed, provided the public health system is well prepared. In order to avoid **laboratory-associated infection**, safety measures are needed and consequently **clinical laboratories** do **not** generally **accept** specimens for culture. However, since clinical management of cases depends on early recognition, there is an **urgent need for diagnostic services**. In addition to its natural occurrence, *F. tularensis* causes great concern as a potential **bioterrorism agen**t. The **present guidelines** on tularaemia (i) provide background information on the disease, (ii) describe the current best practices for its diagnosis and treatment in humans, (iii) suggest measures to be taken in case of epidemics and (iv) provide guidance on how to handle *F. tularensis* in the laboratory. The **target groups** for these guidelines include **clinicians, laboratory personnel**, public health workers, veterinarians, and any other person with an interest in zoonoses.

Key terms: clinical laboratories, bioterrorism agent

Cause and effect: because safety measures are needed in handling tularaemia, many clinical laboratories will not accept specimens; because clinical management requires early recognition, there is an urgent need for diagnosis

The **guidelines** are the result of an **international collaboration**, initiated at a **WHO** meeting in Bath, United Kingdom of Great Britain and Northern Ireland in 2003, continued in Umeå, Sweden, in 2004 and finalized in Geneva, Switzerland, in 2005. Each chapter of the guidelines was developed by a selected group of **scientists with extensive developmental work** and general experience relevant to the field covered. Chairs of each group **met regularly throughout** the process to ensure consistency and for critical review. The document was also subject to internal and external peer reviews. As with many other areas, understanding of the nature of tularaemia and its causative agent is **evolving rapidly** across all aspects discussed in the guidelines, including taxonomy, epidemiology, epizootiology, detection, diagnostics, therapy and prophylaxis. It is envisaged therefore that **modifications to these guidelines will become necessary every three years**.

Key Terms: WHO meeting, Bath, United Kingdom, 2003, Umeå, Sweden, 2004, Geneva, Switzerland, 2005

Cause and effect: multiple meetings with scientists with lots of experience in the field led to guidelines; because understanding of tularaemia and its causes is evolving rapidly, modifications should be made every three years

Main Idea: The passage discusses what is known about the transmission of tularaemia, and the need for rapid diagnosis for clinical management; it sets up the need for guidelines in addressing the disease and how they came about.

7. C is correct. The third paragraph states that "in order to avoid laboratory-associated infection, safety measures are needed and consequently clinical laboratories do not generally accept specimens for culture".

    A: There is no discussion of the difficulty of detection in the passage.

    B: While the second paragraph states that diagnosis can be hindered because of lack of recognition of tularaemia, this is not linked to clinical testing.

    D: It is true that clinical management requires rapid detection, but this is not the reason laboratories don't wish to accept specimens.

8. D is correct. In the first paragraph, the passage states that "there is no human-to-human transmission."

    A, B: Since humans can catch the disease, it is not true that it can only be transmitted between animals, and there is no discussion of how readily it transmits animal to animal.

    C: There is no discussion of human to animal transmission.

9. D is correct. The author states that "the reasons for this temporal variation in the occurrence of outbreaks are not well understood. When, after a long lapse, the first case of a new outbreak appears, the disease may be more or less forgotten and is therefore not easily diagnosed." Later, the passage discusses how important diagnosis is in managing the disease.

    A: The passage focuses only on tularaemia, not all diseases and their relative danger.

    B, C: There is no discussion in the passage of the reasons for temporal variations or for levels of infectivity.

10. B is correct. The passage focuses on why tularaemia needs to be managed and the difficulties it poses, before discussing how the WHO guidelines were developed.

    A, C: Bioterrorism and aerosol-based spread are only very briefly discussed.

    D: While the passage does stress the need for better diagnosis and clinical response, it is too measured to be considered a manifesto; a manifesto is usually a very strong, ideological document that calls people to action about a particular political cause.

11. B is correct. The passage states that due to the fact that "understanding of the nature of tularaemia and its causative agent is evolving rapidly across all aspects discussed in the guidelines . . . it is envisaged . . . that modifications to these guidelines will become necessary every three years." Thus WHO encourages reassessment by scientists with experience, who are described as the developers of the guidelines.

    A: While the passage suggests that reassessment take place every three years, it does not name three years as a waiting period before making changes.

    C: Epizootiology is one of the aspects discussed in the passage, but there is no indication that it should receive special scrutiny.

    D: The passage suggests that tularaemia has potential as a bioterrorist threat, but does not make that the main focus of endeavors.

12. C is correct. Tularaemia can be transmitted to humans "(i) by arthropod bites," as in Choice II, "(ii) by direct contact with infected animals, infectious animal tissues or fluids, (iii) by ingestion of contaminated water or food," as in choice I, "or (iv) by inhalation of infective aerosols."

    III: An animal 25 feet away would be too far too inhale the aerosolized blood.

13. D is correct. The passage states that "the risk posed by tularaemia can be properly managed, provided the public health system is well prepared. In order to avoid laboratory-associated infection, safety measures are needed and consequently clinical laboratories do not generally accept specimens for culture. However, since clinical management of cases depends on early recognition, there is an urgent need for diagnostic services." Thus it is aimed at increasing laboratories willing to diagnose tularaemia, assuming this will lead to more rapid diagnosis and thus better management.

    A: There is no suggestion tularaemia could be prevented.

    B: The passage admits that the reason for temporal spacing is not clear, but still aims itself at clinicians.

    C: The threat of bioterrorism is not linked to clinical practice.

Passage 3 (Questions 14 – 18)

First, as to the science of **numbers**. So far as the acquirements of the **Phoenicians** on this subject are concerned it is impossible to speak with certainty. The magnitude of the commercial transactions of **Tyre** and **Sidon** necessitated a considerable development of **arithmetic**, to which it is probable the name of science might be properly applied. A **Babylonian** table of the numerical value of the **squares** of a series of consecutive integers has been found, and this would seem to indicate that properties of numbers were studied. According to **Strabo** the **Tyrians** paid particular attention to the sciences of numbers, **navigation**, and **astronomy**; they had, we know, considerable commerce with their neighbors and kinsmen the **Chaldaeans**; and **B'ockh** says that they regularly supplied the weights and measures used in Babylon. Now the Chaldaeans had certainly paid some attention to arithmetic and geometry, as is shown by their astronomical calculations; and, whatever was the extent of their attainments in arithmetic, it is almost certain that the Phoenicians were equally proficient, while it is likely that the knowledge of the latter, such as it was, was communicated to the **Greeks**. On the whole it seems probable that the early Greeks were largely indebted to the Phoenicians for their knowledge of practical arithmetic or the art of calculation, and perhaps also learnt from them a few properties of numbers. It may be worthy of note that **Pythagoras** was a Phoenician; and according to **Herodotus**, but this is more doubtful, Thales was also of that race.

Key terms: numbers, Phoenicians, Tyre, Sidon, arithmetic, Babylonian, squares, Strabo, Tyrians, navigation, astronomy, Chaldeans, B'ockh, Greeks, Pythagoras, Herodotus

Contrast: the Chaldeans and Phoenicians were probably similar in their mathematical attainment

Cause and effect: the Greeks were given their math knowledge by the Phoenicians, according to the author; astronomy and commerce led to the development of the theory of numbers and arithmetic in the ancient world.

Geometry is supposed to have had its origin in **land-surveying**; but while it is difficult to say when the study of numbers and calculation—some knowledge of which is essential in any civilized state—became a science, it is comparatively easy to distinguish between the abstract reasonings of geometry and the practical rules of the land-surveyor. Some methods of land-surveying must have been practiced from very early times, but the universal tradition of antiquity asserted that the origin of geometry was to be sought in **Egypt**. That it was not indigenous to **Greece**, and that it arose from the necessity of surveying, is rendered the more probable by the derivation of the word from γη˜, the earth, and μετρέω, I measure. Now the Greek geometricians, as far as we can judge by their extant works, always dealt with the science as an **abstract** one: they sought for theorems which should be **absolutely true**, and, at any rate in historical times, would have argued that to measure quantities in terms of a unit which might have been incommensurable with some of the

magnitudes considered would have made their results mere approximations to the truth. The name does not therefore refer to their practice. It is not, however, unlikely that it indicates the use which was made of geometry among the Egyptians from whom the Greeks learned it. This also agrees with the Greek traditions, which in themselves appear probable; for Herodotus states that the periodical inundations of the **Nile** (which swept away the landmarks in the valley of the river, and by altering its course increased or decreased the taxable value of the adjoining lands) rendered a tolerably accurate system of surveying indispensable, and thus led to a systematic study of the subject by the **priests**.

Key terms: Geometry, land-surveying, Egypt, Greece, abstract, absolutely true, Nile, priests

Contrast: the Greeks dealt with geometry in the abstract, while the Egyptians developed it for practical reasons

Cause and effect: geometry originated from land-surveying; the Egyptians developed geometry to prevent disasters from flooding; the Greeks learned geometry from the Egyptians

We have no reason to think that any special attention was paid to geometry by the **Phoenicians**, or other neighbors of the **Egyptians**. A small piece of evidence which tends to show that the **Jews** had not paid much attention to it is to be found in the mistake made in their sacred books, where it is stated that the circumference of a circle is three times its diameter: the **Babylonians** also reckoned that π **was equal to 3**.

Key terms: Phoenicians, Egyptians, 3, Jews, Babylonians

Contrast: the author believes the Phoenicians didn't know geometry like the Egyptians

Main Idea: The passage presents the history of mathematics and the author identifies groups that developed mathematical ideas and where those ideas were inherited from and how they originated.

14. B is correct. The passage states that "the Chaldaeans had certainly paid some attention to arithmetic and geometry, and, it is almost certain that the Phoenicians were equally proficient, while it is likely that the knowledge of the latter, such as it was, was communicated to the Greeks".

    A, C, D: These are not stated in the passage.

15. C is correct. The passage mentions that the Egyptians were forced to develop a system of land surveying because their survival depended on it. Knowing the land and what plots of land will best be able to produce food based on seasonal or periodic changes will necessitate the development of a geometry.

    A: A land surveying system might be useful to this civilization but not nearly so much as for farmers.

    B: A civilization living thusly would have the food they needed regardless of land surveying.

    D: There would be no need for a land surveying system for the survival of this civilization.

16. A is correct. The passage states that the Egyptians were good at geometry and that the Phoenicians paid less attention to it. The evidence given for this claim is that the Phoenicians thought that the ratio of a circumference of a circle to its diameter was 3. Thus we can assume the Egyptians knew better.

    B: The passage states that the Greeks developed geometrical theory more purely than the Egyptians.

    C: The passage gives no information to support this.

    D: Both groups erroneously believed that π is 3 but there is no reason to think that the Jews inherited it from the Babylonians; they may have come to that conclusion on their own or by borrowing the idea from another culture.

17. C is correct. The passage states that "the universal tradition of antiquity asserted that the origin of geometry was to be sought in Egypt".

18. A is correct. The author states that no neighbors of the Egyptians seemed to be interested in geometry. This would contradict that statement by suggesting that the Phoenicians cared enough about geometry to give a more accurate definition of π than simply rounding it to 3.

Passage 4 (Questions 19 – 25)

At this point you may think that the primary use of **logic** in the **real world** is to **deduce conclusions** from workable premises and to satisfy yourself that conclusions deduced by others are correct. If only it were! **Society** would be far less disposed to panics and other delusions, and politics especially would be an **entirely different thing** if even a majority of the **arguments** that are regularly broadcast across the world **were correct**. Rather, I fear the inverse is true. For every one workable pair of premises that leads to a logical conclusion you meet in newspapers or magazines or other media, you will find five that lead to no conclusion at all. Even when the premises are workable, for every **one** instance where the writer draws a **correct conclusion**, there are **ten** where they draw an **incorrect one**.

Opinion: author thinks most of what you read in the world is bad argumentation, with incorrect conclusions

In the case of the former, you may say, "The **premises** are **fallacious**." In the case of the latter, "The **conclusion** is **fallacious**." The primary use you will find for your new logical skills will actually be in **detecting these two types of fallacies**.

Opinion: author thinks that learning logic helps you spot fallacies, both fallacious premises and fallacious conclusions, rather than deducing conclusions yourself

You can **detect** the first kind, **fallacious premises**, when, after **marking them out** on the larger diagram, you attempt to move those marks to the smaller diagram. You will take the four compartments, one by one, and ask for each one, "What mark can I place here?" For every one, the answer will be, "Nothing." This of course shows that there is **no conclusion at all**. For example: "All soldiers are brave. Some Englishmen are brave. Therefore, some Englishmen are soldiers." This statement looks like a syllogism, with a conclusion drawn from two premises, and might easily fool a less experienced logician, but not you. Rather, you would simply set out the premises and then calmly **proclaim them to be fallacious**: you wouldn't condescend to ask what conclusion the writer professed to find, knowing that no matter what it is, it must be wrong. You would be safe like the wise mother who said, "Mary, go up to the nursery, see what Baby's doing, and tell him not to do it."

Cause and effect: if you attempt to move premises from the larger diagram to the smaller and you cannot discern any marks to put down for them, you have come across fallacious premises; thus you will not condescend to seek the conclusion because, as the premises were false, the conclusion must therefore also be false

You can detect the more difficult to spot second kind, **fallacious conclusions**, only after marking both diagrams, **reading of the correct conclusion**, and then **comparing** it with the **conclusion drawn by the writer**. Keep in mind, however, you ought not to immediately claim a conclusion to be fallacious simply because it is not identical to the correct

one. Rather, **it may be a part of the correct conclusion**, and be correct as far as it goes. In this case, you would call it a **defective conclusion**. Take for example this syllogism: "All unselfish people are generous. No misers are generous. Therefore, no misers are unselfish." These premises, expressed in letters, are as follows: "All not-x are m. No y are m."

Contrast: correct conclusion drawn from marking both diagrams vs the conclusion drawn by the writer, a fallacious conclusion vs a defective conclusion

Cause and effect: if you mark both diagrams and read the correct conclusion, you can compare it with the conclusion drawn by the writer; because a conclusion that is not identical to the correct one may be in part correct, you ought not to dismiss it as incorrect, but rather, as defective

The **correct conclusion** would be, "All not-x are not-y," or in other words, "**All unselfish people are not misers**," while the conclusion by the writer is, "No y are not-x," which is the same as "No not-x are y," and so is part of "All not-x are not-y." In this case, you would simply claim a defective conclusion. The same problem would arise if you were in a bakery and a little boy came in, **put down two pence**, and marched off with a **bun worth a single penny**. You would shake your head and say, "Defective conclusion. Poor chap!" Perhaps at this point you would ask the lady behind the counter whether she would let you eat the bun left behind by that poor chap, and perhaps she would reply, "You shall not!"

Contrast: defective conclusion (no misers are unselfish) vs correct conclusion (all unselfish people are not misers)

Cause and effect: because the conclusion drawn by the writer, no y are not-x, is the same as no not-x are y, then this conclusion is part of the correct conclusion (all not-x are not-y); because of this, you would claim the writer's conclusion as defective

Main Idea: The author addresses that the primary use of skill in logic is to spot the fallacious arguments put forth by others; the author goes into depth about the two types of fallacies, explaining how to detect them and how to deal with them.

19. C is correct. In the third paragraph, the author mentions these diagrams as if out of nowhere, suggesting that they have been mentioned earlier in the text. Moreover, it seems like the use of these diagrams is important and therefore was likely explained to the reader.

20. A is correct. In the second half of the first paragraph, the writer says that one of every five people is able to put together a workable pair of premises, while one of every ten people is able to draw the correct conclusion from correctly laid out premises. Therefore, 20% of people can put together a workable pair of premises, and only 2% of all people can correctly draw a conclusion from those correctly laid out premises. Therefore, more people can put together a workable pair of premises than can accurately draw a conclusion.

21. D is correct. The first syllogism requires less thinking through because we know from the improper putting together of premises no conclusion can be true. However, the second syllogism is partially correct, or is a defective conclusion. Therefore, it requires more looking into, and therefore, warrants the letter formulas where the first syllogism does not.

    A: This is not true.

    B: Rather, the author claims that some people will be fooled by it.

    C: The author does not seem to judge which type of fallacy is more egregious. Moreover, the first type is seemingly more egregious because it entails incorrectly setting up the premises right at the start of the argument.

22. A is correct. As was said before, the first noun is x, the second is y, and the adjective is m. Only Choice A satisfies this formula.

    B: This would translate to: No x are m. All y are not-m. Therefore, all x are y and all y are x.

    C: This would translate to : All x is m. All y is m. Therefore, all x and all y is m.

    D: This would translate to: All x and y are m. All z are not-m. Therefore, all x and y are not-z and all z are not-x and not-y.

23. D is correct. Rather, it can be used this way, but it is not the primary way it is used.

    A, B, C: These three choices are true and mentioned in the passage.

24. B is correct. The passage tells us in paragraph 4 that the second logical fallacy is harder to spot. So statement II is true, because an experienced logician is less likely to be fooled by the first fallacy, but may be fooled by the "harder to spot" second fallacy.

    I, III: Since the second fallacy is trickier, it's more likely to fool a logician, regardless of experience level.

25. B is correct. As the syllogism reads, "All soldiers are brave. Some Englishmen are brave. Therefore, some Englishmen are soldiers." As the pattern goes, the first noun is x, the second is y, and the adjective is m. So, given these rules, the syllogism translates to: All x are m. Some y are m. Therefore, some y are x. (Note: this syllogism has fallacious premises).

    A, C, D: As each of these options contains a negation, they cannot match the passage, as the third paragraph syllogism contains no negatives.

Passage 5 (Questions 26 – 32)

The **jenny**, invented in 1765 by the **weaver James Hargreaves**, was the **first invention** to bring about a radical change in the state of English workers. Instead of one spindle like the spinning-wheel used before, the jenny carried sixteen or eighteen spindles, manipulated by hand by a single workman, making it possible to **deliver more yarn than ever before**. Whereas one weaver used to employ three spinners and had to wait for yarn, there was now **more yarn than could actually be woven** by the available workers. Because of the diminished cost of production, the **price** of woven goods shot **down**, driving the already **increasing demand** for them even higher.

Key terms: jenny, James Hargreaves

Contrast: prior to the spinning jenny, getting spun yarn was the slow step in the process but after it came into use more yarn could be spun than there were weavers to work with it

Cause and effect: the improved production led to a drop in prices and an increase in demand

As such, **more weavers were needed**, and weaver's **wages** also **rose**. Now that the weavers could earn more at their looms, they gradually **abandoned farming**. At that time, a family of four adults and two children (who were often set to spooling) could earn, with eight hour work days, four pounds sterling per week, and oftentimes more if trade was good. In fact, a single weaver could often earn two pounds a week at his loom. Gradually, the **class of farming weavers disappeared**, reshaping itself into the class of weavers who lived entirely upon wages and had no property at all, not even the pretended property. Thus, **they became working-men, proletarians**.

Key terms: proletarians

Cause and effect: the increase in pay for weavers meant that many abandoned their small farms to do weaving full time, for the first time creating a class of workers who relied on wages

The **old relationship** between spinner and weaver was **destroyed**. Up until this historical moment, yarn had been spun and woven under one roof. Now that **both the jenny and the loom required a strong hand**, **men** began to spin as well as weave, and whole families lived by spinning while others laid their superseded spinning-wheels aside, and if they did not have the means to purchase a jenny, were forced to live entirely upon the wages of the father. This split of spinning and weaving **began the division of labor** that has since been perfected.

Cause and effect: the spinning jenny required a strong hand, leading some men to specialize solely in spinning; this started the division of labor and specialization that continues today

While the **industrial proletariat** was birthed from this still imperfect machine, the same machine gave rise to the **agricultural proletariat**. Up to this point, there had been a vast number of small land owners, **yeomen**, who had vegetated in the same unthinking peace as their neighbors, the farming weavers. These yeomen cultivated their land in the **inefficient fashion** of their ancestors and, after remaining stationary from generation to generation, **opposed every change** with the stubbornness characteristic of creatures of habit. Among them were also many small holders, those who had their land handed down from their fathers by hereditary lease of ancient force of custom, and who had held the land as securely as if it had been their own.

Contrast: industrial proletariat vs agricultural proletariat

Opinion: author thinks that the small yeoman farmers were stubborn, resisted change, and continued to work in the old-fashioned and very inefficient methods of the past

When the new industrial workers withdrew from farming, many of these small holdings became idle, and upon them the **new class of large tenants** established themselves, holding fifty to two hundred or more acres. Though they were liable to be turned out by year's end, they **improved tillage** and farming practices to **increase the land's yield**. Therefore, they **could sell produce more cheaply** than the yeomen, for whom nothing remained when their farms no longer supported them but to sell it, buy a jenny or loom, or become a farm laborer. Their inherited slowness and inefficient methods left them no alternative when forced to compete with those who **managed their holdings with sounder principles** and with the advantages bestowed by **large scale farming and capital investment** in the improvement of soil.

Cause and effect: since the new class of weavers and spinners abandoned their small farms, that created room for people to come in and set up large farms, making improvements that increased yield and lowered prices

Main Idea: The author sets out to briefly and generally explain how the invention of the jenny, a device which could spin wool much more efficiently than the spinning-wheel, led to the formation of the proletariat, by driving smaller farmers into industrial jobs.

26.   B is correct. As the author writes in the first paragraph, "Whereas one weaver used to employ three spinners and have to wait for yarn, there was now more yarn than could actually be woven by the available workers."

A: According to the passage, men did not spin wool until after the invention of the jenny.

C: Rather, large tenants appear after invention of the jenny.

D: Again, this happens after the invention of the jenny.

27.   C is correct. The passage asserts that: ". . . there had been a vast number of small land owners, yeomen, who had vegetated in the same unthinking peace . . . cultivated their land in the inefficient fashion of their ancestors . . . opposed every change with the stubbornness characteristic of creatures of habit." So, the word vegetated must be related to staying in an "unthinking peace," remaining stationery, and being stubborn to change. Slow and rooted seem to match this.

A: The author does not seem to be passing judgment on intelligence, but rather, on a type of culture.

B: This seems a bit harsh for the author's actual content and tone.

D: Rather, these two groups are put on the same level.

28.   D is correct. The chain of events described in this passage shows how the new found efficiency of the jenny began to disadvantage workers and began to increase the wealth and holdings of those who could buy large tracts of land, use sounder principles, and invest in the quality of the soil.

A: Not necessarily, for it did drive these working people away from their land and into laboring positions. Moreover, this invention actually led to the birth of the proletariat. Whereas land was more spread out before, after the invention, it is now more concentrated in fewer hands.

B: We don't get a sense if this is true or not, as the passage doesn't discuss the effect of cultural erosion.

C: The word "ought" is too strong here as the author never seems to suggest that the jenny (or any invention) somehow should have not been used or not been invented.

29.   A is correct. As the author writes about the former yeomen, now proletariat, "Their inherited slowness and inefficient methods left them no alternative when forced to compete . . ." This statement explains what makes these new large tenants so successful: sound principles, large scale farming, and capital investment in the improvement of soil.

B: More business savvy, yes. More intelligent–we can't be sure of that.

C: This is true, but the author doesn't use it as an explanation for the success of the large tenant farmers.

D: The price of goods actually went down.

30.   C is correct. Mr. Hargreaves was himself, as we know from the first sentence, a weaver. Therefore, any negative effects inflicted upon weavers are likely to be personal to him. Though wages did go up, these weavers lost their land and therefore became proletariats, and C tells us that the proletariat, or working class, has been often taken advantage of.

A: This is a positive outcome of his invention.

B: This can be seen as positive, and certainly be designing such an efficient machine, he may have expected this and we have no reason to think self-sufficiency was ever a virtue Mr. Hargreaves cared about.

D: Again, by making an efficient machine, it makes sense that he would have expected this as well.

31.   D is correct. The cost shot down.

32.   B is correct. Statement I is true because we know that men only started spinning after the invention of the jenny, because the jenny required a strong hand. Minus men, we are left with women and children. Statement II is true because we know that "Up until this historical moment, yarn had been spun and woven under one roof."

III: This is false because, of course, wool still needed to be spun in order to be woven. The relationship changed; the old relationship was gone, but a new one took its place.

Passage 6 (Questions 33 – 38)

By **directing the activities of the young**, **society** determines their **future**, and therefore, its own future. Because at some later date the young will compose the society of that period, the nature of society will be largely informed by the direction of children's activities in the earlier period. This effect, a cumulative **movement of action** towards a **later result**, is known as **growth**.

Cause and effect: because society determines the future of children by directing their activities, it determines its own future

The **first condition** of growth is **immaturity**. This may seem to be a simple truism, that anything that develops must first be undeveloped. But the prefix "im" actually refers to something **positive**, not merely a lack. To begin, we will look at the words "**capacity**" and "**potentiality**," both having a **double meaning, one negative and one positive**. Capacity can refer to mere receptivity, as in the capacity of a cup. Potentiality may refer to a dormant state: an ability to become something different with the influence of some external force. But capacity also has a power to it, and potentiality has a force to it. So, when we say that **immaturity** is the possibility of growth, we are not so much referring to the absence of things or abilities which may exist later, we are referring to a **positive force** that is present: the very **ability to develop**.

Contrast: growth vs immaturity, capacity vs potentiality, immaturity as an absence of things which may exist later vs immaturity as the ability to develop

Opinion: author thinks immaturity is positive; it represents the power to develop

We tend to view immaturity as a lacking and growth as that which fills the void. This is because we view childhood comparatively and not intrinsically: we treat it as a **lack** because we **compare** it to **adulthood** as a fixed standard, and therefore, our attention is set upon what the child lacks, what he will not have until adulthood. In some cases this **comparison is legitimate**, but if this is our **only way of viewing immaturity**, we may perhaps be guilty of overconfident analysis.

Contrast: viewing childhood comparatively vs viewing it intrinsically

Cause and effect: because we view childhood comparatively and not intrinsically, we tend to view immaturity as a lacking and growth as that which fills the void

Opinion: author says that is legitimate to compare childhood to adulthood, but that shouldn't be the only way to look at it

If children could express themselves articulately, they would tell a different story. Moreover, there is evidence to suggest that **for certain moral or intellectual purposes**, adults ought to **emulate children**. The problem of our assumption that **immaturity** is a **negative** quality is most apparent when we

consider that that it sets up a **static end as a standard**. Within this conception, the completion of growing is an accomplished growth, a state in which we no longer grow, an ungrowth. We can clearly observe the futility of this conception in the fact that **every adult resents** the notion of **no longer having an ability to grow**, and every adult will mourn this loss instead of falling back on all that has been achieved and considering it adequate. Why should there be an unequal measure for adult and child?

Opinion: there are some cases where adults should try to be like children; assuming a static end to growth is a bad thing

Taken in **absolute** and not comparative terms, **immaturity refers to a positive ability: the power to grow**. We do **not** have to **draw out** latent positive activities from a child, as some education doctrines would have it, for where there is life, there are already eager, impassioned activities. Growth is **not** something that is **done to children**. Rather, it is **something they do**. This positive aspect of **immaturity** allows us to understand its two primary traits: **dependence and plasticity**.

Opinion: author thinks that, on its own terms, immaturity is positive in power to grow

Contrast: the idea that growth is something done to children vs the idea that growth is something children do

Cause and effect: immaturity's two defining qualities are dependence and plasticity

It may seem absurd to claim **dependence** as something **positive**, but consider this: if **helplessness** were all there was to dependence, no development would ever take place and children would grow into adults that would need caring for throughout their whole lives. Dependence is accompanied by **growth in ability** and is therefore something constructive.

Opinion: author thinks dependence doesn't just mean helplessness

Cause and effect: if helplessness were the only element of dependence, children would not develop and would need caring for throughout their lives

A child's **plasticity** is his **adaptability** for growth, and it is something quite different than the plasticity of putty. It is **not** so much the ability to change form in accord with **external pressure**, but rather, the **ability to learn from experience**, to **retain** something from one **experience** that will be useful in another. It is the power to modify actions based upon the results of what has happened before. Without this, the acquisition of habits and growth itself would be impossible.

Cause and effect: because a child has plasticity he can learn from past experience and retain useful lessons for later

Contrast: plasticity of a child (learning) vs plasticity that just conforms to external pressure

Main Idea: The passage sets out to demonstrate that "immaturity" is not merely a negative term, but can also be viewed as a positive one; it makes the case that immaturity refers to a potential to grow, and it shows the fallacy of comparing childhood to adulthood as a fixed standard; rather, we ought to view immaturity as a positive condition.

33.   C is correct. The first sentence expresses how children, if they were able, would likely paint a more accurate picture of childhood than adults. The second sentence asserts that there is evidence to support the notion that adults ought to act like children sometimes, meaning there must be something inherently good and worthy about being a child. Moreover, the whole passage has the ongoing theme of a misunderstanding of immaturity, and therefore, childhood.

   A: The passage only suggests that adults should emulate children in some circumstances, not that they are more wise.

   B: Rather, it ought to be viewed intrinsically, or absolutely.

   D: Rather, these statements are somewhat vague and general. They are more focused on the misunderstanding of adults than the actual nature of children.

34.   C is correct. The author writes of immaturity in positive terms, referring to it as a positive force. Moreover, he goes so far as to describe how adults do not take kindly to being told they can no longer grow. For the author, immaturity is the ability to grow and develop; it is the potential that all people, young and old, hold dear.

   A: The author tells us that adults resent the idea that they cannot grow anymore.

   B: Though the author does take issue with one particular type of doctrine, he never says there should be no doctrines.

   D: This is never said. Rather, adults ought to emulate children in some occasions. That doesn't make children adult-like.

35.   B is correct. As the author writes at the beginning of the seventh paragraph, "A child's plasticity is his adaptability for growth . . . [i]t is the power to modify actions based upon the results of what has happened before. Without this, the acquisition of habits and growth itself would be impossible." For the author, plasticity refers to the ability to acquire habits.

   A: Rather, dependence is accompanied by growth in ability.

   C: This is never said. The author is concerned with learning in general, not physical adaptation.

D: This may be somewhat true, but in the terms of the passage, "latent, positive activities" is mentioned earlier, in relation to childhood itself.

36.   A is correct. As the author writes in the fifth paragraph, "We do not have to draw out latent positive activities from a child, as some education doctrines would have it, for where there is life, there are already eager, impassioned activities." Instead of drawing activities out of children, allow them to play how they will and create a curriculum around that.

   B: This choice mirrors what we do NOT have to do, according to the author.

   C: The author believes the relationship between childhood and adulthood ought to be viewed intrinsically, not comparatively.

   D: It seems the author believes these qualities are inherent to children.

37.   C is correct. As the author writes in the third paragraph, "We treat [childhood] as a lack because we compare it to adulthood as a fixed standard." Here, variable is the opposite of fixed.

   A, B, D: These are all true, according to the passage.

38.   D is correct. Items I, II, and III are all true and are discussed explicitly in the passage.

Passage 7 (Questions 39 – 45)

But it is otherwise with **moral laws**. These, in contradistinc-tion to **natural laws**, are **only valid** as laws, insofar as they can be **rationally** established a priori and **comprehended as necessary**. In fact, conceptions and judgments regarding ourselves and our conduct have **no moral significance**, if they contain only what may be learned from **experience**; and when any one is, so to speak, misled into making a mor-al principle out of anything derived from this latter source, he is already in danger of falling into the coarsest and most fatal errors.

Key terms: moral laws; natural laws

Contrast: moral laws, which require a priori establishment and comprehension as to necessity vs natural laws

Cause and effect: basing moral principles on observation leads to the danger of error

If the philosophy of morals were nothing more than a theory of happiness (**eudaemonism**), it would be absurd to search after principles a priori as a foundation for it. For however plausible it may sound to say that reason, even prior to experience, can comprehend by what means we may attain to a lasting enjoyment of the real pleasures of life, yet all that is taught on this subject a priori is either tauto-logical, or is assumed wholly without foundation. It is **only experience that can show what will bring us enjoyment**. The natural impulses directed towards nourishment, the sexual instinct, or the tendency to rest and motion, as well as the higher desires of honour, the acquisition of knowledge, and such like, as developed with our natural capacities, are alone capable of showing in what those enjoyments are to be found. And, further, the **knowledge thus acquired is available for each individual merely in his own way**; and it is only thus he can learn the means by which he has to seek those enjoyments. All specious rationalizing a priori, in this connection, is nothing at bottom but carrying facts of expe-rience up to generalizations by induction (*secundum principia generalia non universalia*); and the **generality** thus attained is **still so limited that numberless exceptions must be allowed to every individual** in order that he may adapt the choice of his mode of life to his own particular inclinations and his capacity for pleasure. And, after all, the individual has really to acquire his prudence at the cost of his own suffering or that of his neighbors.

Key terms: eudaemonism; generalizations by induction

Contrast: belief in necessary principles for a morals based on happiness texts absurdity of such an idea in operation

Cause and effect: because only experience can teach us what causes happiness, a principle of happiness cannot demand rational reasoning; because enjoyment is individual such a theory cannot be universal and may cause suffering of others

But it is quite otherwise with the **principles of morality**. They lay down **commands for every one** without regard to

his particular inclinations, and merely because and so far as he is free, and has a practical reason. Instruction in the laws of morality is not drawn from observation of oneself or of our animal nature, nor from perception of the course of the world in regard to what happens, or how men act. But **reason** commands how we **ought to act**, even although no example of such action were to be found; nor does reason give any regard to the **advantage** which may accrue to us by so acting, and which experience could alone actually show. For, although **reason** allows us to seek **what is for our advan-tage** in every possible way, and although, founding upon the evidence of experience, it may further promise that greater advantages will probably follow on the average from the observance of her commands than from their transgression, especially if prudence guides the conduct, yet the **authority of her precepts as commands does not rest on such con-siderations**. They are used by reason only as counsels, and by way of a counterpoise against seductions to an opposite course, when adjusting beforehand the equilibrium of a partial balance in the sphere of practical **judgment**, in order thereby to secure the decision of this judgment, according to the due weight of the a priori principles of a pure practical reason.

Contrast: advantage by acting vs seductions to an opposite course

Cause and effect: ideally, people use reason to come to prac-tical judgment

Main Idea: The passage differentiates between natural laws, which are based on observation, and moral laws, which should be based on reason and developed as necessary principles; this also means, the author argues, that moral laws are not founded on the principle of happiness nor of advantage and cannot be reasoned out based on experience.

39. C is correct. The passage states that "the principles of morality…lay down commands for every one with-out regard to his particular inclinations, and merely because and so far as he is free, and has a practical reason."

   A: The passage argues that moral laws cannot be based on the principle of happiness, as in choice.

   B: While the passage states moral laws must be rational, it does not argue they derive from practical reasons.

   D: Natural laws are differentiated from moral laws.

40. C is correct. Moral laws, in the passage, are opposed to natural laws, "in so far as they can be rationally established a priori and comprehended as necessary." Additionally, "if they contain only what may be learned from experience" they may lead to bad judgments. Thus moral laws cannot be based on observation, un-like the natural laws to which they are opposed.

   A: Natural and moral laws are compared in terms of their derivation, but not their validity, as in choice A.

B: It is focusing only on experience, not natural laws in total, that can lead to moral errors.

D: Moral, not natural, laws must be derived rationally.

41. A is correct. In the second paragraph, the author objects to "specious rationalizing a priori," which is defined as "carrying facts of experience up to generalizations by induction," adding that "the generality thus attained is still so limited that numberless exceptions must be allowed to every individual in order that he may adapt the choice of his mode of life to his own particular inclinations and his capacity for pleasure." Thus generalization is not valuable when it allows exceptions based on personal inclinations.

B: Moral laws should be derived a priori, according to the passage.

C: This is the opposite of what is stated in the passage.

D: While the author links bad generalizations to causing suffering, preventing suffering is not discussed in the passage.

42. A is correct. The passage argues against using either post facto experience or the principle of happiness.

B: Based on the passage, rationality, or reason, is what commands us to act morally.

C: The passage never discusses the idea of integrating laws which ought to be derived on such different bases.

D: The passage does not dismiss generalizations, just those which allow exceptions.

43. B is correct. The passage argues that "conceptions and judgments regarding ourselves and our conduct have no moral significance, if they contain only what may be learned from experience; and when any one is, so to speak, misled into making a moral principle out of anything derived from this latter source, he is already in danger of falling into the coarsest and most fatal errors." Thus basing actions on the basis of experience in the form of observations, as in the case of the visitor, would be problematic for the author due to the lack of reasoning.

A: In the passage, attending to our own animal nature leads to moral flaws.

C, D: These are both positive, but the passage author would have a negative view of an ethical decision made on the basis of experience and conformity alone.

44. A is correct. Paragraph two, which focuses on eudaemonism, lists "the natural impulses directed towards nourishment," as in choice D, "the sexual instinct," as in choice C, "or the tendency to rest and motion, as well as the higher desires of honour," as in choice B,

as well as "the acquisition of knowledge, and such like, as developed with our natural capacities," as "enjoyments." Choice A is the one not discussed here and thus the credited answer.

45. C is correct. In discussing eudaemonism, the passage states that "all that is taught on this subject a priori is either tautological, or is assumed wholly without foundation. It is only experience that can show what will bring us enjoyment." Thus choice C, in which previous experience is mentioned, is the credited answer.

A: Rational principles are required of moral laws, not connected to tautologies.

B: This is the opposite of what is stated in the passage.

D: Eudaemonism is based upon inclinations, but it is not always tautological according to the passage.

Passage 8 (Questions 46 – 49)

Dogs, pigs, chickens, and carabao appear to have been long in the possession of the **Tinguian** tribe. **Horses, goats, and cattle** are now owned by some of the people, but only the former are of sufficient number to be considered important.

Key terms: dogs, pigs, chickens, carabao, Tinguian tribe, horses, goats, cattle

Opinion: the author believes that horses, goats, and cattle are not found in sufficient number to be considered important to the Tinguian tribe

The dogs are **surly, ill-kept** creatures of **mongrel** breed. They are seldom treated as **pets**, but are kept for **hunting**. Well-fed dogs are considered lazy, and hence they are fed only with a rice gruel, which seems to be neither fattening nor satisfactory. When in the village, the **miserable creatures** wander about under the houses, there to pick up and fight over morsels which may drop from above, or they lie in the ashes of the bonfires, the better to protect themselves from fleas and other enemies. When used in **hunting**, they are kept in leash until the game is started. When released, they **follow the quarry at full cry**, and if the game has been injured, they will seldom give up the chase. It is necessary for the hunters to follow the dogs closely and beat them off a slain animal, **otherwise they will quickly devour it**. They are always **rewarded with a part** of the intestines and some other portions, so that they may be keen for the next hunt.

Key terms: mongrel, pets, hunting

Opinion: the dogs are considered surly, mongrel, miserable creatures

Cause and effect: dogs are fed with rice gruel to keep them thin and desperate on the hunt

Pigs **run at large** throughout the villages or in the neighboring underbrush. They are fed at night close to the dwellings, and thus become at least **half tame**. Many spend the hot hours of mid-day beneath the houses, from which they are occasionally driven by the **irate housewives**, when their squealing and fighting become unbearable. The **domestic** pigs are probably all descended from the **wild stock** with which they still constantly mix. Most of the young pigs are born with **yellow stripes** like the young of the wild, but they lose these marks in a short time. **Castration** of the young males is usually accomplished when the animals are about **two months** old.

Key terms: half tame, irate housewives, domestic, yellow stripes, castration

Opinion: the squealing and fighting of the pigs is considered unbearable by the tribe housewives

Cause and effect: the young pigs have yellow stripes which are lost in adulthood; we are not told whether wild pigs lose the stripes or not

Considerable numbers of chickens are raised. **Nets or coops** are arranged for them beneath the houses, but they run at large during the day time. **Eggs** are an important part of the food supply, but the fowls themselves are **seldom killed or eaten**, except in connection with the ceremonies. The domestic birds closely resemble the **wild fowl** of the neighborhood, and probably are **descended from them**. Except for a few strongly influenced settlements, cock-fighting has no hold upon this people.

Key terms: nets or coops, eggs, wild fowl

Cause and effect: chickens are descended from the wild fowl

The carabao or **water buffalo** is the **most prized** and valuable animal possessed by this tribe. As a rule, it is **handled and petted by the children from the time of its birth**, and hence its **taming** and breaking is a matter of little moment. In the mountain region about **Lakub**, where most of the animals are allowed to run half wild, only the strongest are broken. The animal is driven into an A-shaped pen, and a heavy pole is fastened across its neck just behind the horns. It is thus prevented from using its strength, and is loaded or ridden until it becomes accustomed to the treatment. Carabao are used for **drawing the sleds** and for plowing and harrowing in the lower fields. Should one be seriously injured, it would be killed and eaten; but **strong animals are slaughtered only on very rare** occasions. Wild carabao are fairly abundant in the mountains. They closely resemble the tame stock, and are generally considered to be derived from animals which have escaped.

Key terms: water buffalo, taming, Lakub

Opinion: the author believes the carabao to be the most valuable animal to the tribe

Cause and effect: a carabao will only be eaten if injured; wild carabao are thought to be derived from the tame animals.

Main Idea: the author is describing the significance of animal life to the Tinguian Tribe. It appears that the author is an objective third party. Carabao are the most important of the common animals.

46. D is correct. The passage states that the pigs are cared for but does not mention their purpose. We can assume they are not used as beasts of labor or for hunting. The only reason they would be cared for would be to eat them later on.

   A: The passage mentions that the wild and tame young pigs have yellow stripes. The passage then states that the tame pigs lose the stripes.

   B: The passage states that the pigs are often seen as a nuisance.

   C: The passage states that the young wild pigs have yellow stripes.

47. D is correct. The passage states that the tribes people thought well-fed dogs were lazy, but there is no evidence as to whether they actually are.

   A: The last paragraph explains why the carabao are the most prized.

   B: The passage gives the appearance of the pigs as evidence of their descending from wild stock.

   C: The passage gives an example of who finds the pigs fighting annoying.

48. C is correct. The passage states that water buffalo are only seldom eaten.

   A: The passage states that water buffalo are the most prized and valuable animal possessed by the tribe. This view may or may not be true but doesn't seem very contrary to the author's opinions.

   B: The passage states that the water buffalo are primarily used to pull sleds or be ridden.

   D: This is expressed in the passage.

49. D is correct. The passage suggests that carabao are more respected because of their utility as beasts of labor. The horses goats and cows would be very useful to the tribe in a similar way and thus would probably be treated similar to the way carabao are treated.

   A: The horses, cows, and goats would not be treated like the dogs, since the ill treatment of dogs seems primarily to hinge on keeping them on edge for the hunt.

   B: The pigs are not beasts of burden like horses and goats.

   C: The chickens are purely a source of food, unlike horses, cows, and goats.

Passage 9 (Questions 50 – 53)

We now pass to **Plato's central work**, *The Republic*, which combines the **humor**, the vividly drawn characters, and the **energetic** dialogue of his earlier works with the **more serious**, more constructive, and more statesmanlike **aims** of his later career. The dialogue opens beautifully with Socrates and a companion walking home from a festival at the harbor of Athens when they comes across some friends who convince them to come to the house of **Cephalus**, an old friend. The companions find the old man seated in his court and crowned, such as the custom was, for the celebration of a family sacrifice, and beaming happiness for his **life well spent**.

Contrast: Plato's early work vs his later work

Opinion: author thinks highly of *The Republic* describing it in positive terms

They all discuss the **happiness of old age** that comes for those who have **done good** and not evil, and who are not overly materialistic. To **Cephalus**, the **good life** is a very simple matter, centering around **duty** to God and duty to neighbors, according to what is prescribed and orderly. To him, this is sufficient, but not, of course, to Socrates.

Contrast: Cephalus thinking his simple definition of the good life is sufficient vs Socrates's estimation

Cause and effect: according to Cephalus, if you have done good, have not been overly materialistic, and have been dutiful, you will have a good life

Socrates raises doubts about one's duty in **special circumstances**, and the discussion is taken up not by Cephalus, "who goes away to the sacrifice," but by his son, and by the **Sophist Thrasymachus**, whose point is that the real meaning of justice is interest, and that might is right. With an analogy of the arts, Socrates shows that **might devoid of justice** is mere **weakness**, and that there is honor even among thieves. However, he does concede that the case for law working among individuals is weak, for they have many conflicting influences, chances, and difficulties that can obscure the relationship between action and happiness.

Key terms: the sophist Thrasymachus

Contrast: normal circumstances vs special circumstances, Thrasymachus's understanding of justice vs what Socrates shows

Cause and effect: because Thrasymachus expresses his point about justice and might, Socrates demonstrates with an example that might without justice is weakness

Therefore, for the sake of the debate, Socrates proposes a state in which justice is "writ large" for the community as a whole. Here, the **relationship** between **individual and community** is that of **education and training**, and many strange theories partially drawn from Sparta, including the equal training of men and women and the community of wives,

are woven in. Then, the dialogue shifts, and **Socrates** raises the role of **education** from community training to the **preparation of the soul** for the heavenly life.

Contrast: education as preparation for the community vs as preparation of the soul for the heavenly life

To represent the **earthly life**, Socrates describes men that have been, from birth, **bound by chains in a cave**, with their backs to the light, able only to see shadows cast upon the wall, **shadows** which they take as **the only realities**. Moreover, they can become skilled in interpreting the shadows. If you turn these men to the **true light**, says Socrates, they are overwhelmed and feel as though they have **lost their reality** and will be tempted to **grope back to the familiar darkness** and shadows.

Contrast: shadows vs the true light

Cause and effect: in order to represent the earthly life, Socrates introduces his allegory of the cave; because the men in the cave only see shadows, they consider them the only reality and become skilled at interpreting them; if the men of the cave are released and turned towards the true light, they will be overwhelmed

But if they **patiently struggle** upwards until the sun itself can be seen, through more pain and more dazzling, they at last **reach revelation**. Now, if they **return to the cave**, they will **see poorly** and their fellows will see them as dreamers who have lost their way. Moreover, if these men who have seen heavenly truth **try to enlighten** these children of darkness and shadows, they may be **persecuted or even killed**.

Contrast: reaching revelation vs returning to the cave, men who have seen heavenly truth vs children of darkness and shadows

Cause and effect: if those who made it out try to enlighten the ones who haven't, they may be persecuted or killed

Socrates says the **world will never be right** until those who have had a **glimpse of the sun come back to** the things of the **earth** and order them in accordance with the eternal verities. For this reason, if the perfect life is to be lived on earth, **the philosopher must be king**, and for the training of these ideal rulers, an **ideal education** is required, an education which Plato calls **dialectic**.

Cause and effect: if those who have escaped the cave and seen the sun return to the cave and order the things of earth in accordance with the heavenly things, the world will be right

Main Idea: The passage is a selection from a summary of Plato's Republic, describing the story behind the dialogue and the main ideas it explores, those being, the nature of justice and law, the ability of people to maintain these things themselves, and the nature of the ideal state, up until Socrates's famous allegory of the cave, which demonstrates the difference between the earthly world and the heavenly world. The ideal ruler of an ideal city must experience the heavenly world.

50. D is correct. The fifth and sixth paragraphs describe the allegory of the cave and difficulty of crawling out, seeing the true light, and coming back to deal with those who have only ever seen shadows. In the seventh paragraph, Socrates argues that the world will only be right when those people who have made the difficult journey, those people being philosophers, are able to order the things of earth in accordance with heavenly verities. For this reason, he says that the philosopher must be king in an ideal state. Given the difficulty of this undertaking, it can be assumed that he believes only a very few people can be philosophers in the sense that he means and be able to rule his ideal state.

   A: This is never said, and is perhaps the opposite of the case.

   B: They do, they are coming from different perspectives. The genius of Socrates is to investigate their claims, to engage in dialectic. Maybe he proves them wrong, but that doesn't mean that they don't know what they are talking about.

   C: As the author writes, "there is honor even among thieves." Socrates concedes that "the case for law working among individuals is weak," not nonexistent.

51. A is correct. The introduction of the cave allegory in the fifth paragraph directly follows the shift of the dialogue described at the end of the fourth. The cave allegory is about the tension between the earthly life and the spiritual life, and education is compared to becoming unchained and getting a glimpse of the true light.

   B: It's not really easy to understand, and Socrates's goal is not to demonstrate our misery and suffering, but to demonstrate how we may overcome it.

   C: Though this is true, he is not setting out to prove it; his main goal is to show how one can become educated when education is "the preparation of the soul for the heavenly life."

   D: This is not true or hinted at.

52. B is correct. Again, if dialectic is the education of the philosopher, and it involves escaping from the cave, seeing the true light, and returning to order the things of the cave in accordance with that true light, then dialectic is very difficult. Only a few people will undertake it and even fewer will be successful in this pursuit and worthy of ruling Socrates's ideal state.

   A: Rather, it could be argued that it would be best to teach it to those with an innate quality making them less likely to be stuck. Moreover, Socrates never says it should be taught to some and not all and he does not exclude anyone.

C: Again, this is not said.

D: This is not true; those details are thrown in to demonstrate how Socrates' interlocutors find his ideas about ideal state strange.

53. C is correct. At the end of the sixth paragraph, the author writes, "Moreover, if these men who have seen heavenly truth try to enlighten these children of darkness and shadows, they may be persecuted or even killed." Sounds risky. Note that Socrates does not say these enlightened people should avoid these possibly dangerous cave people. Rather, they should try to order the things of the earth, the cave, in accordance with the eternal verities, or the sun, the true light. So, the enlightened person cannot attempt to directly enlighten his or her former comrades, but rather, should align the rules and the laws of the cave with truth. This must take a certain degree of subtlety, to not come across as someone trying to enlighten the people of the cave. Obviously parents don't want their children persecuted or killed.

   A: Yes, it is very difficult, but if parents want their children to be President, they must have some understanding that it will be difficult.

   B: While that sounds like a good life, if you want to be President, according to this passage, you have to engage with dialectic and go deeper than Cephalus's simple standards for the good life.

   D: Socrates is not a politician, but he is well versed in the art of dialectic, which is, in this passage at least, the primary education for a philosopher, and only philosophers should be ruler or politicians, at least in the ideal state explained here.

SECTION 7
53 Questions, 90 Minutes
Use an answer grid from the back of the book to record your answers

Passage 1 (Questions 1 – 5)

Experienced tuberculosis controllers are keenly aware of the discrepancies between the theory and the reality of finding and treating latent tuberculosis infection (LTBI). Although the guidelines about LTBI appear to be straightforward on the surface, in truth the tasks are challenging, and efficiency and effectiveness are difficult to achieve. In this section, we review the general principles that influence the success of your prevention activities.

The success of your prevention activities is governed by three elements that we all need to balance simultaneously in order to have successful public health interventions. These elements are: (1) finding and accurately diagnosing LTBI, (2) determining the urgency of treatment, and (3) completely treating the patients who have LTBI. Problems in any of these three areas will detract from the success of your activities. For example, if you start a project that finds dozens of at-risk patients who have LTBI but none of the patients start or complete treatment, the project does not contribute to tuberculosis prevention. ARPEs give you a broad overview that helps you to find problems and to strike a balance among the three elements.

Finding and accurately diagnosing LTBI depends on the prevalence rate of LTBI in the population that is under consideration. The prevalence rate refers to how common LTBI is, and it is a population characteristic that reflects the tuberculosis history of the population. The prevalence rate controls how many infected individuals you will discover by testing. This is your yield of LTBI. The minimum prevalence rate for a successful strategy is unknown, but you need to take a critical look at the balance of the three elements if you are testing in a population having an LTBI prevalence rate less than 10 percent. The LTBI prevalence rate also influences the accuracy of the tuberculin skin test. This is because the predictive value of a positive test result depends on the prevalence rate. When the prevalence rate is low, the predictive value of a positive result is also low. For example, when the LTBI prevalence rate falls below 10 percent, most of the patients with positive results from the skin test actually will have false-positive results. Therefore, when the prevalence rate of LTBI is low, most of the patients who are being treated for LTBI are actually not at risk for tuberculosis because they do not even have LTBI. This is wasteful of resources and possibly hazardous to the patients.

The urgency of treatment for LTBI patients depends on how likely they are to get sick with active tuberculosis. If the likelihood of active tuberculosis is high, then the urgency of treatment is high. One example is the patients who have been recently exposed to contagious tuberculosis (i.e., contacts). We also worry about patients who have medical problems that change their immune capacity: co-infection with the human immunodeficiency virus (HIV) is a very serious example. The urgency of treatment is relative. No one can predict which patients with LTBI are going to become sick with tuberculosis. The risk of tuberculosis might be high, medium, or low, and this determines the urgency of

treatment. The current medical condition and the tuberculosis exposure history are factors to consider when determining the urgency of treatment for an individual. The final decision to treat rests with the individual patient and the prescribing provider.

Sometimes the urgency of treatment offsets the concerns about testing a population with a low LTBI prevalence rate. For example, infants who might have been exposed to contagious tuberculosis should be tested even if the exposure was minimal because infection could be very dangerous for them. In this example, the concern about the danger of tuberculosis overrides the low yield of testing.

1. Based on the passage, low yields of LTBI are not a factor when it comes to:

    A. the risks of false positives.

    B. any infant in an affected area.

    C. predicting the likelihood of a particular patient getting sick.

    D. those who have an extremely high risk of infection.

2. The author assumes which of the following when discussing the problems inherent in balancing diagnosing, determining the urgency of treatment, and treatment?

    A. Getting patients to complete treatment is often the most difficult element.

    B. All three elements must be equally balanced for successful treatment.

    C. Finding at-risk patients is of the prime importance in prevention.

    D. Tuberculosis prevention is the primary goal of such interventions.

3. Suppose that physicians reviewed a preventive activity and discovered that many of those treated did not actually have LTBI. Based on the passage, the author would most likely suggest that:

    A. the prevalence rate was most likely in the single digits.

    B. those treated were most likely at a high risk of co-infection due to immune-compromising diseases.

    C. all three elements of prevention had been properly addressed.

    D. since no one can predict who will fall ill with tuberculosis, an extremely aggressive approach is called for.

4. Which of the following would most weaken the author's argument?

    A. The prevalence rate is shown to connect to the number of individuals infected with LTBI discovered by testing.

    B. Experts well versed in the theory of tuberculosis prevention have been found to create ineffective practices.

    C. A program that focused on diagnosing LTBI and treating patients to the exclusion of all other goals was shown to be effective in contributing to tuberculosis prevention.

    D. Tuberculosis has been shown to cause multi-system infections that can spread rapidly after the initial incubation period, although the prevalence of such cases is low.

5. All of the following are factors in the urgency of treatment EXCEPT:

    A. ability to predict those who will actually become sick.

    B. the opinions of the patient and his or her doctor.

    C. co-infection with an immunosuppressant disease.

    D. contact with a contagious patient.

Passage 2 (Questions 6 – 10)

"Revelations," choreographer Alvin Ailey's masterwork, has been in Alvin Ailey American Dance Theater's repertory since its creation in 1960. In that time, the piece has been viewed by more than 23 million people in 71 countries worldwide – more than any other modern dance piece. Created by Ailey when he was 29 years old, the work draws on his recollections of his childhood in the rural south, and his experiences in his small church. Ailey described the memories that informed Revelations as "blood memories" – experiences so strong that they were as present and important to him as the blood running through his veins.

Revelations is divided into three sections, each of which contains several dances. The first section, entitled "Pilgrim of Sorrow," has to do with "the burden of life," said Ailey, and portrays dancers yearning for salvation in the face of their difficulties. Dancers, huddled together with heads bowed, lit by a single spotlight, stretch their open-palmed hands heavenward, only to be pulled back to earth. Dressed in drab, earth-toned garments, the dancers evoke sorrow and hardship, elements of African American life that were particularly familiar to Alvin Ailey, who was raised in segregated Texas in the 1930s by a single mother.

In "Take Me To the Water," the second section of Revelations, the dancers, clad in white, stage a ceremonial baptism. To the sounds of the traditional spiritual "Wade in the Water," dancers move across the stage in motions that represent water – undulating arms, sinuous hips – and yards of billowing blue silk represent the river, in which a pair of dancers is "baptized" by a devotional leader bearing a large umbrella. The baptismal is based on Ailey's recollections of his own baptism, which took place in a pond behind his church. Yet even if you don't share Alvin Ailey's personal experience of baptism, "Take Me To the Water" still speaks of the possibility of transformation: according to one of Ailey's dancers, this section is about "cleansing and changing and becoming someone better."

"Move, Members, Move," the third section, suggests a congregation in church on a hot day. Dancers seem to gossip, fan themselves against the heat, and look about the church – all motions that were deeply familiar to Ailey, and reflected his keen observation of motion and gesture. Costumes are bright yellow, jubilant, and dancers are carried away in joy as they move in sweeping motions across the stage. In this section, too, though, one doesn't need to have had the experience of gospel music in church to feel uplifted– it speaks of "joyous relief," as one dancer put it, and "the sense of just being elated in knowing that there is something bigger than you."

Alvin Ailey once said that one of our country's richest treasures is African American cultural heritage, which he called "sometimes sorrowful, sometimes jubilant, but always hopeful." Judith Jamison, one of the company's principal dancers and later its artistic director, said that Revelations "set a tone for what is human in all of us, no matter where you come from." Revelations captures all these sentiments, which may explain its popularity worldwide. Although Ailey formed his company in 1958 with the intent of providing opportunities for black dancers to express their experience and heritage, the company has always been multiracial, welcoming dancers of all backgrounds, and expresses the deepest facets of human experience. "You sit and watch that ballet," said Jamison, "and you know what it's like to be human."

6. According to the passage, the "story" that Revelations tells can best be described as:

    A. a history of African-American slavery.

    B. an examination of the nature of oppression.

    C. a celebration of the transformative power of religion.

    D. a portrayal of the struggle to attain transcendence and joy in the face of oppression.

7. Which of the following best represents the concept conveyed by "Pilgrim of Sorrow"?

    A. Although life is difficult, hard work allows us to transcend our limitations.

    B. All human beings yearn to connect with others.

    C. People strive to pull themselves out of hardship and difficult circumstances.

    D. The "burden of life" was a concept unique to African-Americans living in the segregated South.

8. A dance critic once said that it was appropriate that Alvin Ailey termed his company an American Dance Theater. What information in the passage best supports this assertion?

    A. Ailey's choreography was more exuberant than that of other dance companies, as is evident in Revelations.

    B. Ailey utilized elements of theater, such as lighting, costume, and set design, to underscore the expressions of his choreography.

    C. Revelations is as popular as the most successful theatrical productions.

    D. Revelations is divided into several sections, and in that way is very much like a play.

9. According to the passage, why is it likely that audiences all over the world can relate to Revelations?

    A. While Revelations speaks specifically of the African-American experience, it taps into universal themes that transcend specific culture.

    B. Dance is a universal art form, which can be appreciated by all people.

    C. Many cultures have oppression and enslavement pervasive in their history.

    D. Ailey's uniquely American message is appealing to nearly all who see Revelations.

10. Suppose a musician were to compose a new score for the third section of Revelations. Based on the passage, which of the following might describe the most appropriate soundscape for that section?

    A. Celebratory music, since the section is joyful and uplifting

    B. Subdued hymns, since the section is set in church

    C. Solemn music, since the piece describes hardship and slavery

    D. Popular music, since Revelations is an immensely popular dance piece

Passage 3 (Questions 11 – 17)

As has been said before, the first duty of the sovereign is to protect his society from the violence or invasion of other independent societies, and this can be performed only with the use of military force. The economic expense of preparing military force in times of peace, and of putting it to use in times of war, is notably different in different periods of society's development.

The second duty of the sovereign is to protect every member of his society from the injustice and oppression that may be posed by every other person in it. In other words, his second duty is the establishment of an exact administration of justice. As with the first duty, this second duty requires very different levels of economic expense in different periods of society's development.

In a nation of hunters, personal property is rare, and what few items do exist do not exceed the value of two to three days of labor. Because of this, there is rarely any established magistrate or administration of justice in this type of nation. Men who have no property can harm each other only in person or in reputation: when one man defames, wounds, or kills another, the attacking man receives no benefits. This is not the case with injuries to property, for in those cases the person who causes the injury takes a benefit that is often equal to the loss of whoever suffers the injury.

The only passions that can prompt a man to attack another's person or reputation are envy, malice, and resentment. The majority of men are infrequently under the influence of these passions, and the very worst of men are swayed by them only occasionally. And though these passions may provide some gratification, they are typically not attended with any real or permanent advantage, and so are commonly restrained by prudential considerations. In this way, even without a civil magistrate to protect them from the injustice of those three passions, men in this nation of hunters may live together with an adequate degree of security.

But in a society with personal property, ambition and avarice in the rich, and the love of present ease and enjoyment in the poor, are passions which lead to the invasion of property. Moreover, these passions are far more steady and universal than the aforementioned three. Because of this, wherever there is great property, as there is in modern society, there is great inequality. For every very rich man there are at least five hundred poor, and the affluence of rich reinforces the indigence of the poor, for the affluence of the rich inspires indignation in the poor. In turn, the poor are driven by want and envy to invade the rich man's possessions.

Only under the shelter of a civil magistrate can the owner of valuable property, acquired by many years or even generations of labor, sleep soundly at night with the knowledge of his and his property's security. At all times, this rich man is surrounded by unknown enemies whom he never provoked, whom he can never appease, and from whose injustice he is protected by the civil magistrate and the administration of justice. Therefore, the accumulation of valuable and extensive property necessitates the establishment of civil government, for where there is no property, or at least no property that exceeds the value of two to three days of labor, civil government is far less necessary.

Naturally, civil government supposes a notable degree of subordination. As the necessity of civil government grows with the continued acquisition of property, the principal causes of subordination, including the social and economic stratification of society, develop simultaneously with the growth of that valuable property.

11. According to the passage, which of the following passions is the most universal and steady?

A. Envy

B. Resentment

C. Avarice

D. Indigence

12. Based upon the passage, it is most likely that the author agrees with which of the following statements?

A. The second duty of a sovereign is the most important.

B. A system of justice can exist without a civil government.

C. Social subordination is inherently unjust.

D. Inequality is inevitable in modern society.

13. The author begins the passage with a mention of the first duty of the sovereign in order to:

A. provide some context and comparison for the argument of the passage.

B. establish the hierarchy of duties a sovereign must learn to employ.

C. posit that internal forces actually pose more danger to society than external.

D. make the comparison between war with other nations and class warfare.

14. Based upon the passage, it can be inferred that the author most believes that the crimes that necessitate a system of justice are:

A. more likely to be motivated by personal vendettas or grudges.

B. of a more violent nature than those crimes which do not necessitate a magistrate.

C. undertaken in the hope of acquiring real, permanent advantage.

D. inspired by passions that are unavoidable and innate to human nature.

15. Suppose a farm has just been built in a small society of hunters, the first of its kind. The man who owns the farm becomes successful growing crops and selling them in a marketplace he also builds. Over time, he builds more farms and more marketplaces that are run by his family and close friends. According to the passage, which of the following statements is true of this scenario?

A. Poor farmers or hunters are likely to attack the farm owner, motivated by envy, malice, and resentment.

B. Poor farmers or hunters are likely to attack the farm, motivated by love of present ease and enjoyment.

C. The farm owner is likely to attack prominent farmers or hunter, motivated by love of present ease and enjoyment.

D. The farm owner is likely to attack prominent farmers or hunters, motivated by malice or resentment.

16. According to the passage, all of the following are direct reasons that a justice system and magistrate must be established EXCEPT:

A. the accumulation of private, valuable property.

B. violent crimes motivated by profit.

C. the gradual stratification of society.

D. the threat of the many poor against the rich few.

17. According to the passage, which of the following statements are true of crime in a nation of hunters?

I. Harm is typically either bodily or reputation-based.

II. The attacker receives as much benefit as the victim loses.

III. It is relatively rare.

A. I only

B. II only

C. I and III only

D. I, II, and III

Passage 4 (Questions 18 – 23)

The birth of a dream is then no mystery. It resembles the birth of all our perceptions. The mechanism of the dream is the same, in general, as that of normal perception. When we perceive a real object, what we actually see—the sensible matter of our perception—is very little in comparison with what our memory adds to it. When you read a book, when you look through your newspaper, do you suppose that all the printed letters really come into your consciousness? In that case the whole day would hardly be long enough for you to read a paper. The truth is that you see in each word and even in each member of a phrase only some letters or even some characteristic marks, just enough to permit you to divine the rest. All of the rest, that you think you see, you really give yourself as an hallucination. There are numerous and decisive experiments which leave no doubt on this point. I will cite only those of Goldscheider and Müller. These experimenters wrote or printed some formulas in common use, "Positively no admission;" "Preface to the fourth edition," etc. But they took care to write the words incorrectly, changing and, above all, omitting letters. These sentences were exposed in a darkened room. The person who served as the subject of the experiment was placed before them and did not know, of course, what had been written. Then the inscription was illuminated by the electric light for a very short time, too short for the observer to be able to perceive really all the letters. They began by determining experimentally the time necessary for seeing one letter of the alphabet. It was then easy to arrange it so that the observer could not perceive more than eight or ten letters, for example, of the thirty or forty letters composing the formula. Usually, however, he read the entire phrase without difficulty. But that is not for us the most instructive point of this experiment.

If the observer is asked what are the letters that he is sure of having seen, these may be, of course, the letters really written, but there may be also absent letters, either letters that we replaced by others or that have simply been omitted. Thus an observer will see quite distinctly in full light a letter which does not exist, if this letter, on account of the general sense, ought to enter into the phrase. The characters which have really affected the eye have been utilized only to serve as an indication to the unconscious memory of the observer. This memory, discovering the appropriate remembrance, i.e., finding the formula to which these characters give a start toward realization, projects the remembrance externally in an hallucinatory form. It is this remembrance, and not the words themselves, that the observer has seen. It is thus demonstrated that rapid reading is in great part a work of divination, but not of abstract divination. It is an externalization of memories which take advantage, to a certain extent, of the partial realization that they find here and there in order to completely realize themselves.

Thus, in the waking state and in the knowledge that we get of the real objects which surround us, an operation is continually going on which is of quite the same nature as that of the dream. We perceive merely a sketch of the object. This sketch appeals to the complete memory, and this complete memory, which by itself was either unconscious or simply in the thought state, profits by the occasion to come out. It is this kind of hallucination, inserted and fitted into a real frame, that we perceive. It is a shorter process: it is very much quicker done than to see the thing itself. Besides, there are many interesting observations to be made upon the conduct and attitude of the memory images during this operation. It is not necessary to suppose that they are in our memory in a state of inert impressions. They are like the steam in a boiler, under more or less tension.

18. Based on the passage, one type of hallucination might be:

    A. florid reinterpretations of prior knowledge.

    B. envisioning printed, rather than oral, phrases that are not there in reality.

    C. a manifestation of unconscious memory.

    D. filling in information to actual perceptions based on previous experience.

19. The author discusses Goldscheider and Müller in order to:

    A. experimentally determine the time necessary to access a memory of a certain phrase.

    B. prove that people read phrases more quickly than they can the letters composing them.

    C. differentiate between perception and memory.

    D. introduce the phenomenon of appropriate remembrance.

20. Which of the following contrasts best expresses a structuring tension of the passage?

    A. Perception vs Reading

    B. Reality vs Hallucination

    C. Dreaming vs Reading

    D. Hallucination vs Dreaming

21. Suppose that experimenters choose to write popular phrases drawn from contemporary fiction with some excluded words, and exposed them to viewers too quickly to be fully read. Based on earlier experiments, it is most likely that:

    A. The viewers would not be able to read the phrases due to an inability to project experience in a hallucinatory form.

    B. The viewers would not be able to read the phrases due to the omission of key letters upon which to build meaning.

    C. The viewers would be able to read the phrases due to the employment of full light as they were exposed to the phrase.

    D. The viewers would be able to read the phrases because they only need to see 8-10 characters of a 40 character phrase.

22. Which of the following letters in a phrase might an observer be sure he saw?

    I. Absent letters

    II. Those seen in full light

    III. One from a language foreign to the observer

    A. I only

    B. III only

    C. I and II only

    D. I and III only

23. The author compares memory images to "steam in a boiler" in order to:

    A. connect physical sensations to abstract ones such as perception.

    B. suggest the active and changeable nature of such impressions.

    C. emphasize the extreme tension felt by a subject trying to recall a submerged memory.

    D. explain why so many subjects try to avoid remembering the content of their dreams.

Passage 5 (Questions 24 – 30)

In October of 1833, Caroline Darwin wrote a letter to her brother Charles aboard *The Beagle*. "I have sent you," she wrote:

". . . a few little books which are talked about by every body at present—written by Miss Martineau who I think had been hardly heard of before you left England. She is now a great Lion in London, much patronized by Ld. Brougham who has set her to write stories on the poor Laws—Erasmus knows her & is a very great admirer & every body reads her little books & if you have a dull hour you can, and then throw them overboard, that they may not take up your precious room."

While the "little books" of which Caroline speaks– Martineau's *Illustrations of Political Economy* (1831), moralistic fairy tales about overpopulation, labor strikes and poorhouses—have indeed been essentially "thrown overboard" in our mental map of the Victorian canon, I argue that they actually speak to an interconnection between evolutionary ideas, liberal ideology, and literature that surfaced regularly throughout the century. The discourses of evolution and liberalism shared a common set of metaphors about the relationship between individual and communal needs, although within evolution the concept that movement between these two states could be generative rather than problematic gained credence more swiftly.

It is commonplace knowledge that Darwin's 1838 re-reading of Thomas Malthus's *An Essay on the Principle of Population* (1798), "crystallized [his observations] into the Darwinian theory" (37), as historian of science Dov Ospovat writes. The most famous dissemination of Malthus's ideas, however, were in the "little books" Caroline Darwin sent her brother. Martineau's popularization of Malthus' theories, encountered at the very moment when Darwin was first observing conditions of scarcity and adaptation, very plausibly primed him to mark this struggle for existence in the first place. While *Principle* was turned, by Darwin, to scientific purposes, the book was written for an explicitly political function. Lord Brougham, the prominent Whig Lord Chancellor, commissioned Martineau, through his Society for The Diffusion of Useful Knowledge, to write them to serve as exemplars of Malthusian economics to justify the reformation of the poor laws that were being heavily debated in parliament at the time.

Karl Marx, of course, famously accused Darwin of "recogniz[ing] amongst beast and plants his English society with its division of labor, competition, opening up of new markets , 'inventions,' and the Malthusian 'struggle for existence,'" adding that Darwin "amuses" him in saying "he is applying the 'Malthusian' theory to plants and animals, as if with Mr. Malthus the whole point were not that he does not apply the theory to plants and animals but only to human beings" (128). Janet Browne points out that Darwin was familiar to Malthusian ideas prior to his voyage: he "came across them in the books by Paley which were a fixed part of the Cam-bridge degree course; and William Whewell discussed them in a paper delivered in 1829 at the Cambridge Philosophical Society" (386). She adds that Charles Lyell, another critical theoretical source for Darwin on his voyage, frequently drew upon Malthus in his work. Thus Martineau's "little book" was not a new idea, but rather re-emphasized a set of principles that he was already accustomed to thinking about as key to observing nature at the very time when he was doing so.

24. Which of the following would most challenge the author's characterization of Malthus's motivations in writing his book?

    A. Before having a change of heart in late middle age, Malthus himself was an ardent supporter of conservative political parties and movements.

    B. Although he did not use the term eugenics, Malthus was known to support programs of "controlled breeding" in human populations in which those in political power would be able to determine who were the "strongest stock of citizens deemed worthy of reproduction to strengthen the national body".

    C. Malthus's work was funded by a political party that opposed the Whigs who went on to commission the subsequent popularization of this theories.

    D. Malthus's letters and journals during the time he was writing the Principle include multiple references to both animal and human populations and Malthus's hope that his ideas would provide those in the natural sciences with an important concept with broad implication.

25. According to the passage, who commissioned Harriet Martineau's works?

    A. Brougham

    B. Erasmus

    C. Malthus

    D. Marx

26. Based on the passage, it can be inferred that Caroline Darwin means which of the following in referring to Martineau as a "lion"?

    A. One who is well known throughout society for her writing and ideas

    B. One who is concerned with ecological issues and species variation

    C. One who serves as an important inspiration for later intellectual advancements

    D. One who is somewhat unapproachable in both demeanor and achievements

27. In discussing the political intentions of Malthus's work, the author assumes which of the following?

    A. It is crucial to divorce everyday content from the principles which may be more widely applicable.

    B. Martineau did not fully understand the import of what she was doing in disseminating Malthus's ideas.

    C. Political and scientific purposes are often identical in their founding principles.

    D. It is possible for works written for one purpose to be crucial in the foundations of another field.

28. Based on the passage, which detail about Martineau's Illustrations of Political Economy would the author find most pertinent?

    A. It employs seemingly childlike metaphors to drive home points about economic reform.

    B. Because it was written for political purposes, Darwin was incorrect in his application of Malthus to nature, as shown by later critics.

    C. It was tremendously popular in London during the time Charles Darwin was abroad.

    D. While given to Darwin at a crucial time of intellectual development, the book did not add any new information to his understanding of populations.

29. Suppose that it was discovered that, while it was in his library, Darwin did not, in fact, re-read Malthus's An Essay on the Principle of Population in 1838. Based on the information in the passage, the author would most likely suggest that:

    A. Dov Ospovat was incorrect in his analysis of the inspiration for Darwinian theory.

    B. Darwin's re-exposure to Malthus's ideas through the medium of Martineau could have helped him develop ideas about population and scarcity.

    C. Darwinian theory has no relation to Malthus's ideas about population.

    D. Darwin had chosen to throw Malthus's work overboard due to storage conditions on the Beagle during his voyage in the early 1830s.

30. Karl Marx objected to Darwin's theory for all of the following reasons EXCEPT that Darwin:

    A. falsely ascribed capitalist values to non-sentient beings.

    B. found justification for competition and inventions in natural circumstances.

    C. ignored the economic conditions that created class struggle.

    D. misrecognized the reasons for which Malthus focused on humans, rather than animals.

Passage 6 (Questions 31 – 35)

By religion, I understand a propitiation or conciliation of powers superior to man which are believed to direct and control the course of nature and of human life. Thus defined, religion consists of two elements, a theoretical and a practical, a belief in powers higher than man and an attempt to propitiate or please them. Of the two, belief clearly comes first, since we must believe in the existence of a divine being before we can attempt to please him. But unless the belief leads to a corresponding practice, it is not a religion but merely a theology; in the language of St. James, "faith, if it hath not works, is dead, being alone." In other words, no man is religious who does not govern his conduct in some measure by the fear or love of God. On the other hand, mere practice, divested of all religious belief, is also not religion. Thus Micah says: "He hath showed thee, O man, what is good; and what doth the Lord require of thee, but to do justly, and to love mercy, and to walk humbly with thy God?" The force by which Christianity conquered the world was drawn from the same high conception of God's moral nature and the duty laid on men of conforming themselves to it.

But if religion involves, first, a belief in superhuman beings who rule the world, and, second, an attempt to win their favor, it clearly assumes that the course of nature is to some extent elastic or variable, and that we can persuade or induce the mighty beings who control it to deflect, for our benefit, the current of events from the channel in which they would otherwise flow. Now this implied elasticity or variability of nature is directly opposed to the principles of magic as well as of science, both of which assume that the processes of nature are rigid and invariable in their operation, and that they can as little be turned from their course by persuasion and entreaty as by threats and intimidation. In magic, indeed, the assumption is only implicit, but in science it is explicit. It is true that magic often deals with spirits, which are personal agents of the kind assumed by religion; but whenever it does so in its proper form, it treats them exactly in the same fashion as it treats inanimate agents, that is, it constrains or coerces instead of conciliating or propitiating them as religion would do. Thus it assumes that all personal beings, whether human or divine, are in the last resort subject to those impersonal forces which control all things, but which nevertheless can be turned to account by anyone who knows how to manipulate them by the appropriate ceremonies and spells. In ancient Egypt, for example, the magicians claimed the power of compelling even the highest gods to do their bidding, and actually threatened them with destruction in case of disobedience. There is a saying everywhere current in India: "The whole universe is subject to the gods; the gods are subject to the spells (mantras); the spells to the Brahmans; therefore the Brahmans are our gods."

This radical conflict of principle between magic and religion sufficiently explains the relentless hostility with which in history the priest has often pursued the magician. The haughty self-sufficiency of the magician, his arrogant demeanor towards the higher powers, and his unabashed claim to exercise a sway like theirs could not but revolt the priest, to whom, with his awful sense of the divine majesty, and his humble prostration in presence of it, such claims and such a demeanor must have appeared an impious and blasphemous usurpation of prerogatives that belong to God alone. And sometimes, we may suspect, lower motives concurred to whet the edge of the priest's hostility. He professed to be the proper medium, the true intercessor between God and man, and no doubt his interests as well as his feelings were often injured by a rival practitioner, who preached a surer and smoother road to fortune than the rugged and slippery path of divine favor.

31. Which of the following statements would the author most likely make?

    A. Faith and works are equally essential to religion.

    B. If a man acts from the love or fear of man, he is religious.

    C. If a man acts from the love or fear of God, he is not religious.

    D. If a man acts concordant with God's will, he is religious.

32. Which of the following best illustrates the difference between theology and religion as outlined in the passage?

    A. Religion is like the belief that a natural disaster is coming and theology is the knowledge that a natural disaster is coming gained from the use of scientific instruments.

    B. Theology is like the belief that a natural disaster is coming and religion is believing that it won't harm you.

    C. Theology is like the belief that there is gold in a mine and religion is mining for it.

    D. Theology is the belief that everything is controlled by fate, religion is believing that everything is controlled by a superhuman being or beings.

33. Which of the following questions is central to the debate in the second paragraph?

    A. Are the forces which govern the world constant and invariable, or changing and elastic?

    B. Are the forces which govern the world conscious and personal, or unconscious and impersonal?

    C. Do magicians and religious people share a belief in powers greater than themselves?

    D. Do magicians and religious people attempt to alter the course of nature?

34. Suppose it were discovered that the author is religious. How would this affect the strength of the author's ideas?

    A. It would not affect the ideas or assertions presented in the passage.

    B. It would explain the author's apparent prejudice against magic.

    C. It would explain the author's apparent prejudice against science.

    D. It would explain the author's assertion of his belief that superhuman powers control the course of nature.

35. Which of the following is supported by the passage?

    A. Science and magic attempt to control the forces of nature that determine the earth's destiny.

    B. Magicians believe in unseeable forces mightier than the gods and that these forces can be controlled.

    C. Magicians believe in unseeable forces mightier than the gods which cannot be controlled.

    D. Religion and magic are similar in their belief that the course of nature is variable.

Passage 7 (Questions 36 – 40)

Sir David Wilkie (1785-1841) has been called the "prince of British genre painters." His father was a minister, and David was placed in the Trustees' Academy in Edinburgh, Scotland in 1799. In 1805 he entered the Royal Academy in London, and was much noticed on account of his "Village Politicians," exhibited the next year. From this time his fame and popularity were established, and each new work was simply a new triumph for him. "The Card Players," "Rent Day," the "Village Festival," and others were rapidly painted and exhibited.

In 1825 Wilkie went to the Continent, and remained three years. He visited France, Germany, Italy, and Spain, and after his return he painted a new class of subjects in a new manner. He made many portraits, and his other works were historical subjects. His most celebrated works in this second manner were "John Knox Preaching," "Napoleon and the Pope at Fontainebleau," and "Peep-o'-Day Boy's Cabin." The portrait of the landscape painter William Daniell is an especially good picture.

In 1830 Wilkie succeeded Sir Thomas Lawrence as painter to the king, as he had been limner to the King of Scotland since 1822. He was not knighted until 1836. In 1840 he visited Constantinople, and made a portrait of the sultan; he went then to the Holy Land and Egypt. While at Alexandria, on his way home, Wilkie complained of illness, and on shipboard, off Gibraltar, he died, and was buried at sea. This burial is the subject of one of Turner's pictures, and is now in the National Gallery.

The name of Landseer is an important one in British art. John Landseer (1761-1852) was an eminent engraver; his son Thomas (1795-1880) followed the profession of his father and arrived at great celebrity in it. Charles, born in 1799, another son of John Landseer, became a painter and devoted himself to a sort of historical genre line of subjects, such as "Cromwell at the House of Sir Walter Stewart in 1651," "Surrender of Arundel Castle in 1643," and various others of a like nature. Charles Landseer travelled in Portugal and Brazil when a young man; he was made a member of the Royal Academy in 1845; from 1851 to 1871 he was keeper of the Academy, and has been an industrious and respected artist. But the great genius of the family was Edwin.

Sir Edwin Landseer (1802-1873) was the youngest son of John Landseer. He received his first drawing lessons from his father, and from a very early age showed a great talent for sketching and that love for the brute creation which have been his chief characteristics as an artist. He had the power to understand his dumb subjects as well as if they spoke some language together, and then he had the ability to fix the meaning of all they had told him upon his canvas, by means of the sketching lines which gave the precise form of it all and by his finishing shades which put in the expression. If his animals were prosperous and gladsome, he represented their good fortune with hearty pleasure; if they were suffering, sad, or bereaved, he painted their woes with a sympathy such as none but a true friend can give.

36. Which of the following are probably true statements according to the passage?

    I. David Wilkie and Charles Landseer were likely members of the Royal Academy at the same time.

    II. Turner was an American painter.

    III. David Wilkie was born in Scotland.

    A. I only

    B. II only

    C. III only

    D. II and III only

37. Which of the following best describes the attitude of the author toward Edwin Landseer? He or she:

    A. is reverential toward Edwin's work.

    B. undervalues Edwin's work.

    C. is approving of Edwin's work.

    D. is disrespectful of Edwin's work.

38. Which of the following is most likely the author's purpose in including the phrase about William Daniell?

    A. To show that David Wilkie was a much better painter of historical subjects than portraits

    B. To show that David Wilkie was a good painter of portraits

    C. To illustrate that David Wilkie had changed the focus of his paintings after returning from Europe

    D. The sentence has no evident purpose in the context of the passage

39. The author mostly likely admires Edwin Landseer because:

    A. he was so prolific during his life.

    B. he was widely regarded as one of the brightest painters of his time in England.

    C. of the style and grace with which the author believed him to paint.

    D. of his preeminence against the backdrop of his less successful brothers.

40. Suppose it were found that Thomas Landseer is most famous for a series of paintings he produced from 1840-1845. Which of the following would be the result of this finding?

    A. It would strengthen the author's argument that the Landseers were a prominent family in British art.

    B. It would strengthen the author's argument that Thomas Landseer was a well-respected painter.

    C. It would weaken the author's argument that Thomas Landseer primarily took after his father.

    D. It would weaken the author's argument that Thomas Landseer was not a very famous artist.

Passage 8 (Questions 41 – 47)

Critics sometimes speak as if the only quality of Michelangelo's genius is a wonderful strength that verges on something singular or strange (in the things of imagination, great strength always does). Certainly, a particular strangeness, like the blossoming of the aloe, is a crucial element of a true work of art, as it is one of great art's indispensible powers that it excites or surprises us. However, it is just as indispensible that it should also charm us and give us pleasure. Therefore, this strangeness must also be sweet. To Michelangelo's true admirers, this is the essence of his work: sweetness meeting strength, pleasure meeting surprise, the energy of conception threatening at every moment to break through the pleasant constructs of form. His art seems to reclaim a sincere loveliness typically found only in simple, natural things. Ex forti dulcedo: from strength comes sweetness.

This allows him to sum up the character of medieval art and make clear that which distinguishes it from classical art: the presence of a convulsive energy, which in less capable hands becomes monstrous or forbidding, and which, even its most masterful iterations, is felt only as a subdued quaintness. Those who feel this sweetness or grace in Michelangelo's work might be at first puzzled if asked where exactly this quality resides. Inventive men such as Victor Hugo, whose work, like Michelangelo's, has either attracted or repelled people by its strength while few have understood its sweetness, have sometimes relieved work of merely moral or spiritual greatness with little aesthetic charms of their own. An example of these lovely accidents or accessories is the butterfly which alights upon the bloodstained barricade in Hugo's *Les Misérables*.

Unlike Hugo, however, Michelangelo's austere genius does not derive its sweetness from such accessories. For him, the natural world has almost no existence. As Herman Grimm said in his *Life of Michelangelo*, "When one speaks of him, woods, clouds, seas, and mountains disappear, and only what is formed by the spirit of man remains behind." Michelangelo traced no flowers like the ones Leonardo dispersed over his gloomiest rocks. He wove nothing like the fretwork of wings and flames that framed Blake's startling conceptions. He painted no forests like the ones with which Titian filled his backgrounds. Rather, he used blank ranges of rocks and dim vegetation as blank as the rocks in order to create a world reminiscent of the first five days of creation.

Indeed, of the whole story of creation, he painted only the creation of the first man and woman, though he feebly, at least for him, depicted the creation of light as well. His genius was of such a quality that it was concerned almost exclusively with the making of man. For him, the making of man was not the last and crowning act of a series of creations, but rather, the first act, the creation of life itself in its most supreme form, off-hand and immediately, in cold, lifeless stone.

With Michelangelo, the beginning of life possesses all the qualities of resurrection: with its gratitude, effusion, and eloquence, it is like the recovery of suspended animation. As fair as the young men of the Elgin marbles are, the Adam of the Sistine Chapel differs from them, lacking that balance and completeness which express a self-contained, independent life. There is something rude and even satyr-like about Adam's languid figure, something almost akin to the hillside on which he lies. His whole form expresses both expectancy and reception, and though he seems to hardly have enough strength to lift his finger to touch that of the creator, he manages to do so, and the mere touch of fingertips is enough.

41. Which of the following statements is true of the final sentence of the passage?

    I. It characterizes human frailty.

    II. It expresses the inability of humans to truly commune with the divine.

    III. It epitomizes the imperfect, honest humanity of Michelangelo's work.

    A. I only

    B. III only

    C. I and II only

    D. I and III only

42. According to the passage, Michelangelo's primary concern in making art was to:

    A. depict the beauty of nature.

    B. depict the making of man.

    C. depict the beauty of man.

    D. depict the duality of life.

43. The author most likely referenced other artists, and particularly Victor Hugo, in order to:

    A. establish Michelangelo's superiority as an artist above all others.

    B. demonstrate how subtle Michelangelo's sense of sweetness is.

    C. delineate Michelangelo's place among the world's greatest artists.

    D. depict just how spare and reserved Michelangelo's work was.

44. Based on the passage, it can be inferred that the author most believes which of the following statements? Michelangelo's particular genius lent him:

    A. and his work a kind of accessibility unparalleled by any other painter.

    B. a passion and a talent that made him the greatest artist of all time.

    C. and his work a kind of undecipherable yet enduringly gratifying mystery.

    D. a passion and a talent that made him a mortal iteration of "the creator."

45. According to the passage, which of the following statements best explains how Michelangelo was able to characterize medieval art, and notably, how it differed from classical art?

    A. He imbued his work with an underlying, nearly uncontrollable energy that he managed to portray as a subdued quaintness.

    B. He imbued his work with a kind of subdued quaintness that managed to bely a hidden sense of foreboding.

    C. He imbued his work not with small aesthetic charms and accessories, but rather, with a foreboding and monstrous energy.

    D. He imbued his work with a surreal understanding of the natural world that managed to improve upon the efforts of his predecessors.

46. Imagine that you have entered an art gallery and that four paintings are featured on the wall. Based upon the passage, which of the following paintings will most likely have been painted by Michelangelo? The one with a male and female figure:

    A. both lifelike and charismatic, standing in a vivid field.

    B. both balanced and complete, standing on a blank range of rocks.

    C. both lifelike and charismatic, standing amidst a drab landscape.

    D. both charismatic and complete, standing amidst a drab landscape, save for the bright red bird alight on the female's hand.

47. All of the following are qualities of Michelangelo's artwork EXCEPT:

    A. a duality of strength meeting sweetness.

    B. a sweetness that is obvious upon second glance.

    C. a sincere loveliness that is typically found in things of nature.

    D. a preoccupation with the creation of man.

Passage 9 (Questions 48 – 53)

From the apparent usefulness of the social virtues, it has readily been inferred by skeptics, both ancient and modern, that all moral distinctions arise from education, and were, at first, invented, and afterwards encouraged, by the art of politicians, in order to render men tractable, and subdue their natural ferocity and selfishness, which incapacitated them for society. This principle, indeed, of precept and education, must so far be owned to have a powerful influence, that it may frequently increase or diminish, beyond their natural standard, the sentiments of approbation or dislike; and may even, in particular instances, create, without any natural principle, a new sentiment of this kind; as is evident in all superstitious practices and observances: but that ALL moral affection or dislike arises from this origin, will never surely be allowed by any judicious enquirer. Had nature made no such distinction, founded on the original constitution of the mind, the words, honorable and shameful, lovely and odious, noble and despicable, had never had place in any language; nor could politicians, had they invented these terms, ever have been able to render them intelligible, or make them convey any idea to the audience.

The social virtues must, therefore, be allowed to have a natural beauty and amiableness, which, at first, antecedent to all precept or education, recommends them to the esteem of uninstructed mankind, and engages their affections. And as the public utility of these virtues is the chief circumstance, whence they derive their merit, it follows, that the end, which they have a tendency to promote, must be some way agreeable to us, and take hold of some natural affection. It must please, either from considerations of self-interest, or from more generous motives and regards.

It has often been asserted, that, as every man has a strong connection with society, and perceives the impossibility of his solitary subsistence, he becomes, on that account, favorable to all those habits or principles, which promote order in society, and insure to him the quiet possession of so inestimable a blessing. As much as we value our own happiness and welfare, as much must we applaud the practice of justice and humanity, by which alone the social confederacy can be maintained, and every man reap the fruits of mutual protection and assistance.

This deduction of morals from self-love, or a regard to private interest, is an obvious thought, and has not arisen wholly from the wanton sallies and sportive assaults of the skeptics. To mention no others, Polybius, one of the gravest and most judicious, as well as most moral writers of antiquity, has assigned this selfish origin to all our sentiments of virtue. But though the solid practical sense of that author, and his aversion to all vain subtleties, render his authority on the present subject very considerable; yet is not this an affair to be decided by authority, and the voice of nature and experience seems plainly to oppose the selfish theory.

We frequently bestow praise on virtuous actions, performed in very distant ages and remote countries; where the utmost subtlety of imagination would not discover any appearance of self-interest, or find any connection of our present happiness and security with events so widely separated from us. A generous, a brave, a noble deed, performed by an adversary, commands our approbation; while in its consequences it may be acknowledged prejudicial to our particular interest.

Where private advantage concurs with general affection for virtue, we readily perceive and avow the mixture of these distinct sentiments, which have a very different feeling and influence on the mind. We praise, perhaps, with more alacrity, where the generous humane action contributes to our particular interest: but the topics of praise, which we insist on, are very wide of this circumstance.

48. Which of the following most accurately reflects the author's opinions on the origin or morals and social virtues?

   A. Morality was formed gradually as an invention of educated society.

   B. Morality is derived from individual self-interest.

   C. Morality is, in part, inherent to the human condition.

   D. Morality is too complex to effectively discuss its origin.

49. Based upon the passage, it can be inferred that the author most likely:

   A. believes that empirical enquiry is the best manner to draw conclusions regarding human behavior.

   B. believes in the divine, and often inexplicable, nature of many human phenomenon.

   C. is partially motivated by his own religious beliefs.

   D. disagrees with the methods and practices of previous writers and philosophers.

50. Based on the passage, it can be inferred that the authors views Polybius as:

   A. writer who he finds to be a keen and practical observer, and who shares his opinions on morality.

   B. writer who he finds to be too calculating and judicious, but nonetheless agrees with his opinions on morality.

   C. writer for whom he has considerable respect, but disagrees with on his opinions on morality.

   D. writer who he finds to be too calculating and judicious, and disagrees with him opinions on morality.

51. The author would most likely agree that which of the following factors contributes to our sense of morality?

   I. Selfish interests

   II. Socially constructed ideals

   III. Inherent disposition towards social virtues

   A. II only

   B. III only

   C. II and III only

   D. I, II, and III

52. Why does the author reference the praise we bestow on "virtuous actions, performed in very distant ages"?

   A. To highlight that our perception of morality is based on historical precedent

   B. To provide an example that is in contrast to the perceived selfish origin of morality

   C. To provide an example that demonstrates the natural origins of morality

   D. To transition the reader to the author's next line of reasoning

53. Which of the following, if true, would most weaken the author's position on the origin of morality and social virtues?

   A. A study indicates that morally conscious individuals report higher levels of satisfaction and personal happiness relative to less morally conscious individuals.

   B. An anthropological study indicates that people never behaved in a moral manner prior to the creation of written language.

   C. A study that indicates that an individual's level of education is correlated to the amount of charitable acts they perform in society.

   D. A study indicates that individuals are more likely to perform virtuous actions if they know that other individuals are watching.

This page intentionally left blank.

SECTION 7

Answer Key

1	D	12	D	23	B	34	A	45	A
2	D	13	A	24	D	35	B	46	C
3	A	14	C	25	A	36	C	47	B
4	C	15	B	26	A	37	A	48	C
5	A	16	C	27	D	38	B	49	A
6	D	17	C	28	D	39	C	50	C
7	C	18	D	29	B	40	C	51	D
8	B	19	D	30	C	41	D	52	B
9	A	20	B	31	A	42	B	53	B
10	A	21	D	32	C	43	B		
11	C	22	C	33	B	44	D		

Passage 1 (Questions 1 – 5)

Experienced tuberculosis controllers are keenly aware of the **discrepancies** between the **theory** and the **reality** of finding and treating **latent tuberculosis infection** (LTBI). Although the guidelines about LTBI appear to be straightforward on the surface, in truth the tasks are challenging, and efficiency and effectiveness are difficult to achieve. In this section, we review the **general principles** that influence the success of your **prevention** activities.

Key terms: latent tuberculosis infection (LTBI)

Contrast: guidelines seem to be straightforward in theory, but are difficult to achieve efficiently and effectively in reality

Cause and effect: following certain guidelines will make prevention more effective

The **success of your prevention** activities is governed by three elements that we all need to balance simultaneously in order to have successful public health interventions. These elements are: (1) **finding** and accurately diagnosing LTBI, (2) determining the **urgency** of treatment, and (3) **completely treating** the patients who have LTBI. Problems in any of these three areas will detract from the success of your activities. For example, if you start a project that finds dozens of at-risk patients who have LTBI but none of the patients start or complete treatment, the project does not contribute to tuberculosis prevention. ARPEs give you a broad overview that helps you to find problems and to strike a balance among the three elements.

Key terms: diagnosing; urgency; completely treating; ARPEs

Cause and effect: not meeting one of the elements means tuberculosis prevention is not occurring

Finding and accurately diagnosing LTBI depends on the **prevalence rate** of LTBI in the population that is under consideration. The prevalence rate refers to how common LTBI is, and it is a population characteristic that reflects the tuberculosis history of the population. The **prevalence rate controls how many infected individuals you will discover** by testing. This is your **yield** of LTBI. The minimum prevalence rate for a successful strategy is **unknown**, but you need to take a **critical look** at the balance of the three elements if you are testing in a population having an LTBI prevalence rate **less than 10 percent**. The LTBI prevalence rate also influences the accuracy of the tuberculin skin test. This is because the predictive value of a positive test result depends on the prevalence rate. When the **prevalence rate is low, the predictive value of a positive result is also low**. For example, when the LTBI prevalence rate falls below 10 percent, most of the patients with positive results from the skin test actually will have false-positive results. Therefore, when the prevalence rate of LTBI is low, most of the patients who are being treated for LTBI are actually not at risk for tuberculosis because they do not even have LTBI. This is **wasteful of resources and possibly hazardous** to the patients.

Key terms: prevalence rate, tuberculin skin test

Cause and effect: prevalence rate affects how many infected individuals you will find; if prevalence rate is low many positives are actually false positives, meaning many of those treated are not infected

The **urgency** of treatment for LTBI patients depends on **how likely they are to get sick with active** tuberculosis. If the likelihood of active tuberculosis is high, then the urgency of treatment is high. One example is the patients who have been **recently exposed** to contagious tuberculosis (i.e., contacts). We also worry about patients who have medical problems that change their immune capacity: co-infection with the human immunodeficiency virus (**HIV**) is a very serious example. The urgency of treatment is relative. No one can predict which patients with LTBI are going to become sick with tuberculosis. The risk of tuberculosis might be high, medium, or low, and this determines the urgency of treatment. The current medical condition and the tuberculosis exposure history are factors to consider when determining the urgency of treatment for an individual. The final decision to treat rests with the individual patient and the prescribing provider.

Key Terms: active tuberculosis

Cause and effect: certain conditions, including exposure to contagious tuberculosis and reduced immune capacity, increase the urgency of treatment although no one can predict who will actually become sick

Sometimes the **urgency** of treatment **offsets** the concerns about testing a population with a **low LTBI prevalence** rate. For example, **infants** who might have been exposed to contagious tuberculosis should be tested even if the exposure was minimal because infection could be very dangerous for them. In this example, the concern about the danger of tuberculosis overrides the low yield of testing.

Cause and effect: urgency of treatment can override concerns about testing low LBTI populations

Main Idea: Prevention of tuberculosis requires finding and treating LTBI (latent tuberculosis infection) and deciding which cases are most urgent; high risk populations increase the urgency of the need for treatment and thus can justify testing normally low yield populations.

1. D is correct. In the passage, it is stated that "sometimes the urgency of treatment offsets the concerns about testing a population with a low LTBI prevalence rate. For example, infants who might have been exposed to contagious tuberculosis should be tested even if the exposure was minimal because infection could be very dangerous for them. In this example, the concern about the danger of tuberculosis overrides the low yield of testing." Thus those with high risks of infection should be tested.

    A: False positives are a reason not to perform test in areas with low yields of LTBI, except in cases of high risk

    B: The passage does not argue that any infant should be tested, as in choice B.

    C: The passage states that "no one can predict which patients with LTBI are going to become sick with tuberculosis."

2. D is correct. The passage focuses on the three elements that need to be balanced to create successful interventions in preventing tuberculosis.

    A: The passage does not identify the most difficult element.

    B: It is not suggested that equal balance is required for an intervention.

    C: Since all elements must be in balance, identifying patients is not of the prime importance.

3. A is correct. According to the passage, "if [the] prevalence rate is low many positives are actually false positives, meaning many of those treated are not infected".

    B, D: The new situation deals with false positives, not who should be treated, or outcomes, as in choices B and D.

    C: Since the situation has a bad outcome, it is not a result of the proper approach, as in choice C.

4. C is correct. The passage states that "(1) finding and accurately diagnosing LTBI, (2) determining the urgency of treatment, and (3) completely treating the patients who have LTBI" are the key elements of treatment and "problems in any of these three areas will detract from the success of your activities." Thus a program that did not focus on all three but was still successful, as in choice C would weaken the author's argument.

    A, B: These are both explicitly stated in the passage, so they do not weaken it.

    D: The course of tuberculosis is not discussed in the passage, making choice D irrelevant.

5. A is correct. The passage states that urgency of treatment depends upon whether "patients . . . have been recently exposed to contagious tuberculosis (i.e. contacts)" as in choice D, whether "patients . . . have medical problems that change their immune system," as in choice C, and adds that "the final decision to treat rests with the individual patient and the prescribing provider," as in choice B. Because "no one can predict which patients with LTBI are going to become sick with tuberculosis," choice A is NOT a factor, making it the credited answer.

Passage 2 (Questions 6 – 10)

"**Revelations**," choreographer **Alvin Ailey's masterwork**, has been in Alvin Ailey American Dance Theater's repertory since its creation in 1960. In that time, the piece has been viewed by more than 23 million people in 71 countries worldwide – **more than any other modern dance piece**. Created by Ailey when he was 29 years old, the work draws on his **recollections of his childhood** in the rural south, and his experiences in his small church. Ailey described the memories that informed Revelations as "blood memories" – experiences so strong that they were as present and important to him as the blood running through his veins.

Key terms: Revelations, Alvin Ailey American Dance Theater, blood memories

Cause and effect: Alvin Ailey based his immensely popular piece Revelations on his memories of his childhood in the rural south

Revelations is divided into **three sections**, each of which contains several dances. The first section, entitled "**Pilgrim of Sorrow**," has to do with "the burden of life," said Ailey, and portrays dancers **yearning for salvation** in the face of their difficulties. Dancers, huddled together with heads bowed, lit by a single spotlight, stretch their open-palmed hands heavenward, only to be pulled back to earth. Dressed in drab, earth-toned garments, the dancers evoke sorrow and **hardship,** elements of African American life that were particularly familiar to Alvin Ailey, who was raised in segregated Texas in the 1930s by a single mother.

Key terms: three sections, Pilgrim of Sorrow, yearning for salvation, hardship

Cause and effect: the first section expresses the dancers' yearning for salvation in the face of difficult lives

In "**Take Me To the Water**," the second section of Revelations, the dancers, clad in white, stage a ceremonial **baptism**. To the sounds of the traditional spiritual "Wade in the Water," dancers move across the stage in motions that represent water – undulating arms, sinuous hips – and yards of billowing blue silk represent the river, in which a pair of dancers is "baptized" by a devotional leader bearing a large umbrella. The baptismal is based on Ailey's recollections of his own baptism, which took place in a pond behind his church. Yet even if you don't share Alvin Ailey's personal experience of baptism," Take Me To the Water" still speaks of the possibility of **transformation**: according to one of Ailey's dancers, this section is about "cleansing and changing and becoming someone better."

Key terms: Take Me To the Water, baptism, transformation

Opinion: even if viewers are not familiar with the ritual of baptism, they understand that Take Me To the Water is a about transformation

"**Move, Members, Move**," the third section, suggests a congregation in **church** on a hot day. Dancers seem to gossip, fan themselves against the heat, and look about the church – all motions that were deeply familiar to Ailey, and reflected his keen observation of motion and gesture. Costumes are bright yellow, **jubilant**, and dancers are carried away in joy as they move in sweeping motions across the stage. In this section, too, though, one doesn't need to have had the experience of gospel music in church to feel uplifted– it speaks of "**joyous relief**," as one dancer put it, and "the sense of just being elated in knowing that there is something bigger than you."

Key terms: Move, Members, Move, church, jubilant, joyous relief

Cause and effect: Ailey represented the experience he'd observed early in his life of joyous relief expressed in church

Opinion: a dancer explains that this celebratory section is about feeling uplifted and elated

Alvin Ailey once said that one of our country's richest treasures is **African American cultural heritage**, which he called "sometimes sorrowful, sometimes jubilant, but always hopeful." Judith Jamison, one of the company's principal dancers and later its artistic director, said that Revelations "set a tone for what is human in all of us, no matter where you come from." Revelations captures all these sentiments, which may explain its **popularity worldwide.** Although Ailey formed his company in 1958 with the intent of providing opportunities for black dancers to express their experience and heritage, the company has always been multiracial, welcoming dancers of all backgrounds, and expresses the deepest facets of **human experience**. "You sit and watch that ballet," said Jamison, "and you know what it's like to be human."

Key terms: African American cultural heritage, popularity worldwide, human experience

Opinion: Ailey thinks that one of the US's richest cultural treasures is the African American cultural heritage

Main Idea: In portraying elements of the African American experience, Revelations captures some of the deepest facets of human experience, which can be understood by people worldwide.

6. D is correct. Revelations speaks of deep human struggles: the struggle against oppression, the possibility of transformation, the desire for transcendence. The three sections of Revelations address each of these themes.

    A: While Revelations is rooted in African-American cultural heritage, describing the piece as a history of African-American slavery is too specific, and misses the more universal human themes the piece puts forth.

    B: The first section portrays oppression, but this choice is too broad.

    C: Choice C overlooks themes of struggle and hardship that the piece includes.

7. C is correct. "Pilgrim of Sorrow," the first section of the piece, shows suffering dancers reaching heavenward, trying to pull themselves out of their misery, as described in paragraph 2.

    A: In this section, no transcendence is achieved – it's all about hardship; also, the passage never suggests that it is hard work that results in transcendence.

    B: It's not connecting with others that the dancers portray in this section, it's simply relief from hardship.

    D: What's notable about Revelations is that while it speaks of historical African-American struggles, it speaks to all humankind. Specifically, the "burden of life" is not unique to certain people at a certain point of history.

8. B is correct. In describing the three sections of Revelations, the author notes that each section includes elements of lighting, costumes, and music to make the expressions of the choreography more effective. That's what correct choice B says. Revelations is indeed exuberant (choice A) and popular (choice C) but the author never suggests that this is what makes it "theater." Similarly, the fact that it is divided into sections is never described as theatrical (choice D).

9. A is correct. Look at the last line of the passage – Judith Jamison's quote. In watching Revelations, she says, the viewer taps into what it's like to be human. The themes of struggle and transcendence are issues that cross cultures, even as the historical particulars center on the African-American experience.

    B, C: Maybe dance is a universal art form, and likely many cultures have some sort of oppression in their histories, but the passage never says this.

    D: The point is that Ailey's message is not uniquely American – it's universal.

10. A is correct. The third section, "Move, Members, Move," takes place in church, and is all about "joyful relief," as one dancer puts it in paragraph 4. So what's most important would be to capture that mood of jubilation. Choice A, "celebratory music," captures this.

    B, C: "Subdued" or "solemn" music would not be in keeping with the joyful mood in section 3 – it would be all wrong!

    D: Whether or not the music is popular is not relevant; what's important is that the music match the spirit of the section.

Passage 3 (Questions 11 – 17)

As has been said before, the **first duty** of the sovereign is to protect his society from the violence or **invasion** of other independent societies, and this can be performed **only** with the use of **military force**. The **economic expense** of preparing military force in times of peace, and of putting it to use in times of war, is **notably different in different periods** of society's development.

Opinion: author thinks a sovereign's first duty is to protect against foreign invasion; cost of military protection varies

The **second** duty of the sovereign is to **protect** every member of his society from the **injustice and oppression** that may be posed by every other person in it. In other words, his second duty is the **establishment of an exact administration of justice**. As with the first duty, this second duty requires **very different levels of economic expense** in different periods of society's development.

Opinion: author thinks a sovereign's second duty is to set up a system of justice

In a **nation of hunters**, **personal property is rare**, and what few items do exist do not exceed the value of two to three days of labor. Because of this, there is rarely any established magistrate or administration of justice in this type of nation. Men who have no property can **harm** each other only in **person** or in **reputation**: when one man defames, wounds, or kills another, the attacking man receives no benefits. This is not the case with injuries to property, for in those cases the person who causes the injury takes a benefit that is often equal to the loss of whoever suffers the injury.

Contrast: injury to person or reputation vs injury to property; benefit taken from causing injury vs loss sustained from suffering injury

Cause and effect: because personal property is rare in a nation of hunters, this type of nation rarely has an established magistrate or administration of justice

The only **passions** that can prompt a man to **attack another's person** or reputation are **envy, malice, and resentment**. The majority of men are infrequently under the influence of these passions, and the very worst of men are swayed by them only **occasionally**. And though these passions may provide some gratification, they are typically not attended with any real or permanent advantage, and so are commonly restrained by prudential considerations. In this way, even without a civil magistrate to protect them from the injustice of those three passions, men in this **nation of hunters** may live together with an **adequate degree of security**.

Opinion: author thinks a nation of hunters doesn't need formal justice systems because attacks are rare

But in a society with personal property, **ambition and avarice** in the rich, and the love of present ease and enjoyment in the poor, are passions which lead to the **invasion of property**. Moreover, **these passions** are far more steady

and **universal** than the aforementioned three. Because of this, wherever there is great property, as there is in modern society, there is **great inequality**. For every very rich man there are at least five hundred poor, and the affluence of rich reinforces the indigence of the poor, for the **affluence of the rich inspires indignation in the poor**. In turn, the poor are driven by want and envy to invade the rich man's possessions.

Contrast: the society of hunters vs a society with lots of property; in the latter the poor resent the wealth of the very few rich people

Only under the **shelter of a civil magistrate** can the owner of valuable property, acquired by many years or even generations of labor, sleep soundly at night with the knowledge of his and his **property's security**. At all times, this rich man is surrounded by unknown enemies whom he never provoked, whom he can never appease, and from whose injustice he is protected by the civil magistrate and the administration of justice. Therefore, the accumulation of valuable and extensive property necessitates the **establishment of civil government**, for where there is no property, or at least no property that exceeds the value of two to three days of labor, civil government is far less necessary.

Cause and effect: the existence of personal property requires a civil government and civil magistrate to protect that property from others

Naturally, **civil government** supposes a **notable degree of subordination**. As the necessity of civil government grows with the continued acquisition of property, the principal causes of subordination, including the social and economic **stratification of society**, develop **simultaneously** with the **growth of that valuable property**.

Cause and effect: because the necessity of civil government grows with the continued acquisition of property, the principal causes of subordination develop simultaneously with the growth of valuable property

Main Idea: A government must protect its people from threats, both external and internal; in a society in which people can amass lots of personal property one constant source of internal threat is the envy and greed of those less fortunate; this threat requires the creation of a civil government, as opposed to a society of hunters in which there is little personal property and no need for such governmental structures.

11. C is correct. In the fifth paragraph, the author introduces the passions that lead to invasion of property in a society with personal property: avarice is one of them. As he writes, ". . . these passions are far more steady and universal than the aforementioned three [envy, malice, resentment]."

12. D is correct. As the author writes in the fifth paragraph, "wherever there is great property . . . there is great inequality." The author further makes this point in the last paragraph, when he writes that "the social and economic stratification of society" develops with the growth of valuable property.

   A: The author does not create an order of importance or preference for these tasks.

   B: The author uses "system of justice" and "civil government" almost synonymously.

   C: The author never makes this claim. He seems to regard it as simply the way things are.

13. A is correct. The passage is about the second duty of the sovereign. The mention of the first duty in the opening paragraph lends context to the passage, as well as comparison: both duties have different economic expenses at different period in a society's development. Furthermore, the opening phrase, "As has been said before," suggests that this first paragraph is being referenced as a kind of set-up for the argument to follow.

   B: Again, the author is not necessarily ranking these duties on a hierarchy of importance. And even if he is implying it, choice A is still a stronger answer.

   C: If indeed the first duty is more important than the second, that would mean protecting against external danger is more important. Ultimately, choice C is just not an argument that is made in the passage.

   D: This argument is not made in the passage.

14. C is correct. The author writes that a system of justice and a magistrate only become necessary in a society in which people can own possessions that are more valuable than two or three days of labor. Moreover, he writes that in the nation of hunters, the passions that motivate crimes are not attended with any real or permanent advantage. In the society of possessions, however, crimes are motivated by passions that are attended with real and permanent advantage (i.e., to acquire possessions).

   A: This is more representative of the crimes committed in the nation of hunters.

   B: Again, this is perhaps more representative of the nation of hunters.

   D: The passions that motivate crime in the society with possessions are linked to the possessions themselves. The author does not describe these possessions in the first type of society. Moreover, he does not clearly say whether they are avoidable or unavoidable.

15. B is correct. The scenario presents a society that transitions from first type of society, the nation of the hunters, to the second type of society, in which possessions are owned. As the author writes in the fifth paragraph, "But in a society with personal property, ambition and avarice in the rich, and the love of present ease and enjoyment in the poor, are passions which lead to the invasion of property." The implication here is that an attack involves "the invasion of property."

   A: These motivations are typical of the nation of hunters.

   C: The rich are more likely to be motivated by avarice and ambition in this society, according to the passage.

   D: Again, these are passions from the other type of society.

16. C is correct. Choices A, B, and D all reflect elements of a society with possessions that necessitate a justice system directly. The stratification of society could be considered an indirect reason. Moreover, as the author writes in the last paragraph, the stratification of society is something happens simultaneously with the growth of valuable property. It is the continued acquisition of property the correlates directly to the necessity of civil government.

17. C is correct. Statement I is made clear in the third paragraph: "Men who have no property can harm each other only in person or in reputation . . ." Statement III is made clear by the fact that prudential considerations often restrain the passions that motivate crime in a nation of hunters. II: This is true of a society with possessions, not a society of hunters.

Passage 4 (Questions 18 – 23)

The **birth of a dream** is then no mystery. It **resembles** the **birth of all our perceptions**. The mechanism of the dream is the same, in general, as that of normal perception. When we perceive a real object, what we actually see—the sensible matter of our **perception**—is **very little** in comparison with what our **memory** adds to it. When you read a book, when you look through your newspaper, do you suppose that all the printed letters really come into your consciousness? In that case the whole day would hardly be long enough for you to read a paper. The truth is that you see in each word and even in each member of a phrase **only some letters** or even some characteristic marks, just enough to permit you to divine the rest. **All of the rest**, that you think you see, you really give yourself as an **hallucination**. There are numerous and decisive experiments which leave no doubt on this point. I will cite only those of **Goldscheider** and **Müller**. These experimenters wrote or printed some formulas in common use, "Positively no admission;" "Preface to the fourth edition," etc. But they took care to write the words incorrectly, changing and, above all, omitting letters. These sentences were exposed in a darkened room. The person who served as the subject of the experiment was placed before them and did not know, of course, what had been written. Then the inscription was illuminated by the electric light for a very short time, too short for the observer to be able to perceive really all the letters. They began by determining experimentally the time necessary for seeing one letter of the alphabet. It was then easy to arrange it so that the observer could not perceive more than **eight or ten letters**, for example, **of the thirty or forty** letters composing the formula. Usually, however, he **read the entire phrase without difficulty**. But that is not for us the most instructive point of this experiment.

Key terms: Goldscheider; Müller

Contrast: what we actually perceive in an object vs what memory adds to it

Cause and effect: experiments proved that people read common phrases much more quickly than they can read all the letters that make them up; the experiments suggests other new findings

If the observer is asked what are the letters that **he is sure of having seen**, these may be, of course, the letters really written, but there may be also absent letters, either letters that we replaced by others or that have simply been omitted. Thus an observer will **see quite distinctly** in full light **a letter which does not exist**, if this letter, on account of the general sense, ought to enter into the phrase. The characters which have really affected the eye have been utilized only to serve as an indication to the unconscious memory of the observer. This memory, discovering **the appropriate remembrance**, i.e., finding the formula to which these characters give a start toward realization, **projects the remembrance** externally in an hallucinatory form. It is this remembrance, and not the words themselves, that the observer has seen.

It is thus demonstrated that **rapid reading** is in great part **a work of divination**, but not of abstract divination. It is an **externalization of memories** which take advantage, to a certain extent, of the partial realization that they find here and there in order to completely realize themselves.

Contrast: what an observer is sure he has seen (memory) vs what is actually there

Cause and effect: when observers see a familiar phrase, their unconscious memory is activated, so they create a hallucination of the phrase in its proper form, believing they have seen it fully; therefore rapid reading is about memory, not abstract divination.

Thus, **in the waking state** and in the knowledge that we get of the real **objects which surround us**, an operation is continually going on which is of **quite the same nature as that of the dream**. We perceive merely a sketch of the object. This sketch appeals to the complete memory, and this complete memory, which by itself was either unconscious or simply in the thought state, profits by the occasion to come out. It is this kind of hallucination, inserted and fitted into a real frame, that we perceive. It is a shorter process: it is **very much quicker** done than to see the thing itself. Besides, there are many interesting observations to be made upon the conduct and attitude of the memory images during this operation. It is not necessary to suppose that they are in our memory in a state of inert impressions. They are like the steam in a boiler, under more or less tension.

Cause and effect: dreams follow the same relation to memory as reading; we experience a sketch but fill in details based on prior memories

Main Idea: The passage stresses that much of reading and dreaming is actually a "hallucination" in the sense that they unconsciously draw upon stored memories to fill out the sketch of what is actually perceived.

18. D is correct. The truth is that you see in each word and even in each member of a phrase only some letters or even some characteristic marks, just enough to permit you to divine the rest. All of the rest, that you think you see, you really give yourself as an hallucination.

19. D is correct. At the end of the first paragraph, the author tells us that the most instructive point of Gold-scheider and Müller's experiment is not that a person can perceive a phrase more quickly than reading an individual letter (choice B), but rather, as in the second paragraph, that we use the "appropriate remembrance" as a sort of hallucination to more quickly process the world of sense information.

20. B is correct. Our memory images (the hallucinations we project onto the world) are not inert. At the end of the passage, we're told that they are in a tension. What would they be in tension with? The actual observations we're making and then projecting the hallucinations on to. We structure our perception of the world in a mix of directly perceiving reality and relying on our memories of such familiar objects.

21. D is correct. These experimenters wrote or printed some formulas in common use, "Positively no admission;" "Preface to the fourth edition," etc. But they took care to write the words incorrectly, changing and, above all, omitting letters. This memory, discovering the appropriate remembrance, i.e., finding the formula to which these characters give a start toward realization, projects the remembrance externally in an hallucinatory form. It is this remembrance, and not the words themselves, that the observer has seen.

22. C is correct. If the observer is asked what are the letters that he is sure of having seen, these may be, of course, the letters really written (II), but there may be also absent letters (I) that have simply been omitted. Thus an observer will see quite distinctly in full light a letter which does not exist, if this letter, on account of the general sense, ought to enter into the phrase.

23. B is correct. The author tells us that, "It is not necessary to suppose that they are in our memory in a state of inert impressions". Since they are not inert, they must be active and changeable.

Passage 5 (Questions 24 – 30)

In October of **1833**, **Caroline Darwin** wrote a letter to her brother **Charles** aboard *The Beagle*. "I have sent you," she wrote:

". . . a few little books which are talked about by every body at present—written by **Miss Martineau** who I think had been hardly heard of before you left England. She is now a great Lion in London, much patronized by **Ld. Brougham** who has set her to write stories on the **poor Laws—Erasmus** knows her & is a very great admirer & every body reads her little books & if you have a dull hour you can, and then throw them overboard, that they may not take up your precious room."

While the "little books" of which Caroline speaks– Martineau's *Illustrations of Political Economy* **(1831)**, **moralistic fairy tales** about **overpopulation**, labor strikes and poorhouses—have indeed been essentially "thrown overboard" in our mental map of the Victorian canon, I argue that they actually speak to an interconnection between **evolutionary ideas, liberal ideology**, and **literature** that surfaced regularly throughout the century. The discourses of evolution and liberalism shared a common set of metaphors about the relationship between individual and communal needs, although within evolution the concept that movement between these two states could be generative rather than problematic gained credence more swiftly.

Key terms: 1833; Caroline Darwin; Charles; Miss Martineau; Ld. Brougham; poor Laws; Erasmus; Illustrations of Political Economy

Opinion: Caroline Darwin felt that Charles might find the *Illustrations* enjoyable; author thinks Martineau's books illustrate important connections between evolution and political ideology

Contrast: popularity of *Illustrations* in the 1830s vs current critical reception

It is commonplace knowledge that Darwin's 1838 re-reading of **Thomas Malthus's** *An Essay on the Principle of Population* **(1798)**, "crystallized [his observations] into the Darwinian theory" (37), as historian of science **Dov Ospovat** writes. The **most famous dissemination of Malthus's ideas**, however, were in the "little books" Caroline Darwin sent her brother. **Martineau's** popularization of Malthus' theories, encountered at the very moment when Darwin was first observing conditions of scarcity and adaptation, very plausibly **primed him to mark this struggle for existence** in the first place. While *Principle* was turned, by Darwin, to scientific purposes, the book was written for an explicitly political function. Lord Brougham, the prominent Whig Lord Chancellor, commissioned Martineau, through his **Society for The Diffusion of Useful Knowledge**, to write them to serve as exemplars of Malthusian economics to justify the reformation of the poor laws that were being heavily debated in parliament at the time.

Key terms: Thomas Malthus' *An Essay on the Principle of Population* (1798), Dov Ospovat, Society for the Diffusion of Useful Knowledge

Opinion: Dov Ospovat argues that Darwin's re-reading of Malthus in 1838 crystallized his observations into Darwinian Theory

Contrast: those who read Malthus vs those who read Martineau; *Principle* used for scientific purposes, but written for political purposes

Cause and effect: Malthus' work helped Darwin to develop his theories of evolution and inspired Martineau's work on political science

Karl Marx, of course, famously accused Darwin of "**recogniz[ing] amongst beast and plants his English society**" with its division of labor, competition, opening up of new markets , 'inventions,' and the Malthusian 'struggle for existence,'" adding that Darwin "amuses" him in saying "he is applying the 'Malthusian' theory to plants and animals, as if with Mr. Malthus the whole point were not that he does not apply the theory to plants and animals but only to human beings" (128). **Janet Browne** points out that Darwin was familiar to Malthusian ideas prior to his voyage: he "came across them in the books by **Paley** which were a fixed part of the Cambridge degree course; and **William Whewell** discussed them in a paper delivered in 1829 at the at the Cambridge Philosophical Society" (386). She adds that **Charles Lyell**, another critical theoretical source for Darwin on his voyage, **frequently drew upon Malthus** in his work. Thus Martineau's "little book" was not a new idea, but rather re-emphasized a set of principles that he was already accustomed to thinking about as key to observing nature at the very time when he was doing so.

Key terms: Karl Marx, Janet Browne, Paley, William Whewell, Charles Lyell

Opinion: Karl Marx thought Darwin uses nature to recognize what is already in English society; Janet Browne thinks Darwin was exposed to Malthus through a number of different writers

Contrast: applying Malthusian theory to plants and animals vs humans

Cause and effect: because Darwin was exposed to Malthus's ideas numerous times, his experience with Martineau simply served to remind him of principles with which he was familiar while he was seeing them in action

Main Idea: The author suggests that Harriet Martineau's Illustrations of Political Economy served as an inspiration in developing Charles Darwin's thinking about evolutionary theory as he was observing physical details about variation and scarcity of resources, particularly in her use of Thomas Malthus's ideas, to which Darwin had been introduced multiple times.

24. D is correct. The passage author asserts that Malthus's book was produced for purely political purposes and it was Darwin who turned the ideas to scientific aims. If Malthus himself had scientific ideas in mind as he was constructing his book, then the author is incorrect to assert that it was purely political.

A, B, C: Each of these choices offer some type of political aim or connection for Malthus's work, which fits the author's characterization.

25. A is correct. According to the passage, "Lord Brougham, the prominent Whig Lord Chancellor, commissioned Martineau, through his Society for The Diffusion of Useful Knowledge".

26. A is correct. Caroline Darwin describes her as "a great Lion in London," stating that "Erasmus knows her & is a very great admirer & every body reads her little books." Thus she is well known and admired for her books.

B: There is no suggestion that Martineau herself was interested in ecology.

C: Caroline Darwin is writing at the time the book was just published, so she can't know her future status as an inspiration.

D: There is no mention in the passage of Martineau's personal demeanor.

27. D is correct. The passage explains the political background that shaped Martineau's work and then shows how it influenced Darwin's thinking in evolution, a different field.

A, C: The passage shows connections, but does not suggest the content must be separated from the principles, or that the principles are identical.

B: There is no discussion of Martineau's understanding of her effect in the passage.

28. D is correct. The passage emphasizes that Darwin was re-exposed to Malthus's ideas, via Martineau, as he was observing natural selection at work, but also that he was aware of these ideas in many forms.

A, C: The passage seeks to connect Malthus, Martineau and Darwin, not just focus on the effects and popularity of Martineau, as in choices A and C.

B: The passage does not argue that Darwin incorrectly applied Malthus, though it does cite Marx's thoughts on the matter.

29. B is correct. The author writes that while "it is commonplace knowledge that Darwin's 1838 re-reading of Thomas Malthus' An Essay on the Principle of Population (1798), "crystallized [his observations] into the Darwinian theory" (37), as historian of science Dov Ospovat writes[,] the most famous dissemination of Malthus's ideas, however, were in the "little books" Caroline Darwin sent her brother. Martineau's popularization of Malthus' theories, encountered at the very moment when Darwin was first observing conditions of scarcity and adaptation, very plausibly primed him to mark this struggle for existence in the first place." Thus choice B, which focuses on the availability of ideas through Martineau, is the credited answer.

A: The passage is not focused on Ospovat's analysis.

C: Because Martineau, and others, disseminated Malthus's ideas, there could still be a connection even if Darwin did not re-read Malthus directly.

D: While Caroline Darwin suggests Charles can "throw the books overboard," there is no evidence Charles did so.

30. C is correct. The final paragraph states that Karl Marx "famously accused Darwin of 'recogniz[ing] amongst beast and plants his English society with its division of labor, competition, opening up of new markets , 'inventions,' and the Malthusian 'struggle for existence,'" as in choices A and B, and adds that Darwin "'amuses' him in saying 'he is applying the 'Malthusian' theory to plants and animals, as if with Mr. Malthus the whole point were not that he does not apply the theory to plants and animals but only to human beings,'" as in choice D. There's no discussion of economic conditions, as in C.

Passage 6 (Questions 31 – 35)

By religion, I understand a propitiation or **conciliation** of powers superior to man which are believed to direct and control the **course of nature** and of human life. Thus defined, religion consists of two elements, a **theoretical** and a **practical**, namely, a belief in powers higher than man and an attempt to propitiate or please them. Of the two, belief clearly comes first, since we must believe in the existence of a divine being before we can attempt to please him. But unless the belief leads to a corresponding practice, it is not a religion but merely a **theology**; in the language of St. James, "faith, if it hath not works, is dead, being alone." In other words, no man is religious who does not govern his conduct in some measure by the fear or love of God. On the other hand, mere practice, divested of all religious belief, is also not religion. Thus **Micah** says: "He hath showed thee, O man, what is good; and what doth the Lord require of thee, but to do justly, and to love mercy, and to walk humbly with thy God?" The force by which Christianity conquered the world was drawn from the same high conception of God's moral nature and the duty laid on men of conforming themselves to it.

Key terms: Micah

Opinion: the author defines religion as the belief in superhuman powers and the attempt at pleasing them to influence the course of nature

Contrast: religion is contrasted to theology, the theoretical to the practical aspect of religion

Cause and effect: the true practice of religion requires action based on the beliefs espoused

But if religion involves, first, a **belief in superhuman beings** who rule the world, and, second, an attempt to win their favor, it clearly **assumes that the course of nature is to some extent elastic** or variable, and that we can persuade or induce the mighty beings who control it to deflect, for our benefit, the current of events from the channel in which they would otherwise flow. Now this **implied elasticity** or variability of nature is **directly opposed to the principles of magic as well as of science**, both of which assume that the processes of nature are rigid and invariable in their operation, and that they can as little be turned from their course by persuasion and entreaty as by threats and intimidation. In magic, indeed, the assumption is only implicit, but in science it is explicit. It is true that **magic** often deals with **spirits**, which are personal agents of the kind assumed by religion; but whenever it does so in its proper form, it treats them exactly in the same fashion as it treats inanimate agents, that is, it **constrains or coerces instead of conciliating or propitiating them as religion would do.** Thus it assumes that all personal beings, whether human or divine, are in the last resort **subject to those impersonal forces** which control all things, but which nevertheless can be turned to account by anyone who knows how to manipulate them by the appropriate ceremonies and spells. In **ancient Egypt**, for example, the magicians claimed the power of

compelling even the highest gods to do their bidding, and actually **threatened them with destruction** in case of disobedience. There is a saying everywhere current in **India**: "The whole universe is subject to the gods; the gods are subject to the spells (mantras); the spells to the Brahmans; therefore the Brahmans are our gods."

Key terms: superhuman, Egypt, Brahmans

Contrast: the belief of magic and science is that impersonal forces dictate the course of nature

Cause and effect: magicians attempt to control the impersonal forces; in this way they can control the gods, who are also subject to these forces

This radical conflict of principle between magic and religion sufficiently explains the relentless **hostility** with which in history the priest has often pursued the magician. The haughty **self-sufficiency** of the magician, his **arrogant** demeanor towards the higher powers, and his unabashed claim to exercise a sway like theirs could not but revolt the priest, to whom, with his awful sense of the **divine majesty**, and his **humble prostration** in presence of it, such claims and such a demeanor must have appeared an impious and blasphemous usurpation of prerogatives that belong to God alone. And sometimes, we may suspect, **lower motives** concurred to whet the edge of the priest's hostility. He professed to be the proper medium, the true intercessor between God and man, and no doubt his interests as well as his feelings were often injured by a rival practitioner, who preached a surer and smoother road to fortune than the rugged and slippery path of divine favor.

Opinion: the author believes that the priest's hostility towards magicians is a natural result of their differences and may also be attributed to a feeling of personal injury held by the priests

Cause and effect: the differing beliefs of magicians and religious people lead to hostility between them

Main Idea: The main idea of the passage is to analyze the belief systems of those who practice magic and those who are religious; religion is defined, their differences are explained and the conclusion is drawn from this that a church's hostility towards magicians is a natural result.

31. A is correct. The author clearly states that faith without works is not religion and that works without faith is not religion.

    B: A man must believe in God and act out of belief in God to be religious.

    C: If a man acts from the love or fear of God, he is religious if he does what God would have him do.

    D: This is not always true, he must believe in God as well.

32. C is correct. The passage develops the idea that theology is a belief and religion is acting in accordance with the belief.

    A: Theology is not founded in scientific observation.

    B: According to the author, religion entails some sort of action rather than just belief.

    D: Theology is not the belief that everything is controlled by fate.

33. B is correct. The second paragraph deals primarily with the differing views regarding the forces that control the course of nature. Magicians and scientists believe these powers are unconscious and impersonal, that they do not answer to the wishes of mankind. Religious people are said to believe in conscious and personal beings that control the world.

    A: This would be correct if it said "is the course of nature constant or changing?" but we're talking about the forces which govern nature.

    C: This is not up for debate, no belief to the contrary is ever expressed.

    D: This is not up for debate, it is simply explained.

34. A is correct. The author appears to be approaching the passage information with little or no bias.

    B, C: The author has no apparent prejudice against magic or science.

    D: The author never states his or her own belief.

35. B is correct. The author states that magicians believe in impersonal forces to which all beings are subject but that these forces can be controlled.

    A: Science is not said to control the forces of nature.

    C: The opposite is true.

    D: This is not true, as religion thinks the course of nature is variable but magic sees nature as rigid and invariable.

Passage 7 (Questions 36 – 40)

Sir **David Wilkie** (1785-1841) has been called the "**prince of British genre painters.**" His father was a minister, and David was placed in the Trustees' Academy in **Edinburgh, Scotland** in 1799. In 1805 he entered the Royal Academy in London, and was much noticed on account of his "Village Politicians," exhibited the next year. From this time his fame and popularity were established, and **each new work was simply a new triumph for him**. The "Card Players," "Rent Day," the "Village Festival," and others were rapidly painted and exhibited.

Key Terms: David Wilkie, Trustees' Academy, Royal Academy, Village Politicians

Cause and effect: David Wilkie became famous for his "Village Politicians" after which he had a string of triumphs and was called the prince of British genre painters

In 1825 Wilkie went to the **Continent**, and remained three years. He visited France, Germany, Italy, and Spain, and after his return he **painted a new class** of subjects in a **new manner**. He made many **portraits**, and his other works were **historical subjects**. His most celebrated works in this second manner were "John Knox Preaching," "Napoleon and the Pope at Fontainebleau," and "Peep-o'-Day Boy's Cabin." The portrait of the landscape painter William **Daniell** is an especially good picture.

Contrast: David Wilkie painted different subjects after returning from mainland Europe

Cause and effect: David Wilkie's travels in Europe may have influenced his painting

In 1830 Wilkie succeeded **Sir Thomas Lawrence** as **painter to the king**, as he had been limner to the **King of Scotland** since 1822. He was not **knighted** until 1836. In 1840 he visited Constantinople, and made a portrait of the sultan; he went then to the Holy Land and Egypt. While at Alexandria, on his way home, Wilkie complained of illness, and on shipboard, off Gibraltar, he died, and was buried at sea. This burial is the subject of one of Turner's pictures, and is now in the National Gallery.

Key Terms: Thomas Lawrence, painter to the king, knighted, Constantinople, Alexandria, Gibraltar, National Gallery

Cause and effect: David died as a result of an illness near Gibraltar

The name of **Landseer** is an important one in British art. **John Landseer** (1761-1852) was an eminent **engraver**; his son **Thomas** (1795-1880) followed the profession of his father and arrived at great celebrity in it. **Charles**, born in 1799, another son of John Landseer, became a **painter** and devoted himself to a sort of **historical genre** line of subjects, such as "Cromwell at the House of Sir Walter Stewart in 1651," "Surrender of Arundel Castle in 1643," and various others of a like nature. Charles Landseer travelled in Portugal and Brazil when a young man; he was made a member

of the **Royal Academy** in 1845; from 1851 to 1871 he was keeper of the Academy, and has been an industrious and respected artist. But the great genius of the family was Edwin.

Key Terms: Landseer, John, engraver, Thomas, Charles, historical genre, Royal Academy

Contrast: Thomas and John were both engravers, Charles was a painter

Sir **Edwin Landseer** (1802-1873) was the youngest son of John Landseer. He received his first drawing lessons from his father, and from a very early age showed a great talent for sketching and that love for the brute creation which have been his chief characteristics as an artist. He had the power to understand his dumb subjects as well as if they spoke some **language** together, and then he had the ability to fix the meaning of all they had told him upon his canvas, by means of the sketching lines which gave the **precise form** of it all and by his finishing shades which put in the **expression**. If his **animals** were **prosperous** and gladsome, he represented their good fortune with hearty pleasure; if they were **suffering**, sad, or bereaved, he **painted their woes** with a sympathy such as none but a true friend can give.

Opinion: the author believes Edwin to be the greatest artist in the Landseer family

Contrast: Edwin is a painter of nature and animals unlike Charles

Cause and effect: Edwin is said to be able to speak some language with his subjects, give precise form and impressive expressions to his sketches; these are apparently the reasons the author thinks Edwin so great

Main Idea: This passage provides a history of a short time in British art; there are several artists mentioned along with their most prominent works; the Landseer family was important in British art, especially Edwin Landseer.

36. C is correct. The passage states that David Wilkie was limner to the King of Scotland and that he attended academy in Scotland at and early age. This implies that he was a Scottish citizen.

   I: David Wilkie died in 1841 and Charles Landseer joined the Royal Academy in 1845.

   II: Turner is most likely a British painter. The author seems to be concerned only with British art history and the fact that Turner painted David Wilkie's death implies more than anything that he is British.

37. A is correct. The author prescribes greatness to Edwin Landseer and states that his skill was not merely in portraying nature but in understanding it and developing connections with his subjects. The author is adoring of Edwin's expertise.

   B, D: The author has a strongly positive view of Edwin Landseer's work, not a negative one.

   C: While this is positive, the word "approving" fails to capture the strongly positive view the author has. The author uses phrases like "great genius", "great talent", and "true friend".

38. B is correct. It seems the author wanted to include an example of Wilkie's portrait work after giving three examples of his work with historical subjects. The author thus included the phrase to illustrate that Wilkie was a good portrait painter in addition to being famous for the other paintings mentioned in the paragraph.

   A: The author does not necessarily want to argue that David Wilkie's historical paintings were better than his portrait paintings.

   C: The author had already made this point. The phrase about William Daniell was not evidence of this, it was simply a statement of Wilkie's accomplishment.

   D: It has a purpose as explained above.

39. C is correct. The passage states that Edwin Landseer had the power to understand the subjects he painted and give deep expression to his paintings. The author lingered on the point of Edwin's talent and appears to believe he is great because of it.

   A: The author may admire Edwin for this but it is not as good a choice as C.

   B: The author does not admire Edwin because others did

   D: There is no evidence in the passage to support this.

40. C is correct. The passage states that Thomas Landseer took after his father who was an engraver. Thomas was best known for his engravings. If he were most famous for paintings, the author's statement would lose validity.

Passage 8 (Questions 41 – 47)

Critics sometimes speak as if the **only quality of Michelangelo's genius** is a **wonderful strength** that verges on something singular or strange (in the things of imagination, great strength always does). Certainly, a particular **strangeness**, like the blossoming of the aloe, is a crucial element of a true work of art, as it is one of great art's indispensible powers that it excites or surprises us. However, it is just as indispensible that it should also **charm** us and give us **pleasure**. Therefore, this strangeness must also be sweet. To **Michelangelo's true admirers**, this is the essence of his work: **sweetness meeting strength**, pleasure meeting surprise, the energy of conception threatening at every moment to break through the pleasant constructs of form. His art seems to reclaim a sincere loveliness typically found only in simple, natural things. Ex forti dulcedo: from strength comes sweetness.

Opinion: author thinks those who are true fans of Michelangelo appreciate both surprising strangeness and charming pleasure

This allows him to sum up the character of medieval art and make clear that which distinguishes its from classical art: the presence of a **convulsive energy**, which in less capable hands becomes monstrous or forbidding, and which, even its most masterful iterations, is felt only as a subdued quaintness. Those who feel this **sweetness or grace in Michelangelo's work** might be at first puzzled if asked **where exactly this quality resides**. Inventive men such as Victor **Hugo**, whose work, like Michelangelo's, has either attracted or repelled people by its strength while few have understood its sweetness, have sometimes relieved work of merely moral or **spiritual greatness** with **little aesthetic charms** of their own. An example of these lovely accidents or accessories is the butterfly which alights upon the bloodstained barricade in Hugo's *Les Misérables*.

Contrast: Michelangelo's work has a convulsive energy vs has a sweetness

Opinion: author thinks other great artists, such as Hugo, have inserted little aesthetic charms (like a butterfly) in works that are otherwise focused on moral/spiritual greatness

Unlike Hugo, however, **Michelangelo's austere genius** does **not** derive its sweetness from such **accessories**. For him, the natural world has almost no existence. As Herman **Grimm** said in his *Life of Michelangelo*, "When one speaks of him, woods, clouds, seas, and mountains disappear, and **only** what is formed by the **spirit of man** remains behind." Michelangelo traced no flowers like the ones **Leonardo** dispersed over his gloomiest rocks. He wove nothing like the fretwork of wings and flames that framed **Blake's** startling conceptions. He painted no forests like the ones with which **Titian** filled his backgrounds. Rather, he used blank ranges of rocks and dim vegetation as blank as the rocks in order to create a world reminiscent of the first five days of creation.

Contrast: others use little touches to give sweetness to their work, but Michelangelo's work is austere and has no little touches

Opinion: author thinks Michelangelo is concerned only with the spirit of humanity and has no particular interest in the natural world

Indeed, of the **whole story of creation**, he painted **only** the creation of the first **man and woman**, though he feebly, at least for him, depicted the creation of light as well. His genius was of such a quality that it was concerned almost exclusively with the making of man. For him, the making of man was **not the last** and crowning act of a series of creations, but rather, **the first act, the creation of life itself** in its most supreme form, off-hand and immediately, in cold, lifeless stone.

Opinion: author thinks Michelangelo shows his interest solely in humanity and his disregard for the natural world by depicting the entire act of God's creation as consisting only in the creation of humans

With Michelangelo, the beginning of life possesses all the qualities of resurrection: with its gratitude, effusion, and eloquence, it is like the recovery of suspended animation. As **fair** as the young **men** of the **Elgin marbles** are, the **Adam of the Sistine Chapel** differs from them, lacking that balance and completeness which express a self-contained, independent life. There is something **rude and even satyr-like about Adam's languid figure**, something almost akin to the hillside on which he lies. His whole form expresses both **expectancy and reception**, and though he seems to hardly have enough strength to lift his finger to touch that of the creator, he manages to do so, and the mere touch of fingertips is enough.

Cause and effect: because Michelangelo's Adam has something rude and satyr-like about his languid form, he differs from the young men of the Elgin marbles

Main Idea: The author's intention is to expand the reader's appreciation of Michelangelo and his work; Michelangelo's sweetness is hard to locate; Michelangelo's work is concerned almost exclusively with the creation of man

41. D is correct. I, III: Surely the fact that Adam has barely enough strength to touch the his finger to the creator's is a sign of some kind of frailty. Moreover, this final sentence captures how imperfect Michelangelo's humans are, honestly portraying this rude man, this man that is one with the hill he lies on, this man who is both expectant and receiving. Michelangelo's greatest strength is his ability to portray humanity honestly.

   II: This is not true: the image of Adam touching his finger to God's is the ultimate testament to the hope and desire to commune with the divine.

42. B is correct. In the fourth paragraph, the author writes, "His genius was of such a quality that it was concerned almost exclusively with the making of man."

   A: This is the opposite of the case.

   C: Rather, Michelangelo's subjects have something rude and imperfect about them.

   D: This is never directly said, though Michelangelo does have that ability to meet sweetness and strength in his work. This may be more related to interpretation than intention. In as much as the making of man relies upon dualities, it could be considered true. But the making of man is his dominant preoccupation.

43. B is correct. Hugo used "little aesthetic charms" like "the butterfly which alights upon the blood-stained barricade..." His sense of sweetness comes from these accessories. Michelangelo's, however, does not.

   A: It is not necessarily true that the author believes Michelangelo is the greatest of all artists.

   C: He is perhaps doing this, but the allusions are more overtly used to compare style and use of subtlety.

   D: The key here is "particularly Victor Hugo." The Hugo reference is all about that sense of subtlety, though the comparisons do illustrate how spare the master's works were.

44. D is correct. "His genius was of such a quality that it was concerned almost exclusively with the making of man." "For him, the making of man was...the first act, the creation of life itself in its most supreme form, offhand and immediately, in cold, lifeless stone." "The beginning of life possess all the qualities of resurrection... it is like the recovery of suspended animation." With sentences like these, the author is painting a certain picture of the master, depicting him as almost god-like in his creative power and his ability to conjure up life itself in stone and on canvas.

A: Rather, his work may have a kind of inaccessibility. After all, the passage begins with a mention of critics who do not fully grasp the artist. Moreover, there is this sentence: "Those who feel this sweetness or grace in Michelangelo's work might be at first puzzled if asked where exactly this quality resides."

B: It is never said that Michelangelo is the greatest artist of all time, though this author may actually feel that way, given his gushing over his subject.

C: Enduring gratifying, perhaps, but it does not seem to be undecipherable, perhaps just not easily decipherable. The whole passage is about deciphering the mystery.

45. A is correct. As the author opens the second paragraph, "This allows him to sum up the character of medieval art and make clear that which distinguishes its from classical art: the presence of a convulsive energy, which in less capable hands becomes monstrous or forbidding, and which, even its most masterful iterations, is felt only as a subdued quaintness." In Choice A, the word convulsive has been substituted for "nearly uncontrollable energy". It's that high energy meeting pleasant form.

B: Misses the mark, as the underlying element is less foreboding and more just energetic.

C: Rather, the less capable hands made this convulsive energy monstrous.

D: Rather, he almost ignored the natural world.

46. C is correct. The accounts for the lack of detail and character in the background or in nature, as well as the more idiosyncratic style with which he conjured humans on the canvas.

A: The vivid field is the no-go.

B: The balanced and complete is the no-go: the men of the Elgin marbles are balanced and complete, not the subjects of Michelangelo.

D: The "complete" and the "bright red bird" don't fit the author's characterization of Michelangelo.

47. B is correct. The sweetness is perhaps never obvious. It is not as if a second glance will reveal it. It is something illusory and mysterious, yet undeniably present.

A, C, D: These are all true and expressed clearly in the passage.

Passage 9 (Questions 48 – 53)

From the apparent **usefulness of the social virtues**, it has readily been inferred by skeptics, both ancient and modern, that **all moral distinctions arise from education**, and were, at first, invented, and afterwards encouraged, by the art of politicians, in order to render men tractable, and subdue their natural ferocity and selfishness, which incapacitated them for society. This principle, indeed, of precept and education, must so far be owned to have a **powerful influence**, that it may frequently increase or diminish, beyond their natural standard, the sentiments of approbation or dislike; and may even, in particular instances, **create, without any natural principle, a new sentiment** of this kind; as is evident in all **superstitious** practices and observances: But that ALL moral affection or dislike arises from this origin, will **never** surely be **allowed** by any judicious enquirer. Had nature made no such distinction, founded on the original constitution of the mind, the words, honorable and shameful, lovely and odious, noble and despicable, had never had place in any language; nor could politicians, had they invented these terms, ever have been able to render them intelligible, or make them convey any idea to the audience.

Opinion: skeptics believe that morality arises from education; the author believes there is also an inherent aspect to morality, or else that original construction would have no basis or meaning

Contrast: the origin of morality as entirely constructed, or based on inherent qualities

Cause and effect: morality is influenced by social expectations, but could only be constructed if we already had an inherent disposition towards it

The **social virtues** must, therefore, be allowed to have a **natural beauty and amiableness**, which, at first, antecedent to all precept or education, recommends them to the **esteem of uninstructed mankind**, and engages their affections. And as the public utility of these virtues is the chief circumstance, whence they derive their merit, it follows, that the end, which they have a tendency to promote, must be some way agreeable to us, and take hold of some natural affection. It **must please**, either from considerations of **self-interest, or** from more **generous motives** and regards.

Opinion: author believes that social virtues and morality must have an inherent attractiveness

Cause and effect: the inherent attractiveness of social virtues must precede further education and definition of morality

It has often been asserted, that, as **every man has a strong connection with society**, and perceives the impossibility of his solitary subsistence, he becomes, on that account, **favorable** to all those habits or **principles**, which **promote** order in **society**, and insure to him the quiet possession of so inestimable a blessing. As much as we value our own happiness and welfare, as much must we applaud the practice of justice and humanity, by which alone the social confederacy

can be maintained, and every man reap the **fruits of mutual protection** and assistance.

Opinion: others assert morality is derived from mutual benefits in society

Cause and effect: if you act virtuously, you will receive the individual benefits and mutual protection assured by society

This deduction of **morals from self-love**, or a regard to private interest, is an **obvious thought**, and has not arisen wholly from the wanton sallies and sportive assaults of the skeptics. To mention no others, **Polybius**, one of the gravest and most judicious, as well as most moral writers of antiquity, has assigned this selfish origin to all our sentiments of virtue. But though the solid practical sense of that author, and his aversion to all vain subtleties, render his authority on the present subject very considerable; yet is **not this an affair to be decided by authority**, and the voice of **nature** and **experience** seems **plainly to oppose the selfish theory**.

Key terms: Polybius

Opinion: Polybius argued that the origin of all morality derived from self-interest; the author clearly respects Polybius and his practicality, argues that experiences oppose this theory

We frequently bestow **praise on virtuous actions**, performed in very **distant ages** and remote countries; where the utmost subtlety of imagination would **not** discover **any** appearance of **self-interest**, or find any connection of our present happiness and security with events so widely separated from us. A **generous**, a brave, a noble deed, performed by an **adversary**, commands our **approbation**; while in its consequences it may be acknowledged prejudicial to our particular interest.

Contrast: selfish origin of virtues vs unselfish, inherent origin

Opinion: author argues the fact that we praise virtuous acts, even if they harm our particular interests, indicates that the origin of morality cannot be derived from purely selfish interests

Cause and effect: we praise virtuous actions that do not offer us any benefit, therefore the origin of our morality can't be purely selfish in nature

Where **private advantage** concurs with general affection for **virtue**, we readily **perceive** and avow the mixture of these **distinct sentiments**, which have a **very different feeling and influence on the mind**. We praise, perhaps, with more alacrity, where the generous humane action contributes to our particular interest: But the topics of praise, which we insist on, are very wide of this circumstance.

Opinion: author argues that while we are potentially more inclined to virtuous sentiments that benefit us, that is not the full scope

Main Idea: The author believes that the origin of our sense of morality and virtue, while influenced by social expectations and to some extent selfish interests, must also derive from a natural and inherent sense of morality.

48.   C is correct. The idea that a sense of morality is inherent to humans is one of the main ideas of the passage, and there are many instances in the passage in which the author argues for this line of reasoning.

   A: The author states that morality could not have been constructed by educated society unless it had a natural basis (bottom of paragraph one).

   B: The author states that morality cannot be derived from self-interest.

   D: This is not stated in the passage.

49.   A is correct. The language the author uses throughout the passage indicates that the author believes in drawing conclusions in a practical, judicious manner. In the first paragraph he states "But that ALL moral affection or dislike arises from this origin, will never surely be allowed by any judicious enquirer", and later in the passage he praises Polybius for his grave and judicious manner.

   B, C: The author never mentions religious beliefs.

   D: The author praises the critical and practical manner of Polybius.

50.   C is correct. Polybius argues that the origins of morality derive from selfish interests, which runs in contrast to the author's argument that morality must be in part natural to humanity. The author, however, praises the practical and judicious way that Polybius came to his conclusions.

   A, B: The author and Polybius differ on their views of morality.

   D: The author praises Polybius.

51.   D is correct. I: While the author believes that the origin of our morality can't be purely from selfish interests, he understands that selfish interests do play some role in our morality. II: This is also accurate. In the first paragraph the author states, "This principle, indeed, of precept and education, must so far be owned to have a powerful influence", so he also acknowledges that morality and social virtues are certainly influenced by what we are taught. III: Finally, this is also accurate. This is the main idea of the passage, that some part of our sense of morality and social virtue must have had an inherent or natural origin.

52.   B is correct. The author uses the example of the praise we bestow on virtuous actions, both performed in distant ages and remote locations, as evidence that our morality can't be selfish in origin.

   A: This is in contrast to what the text states, and is also in opposition to the author's main point.

   C: This is consistent with the passage, however the praise we bestow on remote virtuous actions is not an example of that argument.

   D: The praise is being used as a specific example of a previously established argument, and is not transitioning the reader to a new line of reasoning.

53.   B is correct. The author asserts that morality stems from a natural human disposition, and furthermore that it could not have been constructed without that initial predisposition. A study that indicated that people never behaved in a moral manner prior to the creation of written language, therefore, would be very problematic for his argument.

   A: This study could be construed to indicate that people are making moral choices because they benefit them as individuals, but the argument is weak and not directly in contradiction to the author's views on the origins of morality.

   C: This study seems to indicate that our level of education affect our sense of morality, but there are many complicating factors that could contribute to the result, and furthermore the author acknowledges that education does have a strong influence on our sense of social virtue.

   D: This study could also be construed to indicate that people have a selfish motivation for acting in a moral manner, but it too is based on a weak argument and does not contradict the author's views.

SECTION 8
53 Questions, 90 Minutes
Use an answer grid from the back of the book to record your answers

Passage 1 (Questions 1 – 7)

Shakespeare understood that tradition could supply a better fable than invention ever could, and in his day, the petulant demand for originality was not nearly so pressed. There was no literature for the masses: the cheap press and universal reading were simply unknown. When he appears in widely illiterate times, a great poet absorbs into his work all the light that is anywhere radiating. Because it his duty to bring every intellectual gem and every flower of sentiment to the people, he comes to value his memory equally with his invention. Therefore, he cares little about from where his thoughts derive: whether they come from translation, tradition, travel, or inspiration, they are all equally welcome to his uncritical audience.

Other men say wise things as well as he does, but they also say many foolish things, and do not actually know when they have spoken wisely. The great poet knows the sparkle of the true stone and puts it in its right and lofty place whenever he finds it. Such is the position of Homer, and perhaps of Chaucer and Saadi, for they three felt that all wit was their wit. As much as they are poets, they are librarians and historiographers: each was heir and dispenser of all the tales of the world. As Milton, another such poet wrote, "Presenting Thebes' and Pelops' line / And the tale of Troy divine."

The influence of Chaucer is clear in all our early literature, and more recently, Pope, Dryden, and many others have been quite beholden to him. One is charmed by this opulence that feeds so many pensioners. Yet, Chaucer himself was a prolific borrower, drawing always from writers who themselves borrowed. One of those from whom he borrows is Gower, who he uses like a stone-quarry out of which he might build his own house. This theft he commits with an apology, that what he takes has no worth where he found it, but the greatest where he leaves it. Indeed, it has essentially become a rule in literature that a writer, once having proven himself capable of original writing, is from thenceforth entitled to steal from the work of others at his own discretion. A thought is the property of the person who can entertain it and who can adequately place it. At first, a certain awkwardness marks the use of a borrowed thought, but as soon as we have learned what to do with it, it becomes our own.

In this way, all originality is relative and every thinker is retrospective. The educated lawmakers at Westminster or in Washington speak and vote for thousands. Every senator has his constituency and is connected to it through invisible channels. Through these, the senator is made aware of the wishes of the people with evidence, anecdotes, and estimates. As Sir Robert Peel and Mr. Webster vote for thousands, so do Locke and Rousseau think for thousands, and so were there foundations all around Homer and Chaucer and Milton from which they drew: friends, lovers, books, traditions, and proverbs, all perished, which if seen would contribute to reducing our sense of wonder.

Does the great poet speak with authority? Does he ever feel himself outmatched? This appeal is to the consciousness of the writer. Is there some oracle in his breast that can be asked about any thought or thing and whether it be true or false, and to have the answer, and to rely on that? All the debts that such an artist could ever owe to other wits would never disturb his consciousness of originality, because the ministrations of books, and yes, even of other minds, are like a whiff of smoke to that most private reality with which he has conversed.

1. Besides Shakespeare, who of the following does the author most likely consider to be the greatest poet?

   A. Milton

   B. Homer

   C. Chaucer

   D. Saadi

2. Which of the following statements most accurately epitomizes the author's argument in the fourth paragraph?

   A. Though it may not seem like it, politicians and thinkers and artists are always indirectly taking commands and dictation from the people.

   B. Great doers and thinkers often receive their inspirations through unseen channels.

   C. Great poets and philosophers rule the world of art as politicians rule their respective nations.

   D. If we were to know all the sources that inform the actions and thoughts of great people, we'd be filled with a sense of wonder.

3. Based upon the passage, which of the following statements is the author most likely to believe?

   A. Today, readers believe that the work of poets ought to be original.

   B. Chaucer is the most influential writer in the English language.

   C. Of the authors mentioned, Milton's work covered the broadest spectrum.

   D. Chaucer alluded to and drew from Gower out of a deep appreciation.

4. In the final paragraph, what does the author most likely mean when he refers to "that most private reality with which he has conversed?"

   A. His original, creative genius

   B. God

   C. The oracle in his breast

   D. The power he takes from unoriginal ideas

5. Suppose a young theatre maker interested in adapting Shakespeare's Julius Caesar through the lens of Pre-World War II fascism. After doing some research, the young theatre maker discovers that this was the approach Orson Welles took with his 1937 production of the play. According to the passage, at what point can this young theatre maker call this Caesar-as-fascist-allegory his own?

   A. Once she has fully understood how the play speaks about the circumstances that give rise to fascism and learned how to execute the production.

   B. Once she has done her homework and fully studied why Welles originally undertook the project in this specific way instead of another way.

   C. Once she has thoroughly studied the history of the circumstances leading up to World War II and why and how fascism took hold.

   D. Once she has studied and learned through experience how to adapt a play out of its original context and into another, closer to modern one.

6. Based upon the passage, all of the following statements about Shakespeare are true EXCEPT:

   A. he knew that the best fables were traditional.

   B. he wrote his plays and poetry for the masses.

   C. he was quite careful about where his thoughts came from.

   D. he is to be considered alongside the likes of Homer and Chaucer.

7. Based upon the passage, which of the following statements are true?

   I. Any thought can be owned by a variable number of people.

   II. The more we know about a work of art's influences, the less amazed by it we are.

   III. To the poet or thinker, memory is actually more important than invention.

   A. I only

   B. II only

   C. I and II only

   D. II and III

Passage 2 (Questions 8 – 12)

When nurse Kaci Hickox returned to the United States after a month-long volunteer stay caring for Ebola patients in Sierra Leone, she did not receive a hero's welcome. Instead, she was quarantined, isolated in an unheated tent with no running water outside of a Newark, New Jersey hospital. Despite the fact that she had tested negative for the Ebola virus and exhibited no symptoms, Hickox was placed in a state-mandated 21-day quarantine, ordered by New Jersey Governor Chris Christie. Hickox loudly protested, and after several days was allowed to leave the tent and return by car to her home in Maine, where under that state's law she was supposed to remain quarantined in her home. However, Hickox refused that quarantine as well, stating that she was of no risk to others. She did, however, abide by the Center for Disease Control's requirements for daily self monitoring.

Hicox's case has brought to the fore legal and ethical quandaries surrounding the appropriateness of quarantine in controlling the possibility of Ebola spreading to the United States. Those who say that mandatory quarantine is a reasonable and effective way to contain Ebola state that constraining the individual liberties of relatively few individuals is a small price to pay for the health and safety of potentially thousands – even millions – of people.

While this stance might seem clear and commonsensical, opponents have raised numerous compelling objections. Although states are allowed to impose quarantines, such measures are intended to be used only when less restrictive options to control a disease outbreak are deemed ineffective or are unavailable. And according to the CDC, less restrictive measures, such as strict daily self monitoring, are available, and are effective. Still, the governors of several states – New York and New Jersey among them – have imposed 21-day quarantines on people returning from the West African countries where Ebola is epidemic.

Critics of the quarantine say that it addresses political agendas rather than public health issues. Quarantining health workers, say critics, is a way of addressing public fear, but paradoxically, doing so increases fear of the very condition it is supposed to contain. Moreover, when politicians enforce quarantines, they are saying to the public that they do not trust public health officials, and they doubt the integrity and judgment of doctors and nurses. This creates a dangerous situation in which panicked individuals are less likely to listen to sound medical advice than to recommendations coming from less knowledgeable politicians. Equally important is the message that draconian quarantine conditions send to health workers. The efforts of volunteers are key to treating Ebola patients and containing the spread of the disease in West Africa. But if volunteers know that they will face a three-week quarantine on their return, they will be less likely to go to stricken African countries and take on the heroic and arduous task of caring for Ebola patients there.

Hickox's quarantine was a near-incarceration, but others who are suspected of exposure to the Ebola virus are quarantined at home, or agree to follow daily self monitoring protocols. Home quarantine and self monitoring are based on the honor system; it's not clear what the ramifications are for those who break quarantine, as Hickox did, or who don't monitor diligently. And therein lies a key issue: is the honor system enough? Do we trust others to be responsible for their own health, when it might impact our own? Do we trust healthcare workers to self monitor, but not others? Or do we want politicians and law enforcement officials to step in and enact quarantines as they did with Kaci Hickox?

8. Which of the following most likely reflects the author's point of view?

   A. Quarantine represents political, not health, agendas, and thus is never warranted.

   B. Despite its appearance of extremism, quarantine is the most reliable way to contain the possible spread of Ebola.

   C. In most circumstances, healthcare workers returning from Ebola-stricken countries should be subjected to daily self-monitoring, but not necessarily quarantine.

   D. Placing healthcare workers exposed to Ebola under quarantine may be unfortunate, but ultimately reassures the public of its safety.

9. According to the passage, what might a proponent of quarantine believe?

   A. Although it is unfortunate that an individual's personal liberty may be limited, quarantine represents a necessary step to protect the community.

   B. It is wrong to describe quarantine as an imposition on individual rights.

   C. Healthcare authorities, not politicians, need to make policy decisions regarding possible quarantines.

   D. Less restrictive measures, such as daily monitoring, should be used in place of quarantine whenever possible.

10. Which of the following provides another example of the conflict described in paragraph 2?

    A. All passengers arriving from other countries are given brief health exams at international airports.

    B. Although a small number will have adverse reactions, all children are required to have measles vaccines.

    C. Individuals of some ethnic groups, but not others, are stopped for questioning by police.

    D. Healthcare workers are permitted to self-monitor for symptoms of Ebola, but other individuals exposed to the virus must be quarantined.

11. Which of the following historical events might be seen as analogous to the mandatory quarantine enacted by Governor Chris Christie?

    A. The "don't ask, don't tell" policy, through which the U.S. military opted not to ask personnel about their sexual orientation, despite prohibitions against gays serving in the military

    B. The internment of Japanese Americans in WWII, a policy by which innocent U.S. citizens were imprisoned for the sake of national security during wartime

    C. The Patriot Act of 2001, which expanded government access to business and personal records in order to protect the United States from terrorism

    D. The Affordable Care Act, a controversial legislative effort to provide health insurance to all Americans

12. Suppose a healthcare worker returns to the U.S. after caring for Ebola patients in Africa. According to the passage, if the worker is exhibiting no symptoms of Ebola, what does the CDC recommend?

    A. Varying, according to the state in which the worker lives

    B. 21-day quarantine in a healthcare facility

    C. Quarantine at home, with reporting done on an as-needed basis

    D. Daily self monitoring during the 21-day period of contagion

Passage 3 (Questions 13 – 19)

Wishing to adopt a style of speechmaking in line with his arrogantly superior manner and lofty spirit, Pericles made liberal use of the instrument his old teacher Anaxagoras had given him, coloring his sweeping oratory with natural philosophy. As Plato called it, his "lofty intelligence and power of universal consummation," in addition to his natural advantages, allowed him to surpass all others in this art, adding apt illustrations drawn from physical science to his oratory.

It is for this reason that some believe he was nicknamed the Olympian. Though some cite his improvement of the city with new, beautiful buildings, and others cite his power as a politician and a general, the comedies of that time, when they allude to him, either in earnest or in jest, always seem to think that the name was given to him for his way of speaking, referring to his "thundering and lightning" and his "rolling fateful thunders from his tongue."

One saying of Thucydides, also jestingly testifying to Pericles's eloquence, has also been preserved. As the leader of the conservative party, Thucydides long struggled to hold his own against Pericles in debate. One day, the king of Sparta asked him who was a better wrestler. Thucydides answered, "When I throw him in wrestling, he beats me by proving that he never was down, and making the spectators believe him."

For all this, however, Pericles was highly cautious of his words, and whenever he ascended to the tribune to speak, he first always prayed to the gods that nothing inappropriate would escape his lips. Besides the legislative measures he brought forward, he left no writings, and very few of his sayings are recorded. One of these, poignantly, was that "he saw war coming upon Athens from Peloponnesus." As Stesimbrotus tells us, Pericles was giving a public funeral oration over those lost at Samos, and he said that the fallen had become immortal, even as the gods, for though we do not see the gods, we conceive their immortality through the respect we pay them and the blessings we receive from them, and the same is true for those who have died for their country.

As Thucydides represents it, the constitution under Pericles was a democracy in name but an aristocracy in practice, for the government was run by one leading citizen. As many writers tell us, due to grants of land abroad, indulgent entertainments, and payments for services, the people during his administration fell into bad habits and became extravagant, instead of sober and hardworking as they had been before. We shall now consider the history of this change.

First of all, Pericles had to compete with Kimon and transfer the affections of the people from this rival to himself. Because he wasn't as rich as Kimon, who used to give a daily dinner for the Athenian poor, clothe the elderly, and remove the fences from his property so that the poor might gather fruit, Pericles turned his attention to distributing the public funds among the people. By putting on public spectacles, as well as paying citizens to serve as jurymen and in other public offices, Pericles soon won the people to his side.

With the people, he was able to lead an attack upon the Senate of the Areopagus, of which he himself was not a member. Upon destroying it, Pericles made Ephialtes bring forward a bill that would restrict the Senate's judicial powers. Meanwhile, he succeeded in banishing Kimon, labeling him as a friend of Sparta and a hater of the Athenian people, even though he was second to none in birth or fortune, had won crucial victories over the Persians, and filled Athens with great spoils of war. This was how great the power of Pericles was with the common people.

13. According to the passage, why did Pericles adopt his particular style of speechmaking?

   A. Because it was in line with his innate character

   B. Because he had been taught by a great master

   C. Because it allowed him to gain influence over the people

   D. Because it was the opposite of that used by Kimon

14. Based upon the passage, it can be inferred that the author believes which of the following explanations for the Pericles' nickname, "the Olympian?"

   A. He was inordinately powerful both as a politician and a general.

   B. He was a great contributor to the physical renewal of Athens.

   C. His way of speaking was pompous, eloquent, and to comedians, god-like.

   D. He was able to achieve greatness even without the wealth that Kimon possessed.

15. Which of the following is most likely the reason why the author first introduces Thucydides to the passage?

   A. To further demonstrate the political genius, and divisiveness, of Pericles

   B. To further illustrate how persuasive Pericles could be in his oratory

   C. To introduce the surprising notion that Pericles was cautious with his words

   D. To introduce the idea of Athens being a democracy in name and an aristocracy in practice

16. According to the passage, which of the following is the most effective way to win over the common people?

   A. By winning wars and bring back spoils

   B. By throwing parties and employing people

   C. By feeding the poor and clothing the elderly

   D. By making the most excellent speeches

17. Suppose that Pericles and a political rival were having a debate, and that the rival brought up a crime from Pericles' past, the theft of several loaves bread from the market that he committed as an adolescent. Based upon the passage, how would Pericles most likely respond?

   A. He would undermine the credibility of his opponent with a fake story and the crowd would believe him.

   B. He would argue that all people make mistakes and this mistake was very minor.

   C. He would argue that the theft was right given his circumstances and that the opponent should know that.

   D. He would convince the crowd that he never committed such a crime and they would believe him.

18. According to the passage, all of the following are qualities of Pericles EXCEPT:

   A. intelligence.

   B. pompousness.

   C. carelessness.

   D. ruthlessness.

19. According to the passage, which of the following are characteristics of Kimon?

   I. Military might

   II. Magnanimity and wealth

   III. Greed

   A. I and II only

   B. I and III only

   C. II and III only

   D. I, II, and III

Passage 4 (Questions 20 – 24)

Economists have long considered knowledge and health as forms of human capital that people invest in by increasing their education and improving their health. Thus, the returns to health spending can be assessed by treating the resulting "health" as a capital good. Schultz (1961) writes that an individual's acquisition of skills and knowledge is the means by which people enhance their welfare, similar to the way in which a business invests in physical capital to increase production and profits.

Based on this point of view, spending on medical treatments (and other activities that improve one's health) is an investment that provides a stream of benefits in the future. Assessing whether today's expenditures on medical treatments are in some sense "worth it" requires that one properly account for the costs and benefits of that spending. The benefits can be far-reaching (in terms of time and those affected, and viewing health as a capital good facilitates analyzing the various channels of improvement. As Mushkin points out, "Viewing expenditures for health programs as an investment helps to underscore the contributions of health programs to expansion of income and economic growth" (Mushkin 1962, 143).

Perhaps the most obvious benefit from investments in health care is the direct increases in welfare, or well being, that accrue to individuals when their health improves. These welfare gains are realized in the form of reduced mortality and improvements in an individual's quality of life. With respect to timing, the benefits occur not only at the time of treatment but also into the future. Additionally, these welfare gains accrue potentially not just to the patient but also to those around him. For example, when a person is vaccinated, both the individual and members of his community benefit from that vaccination.

Other benefits from health spending have a more indirect effect on an individual's welfare. Consider the common belief that a major potential benefit from preventive health care expenditures today may be a substantial reduction in health care costs in the future. Some of these benefits accrue directly to the patient—reduced out-of-pocket expenditures for health care in the future—while others accrue to society as a whole—a healthier population demands less private and government insurance-related resources. Benefits from preventive care may be significant since it is thought to be less costly than treating advanced diseases. However, an extension of the average life span results in a larger aged population—a population that consumes a larger percentage of health services while achieving less productive returns to their health investment.

Another potentially important indirect benefit of improved health is the effects on macroeconomic conditions from a healthier population. For example, health spending today improves both the quantity of the labor force and the quality of the workers. Healthier workers are more productive because of an extension of the working age, fewer sick days,

and a decline in the loss of labor from disease or death (which reduces the costs of hiring and training associated with replacing that lost labor). In addition to greater productivity, a healthier (and longer living) population consumes more nonhealth-related expenditures, thereby boosting economic growth.

While the benefits seem intuitive, quantifying them is difficult. A National Academies Panel noted, "Health cannot be purchased directly and …There is no market equivalent to help us answer valuation questions, so one must turn to other methods" (Abraham and Mackie 2005, 117). We may be able to identify a drop in the number of sick days taken by individuals, thereby increasing productivity, but we cannot quantify the increase in their welfare. Therefore, it is difficult to estimate the entire return to investments in health care services. In addition, a distortion of the demand for health care services exists because most people do not face the full cost of the service; private or public insurance programs subsidize most health care costs. Nevertheless, academic work has applied a multitude of approaches to value the returns to improvements in health. Although the estimates vary depending on the methods and data, all existing work suggests that these benefits can be quite high.

20. What is the purpose of the discussion of vaccination?

    A. To give an example of a health care initiative that promotes public health at the expense of the individual

    B. To give an example of how health care benefits have grown more dramatic

    C. To give an example of how modern medicine has advanced to better treat deadly diseases

    D. To give an example of how health care benefits oneself and those surrounding oneself

21. Suppose it were found that an increase in health care spending over the last few years has corresponded with an increase in unemployment. How would this information affect the author's claims?

    A. It would disagree with the author's assertion that medical spending would improve the quality of workers.

    B. It would not disagree with the author's assertion that medical spending would increase the quantity of workers.

    C. It would directly disagree with the assertion that medical spending would result in more workers.

    D. It would agree with the assertion that medical spending would improve the health of the economy.

22. Which of the following would the author argue to be a benefit in investing in the knowledge and education of the population?

    A. Increased quantity of labor force

    B. Increased quality of labor force

    C. Decreased working age and decline in loss of labor

    D. Decreased wages for labor force

23. With which of the following statements would the author most likely agree?

    A. It is easier to measure return on investments in knowledge than investments in health.

    B. It is easier to measure benefits from investment in health care on the economy than on population health.

    C. It is easier to measure the benefits from investment in health care than the costs of investment in health care.

    D. It is easier to measure the costs of investments in knowledge than costs of investments in health.

24. Which of the following best describes the passage?

    A. A treatise on economics from the viewpoint of cost/benefit analysis to the medical professionals

    B. A treatise on economics in the private sector with emphasis on the impact of insurance companies on the health of the population

    C. A treatise on health care filtered through the principles of economics

    D. A treatise on the effects of health care investment from the viewpoint of those insurance companies that bear the brunt of health care costs

Passage 5 (Questions 25 – 30)

Though experience be our only guide in reasoning concerning matters of fact, it must be acknowledged that this guide is not altogether infallible, but in some cases is apt to lead us into errors. One, who in our climate, should expect better weather in any week of June than in one of December, would reason justly, and conformably to experience; but it is certain, that he may happen, in the event, to find himself mistaken. However, we may observe, that, in such a case, he would have no cause to complain of experience; because it commonly informs us beforehand of the uncertainty, by that contrariety of events, which we may learn from a diligent observation. All effects follow not with like certainty from their supposed causes. Some events are found, in all countries and all ages, to have been constantly conjoined together: others are found to have been more variable, and sometimes to disappoint our expectations; so that, in our reasonings concerning matter of fact, there are all imaginable degrees of assurance, from the highest certainty to the lowest species of moral evidence.

A wise man, therefore, proportions his belief to the evidence. In such conclusions as are founded on an infallible experience, he expects the event with the last degree of assurance, and regards his past experience as a full *proof* of the future existence of that event. In other cases, he proceeds with more caution. He weighs the opposite experiments; he considers which side is supported by the greater number of experiments; to that side he inclines, with doubt and hesitation; and when at last he fixes his judgment, the evidence exceeds not what we properly call *probability*. All probability, then, supposes an opposition of experiments and observations, where the one side is found to overbalance the other, and to produce a degree of evidence, proportioned to the superiority. A hundred instances or experiments on one side, and fifty on another, afford a doubtful expectation of any event; though a hundred uniform experiments, with only one that is contradictory, reasonably beget a pretty strong degree of assurance. In all cases, we must balance the opposite experiments, where they are opposite, and deduct the smaller number from the greater, in order to know the exact force of the superior evidence.

A miracle is a violation of the laws of nature; and as a firm and unalterable experience has established these laws, the proof against a miracle, from the very nature of the fact, is as entire as any argument from experience can possibly be imagined. Nothing is esteemed a miracle, if it ever happens in the common course of nature. It is no miracle that a man, seemingly in good health, should die all of a sudden: because such a kind of death, though more unusual than any other, has yet been frequently observed to happen. But it is a miracle, that a dead man should come to life; because that has never been observed in any age or country. There must, therefore, be a uniform experience against every miraculous event, otherwise the event would not merit that appellation. And as a uniform experience amounts to a proof, there is here a direct and full *proof*, from the nature of the fact, against the existence of any miracle; nor can such a proof be destroyed, or the miracle rendered credible, but by an opposite proof, which is superior.

The plain consequence is "That no testimony is sufficient to establish a miracle, unless the testimony be of such a kind, that its falsehood would be more miraculous, than the fact, which it endeavors to establish; and even in that case there is a mutual destruction of arguments." When anyone tells me that he saw a dead man restored to life, I immediately consider with myself, whether it be more probable that this person should either deceive or be deceived, or that the fact, which he relates, should really have happened. I weigh the one miracle against the other; and according to the superiority, which I discover, I pronounce my decision, and always reject the greater miracle. If the falsehood of his testimony would be more miraculous than the event which he relates; then, and not till then, can he pretend to command my belief or opinion.

25. According to the passage, the author believes that:

   A. men who proclaim to have witnessed miracles are untrustworthy.

   B. evidence for an outcome is based on the probability of opposite outcomes.

   C. there are events that can be interpreted beyond the confines of reason.

   D. prior experiences dictate future results.

26. It can be inferred from the passage that the author:

   A. would choose to believe scientific reasoning in all circumstances.

   B. does not believe in a divine presence.

   C. frequently distrusts the accounts of others.

   D. believes in a divine presence, but cannot trust in the accounts of miraculous events.

27. A new scientific study is released that contradicts our prior knowledge on the subject. Based on the passage, the author would most likely:

   A. be skeptical of the personal credibility of the authors of the study.

   B. only evaluate the probability that the new evidence is correct in comparison to his prior knowledge.

   C. continue to believe the prior knowledge until a satisfactory number of studies confirm the new result.

   D. withhold judgment until he can see the results for himself.

28. Which of the following is closest to the author's viewpoint on miracles?

   A. Miracles are a philosophical impossibility according to the principles of reason.

   B. A miraculous event can only be explained by forces beyond human reason.

   C. Miracles, however possible, are incredibly unlikely.

   D. Miracles, if confirmed, would provide evidence for a divine influence.

29. The overall tone of the passage can be described as:

   A. esoteric, but relatable.

   B. erudite, but conversational.

   C. logical, but inquisitive.

   D. colloquial, but informative.

30. Which of the following statements, if true, would weaken the author's argument?

   A. A miracle is witnessed by a great number of trustworthy, reasonable individuals.

   B. A miraculous event is consistently observed under rigorous empirical observation.

   C. Our current understanding of the physical laws of nature, based on empirical observation, is proven to be inaccurate.

   D. None of the above

Passage 6 (Questions 31 – 36)

It is a common weakness of mankind to be caught by an idea and captivated by a phrase. To rest therewith content and to neglect the carrying of the idea into practice is a weakness still more common. It is this frequent failure of reformers to reduce their theories to practice, their tendency to dwell in the cloudland of the ideal rather than to test it in action, that has often made them distrusted and unpopular.

With our forefathers the phrase "mens sana in corpore sano" was a high favorite. It was constantly quoted with approval by writers on hygiene and sanitation, and used as the text or the finale of hundreds of popular lectures. And yet we shall seek in vain for any evidence of its practical usefulness. Its words are good and true, but passive and actionless, not of that dynamic type where words are "words indeed, but words that draw armed men behind them."

Our age is of another temper. It yearns for reality. It no longer rests satisfied with mere ideas, or words, or phrases. The modern Ulysses would drink life to the dregs. The present age is dissatisfied with the vague assurance that the Lord will provide, and, rightly or wrongly, is beginning to expect the state to provide. And while this desire for reality has its drawbacks, it has also its advantages. Our age doubts absolutely the virtues of blind submission and resignation, and cries out instead for prevention and amelioration. Disease is no longer regarded, as Cruden regarded it, as the penalty and the consequence of sin. Nature herself is now perceived to be capable of imperfect work. Time was when the human eye was referred to as a perfect apparatus, but the number of young children wearing spectacles renders that idea untenable to-day.

Meanwhile the multiplication of state asylums and municipal hospitals, and special schools for deaf or blind children and for cripples, speaks eloquently and irresistibly of an intimate connection between civics and health. There is a physical basis of citizenship, as there is a physical basis of life and of health; and any one who will take the trouble to read even the Table of Contents of this book will see that for Dr. Allen prevention is a text and the making of sound citizens a sermon. Given the sound body, we have nowadays small fear for the sound mind. The rigid physiological dualism implied in the phrase "mens sana in corpore sano" is no longer allowed. Today the sound body generally includes the sound mind, and vice versa. If mental dullness be due to imperfect ears, the remedy lies in medical treatment of those organs, not in education of the brain. If lack of initiative or energy proceeds from defective aeration of the blood due to adenoids blocking the air tides in the windpipe, then the remedy lies not in better teaching but in a simple surgical operation.

Shakespeare, in his wildwood play, saw sermons in stones and books in the running brooks. We moderns find a drama in the fateful lives of ordinary mortals, sermons in their physical salvation from some of the ills that flesh is heir to, and books--like this of Dr. Allen's--in striving to teach man-kind how to become happier, and healthier, and more useful members of society.

Dr. Allen is undoubtedly a reformer, but of the modern, not the ancient, type. He is a prophet crying in our present wilderness; but he is more than a prophet, for he is always intensely practical, insisting, as he does, on getting things done, and done soon, and done right.

31. Which of the following best describes the author's attitude towards Dr. Allen?

    A. Objective approval

    B. Admiration

    C. Skepticism

    D. Indebtedness

32. Which of the following is a reason that the author might give for the fact that ancient reformers took less action to enact their reforms?

    A. They didn't believe that their theories would work in practice.

    B. They lacked the motivation to do physical labor.

    C. Their societies placed less emphasis on the importance of moving theories into action.

    D. Their societies were not interested in improving.

33. Which of the following is most likely the subject of Dr. Allen's book?

    A. Public health as it relates to civic matters

    B. Mental illnesses

    C. The physiology of mental health

    D. The difference between ancient and modern reformers

34. Suppose none of Dr. Allen's reforms were ever enacted. How might the author's view towards Dr. Allen change?

    A. Dr. Allen would be less popular and trusted.

    B. Dr. Allen would still be viewed as an effective reformer.

    C. Dr. Allen would be classified as an ancient reformer.

    D. Dr. Allen would be classified as a medical reformer but not a civic reformer.

35. What is the author's purpose in discussing the phrase "mens sana in corpore sano" and how it's been interpreted and acted on throughout the ages?

    A. To illustrate that mental illnesses are just another form of bodily illnesses

    B. To illustrate that ancient reformers were satisfied with dealing in hypotheticals

    C. To illustrate the difference between ancient and modern times in dealing with public health problems

    D. To illustrate that modern reformers are all focused on improving public health

36. What did the author mean by the phrase "given the sound body, we have nowadays small fear for the sound mind"?

    A. People with mental illnesses are no longer as feared as they once were.

    B. Nowadays, we understand that mental illnesses do not result from personal sin.

    C. Mental illness itself is much more prevalent in today's society.

    D. Mental illnesses can be explained as failures of the body's physical systems.

Passage 7 (Questions 37 – 41)

You observe, I have hitherto spoken of the power of Athena, as over painting no less than sculpture. But her rule over both arts is only so far as they are zoographic;—representative, that is to say, of animal life, or of such order and discipline among other elements, as may invigorate and purify it. Now there is a specialty of the art of painting beyond this, namely, the representation of phenomena of color and shadow, as such, without question of the nature of the things that receive them. I am now accordingly obliged to speak of sculpture and painting as distinct arts: but the laws which bind sculpture, bind no less the painting of the higher schools, which has, for its main purpose, the showing of beauty in human or animal form; and which is therefore placed by the Greeks equally under the rule of Athena, as the Spirit, first, of Life, and then of Wisdom in conduct.

First, I say, you are to "see Pallas" in all such work, as the Queen of Life; and the practical law which follows from this, is one of enormous range and importance, namely, that nothing must be represented by sculpture, external to any living form, which does not help to enforce or illustrate the conception of life. Both dress and armor may be made to do this, by great sculptors, and are continually so used by the greatest. One of the essential distinctions between the Athenian and Florentine schools is dependent on their treatment of drapery in this respect; an Athenian always sets it to exhibit the action of the body, by flowing with it, or over it, or from it, so as to illustrate both its form and gesture; a Florentine, on the contrary, always uses his drapery to conceal or disguise the forms of the body, and exhibit mental emotion; but both use it to enhance the life, either of the body or soul; Donatello and Michelangelo, no less than the sculptors of Gothic chivalry, ennoble armor in the same way; but base sculptors carve drapery and armor for the sake of their folds and picturesqueness only, and forget the body beneath. The rule is so stern, that all delight in mere incidental beauty, which painting often triumphs in, is wholly forbidden to sculpture;—for instance, in painting the branch of a tree, you may rightly represent and enjoy the lichens and moss on it, but a sculptor must not touch one of them: they are inessential to the tree's life,—he must give the flow and bending of the branch only, else he does not enough "see Pallas" in it.

Or, to take a higher instance, here is an exquisite little painted poem, by Edward Frere; a cottage interior, one of the thousands which within the last two months have been laid desolate in unhappy France. Every accessory in the painting is of value—the fireside, the tiled floor, the vegetables lying upon it, and the basket hanging from the roof. But not one of these accessories would have been admissible in sculpture. You must carve nothing but what has life. "Why?" you probably feel instantly inclined to ask me.—You see the principle we have got, instead of being blunt or useless, is such an edged tool that you are startled the moment I apply it. "Must we refuse every pleasant accessory and picturesque detail, and petrify nothing but living creatures?" Even so: I would not assert it on my own authority. It is the Greeks who say it, but whatever they say of sculpture, be assured, is true.

37. Based on the passage it can be assumed that Donatello's depiction of armor:

    A. is completely unlike that of the Athenian school.

    B. focuses on a delight in aesthetic beauty and detail.

    C. makes use of detail to enhance the depiction of life.

    D. seeks to exhibit the action of the body through detail.

38. How does the author support his assertions about sculpture only depicting details of life?

    A. Greek scriptures on sculpture must be obeyed.

    B. The principle that is least blunt or useless is the most viable.

    C. Personal authority is the only principle when it comes to art.

    D. Scriptures on sculpture oppose those of other art forms.

39. In discussing both painting and sculpture, the author's intention is to:

    A. suggest that an emphasis on life and form is a natural offshoot of the material conditions of sculpting.

    B. show the shared roots, in Greek culture, of both art forms.

    C. argue that sculpture shares no principles with painting.

    D. demonstrate that the principles of sculpture preclude certain elements that are admirable in painting.

40. Suppose that a painting demonstrated such mastery of color and shading in a woman's dress and jewelry that viewers swear it was painted from life. The author would most likely state that:

    A. painting ought to focus on beauty in human or animal form, not accouterments.

    B. this mastery marks the painting as under the rule of Pallas.

    C. such an emphasis is what separates sculpture from painting.

    D. painting of the higher schools focuses on enjoyment of incidental beauties.

41. Suppose a sculpture of a whale was receiving praise for the depiction of the various barnacles on its body. The author of the passage would most likely state that:

    A. the contrast between extremely large and extremely small counters the intention of good sculpture.

    B. such an emphasis on externals is inadmissible in sculpture.

    C. the delight caused by the beauty of the barnacles justifies the sculptor's choice to include them.

    D. such exquisite details elevate sculpture to the level of poetry.

Passage 8 (Questions 42 – 48)

The primary belief of Christianity concerns the Unity of the Trinity: the Father is God, the Son is God, the Holy Spirit is God. Therefore, Father, Son, and Holy Spirit are one God, not three. The principle of this union is absence of difference. Some, however, by ranking the elements of the Trinity by merit, break it up and convert it to plurality. We shall now explore why this is misguided.

Speculative science may be divided into three different kinds: Physics, Mathematics, and Theology. To begin, Physics studies motion and is neither abstract nor separable, for its primary concern is with the forms of bodies and their constituent matter. Realistically, these forms cannot be separated from their bodies, or matter. As these bodies are in motion, form takes on the movement of the particular thing to which it is attached. For example, earth tends downwards and fire tends upwards. Mathematics does not deal with motion and is not abstract: its interest is in the forms of bodies apart from matter, and therefore apart from movement. However, because these forms are ultimately connected with matter, they cannot be truly separated from bodies.

Because the Divine Substance is without either matter or motion, Theology does not deal with motion and is both abstract and separable. In Physics, we must use scientific concepts, in Mathematics, systematical, and in Theology, intellectual. In Theology, we aim to not be distracted by imaginations and to simply recognize and appreciate that Form which is pure form and no image, which itself is Being and the source of Being. Everything owes its being to it.

A statue is not a statue because of the brass that makes up its matter, but because of the form through which the likeness of a living thing is impressed upon it. Likewise, the brass itself is not brass because of the earth that is its matter, but because of its form. In the same way, earth is not earth because it is matter, but because of its dryness and weight, which are forms. Nothing is said to be because it has matter, but rather, because it has form.

However, the Divine Substance is form without matter and because of this, is One, and is its own essence. All other things are not their own essences: every other thing takes its being from the things of which it is composed, from its parts. It is this *and* that, its parts in conjunction. It is not this *or* that. For example, man consists of body *and* soul, not body *or* soul. Therefore, man is not his own essence.

On the other hand, that which consists not of this and that, but only this, is truly its own essence, and is therefore beautiful and stable, being grounded in nothing. Therefore, the thing in which there is no number, in which nothing is present except for its own essence, is truly One. Moreover, it cannot become the substrate of anything, for it is pure form and pure forms cannot have substrates.

If humanity, like other forms, is a substrate for accidents (happenings), it does not receive these accidents because it exists, but rather, because matter is subjected to it. Indeed, humanity seems to appropriate the accidents which actually belong to the matter underlying its very conception. Form without matter cannot be a substrate and also cannot have its essence in matter. Otherwise, it would be a reflection, not a form.

From the forms which are outside of matter come the forms which are in matter and make up bodies. In reality, we mislabel these entities that reside in bodies when we call them forms: they are mere images resembling those forms which are not embodied in matter. In God, then, there is no difference, no plurality from difference, no multiplicity from accidents, and therefore, no number: the Holy Trinity is one God.

42. According to the passage, which of the following statements accurately describe the study of Physics?

   I. It is concerned with motion.

   II. It is equally concerned with form and matter.

   III. Because matter is in motion, form takes on motion.

   A. I only

   B. I and II only

   C. II and III only

   D. I, II, and III

43. According to the passage, which of the following accurately describes the principle underlying the Christian notion of the Unity of the Trinity?

   A. The plurality of difference

   B. The absence of difference

   C. The unity of difference

   D. The difference between form and matter

44. The author most likely introduces the first two speculative sciences in order to:

   A. help characterize the nature of theology.

   B. help prove their inferiority to theology.

   C. establish a scientific approach to theology.

   D. help prove their superiority to theology.

45. According to the passage, which of the following statements about Mathematics is true?

   A. Mathematics deals with motion and can be abstract.

   B. Mathematics does not deal with matter or motion and is abstract.

   C. Mathematics studies motion and is concrete and separable.

   D. Mathematics is concrete and does not deal with motion.

46. Based upon the passage, it can be assumed that the author believes which of the following statements?

   A. The notion of the Holy Trinity representing one God can be explained in intellectual terms.

   B. Physics and Mathematics are more practical than Theology, and therefore, more useful.

   C. We can use scientific and systematic as well as intellectual concepts to study the nature of the Divine.

   D. There are many interpretations of the nature of the Holy Trinity and all of them are legitimate.

47. Suppose a student was trying to decide whether to pursue further education and a career in either Mathematics, Physics, or Theology. This student has an excellent imagination and a penchant for a methodical approach to study and work. Moreover, if asked to choose between the two, this student would say she was more interested in forms than matter. According to the passage and its context, which of the following disciplines ought the student to pursue?

   A. Mathematics

   B. Physics

   C. Theology

   D. Mathematics and Theology

48. All of the following statements about the relationship between form and matter are true EXCEPT:

   A. a statue is a statue because of the likeness of a living thing that it displays.

   B. earth is earth because of its dryness, weight, and coarseness.

   C. water is water because of its wetness, weight, and other properties.

   D. brass is brass because it is made up of brass.

Passage 9 (Questions 49 – 53)

The time, it is to be hoped, is gone by, when any defense would be necessary of the "liberty of the press" as one of the securities against corrupt or tyrannical government. No argument, we may suppose, can now be needed, against permitting a legislature or an executive, not identified in interest with the people, to prescribe opinions to them, and determine what doctrines or what arguments they shall be allowed to hear. This aspect of the question, besides, has been so often and so triumphantly enforced by preceding writers, that it need not be specially insisted on in this place. Though the law of England, on the subject of the press, is as servile to this day as it was in the time of the Tudors, there is little danger of its being actually put in force against political discussion, except during some temporary panic, when fear of insurrection drives ministers and judges from their propriety; and, speaking generally, it is not, in constitutional countries, to be apprehended that the government, whether completely responsible to the people or not, will often attempt to control the expression of opinion, except when in doing so it makes itself the organ of the general intolerance of the public. Let us suppose, therefore, that the government is entirely at one with the people, and never thinks of exerting any power of coercion unless in agreement with what it conceives to be their voice. But I deny the right of the people to exercise such coercion, either by themselves or by their government. The power itself is illegitimate. The best government has no more title to it than the worst. It is as noxious, or more noxious, when exerted in accordance with public opinion, than when in opposition to it. If all mankind minus one were of one opinion, and only one person were of the contrary opinion, mankind would be no more justified in silencing that one person, than he, if he had the power, would be justified in silencing mankind. Were an opinion a personal possession of no value except to the owner; if to be obstructed in the enjoyment of it were simply a private injury, it would make some difference whether the injury was inflicted only on a few persons or on many. But the peculiar evil of silencing the expression of an opinion is, that it is robbing the human race, posterity as well as the existing generation; those who dissent from the opinion, still more than those who hold it. If the opinion is right, they are deprived of the opportunity of exchanging error for truth: if wrong, they lose, what is almost as great a benefit, the clearer perception and livelier impression of truth, produced by its collision with error.

It is necessary to consider separately these two hypotheses, each of which has a distinct branch of the argument corresponding to it. We can never be sure that the opinion we are endeavoring to stifle is a false opinion; and if we were sure, stifling it would be an evil still.

First: the opinion which it is attempted to suppress by authority may possibly be true. Those who desire to suppress it, of course deny its truth; but they are not infallible. They have no authority to decide the question for all mankind, and exclude every other person from the means of judging. To refuse a hearing to an opinion because they are sure that it is false is to assume that their certainty is the same thing as absolute certainty. All silencing of discussion is an assumption of infallibility. Its condemnation may be allowed to rest on this common argument, not the worse for being common.

Let us now pass to the second division of the argument, and dismissing the supposition that any of the received opinions may be false, let us assume them to be true, and examine into the worth of the manner in which they are likely to be held, when their truth is not freely and openly canvassed. However unwillingly a person who has a strong opinion may admit the possibility that his opinion may be false, he ought to be moved by the consideration that however true it may be, if it is not fully, frequently, and fearlessly discussed, it will be held as a dead dogma, not a living truth.

49. With which of the following statements would the author most likely agree?

   A. To obtain truth is the noblest goal of discussion

   B. A non-constitutional government has the right to manipulate what the public hears

   C. The silencing or misconstruing of another's opinion is akin to physically abusing them

   D. The people of a society have the responsibility to overthrow a government that attempts to mold their opinions

50. To what is the author referring when he or she speaks of "this aspect of the question" in the first paragraph?

   A. The question of whether it is lawful to print slanderous materials about a government

   B. The question of whether the voice of many should outweigh the voice of one

   C. The question of whether people are free to say what they will and require newspapers to publish these opinions

   D. The question of whether governments should have the right to control opinions seen by the masses

51. What is the purpose of the analogy made between a personal opinion and a personal possession?

   A. To demonstrate that harming a possession only harms the possessor but obstructing an opinion harms everyone

   B. To show that the obstruction of an opinion is more hurtful to the dissenter than to the holder of the opinion

   C. To illustrate that the obstruction of the opinion of many is more hurtful than obstructing that of one

   D. To show that if a right opinion is silenced, the human race is at a loss

52. Which of the following are most likely NOT sentiments espoused by the author?

   I. Truth is relative depending on your point of view

   II. Every opinion can be backed by evidence

   III. Every opinion deserves to be considered

   A. I only

   B. III only

   C. I and II only

   D. II and III only

53. If the author believes that absolute truth exists, which of the following ideas expressed by the author could be used as a counterargument?

   A. One should always doubt one's convictions

   B. Truth that is not frequently discussed will be considered dead dogma

   C. No opinion held by the majority is infallible

   D. No man can know a thing with absolute certainty

This page intentionally left blank.

SECTION 8

Answer Key

1	B	12	D	23	B	34	A	45	D
2	B	13	A	24	C	35	C	46	A
3	A	14	C	25	B	36	D	47	A
4	C	15	B	26	A	37	C	48	D
5	A	16	B	27	B	38	A	49	A
6	C	17	D	28	A	39	D	50	D
7	C	18	C	29	C	40	C	51	A
8	C	19	A	30	D	41	B	52	C
9	A	20	D	31	B	42	D	53	D
10	B	21	B	32	C	43	B		
11	B	22	B	33	A	44	A		

Passage 1 (Questions 1 – 7)

Shakespeare understood that **tradition** could supply a **better fable** than ever invention could, and in his day, the **petulant demand for originality** was not nearly so much pressed. There was no literature for the masses: the cheap press and **universal reading** were simply unknown. When he appears in widely illiterate times, a great poet absorbs into his work all the light that is anywhere radiating. Because it his duty to bring every intellectual gem and every flower of sentiment to the people, he comes to value his **memory** equally with his **invention**. Therefore, he **cares little** about from where his thoughts **derive**: whether they come from translation, tradition, travel, or inspiration, they are all equally welcome to his **uncritical audience**.

Opinion: author thinks Shakespeare pulled from many sources without worrying about originality; author thinks demand for originality is "petulant"

Other men say wise things as well as he does, but they also say many foolish things, and do not actually know when they have spoken wisely. The great poet knows the sparkle of the true stone and puts it in its right and lofty place whenever he finds it. Such is the position of **Homer**, and perhaps of **Chaucer** and **Saadi**, for they three felt that **all wit was their wit**. As much they are poets, they are **librarians** and **historiographers**: each was **heir** and **dispenser** of all the tales of the world. As **Milton**, another such poet wrote, "Presenting Thebes' and Pelops' line / And the tale of Troy divine."

Key terms: Homer, Chaucer, Saadi, Milton

Opinion: author appreciates great authors who took tales from wherever they could find the "sparkle of true stone" and used it

The influence of **Chaucer** is clear in all our early literature, and more recently, **Pope**, **Dryden**, and many others have been quite **beholden to him**. One is charmed by this opulence that feeds so many pensioners. Yet, **Chaucer himself** was a **prolific borrower**, drawing always from writers who themselves borrowed. One of those from whom he borrows is **Gower**, who he uses like a stone-quarry out of which he might build his own house. This theft he commits with an apology, that what he takes has **no worth where he found it**, but the **greatest where he leaves it**. Indeed, it has essentially become a rule in literature that a writer, once having proven himself **capable of original writing**, is from thenceforth **entitled to steal** from the work of others at his own discretion. A **thought** is the **property of the person** who can entertain it and who **can adequately place** it. At first, a certain awkwardness marks the use of a borrowed thought, but as soon as we have learned what to do with it, it becomes our own.

Key terms: Chaucer, Pope, Dryden, Gower

Opinion: author extends his idea to even say the idea belongs to the person who uses it well, not the person who thought it up

In this way, all **originality is relative** and **every thinker is retrospective**. The educated lawmakers at Westminster or in Washington speak and vote for thousands. Every senator has his **constituency** and is connected to it through invisible channels. Through these, the senator is made **aware of the wishes of the people** with evidence, anecdotes, and **estimates**. As Sir Robert **Peel** and Mr. **Webster** vote for thousands, so do **Locke** and **Rousseau** think for thousands, and so were there **foundations** all around Homer and Chaucer and Milton **from which they drew**: friends, lovers, books, traditions, and proverbs, all perished, which if seen would contribute to reducing our sense of wonder.

Key terms: Sir Robert Peel, Mr. Webster, Locke, Rousseau

Opinion: author sees a parallel between representatives in government and philosophers and poets who draw from many sources to help keep our sense of wonder

Does the great poet speak with authority? Does he ever feel himself outmatched? This appeal is to **the consciousness of the writer**. Is there some oracle in his breast that can be asked about any thought or thing and whether it be true or false, and to have the answer, and to rely on that? All the **debts** that such an artist could ever owe to **other wits** would never disturb his **consciousness of originality**, because the **ministrations of books**, and yes, even of **other minds**, are like a **whiff of smoke** to that **most private reality** with which he has conversed.

Cause and effect: the author asserts that writers are not troubled when borrowing from other books as they create their own work

Main Idea: The author asserts that great poets actively borrow from other sources, for ideas can be owned by anyone who knows how to properly use them; Shakespeare and others are set apart not because of their originality, but because they can tell whether a thing is wise or not, and have an inner oracle.

1. B is correct. With Shakespeare out of the running, we can turn to the second paragraph: "Such is the position of Homer, and perhaps of Chaucer and Saadi . . ." So, Homer is definitely in this position while Chaucer and Saadi are "perhaps" in this position. And, as Milton is mentioned offhandedly at the end of the paragraph, we see that the author would credit Homer as the greatest of these poets.

2. B is correct. Just like lawmakers, connected to their constituencies, vote for thousands, great philosophers are also connected and think for thousands, while great poets are also connected and write for thousands. All of these people are either great doers or thinkers who are connected through invisible channels "which if seen would contribute to reducing our sense of wonder."

   A: They are not taking commands as much as they are taking inspiration.

   C: This is a less clear comparison. Politicians legislate while poets and philosophers create: they contribute content to the world while politicians attempt to organize and manage their countries.

3. A is correct. In Shakespeare's day, "the petulant demand for originality was not nearly so much pressed." This is in comparison to now, when there is a petulant demand for originality that is pressed.

   B: What about Shakespeare? We never see any claim of supremacy made.

   C: This is not necessarily true.

   D: Rather, we get the sense that Chaucer did not appreciate Gower, as he committed the theft of Gower's ideas with the "apology" that what he took had no worth where he found it.

4. C is correct. The last sentence answers the question posed directly before it: "Is there some oracle in his breast that can be asked about any thought or thing and whether it be true or false, and to have the answer, and to rely on that?" The answer is yes, because this is what sets a great artist apart. Ideas from books and other people are insubstantial in comparison to "that most private reality with which he has conversed". This is what sets the genius apart, not his ideas, but the ability to know which ones are true or not, which ones are wise or not.

   A: The author's main idea seems to go against the importance of originality.

   B: It is not said directly God, but rather, an oracle.

   D: The power comes from this oracle in his chest that allows him to judge accurately.

5. A is correct. For his answer, we zoom into the second to last sentence of the third paragraph which states: "A thought is the property of the person who can entertain it and who can adequately place it." This is the only sentence of the paragraph that clearly defines how a person can "own" a thought. A person must be able to entertain, or understand a thought, and also know how to place it. Therefore, choice A, in which the theatre maker understands how the play connects with the chosen theme or conceit, as well as she understands how to place that idea into execution, is correct.

   B: Welles's motives are not necessary for her to know, given the what the passage has to say.

   C: But what about the play? She cannot just study context.

   D: In this option, she doesn't learn about the context of pre WW2 Europe or the play, but rather, how to generally adapt a play. So, she would own this idea, but not the idea expressed in the question.

6. C is correct. Rather, as the author writes in the last sentence of the first paragraph, "he cares little about from where his thoughts derive."

   A, B, D: All of these are true.

7. C is correct. I: This is true because anyone who can entertain an idea and who can adequately place it can own it. This means, however many people satisfy this demand will "own" the idea. II: This is true because the last sentence of the fourth paragraph makes it clear that if the invisible connections between artists and poets and their sources were seen, this would "contribute to reducing our sense of wonder."

   III: This is false because, as the author writes of the great poet, ". . . he comes to value his memory equally with his invention."

Passage 2 (Questions 8 – 12)

When nurse **Kaci Hickox** returned to the United States after a month-long volunteer stay **caring for Ebola** patients in Sierra Leone, she did not receive a hero's welcome. Instead, she was **quarantined**, isolated in an unheated tent with no running water outside of a Newark, **New Jersey** hospital. Despite the fact that **she had tested negative for the Ebola virus** and exhibited **no symptoms**, Hickox was placed in a state-mandated 21-day quarantine, ordered by New Jersey Governor Chris **Christie**. Hickox loudly protested, and after several days was allowed to leave the tent and return by car to her home in Maine, where under that state's law she was supposed to remain quarantined in her home. However, Hickox **refused that quarantine** as well, stating that she was of no risk to others. **She did**, however, abide by the **Center for Disease Control's** requirements for **daily self monitoring**.

Key terms: Kaci Hickox, Ebola, quarantine, Center for Disease Control, self monitoring

Cause and effect: nurse Kaci Hickox refused to remain in quarantine after returning from treating Ebola patients in West Africa

Hicox's case has brought to the fore **legal** and **ethical** quandaries surrounding the appropriateness of **quarantine** in controlling the possibility of Ebola spreading to the United States. Those who say that mandatory quarantine is a reasonable and effective way to contain Ebola state that **constraining the individual liberties** of relatively few individuals is a small price to pay for the **health and safety of potentially thousands** – even millions – of people.

Key terms: legal and ethical quandaries, mandatory quarantine, individual liberties

Opinion: proponents of quarantine say that temporary loss of liberty for a few is a reasonable price for the health and safety of the community

While this stance might seem clear and commonsensical, opponents have raised **numerous compelling objections**. Although states are allowed to impose quarantines, such measures are intended to be used **only when less restrictive options** to control a disease outbreak are deemed ineffective or are **unavailable**. And according to the CDC, less restrictive measures, such as strict **daily self monitoring**, are available, and are effective. Still, the governors of several states – New York and New Jersey among them – have imposed 21-day quarantines on people returning from the West African countries where Ebola is epidemic.

Key terms: objections, less restrictive options, people returning from West Africa

Opinion: critics say less restrictive options like self monitoring are effective and more appropriate than quarantine

Contrast: some states imposing quarantines, despite the CDC's recommendations

Critics of the quarantine say that it addresses **political agendas rather than public health issues**. Quarantining health workers, say critics, is a way of addressing public fear, but **paradoxically**, doing so **increases fear** of the very condition it is supposed to contain. Moreover, when politicians enforce quarantines, they are saying to the public that they **do not trust public health officials**, and they doubt the integrity and judgment of doctors and nurses. This creates a dangerous situation in which panicked individuals are less likely to listen to sound medical advice than to recommendations coming from less knowledgeable politicians. Equally important is **the message** that draconian quarantine conditions **send to health workers**. The efforts of volunteers are key to treating Ebola patients and containing the spread of the disease in West Africa. But if volunteers know that they will face a three-week quarantine on their return, they will be less likely to go to stricken African countries and take on the heroic and arduous task of caring for Ebola patients there.

Key terms: critics, political agendas, public fear, volunteers

Opinion: critics say quarantine represents political interests, increases fear, and discourages volunteerism

Hickox's quarantine was a **near-incarceration**, but others who are suspected of exposure to the Ebola virus are quarantined at home, or agree to follow daily self monitoring protocols. Home quarantine and self monitoring are based on the honor system; it's not clear what the ramifications are for those who break quarantine, as Hickox did, or who don't monitor diligently. And therein lies a key issue: **is the honor system enough**? Do we trust others to be responsible for their own health, when it might impact our own? Do we trust healthcare workers to self monitor, but not others? Or do we want politicians and law enforcement officials to step in and enact quarantines as they did with Kaci Hickox?

Key terms: honor system, trust

Opinion: home quarantine and self monitoring work on the honor system, which raises additional issues

Main Idea: Quarantine is a complex issue, and less extreme options, such as monitoring, should be used in its stead in most cases.

8.   C is correct. The author's attitude toward quarantine comes through most clearly in paragraph 3: quarantine should be used when less restrictive measures are not effective or available.

   A: Quarantine may represent a political agenda, but to say it is never warranted is too extreme.

   B: The author mentions several objections to quarantine and does not embrace it without reservation.

   D: Quite the opposite – the author says that quarantine worries, not reassures, the public of its safety.

9.   A is correct. The views of proponents of quarantine are summarized in paragraph 2; that limiting individual liberties is a small and necessary price to pay for safeguarding the health of many.

   B: Even proponents of quarantine admit it is an imposition on individuals – a necessary imposition.

   C: According to this passage, proponents are okay with politicians making the decisions.

   D: This choice represents the belief of critics of quarantine.

10.   B is correct. The conflict described in paragraph 2 is between individual rights and the health and safety of the community. The example in choice B – requiring all children to get measles vaccines despite the likelihood that a small number will have adverse reactions – is similar.

11.   B is correct. Correct choice B describes another situation in which the rights and liberty of a few (actually, not so few) are constrained in the name of the safety of the larger group. None of the other choices reflect that model.

12.   D is correct. In paragraphs one and three, we learn that the CDC favors regular self monitoring for healthcare workers who are asymptomatic of Ebola.

   A: Policies regarding quarantine do indeed vary by state, but that is different from the CDC's recommendation, which is not state-specific.

   B: This is only recommended by the CDC if less restrictive measures are ineffective or unavailable.

   C: The CDC recommends "strict daily self monitoring" – not monitoring on an "as-needed basis."

Passage 3 (Questions 13 – 19)

Wishing to adopt a style of **speechmaking** in line with his **arrogantly superior manner and lofty spirit**, **Pericles** made liberal use of the instrument his old teacher **Anaxagoras** had given him, coloring his sweeping oratory with natural philosophy. As Plato called it, his "lofty intelligence and power of universal consummation," in addition to his **natural advantages**, allowed him to **surpass all others in this art**, adding apt illustrations drawn from physical science to his oratory.

Cause and effect: because of his natural advantages and arrogantly superior manner, Pericles adopted a style of speechmaking that was suited to him and became one of the greatest speechmakers

It is for this reason that some believe he was **nicknamed the Olympian**. Though some cite him improvement of the city with **new**, beautiful **buildings**, and other cite his power as a **politician and a general**, the comedies of that time, when they allude to him, either in earnest or in jest, always seem to think that the name was given to him **for his way of speaking**, referring to his "**thundering and lightning**" and his "rolling fateful thunders from his tongue."

Opinion: Pericles was called the Olympian and the author seems to think it was because of his manner of speaking, although others attributed the nickname to his skills as a politician, or his improvements to the city with new buildings

One saying of **Thucydides**, also **jestingly testifying to Pericles's eloquence**, has also been preserved. As the leader of the conservative party, Thucydides long struggled to hold his own against Pericles in debate. One day, the king of Sparta asked him who was a better wrestler. Thucydides answered, "**When I throw him in wrestling, he beats me by proving that he never was down, and making the spectators believe him.**"

Opinion: Thucydides was a rival of Pericles and jokes that Pericles could convince people that he'd won a wrestling match that he'd actually lost

For all this, however, Pericles was **highly cautious of his words**, and whenever he ascended to the tribune to speak, he first always prayed to the gods that nothing inappropriate would escape his lips. Besides the legislative measures he brought forward, **he left no writings**, and very **few of his sayings** are recorded. One of these, poignantly, was that "he saw war coming upon Athens from Peloponnesus." As **Stesimbrotus** tells us, Pericles was giving a public funeral oration over those lost as **Samos**, and he said that the fallen had become immortal, even as the gods, for though we do not see the gods, we conceive their immortality through the respect we pay them and the blessings we receive from them, and the same is true for those who have died for their country.

Contrast: despite his eloquence, Pericles was cautious with his speech and oddly he left behind very little in the way of writings or recordings of his sayings

As Thucydides represents it, the constitution **under Pericles** was a democracy in name but an **aristocracy** in practice, for the government was run by one leading citizen. As many writers tell us, due to grants of land abroad, **indulgent entertainments, and payments for services**, the people during his administration **fell into bad habits** and became extravagant, instead of sober and hardworking as they had been before. We shall now consider the history of this change.

Opinion: Thucydides criticized the government under Pericles as an aristocracy rather than a democracy and blamed Pericles for the indulgent bad habits developed by the people

First of all, Pericles had to **compete with Kimon** and transfer the affections of the people from this rival to himself. Because he wasn't as rich as **Kimon, who used to give a daily dinner for the Athenian poor**, clothe the elderly, and remove the fences from his property so that the poor might gather fruit, Pericles turned his attention to **distributing the public funds among the people**. By putting on public **spectacles**, as well as **paying** citizens to serve as jurymen and in other public offices, Pericles soon won the people to his side.

Contrast: Pericles vs Kimon, Kimon's wealth and magnanimity vs Pericles' cunning and (essentially) bribery

With the people, he was able to lead an **attack upon the Senate of the Areopagus**, of which he himself was not a member. Upon **destroying it**, Pericles made **Ephialtes** bring forward a bill that would **restrict the Senate's judicial powers**. Meanwhile, he succeeded in **banishing Kimon**, labeling him as a friend of Sparta and a hater of the Athenian people, even though he was second to none in birth or fortune, had won crucial victories over the Persians, and filled Athens with great spoils of war. This was how great the power of Pericles was with the common people.

Cause and effect: because he had the people on his side, Pericles was able to lead a successful attack against the Senate; because of his rivalry with Kimon, and because he was able to gain the affections of the people, Pericles banished Kimon, even though he was perhaps the most well respected man in Athens

Main Idea: The passage aims to convey how persuasive Pericles was in his speechmaking, and how cunning and decisive he was in his actions; the negative results of his rule are also mentioned, but in less clear terms.

13. A is correct. In the very first sentence of the passage, the author writes, "Wishing to adopt a style of speech-making in line with his arrogantly superior manner and lofty spirit . . ."

 B: This is true, but not the primary reason.

 C: Also true, but not the primary reason as stated in the passage.

 D: It is never made clear what Kimon's style is.

14. C is correct. The author gives most preference to the notion that the nickname came from his style of speaking, which the comedians noted was "thundering and lightening." The use of "though," as in, though some cite this reason or that, implies a kind of: "actually, it was this . . ."

 A: True, but not the reason given most credence by the author.

 B: True, but again, not the primary reason.

 D: True, but this is not even one of the arguments for the nickname made.

15. B is correct. The first introduction of Thucydides is in the third paragraph, and the author continues the jesting depiction of Pericles's eloquence with Thucydides's anecdote. It was in jest, but it also showed, albeit hyperbolically, just how persuasive Pericles could be.

 A, D: These ideas don't show up until the fifth paragraph.

 C: Rather, this notion is introduced after the anecdote.

16. B is correct. As the author writes at the end of the sixth paragraph, "By putting on public spectacles, as well as paying citizens to serve as jurymen an in other public office, Pericles soon won the people to his side." In other words, he threw parties and employed people.

 A: Kimon won wars and brought back spoils, but he got booted!

 C: Kimon did this too. A lot of good it did him!

 D: Well, Pericles did do this, but according to the passage, he doesn't win the people of Athens away from Kimon until he throws parties and employs people.

17. D is correct. This answer is drawn from the first Thucydides anecdote, in which even though Thucydides has thrown Pericles, Pericles proves with oratory that he was actually not thrown and that he actually won. So, the closest of these choices to mirror this is Choice D, the only option in which Pericles fakes what happened.

 A, B, C: All of these choices are less reflective of the Thucydides anecdote.

18. C is correct. At the top of the fourth paragraph, the author writes, "For all this, however, Pericles was highly cautious of his words . . ." This implies that Pericles was very careful about what he did (he also, very carefully, seems to choose the perfect style of oratory, and to choose the perfect way to win the people). His actions may ultimately prove careless if they undermine the city, but as it is the antonym of deliberate, it cannot stand here: Pericles was VERY deliberate.

 A, B, D: These are true of Pericles as the passage portrays him.

19. A is correct. I, II: Kimon won several victories over the Persians, was second to none in fortune, and gave freely of his own. So, he display military might, wealth, and magnanimity (a.k.a generosity), but not greed. III: Because he gave freely of his fortune, Kimon was not greedy.

Passage 4 (Questions 20 – 24)

Economists have long considered **knowledge** and **health** as forms of **human capital** that people invest in by increasing their education and improving their health. Thus, the returns to health spending can be assessed by treating the resulting "health" as a **capital good**. Schultz (1961) writes that an individual's acquisition of skills and knowledge is the means by which people enhance their welfare, similar to the way in which a business invests in physical capital to increase production and profits.

Key terms: economists, knowledge, health, human capital, capital good

Opinion: the author believes that knowledge and health are forms of capital

Cause and effect: the acquisition of health and knowledge enhances welfare

Based on this point of view, spending on **medical treatments** (and other activities that improve one's health) is an investment that provides a stream of benefits in the future. Assessing whether today's expenditures on medical treatments are in some sense "worth it" requires that one properly account for the costs and benefits of that spending. The benefits can be far-reaching (in terms of time and those affected., and viewing health as a capital good facilitates analyzing the various channels of improvement. As Mushkin points out, "Viewing expenditures for health programs as an investment helps to underscore the contributions of health programs to expansion of income and economic growth" (Mushkin 1962, 143).

Key terms: medical treatments, worth it, far-reaching, expansion of income and economic growth

Opinion: the author states that one must account for the costs and benefits of medical treatments

Contrast: knowledge and health are different from other forms of capital in that they cannot be easily measured

Cause and effect: the benefits of health from medical treatments affect many for a long time; health programs promote expansion of income and economic growth

Perhaps the most obvious benefit from investments in health care is the direct **increases in welfare**, or **well being**, that accrue to individuals when their health improves. These welfare gains are realized in the form of **reduced mortality** and improvements in an individual's **quality of life**. With respect to timing, the benefits occur not only at the time of treatment but also into the future. Additionally, these welfare gains accrue potentially not just to the patient but also to those around him. For example, when a person is **vaccinated**, both the individual and members of his community benefit from that vaccination.

Key terms: increases in welfare, well being, reduced mortality, quality of life, vaccinated

Opinion: the author states that the most obvious benefit of health care is wellness, i.e. higher quality of life

Cause and effect: benefits to a patient affect those around him or her

Other benefits from health spending have a more indirect effect on an individual's welfare. Consider the common belief that a major potential benefit from preventive health care expenditures today may be a substantial **reduction in health care costs** in the future. Some of these benefits accrue directly to the patient—reduced out-of-pocket expenditures for health care in the future—while others accrue to society as a whole—a healthier population demands less private and government insurance-related resources. Benefits from **preventive care** may be significant since it is thought to be less costly than treating advanced diseases. However, an extension of the average life span results in a **larger aged population**—a population that consumes a larger percentage of health services while achieving less productive returns to their health investment.

Key terms: reduction in health care costs, preventive care, larger aged population

Contrast: there are benefits of health care that directly effect an individual and those that do so indirectly, such as reduction in health care costs in the future

Cause and effect: health care reduces the cost of health care in the future for everyone; preventive care is cheaper than treatment of disease, however more people living to old age can increase costs

Another potentially important indirect benefit of improved health is the effects on **macroeconomic conditions** from a healthier population. For example, health spending today improves both the quantity of the **labor force** and the **quality of the workers**. Healthier workers are more productive because of an extension of the **working age**, **fewer sick days**, and a decline in the **loss of labor** from disease or death (which reduces the costs of hiring and training associated with replacing that lost labor). In addition to greater productivity, a healthier (and longer living) population consumes more **nonhealth-related expenditures**, thereby boosting economic growth.

Key terms: macroeconomic conditions, labor force, quality of workers, working age, fewer sick days, loss of labor, nonhealth-related expenditures

Opinion: the author believes that investment in health care affects the economic condition of society

Cause and effect: health spending results in more and better workers that can spend money on things other than health care, promoting economic growth

While the benefits seem intuitive, **quantifying** them is difficult. A National Academies Panel noted, "Health cannot be purchased directly and …There is no market equivalent to help us answer valuation questions, so one must turn to other methods" (Abraham and Mackie 2005, 117). We may be able to identify a drop in the number of sick days taken by individuals, thereby increasing productivity, but we cannot quantify the increase in their welfare. Therefore, it is difficult to estimate the entire **return to investments** in health care services. In addition, a distortion of the demand for health care services exists because most people do not face the full cost of the service; private or public insurance programs **subsidize** most health care costs. Nevertheless, academic work has applied a multitude of approaches to value the returns to improvements in health. Although the estimates vary depending on the methods and data, all existing work suggests that these benefits can be quite high.

Key terms: quantifying, return to investments, subsidize

Contrast: the benefits of health care are difficult to quantify

Cause and effect: insurance programs cause a distortion in the demand for health care services because they prevent people from facing the full cost of the service

Main Idea: The main idea of the passage is to present medical spending as an investment in the human capital of health; the benefits of health care spending are analyzed from an economic standpoint.

20. D is correct. The example is given directly after the discussion of health care benefits helping those who do not directly receive the care.

A: Vaccination can best be described as a benefit for the vaccinated individual, not a cost.

B, C: There is no discussion of these topics.

21. B is correct. Unemployment would not be solved by an increase in the labor force, which increase the author claims would occur. It is true that the author states that the overall health of the labor force would increase but a problem like unemployment is likely not within the scope of the author's claims. Certainly, increased unemployment could mean there is a larger labor force.

A: The quality of workers is not the issue here.

C: This is the opposite of the correct answer since the new information in the question would not disagree with the author.

D: The health of the economy is not improved if unemployment rises.

22. B is correct. The author states that investing in healthcare will provide a better quality of worker. Likewise, investing in their education will likely have a similar effect.

A, C, D: There is no reason to think that more education would have a significant effect on these variables.

23. B is correct. The author states that it is difficult to measure the benefits of health care in terms of healthiness of the population. It is easier to measure how much money might be saved in the future or other economic variables.

A, D: Measuring investments in knowledge is outside the scope of the passage.

C: The opposite is true.

24. C is correct. The passage is about health care but viewed from an economic point of view.

A, B: The subject matter is health care spending, not economics itself.

D: The view point of insurance companies is only briefly mentioned.

Passage 5 (Questions 25 – 30)

Though **experience be our only guide** in reasoning concerning matters of fact it must be acknowledged that this guide is not altogether infallible, but in some cases is apt to **lead us into errors**. One, who in our climate, should expect better weather in any week of June than in one of December, would reason justly, and conformably to experience; but it is certain, that he **may** happen, in the event, to find himself **mistaken**. However, we may observe, that, in such a case, he would have no cause to complain of experience; because it commonly informs us beforehand of the uncertainty, by that contrariety of events, which we may learn from a diligent observation. All effects follow not with like certainty from their supposed causes. **Some events** are found, in all countries and all ages, to have been **constantly** conjoined together: Others are found to have been more **variable**, and sometimes to disappoint our expectations; so that, in our reasonings concerning matter of fact, there are all imaginable degrees of assurance, from the highest certainty to the lowest species of moral evidence.

Key terms: experience be our only guide, uncertainty, diligent observation, degrees of assurance

Contrast: events that are constantly conjoined vs events that are more variable (such as the weather)

A wise man, therefore, **proportions his belief to the evidence**. In such conclusions as are founded on an infallible experience, he expects the event with the last degree of assurance, and regards his past experience as a full *proof* of the future existence of that event. In other cases, he proceeds with more caution. He weighs the opposite experiments; he considers which side is supported by the greater number of experiments; to that side he inclines, with doubt and hesitation; and when at last he fixes his judgment, the evidence exceeds not what we properly call *probability*. All probability, then, supposes an opposition of experiments and observations, where the one side is found to overbalance the other, and to produce a degree of evidence, proportioned to the superiority. A hundred instances or experiments on one side, and fifty on another, afford a doubtful expectation of any event; though a hundred uniform experiments, with only one that is contradictory, reasonably beget a pretty strong degree of assurance. In all cases, we must **balance the opposite experiments**, where they are opposite, and deduct the smaller number from the greater, in order to know the exact force of the superior evidence.

Key terms: proportions his belief to the evidence, probability, balance the opposite experiments

Opinion: the author believes that wise individuals vary their expectations based on the probability of one outcome occurring over another

Cause and effect: the outcome of an event will be determined by the probability of the event as well as the opposite outcomes, and therefore an individual should vary his or her amount of assurance regarding that event

A **miracle** is a **violation of the laws of nature**; and as a firm and unalterable experience has established these laws, the proof against a miracle, from the very nature of the fact, is as entire as any argument from experience can possibly be imagined. Nothing is esteemed a miracle, if it ever happens in the common course of nature. It is no miracle that a man, seemingly in good health, should die all of a sudden: because such a kind of death, though more unusual than any other, has yet been frequently observed to happen. But it is a **miracle**, that a **dead man should come to life**; because that has **never been observed** in any age or country. There must, therefore, be a uniform experience against every miraculous event, otherwise the event would not merit that appellation. And as a uniform experience amounts to a proof, there is here a direct and full *proof*, from the nature of the fact, **against the existence of any miracle**; nor can such a proof be destroyed, or the miracle rendered credible, but by an opposite proof, which is superior.

Key terms: miracle, full proof, miracle rendered credible, opposite proof

Opinion: the author believes that because a miracle, by definition, is a violation of the laws of nature, there is already a direct and complete proof against its existence

Cause and effect: a miracle is violation of the observed laws of nature, yet as a result there is as complete and direct a proof as possible against their existence

The plain consequence is "That **no testimony is sufficient to establish a miracle**, unless the testimony be of such a kind, that its falsehood would be more miraculous, than the fact, which it endeavors to establish; and even in that case there is a mutual destruction of arguments." When anyone tells me that he saw a **dead man restored to life**, I immediately consider with myself whether it be **more probable** that this person should either **deceive** or be deceived, or that the fact, which he relates, should **really have happened**. I weigh the one miracle against the other; and according to the superiority, which I discover, I pronounce my decision, and **always reject the greater miracle**. If the falsehood of his testimony would be more miraculous than the event which he relates; then, and not till then, can he pretend to command my belief or opinion.

Key terms: establish a miracle, falsehood would be more miraculous, superiority, reject the greater miracle

Contrast: the miraculous nature of an event vs the miraculous nature of the falsehood of said event

Cause and effect: all conclusions must be based on reason and probabilities, therefore before a miracle can be accepted it must be deemed that the odds of the reported miracle being false must be more miraculous than the full proof of prior experience

Main Idea: Conclusions must be based on observation, reason, and the probability of one outcome occurring relative to another; as a result miracles, which defy all past observation, can only be deemed credible if it would be likely that evidence supporting a miracle was more substantive than the evidence against it; the author implies strongly that, given this hurdle, no miracle can be believed to have occurred.

25.   B is correct. The author states that a reasonable individual bases his or her expectation for an outcome on the balance between the probability of that outcome and the other possibilities.

    A: The author states that individuals who witness miracles aren't necessarily liars, but could have been deceived by their senses.

    C: The author believes that reason is the only guide to determining outcomes.

    D: The author argues that prior experiences dictate an understanding of the probability of a given outcome, not the outcome itself.

26.   A is correct. The author states that "experience is our only guide", and furthermore the main idea of the passage is that reasoning and the probability of a certain outcome must be used to evaluate events.

    B, D: Although the subject matter relates to miracles, the author's belief in a divine presence (or lack thereof) is never discussed in the passage.

    C: The author would evaluate the likelihood that the accounts of others' were true or false, however it cannot be inferred that he frequently distrusts others.

27.   B is correct. The author believes that the credibility of a reported finding can only be determined by comparing the likelihood of that event being accurate versus the likelihood that the finding is inaccurate.

    C: A single study that left no room for any doubt regarding its results would not need further study in the eyes of the author, as the likelihood of the finding being incorrect would therefore be smaller than the likelihood of our previous understanding being incorrect.

    A, D: These conclusions assume too much regarding the author's beliefs – all we know is that the author would weigh all of the evidence available to him.

28.   A is correct. This is a difficult question, however the author states that since miracles are by definition a violation of the laws of nature, the proof against their existence is therefore also as full and complete as possible. He also argues that to establish credibility for a miracle the likelihood of the event being false must be more miraculous than the event itself, but since the proof against it is as complete as possible this is an impossibility.

    B, D: The author never discusses divine reasoning, and furthermore believes that experience and reason is "our only guide".

    C: The author would most likely conclude that miracles are an impossibility according to the principles of reason.

29.   C is correct. The author's arguments are all based on the principles of reason, and the purpose of the passage is to investigate, and challenge, our conception of miracles. The tone of the passage could therefore be described as both logical and inquisitive.

    A: It is impossible for a passage to be both esoteric and relatable, as they are close to antonyms.

    B, D: The tone of the passage is not conversational nor colloquial as that would mean the passage has a non-academic feel with the author speaking in a more casual voice, whereas this passage is a very philosophical, academic work.

30.   D is correct. The author believes that the credibility of an event that contradicts our experiences must be judged based upon the probability that the outcome occurred versus the probability that the outcome was falsely reported. Neither A, B nor C stand to contradict that argument, instead they merely demonstrate methods that would strengthen the evidence for the credibility of the miraculous event.

Passage 6 (Questions 31 – 36)

It is a common **weakness of mankind to be caught by an idea and captivated by a phrase**. To rest therewith content and to **neglect the carrying of the idea into practice is a weakness** still more common. It is this frequent **failure** of reformers to reduce their theories to practice, their tendency to dwell in the cloudland of the ideal rather than to test it in action, that has often made them **distrusted** and **unpopular**.

Opinion: the author believes that reformers must bring their reforms to action

Cause and effect: being caught by an idea or neglecting to carry an idea into practice is a weakness; also, this failure causes reformers to be distrusted and unpopular

With our forefathers the phrase "**mens sana in corpore sano**" was a high favorite. It was constantly quoted with approval by writers on hygiene and sanitation, and used as the text or the finale of hundreds of popular lectures. And yet we shall **seek in vain for any evidence of its practical usefulness**. Its words are good and true, but passive and actionless, not of that dynamic type where words are "words indeed, but words that draw armed men behind them."

Key terms: mens sana in corpore sano

Opinion: ancient reformers were inept at bringing reforms into practice

Cause and effect: a case is presented which shows the author's point that ancient reformers were passive and actionless

Our age is of another temper. It yearns for **reality**. It no longer rests satisfied with mere ideas, or words, or phrases. The modern Ulysses would drink life to the dregs. The present age is dissatisfied with the vague assurance that the Lord will provide, and, rightly or wrongly, is beginning to expect the state to provide. And while this **desire for reality has its drawbacks, it has also its advantages**. Our age **doubts absolutely the virtues of blind submission and resignation**, and cries out instead for prevention and amelioration. Disease is no longer regarded, as Cruden regarded it, as the penalty and the consequence of sin. **Nature herself is now perceived to be capable of imperfect work**. Time was when the human eye was referred to as a perfect apparatus, but the number of young children wearing spectacles renders that idea untenable to-day.

Opinion: modern reformers do not have the same problem that ancient reformers did

Contrast: our day is contrasted to ancient times; nowadays, reformers must call for their theories to be placed into practice and society demands that reforms be attempted

Cause and effect: as a result of our day's desire for reality, we do not submit blindly to authority and have more scientific knowledge

Meanwhile the multiplication of state asylums and **municipal hospitals, and special schools** for deaf or blind children and for cripples, **speaks eloquently** and irresistibly of an intimate **connection between civics and health**. There is a physical basis of **citizenship**, as there is a physical basis of life and of health; and any one who will take the trouble to read even the **Table of Contents of this book will see that for Dr. Allen prevention is a text and the making of sound citizens a sermon**. Given the sound body, we have nowadays small fear for the sound mind. The rigid physiological dualism implied in the phrase "mens sana in corpore sano" is no longer allowed. To-day the sound body generally includes the sound mind, and vice versa. If mental dullness be due to imperfect ears, the remedy lies in medical treatment of those organs, not in education of the brain. If lack of initiative or energy proceeds from defective aeration of the blood due to adenoids blocking the air tides in the windpipe, then the remedy lies not in better teaching but in a simple surgical operation.

Opinion: the main opinion expressed here is that Dr. Allen is attempting to make "sound citizens" and is a modern reformer

Contrast: the modern approach to the phrase "mens sana in corpore sano" is contrasted to the ancient reformers' approach

Cause and effect: the fact that civics and health are becoming more intertwined is evidenced by several things mentioned at the beginning of the paragraph

Shakespeare, in his wildwood play, saw sermons in stones and books in the running brooks. We moderns find a drama in the fateful lives of ordinary mortals, **sermons** in their physical salvation from some of the ills that flesh is heir to, and **books**--like this of Dr. Allen's--in striving to teach mankind how to become **happier**, and **healthier**, and **more useful members of society.**

Opinion: the author tells us that Dr. Allen's book strives to teach mankind to become happier, healthier, and more useful members of society

Dr. Allen is undoubtedly a **reformer**, but of the **modern**, not the ancient, type. He is a **prophet** crying in our present wilderness; but he is more than a prophet, for he is always intensely practical, insisting, as he does, on getting things done, and done soon, and done right.

Contrast: the modern reformer is further contrasted to the ancient reformer

Cause and effect: Dr. Allen is a modern reformer because he gets things done

Main Idea: The main idea is that Dr. Allen is as modern reformer who insists that his reforms are practiced, and that he strives for the making of sound and healthy citizens; the whole passage is the opinion of another man who is reviewing Dr. Allen's book.

31. B is correct. This question asks us to analyze the author's attitude in the passage. It is evident from how the author views ancient reformers as distrusted and unpopular that he has a lack of admiration for them. Conversely, the author presents Dr. Allen's motives and actions as purely altruistic and with humanity's betterment as his goal. The author esteems Dr. Allen highly.

    A: The author approves of Dr. Allen but does so emphatically and with emotion.

    C: The author is not skeptical of Dr. Allen but of ancient reformers.

    D: The author does not express that Dr. Allen has in some way improved his own life personally or that he is indebted to Dr. Allen.

32. C is correct. This question asks us to determine what reason the author might give for the distinction he noticed between ancient and modern reformers. The author states that the emphasis of the change is primarily a societal change. This means that he might agree that it wasn't necessarily all on the reformers themselves, but the times they lived in that prevented them from enacting reforms.

    A, B: There is no indication that reformers didn't believe in their own reforms or were simply lazy.

    D: This is unlikely, as the passage never indicates that their whole societies weren't interested in improving.

33. A is correct. The passage is a foreword to a book written by Dr. Allen. This states that upon looking at the table of contents, one realizes that Dr. Allen strives for the "making of sound citizens." Later we learn that the book treats the subject of citizenship and making useful and healthy members of society.

    B: The example of the difference between ancient and modern reformers uses mental illnesses and their treatment as an illustration. This does not mean that Dr. Allen's book is about mental illnesses.

    C: There is no evidence that Dr. Allen's book would talk about mental health more than any other aspect of health.

    D: This subject is treated by the author as a means to illustrate what type of reformer Dr. Allen is.

34. A is correct. This question asks us to determine how the author would view learning that Dr. Allen was not successful in bringing about change. The author would likely view Dr. Allen as more similar to ancient reformers, stuck in ideas. The author states that ancient reformers are distrusted and unpopular.

    B: This is not true because modern reformers are those who bring their reforms into action.

    C: This does not make sense because he is not from ancient times.

    D: The passage doesn't hinge on the distinction between medical and civic reformers.

35. C is correct. This question asks us to analyze the author's purpose for speaking about the phrase "mens sana in corpore sano". The author first mentions it to show how ancient reformers' theories were seldom brought into practice. Later, he brings it up to show how modern reforms have been enacted and knowledge obtained that allows humanity to effectively understand and act on the words in the phrase. It is a tool to bring out the contrast in the two types of reformers.

    A: This choice is too confined.

    B: This choice deals with only half of the discussion of the phrase.

    D: This choice is unfounded in passage information.

36. D is correct. This question asks us to interpret the author's meaning. When the author wrote this phrase, he was speaking of how the mind and body are connected, mentioning both failure of the ears and overly large adenoids as examples of bodily defects creating what appears to be a mental problem.

    A: The author was not speaking of actually fearing people.

    B: The author was not speaking of this phenomenon when he wrote the phrase.

    C: The author was not talking about the prevalence of mental illness.

Passage 7 (Questions 37 – 41)

You observe, I have hitherto spoken of the power of **Athena**, as over **painting** no less than **sculpture**. But her rule over **both arts is only** so far as they are **zoographic**;—representative, that is to say, of animal life, or of such order and discipline among other elements, as may invigorate and purify it. Now there is a specialty of the art of painting beyond this, namely, the representation of phenomena of **color and shadow**, as such, without question of the nature of the things that receive them. I am now accordingly obliged to speak of sculpture and painting as distinct arts: but the laws which bind sculpture, bind no less the painting of the higher schools, which has, for its **main purpose**, the **showing beauty** in human or animal form; and which is therefore placed by the **Greeks** equally under the rule of Athena, as the Spirit, first, of Life, and then of Wisdom in conduct.

Key terms: Athena, zoographic, Greeks

Contrast: painting's focus on color and shadow vs painting's purely on representation of life

Cause and effect: great painting, because it focuses on showing beauty in human or animal form, is, like sculpture, under the rule of Athena

First, I say, you are to **"see Pallas" in all such work**, as the Queen of Life; and the practical law which follows from this, is one of enormous range and importance, namely, that nothing must be represented by **sculpture**, external to any living form, which does not help to **enforce or illustrate the conception of life**. Both dress and armor may be made to do this, by great sculptors, and are continually so used by the greatest. One of the essential distinctions between the Athenian and Florentine schools is dependent on their **treatment of drapery** in this respect; an **Athenian** always sets it to exhibit the **action of the body**, by flowing with it, or over it, or from it, so as to illustrate both its form and gesture; a **Florentine**, on the contrary, always uses his drapery to conceal or disguise the forms of the body, and exhibit **mental emotion**; but both use it to enhance the life, either of the body or soul; **Donatello** and **Michelangelo**, no less than the sculptors of Gothic chivalry, ennoble armor in the same way; but **base sculptors** carve drapery and armor for the sake of their folds and picturesqueness only, and **forget the body** beneath. The rule is so stern, that all delight in mere incidental beauty, which painting often triumphs in, is wholly forbidden to sculpture;—for instance, in painting the branch of a tree, you may rightly represent and enjoy the lichens and moss on it, but a sculptor must not touch one of them: they are inessential to the tree's life,—he must give the flow and bending of the branch only, else he does not enough "see Pallas" in it.

Key terms: Pallas, Athenian, Florentine, Donatello, Michelangelo

Contrast: Athenian emphasis on movement of body vs Florentine emphasis on concealment and mental emotion vs base sculptors emphasis on details of drapery instead

of body it covers; painting's ability to delight in incidental beauty vs need for sculpture to focus on form of life only

Cause and effect: because sculpture is focused purely on Pallas, nothing can be depicted in sculpture that is not focused on the depiction of life

Or, to take a higher instance, here is an exquisite little painted poem, by **Edward Frere**; a cottage interior, one of the thousands which within the last two months have been laid desolate in unhappy France. **Every accessory in the painting** is of **value**—the fireside, the tiled floor, the vegetables lying upon it, and the basket hanging from the roof. But **not one** of these accessories would have been **admissible in sculpture**. You must carve nothing but what has life. "Why?" you probably feel instantly inclined to ask me.—You see the principle we have got, instead of being blunt or useless, is such an edged tool that you are startled the moment I apply it. "Must we refuse every pleasant accessory and picturesque detail, and petrify nothing but living creatures?" Even so: I would not assert it on my own authority. It is the **Greeks** who say it, but **whatever they say of sculpture, be assured, is true**.

Key terms: Edward Frere, Greeks

Contrast: the inclusion of accessories and details in painting vs the refusal of such details in sculpture

Cause and effect: because the Greeks said sculpture must focus on living creatures only, it must feature living creatures only

Main Idea: The passage stresses the principle of only showing living things in sculpture, regardless of other aesthetic pleasures, due to Greek principles.

37. C is correct. In the second paragraph, the author says that both the Athenian and Florentine schools use drapery "to enhance the life, either of the body or soul" and adds that "Donatello and Michelangelo, no less than the sculptors of Gothic chivalry, ennoble armor in the same way."

    A: The passage suggests that Donatello treats armor "in the same way" as the Florentines do drapery, not differently.

    B: There is no emphasis of aesthetic beauty in the passage.

    D: While the passage states that "an Athenian always sets it to exhibit the action of the body," Donatello is compared to a Florentine who "uses his drapery to conceal or disguise the forms of the body, and exhibit mental emotion," eliminating choice D.

38. A is correct. After stressing that sculpture can only depict that which is alive, the author admits that the rule is strict, but states, "I would not assert it on my own authority. It is the Greeks who say it, but whatever they say of sculpture, be assured, is true."

    B: The author states that the insistence on depicting what is alive is a tool that might seem "blunt or useless," but does not specifically compare that to other, more workable, theories.

    C: The author says this principle should not be taken on personal authority.

    D: Other art forms are not discussed in this part of the passage.

39. D is correct. Throughout the passage, the author focuses on the principle of only portraying life in sculptures. When painting is discussed, it is contrasted with sculpture in terms of the kind of details of non-living elements it can have that sculpture cannot.

    A, B: Neither the material conditions of painting nor the roots of the art forms are discussed in the passage.

    C: The passage shows some differences in the forms, but states that "the painting of the higher schools ... has, for its main purpose, the showing beauty in human or animal form," suggesting a comparison as opposed to choice C.

40. C is correct. The author states that painting specializes in "the representation of phenomena of color and shadow," and often "triumphs" in "delight in mere incidental beauty." Thus a focus on color and detail, as with the dress and jewelry, is the credited answer.

    A: Incidental beauty, such as accouterments, or extras, are allowed in painting, eliminating choice A.

    B: It is "showing beauty in human or animal form" in paintings which "is therefore placed by the Greeks equally under the rule of Athena," (also called Pallas in the passage), not emphasis on details like clothing and jewelry.

    D: The author states that the highest schools of painting are still connected with representing life, not incidental beauties, as in choice D.

41. B is correct. The passage stresses the rule of portraying life only, arguing that "the rule is so stern, that all delight in mere incidental beauty, which painting often triumphs in, is wholly forbidden to sculpture;—for instance, in painting the branch of a tree, you may rightly represent and enjoy the lichens and moss on it, but a sculptor must not touch one of them: they are inessential to the tree's life." The barnacles on the whale can be read as equivalent to lichen or moss: interesting, but not "essential to . . . life," and this not allowed.

    A, C: The passage does not discuss size contrasts, or whether delight justifies artistic decisions.

    D: While the author refers to a work as a "painted poem," there is no discussion of elevating sculpture to poetry.

Passage 8 (Questions 42 – 48)

The **primary belief of Christianity** concerns the **Unity of the Trinity**: the Father is God, the Son is God, the Holy Spirit is God. Therefore, Father, Son, and Holy Spirit are **one God, not three**. The principle of this union is absence of difference. Some, however, by **ranking** the elements of the Trinity by **merit**, **break it up** and convert it to plurality. We shall now explore why this is **misguided**.

Key terms: Unity of the Trinity

Contrast: understanding the Holy Trinity as one god vs understanding it as three gods

Opinion: author thinks that breaking up the Holy Trinity and ranking them is wrong

Speculative science may be divided into three different kinds: **Physics, Mathematics, and Theology**. To begin, **Physics** studies motion and is **neither abstract nor separable**, for its primary concern is with the forms of bodies and their constituent matter. Realistically, these forms cannot be separated from their bodies, or matter. As these bodies are in motion, form takes on the movement of the particular thing to which it is attached. For example, earth tends downwards and fire tends upwards. **Mathematics** does not deal with motion and is **not abstract**: its interest is in the **forms** of bodies **apart from matter**, and therefore apart from movement. However, because these forms are ultimately connected with matter, they **cannot be truly separated** from bodies.

Key terms: Physics, Mathematics, Theology

Contrast: forms of bodies vs their constituent matter, Physics dealing with motion vs Mathematics not dealing with motion

Cause and effect: the primary concern of Physics is to study motion, so it is neither abstract nor separable; Mathematics is interested in the forms of bodies, so it is not interested in movement; because forms are always connected with matter, they cannot truly be separated from bodies

Because the **Divine Substance** is **without** either **matter** or **motion**, **Theology** does not deal with motion and is both **abstract and separable**. In Physics, we must use scientific concepts, in Mathematics, systematical, and in Theology, intellectual. In Theology, we aim to **not** be distracted by **imaginations** and to simply recognize and appreciate that Form which is **pure form and no image**, which itself is Being and the source of Being. Everything owes its being to it.

Key terms: Divine Substance

Contrast: scientific concepts vs systematical concepts vs intellectual concepts

Cause and effect: because the Divine Substance has neither matter nor motion, Theology does not deal with motion and is both abstract and separable

A **statue** is **not** a statue because of the **brass** that makes up its matter, **but because** of the **form** through which the likeness of a living thing is impressed upon it. Likewise, the **brass** itself **is** not **brass** because of the earth that is its matter, but **because of its form**. In the same way, earth is not earth because it is matter, but because of its dryness and weight, which are forms. Nothing is said to be because it has matter, but rather, because it has form.

Contrast: being made of brass vs having the likeness of a living thing

Cause and effect: a statue is a statue because it looks like a living thing; brass is brass because of its form, not because of the earth that is its matter

However, **the Divine Substance** is **form without matter** and because of this, is One, and **is its own essence**. **All** other things are **not their own essences**: every other thing takes its being from the things of which it is composed, from its parts. It is this *and* that, its **parts in conjunction**. It is not this *or* that. For example, **man** consists of **body *and* soul,** not body *or* soul. Therefore, man is not his own essence.

Contrast: Divine Substance being its own essence vs all other things not being so

Cause and effect: because only the Divine Substance is form without matter, it is One and is its own essence

On the other hand, that which consists not of this and that, but only this, is truly its own essence, and is therefore **beautiful and stable**, being **grounded in nothing**. Therefore, the thing in which there is no number, in which nothing is present except for its own essence, is truly One. Moreover, it **cannot** become the **substrate of anything**, for it is pure form and pure forms cannot have substrates.

Cause and effect: the Divine Substance is grounded in nothing but its own essence and cannot serve as the substrate of anything else (e.g. you can't make a statue out of the Divine Substance)

If **humanity**, like other forms, is a substrate for accidents (**happenings**), it does not receive these accidents because it exists, but rather, because **matter is subjected to it**. Indeed, humanity seems to appropriate the accidents which actually belong to the matter underlying its very conception. Form without matter cannot be a substrate and also **cannot have its essence in matter**. Otherwise, it would be a **reflection**, not a form.

Cause and effect: things happen to humanity which we want to take credit for, but actually things happen to humanity simply because humans are made of matter, and accidents (happenings) are what happens to matter; the Divine Substance cannot have its essence in matter because then it would just be a reflection

From the **forms** which are **outside of matter** come the **forms** which are **in matter** and make up bodies. In reality, we mislabel these entities that **reside in bodies** when we call them forms: they are mere **images resembling those forms** which are not embodied in matter. **In God**, then, **there is**

no difference, no plurality from difference, no multiplicity from accidents, and therefore, **no number**: the Holy Trinity is one God.

Contrast: forms outside of matter vs forms in matter, one God vs plurality

Cause and effect: forms exist outside matter (e.g. a pure idea of a triangle) so matter itself is only an image of a form (e.g. a triangular rock is just an image of the pure idea of triangle); because God has no matter, He is only form, and because of this, has no differences, no plurality

Main Idea: The author sets out to prove that the Holy Trinity is in fact one God. In order to do this, he introduces a comparison of the three speculative sciences and what characterizes them. From here, he seeks to show that all things on Earth consist of parts, whereas the divine, which is form without matter has unity and no differences within it.

42. D is correct. Items I, II, and III are true and are all mentioned in the second paragraph.

43. B is correct. As the author writes of the Holy Trinity in the first paragraph, "The principle of this union is absence of difference."

   D: The Divine Substance has only form, not matter.

44. A is correct. The first paragraph introduces the point of the passage: to prove that those who break up the Holy Trinity and convert it into a plurality are misguided. This already suggests that the mentions of Physics and Mathematics are meant to further the theological argument being made.

   B, D: The author never claims to rank these speculative sciences.

   C: We take a scientific approach to Physics and a systematical approach to Mathematics. For Theology, we must use intellectual concepts. Here, the divine cannot be studied scientifically, but rather, intellectually.

45. D is correct. As the author writes in the second paragraph, "Mathematics does not deal with motion and is not abstract." Here, the opposite of abstract is concrete.

   A, B: Mathematics is not abstract.

   C: Math does not deal with motion.

46. A is correct. The author tries to prove the Holy Trinity is one. He uses an intellectual process to make his case.

   B: This point is never made.

   C, D: These are the opposite of the author's view.

47. A is correct. In the second paragraph: "Mathematics does not deal with motion and is not abstract: its interest is in the forms of bodies apart from matter". So, Mathematics is concerned with forms and not matter, which would appeal to this student. In the third paragraph, the author writes that in Mathematics, we must use systematic concepts. Here, methodical is a synonym for systematic. Lastly, in the third paragraph we see that imaginations distract from the study of Theology, but no mention of them is made in regards to Physics or Mathematics.

   B: Physics is concerned with form and matter.

   C, D: Theology is concerned with just form, yes, but also, the imagination might get in the way. Plus, the approach to Theology must be intellectual, not systematic/methodical.

48. D is correct. A thing is not a thing because of its matter, but because of its form. The rest of the choices are true, and Choice C, with the mention of water, is an extrapolation the example referenced in Choice B.

Passage 9 (Questions 49 – 53)

The time, it is to be hoped, is gone by, when any defense would be necessary of the "**liberty of the press**" as one of the **securities against corrupt** or tyrannical **government**. No argument, we may suppose, can now be needed, against permitting a legislature or an executive, not identified in interest with the people, to prescribe opinions to them, and determine what doctrines or what arguments they shall be allowed to hear. This aspect of the question, besides, has been so often and so triumphantly enforced by preceding writers, that it need not be specially insisted on in this place. Though the **law of England**, on the subject of the press, **is as servile to this day** as it was in the time of the **Tudors**, there is little danger of its being actually put in force against political discussion, except during some temporary panic, when fear of insurrection drives ministers and judges from their propriety; and, speaking generally, it is not, in constitutional countries, to be apprehended that the government, whether completely responsible to the people or not, will often attempt to control the expression of opinion, except when in doing so it makes itself the organ of the general intolerance of the public. Let us suppose, therefore, that the government is entirely at one with the people, and never thinks of exerting any power of **coercion** unless in agreement with what it conceives to be **their voice**. But **I deny the right of the people** to exercise such coercion, either by themselves or by their government. The power itself is **illegitimate**. The best government has no more title to it than the worst. It is as **noxious**, or more noxious, when exerted in accordance with public opinion, than when in opposition to it. If all mankind minus one were of one opinion, and only one person were of the contrary opinion, mankind would be no more justified in silencing that one person, than he, if he had the power, would be justified in silencing mankind. Were an opinion a **personal possession** of no value except to the owner; if to be obstructed in the enjoyment of it were simply a private injury, it would make some difference whether the injury was inflicted only on a few persons or on many. But the **peculiar evil of silencing the expression of an opinion** is, that it is robbing the human race, posterity as well as the existing generation; those who dissent from the opinion, still more than those who hold it. If the opinion is **right**, they are deprived of the opportunity of exchanging error for truth: if **wrong**, they lose, what is almost as great a benefit, the clearer perception and livelier impression of truth, produced by its collision with error.

Key terms: liberty of the press, government, England, Tudors, coercion, their voice, illegitimate, noxious, personal possession, right, wrong.

Opinion: the author supports freedom of speech and the press, even if the opinion being expressed is by a single person and everyone else agrees that they would prefer that person be silenced

Contrast: modern English law is compared to that in place in the time of the Tudors; there is a contrast drawn between personal opinions and personal possessions, between right

opinions and wrong opinions, between the opinion of many versus the opinion of one, and the coercion of people by their governments whether it be with the voice of the people or against

Cause and effect: for a government to coerce its people, in whatever degree it does so, is unlawful; to dismiss, silence, or obstruct another's opinion is unlawful

It is necessary to consider separately these two hypotheses, each of which has a distinct branch of the argument corresponding to it. We can never be sure that the opinion we are endeavoring to stifle is a **false opinion**; and if we were sure, **stifling it would be an evil still**.

Opinion: author thinks it is evil even to try and stifle a false opinion

First: the opinion which it is attempted to suppress by authority may possibly be **true**. Those who desire to suppress it, of course deny its truth; but they are not **infallible**. They have no authority to decide the question for all mankind, and exclude every other person from the means of judging. To refuse a hearing to an opinion, because they are sure that it is false, is to assume that their certainty is the same thing as **absolute** certainty. **All silencing of discussion is an assumption of infallibility**. Its condemnation may be allowed to rest on this common argument, not the worse for being common.

Contrast: there is a contrast between certainty and absolute certainty; no one can obtain absolute certainty

Opinion: the author considers how one should approach the belief that another person's opinion is false; one should recognize that they cannot have absolute certainty

Let us now pass to the second division of the argument, and dismissing the supposition that any of the received opinions may be **false**, let us assume them to be true, and examine into the worth of the manner in which they are likely to be held, when their truth is not freely and openly canvassed. However unwillingly a person who has a strong opinion may admit the possibility that his opinion may be false, he ought to be moved by the **consideration that however true it may be, if it is not fully, frequently, and fearlessly discussed**, it will be held as a **dead dogma**, not a **living truth**.

Contrast: there is a distinction between truth, dead dogma, and living truth

Cause and effect: truth must be frequently discussed to remain lively

Main Idea: The main idea of the passage is that the liberty of free speech is sacred and should not be suppressed by governments of individuals; one most consider all sides of an argument and recognize one's own fallibility; it is in vigorously debating one's opinions that they are kept as living truth rather than dead dogma.

49.   A is correct. The last sentence of the first paragraph gives us a hint. The author states that to exchange error for truth is a great opportunity, even more so when it is done by forceful collision with the truth. This tells us that the author believes it important to obtain truth through our interactions.

    B: The author would disagree with this.

    C: This could be true but lacks the evidence that A has. It is more reasonable to say that the silencing of an opinion is akin to theft of property.

    D: The author may or may not believe this, as he does not discuss overthrowing governments.

50.   D is correct. The phrase in question occurs directly after the discussion of how governments should not be allowed to prescribe opinions to the people or decide what they are able to hear.

    A: This is not mentioned.

    B: This is talked about later on in the paragraph.

    C: The author never addresses the idea that a newspaper might be obligated to publish the opinion of any person.

51.   A is correct. The author states that if the analogy were to be made, it would immediately follow that "it would make some difference whether the injury was inflicted only on a few persons or on many." That is, when harming a possession, there is moral weight to the consideration of whether you're harming the possession of one person or many people. By contrast, when you obstruct an opinion, it doesn't matter if you're blocking one person's opinion or the majority opinion – in either case you rob the entire human posterity of access to that opinion.

    B: This sentiment is expressed later, but not in connection with the parallel drawn between opinions and possessions.

    C: This is the opposite of the author's opinion.

    D: This sentiment is expressed later, but not in connection with the parallel drawn between opinions and possessions.

52.   C is correct. The passage states that some opinions are right and others wrong. This implies that the author believes that truth is not relative and can be discovered. The author advocates in the passage that thoughtful consideration be given to every opinion and that each person consider the fallibility of their own opinions. He or she doesn't make mention of whether certain opinions can be backed by evidence.

III: The author states that everybody has the right to their opinions and to not be obstructed in their enjoyment of them.

53.   D is correct. The passage states that no man can know a thing with absolute certainty. This seems to clash with the author's classification of some opinions as true or right, almost as if to say they are universally correct.

    A: This idea is not expressed in the passage.

    B: This does not preclude that absolute truth exists. This deals more with how a true idea would be perceived as dead dogma.

    C: This idea is not expressed in the passage. The author never links how true an idea is with whether or not the majority of people believe it to be true.

SECTION 9

53 Questions, 90 Minutes

Use an answer grid from the back of the book to record your answers

Passage 1 (Questions 1 – 6)

Put shortly, there are two views. One, that man is intrinsically good, spoilt by circumstance; and the other that he is intrinsically limited, but disciplined by order and tradition to something fairly decent. To the one party man's nature is like a well, to the other like a bucket. The view which regards man as a well, a reservoir full of possibilities, I call the romantic; the one which regards him as a very finite and fixed creature, I call the classical.

I must now shirk the difficulty of saying exactly what I mean by romantic and classical in verse. I can only say that it means the result of these two attitudes towards the cosmos, towards man, insofar as it gets reflected in verse. The romantic, because he thinks man infinite, must always be talking about the infinite; and as there is always the bitter contrast between what you think you ought to be able to do and what man actually can, it always tends to be gloomy.

What I mean by classical in verse is this. That even in the most imaginative flights there is always a holding back, a reservation. The classical poet never forgets this finiteness, this limit of man. He remembers always that he is mixed up with earth. He may jump, but he always returns back; he never flies away into the circumambient gas. You might say if you wished that the whole of the romantic attitude seems to crystallize in verse round metaphors of flight. Hugo is always flying, flying over abysses, flying up into the eternal gases. The word infinite in every other line.

In the classical attitude you never seem to swing right along to the infinite nothing. If you say an extravagant thing which does exceed the limits inside which you know man to be fastened, yet there is always conveyed in some way at the end an impression of yourself standing outside it, and not quite believing it, or consciously putting it forward as a flourish. You never go blindly into an atmosphere more than the truth, an atmosphere too rarefied for man to breathe for long. You are always faithful to the conception of a limit. It is a question of pitch; in romantic verse you move at a certain pitch of rhetoric which you know, man being what he is, to be a little high-falutin. The kind of thing you get in Hugo or Swinburne. For an example of the opposite thing, a verse written in the proper classical spirit, take the song from *Cymbeline*. Take the last two lines:

'Golden lads and girls all must,

Like chimney sweepers come to dust.'

The thing that I think quite classical is the word "lad". Your modern romantic could never write that. He would have to write "golden youth", and take up the thing at least a couple of notes in pitch.

The essence of poetry to most people is that it must lead them to a beyond of some kind. Verse strictly confined to the earthly and the definite (Keats is full of it) might seem to them to be excellent writing, excellent craftsmanship, but not poetry. So much has romanticism debauched us, that,

without some form of vagueness, we deny the highest. The thing has got so bad now that a poem which is all dry and hard, a properly classical poem, would not be considered poetry at all.

In the classic it is always the light of ordinary day, never the light that never was on land or sea. It is always perfectly human and never exaggerated:man is always man and never a god. But the awful result of romanticism is that, accustomed to this strange light, you can never live without it. Its effect on you is that of a drug.

1. Which of the following best describes the author's view of romantic verse?

    A. Romantic verse expresses the human quest for order amidst the chaos.

    B. It is superior to classical verse because it is infinite in its possibilities.

    C. It is inferior to classical verse in its craftsmanship.

    D. It is unrealistic and unappealing in its habitual reaching for the sublime.

2. Given the viewpoint that the author puts forth about classicism, what does the author think about "a poem which is all dry and hard" (paragraph 5)?

    A. It is lacking in the transcendence that is essential to poetry.

    B. Its problem is that it is confined to the earth.

    C. It is free of the light of the ordinary.

    D. It is satisfying in its definiteness and restraint.

3. Consider the following lines of poetry: "When love has fused and mingled two beings in a sacred and angelic unity, the secret of life has been discovered so far as they are concerned; they are no longer anything more than the two boundaries of the same destiny; they are no longer anything but the two wings of the same spirit." Based on information in the passage, which of the following would best describe the poem?

    A. Because it focuses on love, it would be categorized as romantic verse.

    B. Its focus on the infinite and otherworldly would categorize it as of the romantic tradition.

    C. Since the theme of love is timeless, it would be categorized as classical.

    D. Since classical verse is about the limits of human beings, and romantic is about infinite spirit, the poem fits neither category.

4. Which of the following best explains the analogy of the well and the bucket that the author describes in paragraph 1?

    A. It is a way of distinguishing between two different views of human nature.

    B. It is a means of expressing the author's preference for romantic verse.

    C. It describes a dichotomy between philosophy and poetry.

    D. It contrasts with metaphors of flight the author uses in paragraph 3.

5. What mistake does the author suggest that most people make in their conception of poetry?

    A. They think that poetry is either romantic, or classical.

    B. They conceive of human nature as a bucket, rather than as a well.

    C. They assume that poetry must take us beyond the ordinary.

    D. They expect that poetry will be gloomy.

6. Of the following, what does the author most likely mean when he says "once you become accustomed to this strange light, you can never live without it"?

    A. Readers of romantic verse become habituated to the pursuit of pleasure.

    B. If readers become accustomed to the exaggerations of romantic poetry, they will cease to appreciate the restraint of classicism.

    C. Readers of romantic poetry begin to imagine themselves as idealized or perfect.

    D. If readers fall under the spell of romantic verse, they are more likely to seek vices such as drugs.

Passage 2 (Questions 7 – 13)

None of the Italian masters has ever taken such a firm hold of the popular imagination as Raphael. While others wax and wane in esteem as they are praised by one generation and disparaged by the next, Raphael continues to be held as the most favored painter in Christendom. Though his work is subjected to severe criticism, the passing centuries do not dim his fame. Rather, he remains, as he began, the first love of the people.

His subjects are nearly all cheerful, for he mostly exercised his skill on scenes that were agreeable to contemplate. As such, he was preeminently the artist of joy, so pain and ugliness were strangers to his work. This quality in him can be attributed not only to his pleasure-loving nature, but also to the great influence made upon him by the rediscovery of the Greeks, which happened in his day, for the Greeks dealt instinctively with objects of delight.

Just as Raphael's work is compassionate to our hearts, it is equally so to our minds, requiring neither strenuous feelings nor too much thinking. Just like his subjects do not overtax our sympathies with harrowing emotions, his art does not overtax our understanding with complicated effects. His works appear so simple that they seem to require no significant intellectual effort and no technical knowledge to enjoy. He does all the work for us. It was not his way to show what difficult things he could with his work, but rather, he made great art seem to be the easiest thing in the world. Of course, this ease was the result of pure mastery, the mastery that enabled him to arrange the fifty-two figures of *The School of Athens* and the three figures of *The Madonna of the Chair* so simply and unobtrusively that we are lead to imagine such undertakings as mundane. Yet in both cases, he solves essentially difficult problems of composition with a success scarcely paralleled.

Even Raphael rarely achieved the same kind of success twice: *The Parnassus* lacks the variety of *The School of Athens*, though the individual figures have a similar grace, and *The Fire in the Borgo* possesses parts equal in beauty to any in the previous two works, but lacks the unity of either. Moreover, though *The Parnassus* and *The Liberation of Saint Peter* show a masterly adaptation to a severely awkward space, *The Transfiguration* fails to solve a much easier composition problem.

Though he instinctually preferred the Greek style of statuesque repose to the portrayal of action, Raphael showed himself capable of both. The charge of avenging spirits upon Heliodorus is just as impressive as the Hellenic calm of his Parnassus. The vigorous realism of Peter when he is called from his fishing to the apostleship matches the visionary idealism of the angel-led Peter. The alert activity of the swiftly moving *Sistine Madonna* perfectly complements the brooding quiet of *The Madonna of the Chair*.

Great though Raphael's achievements were in a many directions, he is most remembered for his Madonnas, those works which best expressed the individuality of his genius. He never ceased to be fascinated by the sweet mystery of motherhood, and so he plumbed the depths of maternity time and time again, always making some new discovery.

The Madonna of the Chair most emphasizes the physical instincts of maternity. As Taine wrote, "She bends over the child with the beautiful action of a wild animal." Like a mother creature instinctively protecting her young, she gathers him in her embrace as if to shield him from some imminent danger. On the other hand, the *Sistine Madonna* is the most spiritual of Raphael's works, a perfect embodiment of womanhood, her love transfigured by the spirit of sacrifice. Forgetful of self and obedient to heaven, she bears her son forth for the good of humanity.

7. Which of the following works did Raphael NOT paint?

    A. The Fire in the Borgo

    B. The Heliodorus

    C. The Parnassus

    D. Sistine Madonna

8. Based upon the passage, which of the following statements most accurately describes the point the author is trying to make in the fourth paragraph?

    A. Even Raphael was often prone to inconsistencies in his work.

    B. Some of Raphael's great successes are unparalleled, even by himself.

    C. Raphael may have ultimately been stretched too thin, except in his Madonnas.

    D. Not at all of Raphael's works make the artistry of painting look easy.

9. Based upon the passage, which of the following paintings of Raphael's would the author claim to be his most popular?

    A. The Heliodorus

    B. The Liberation of Saint Peter

    C. The School of Athens

    D. The Madonna of the Chair

10. Based upon the passage, which of the following is most likely the intended meaning of the word "Hellenic" in the fifth paragraph?

    A. Peaceful

    B. Statuesque

    C. Greek

    D. Classical

11. Suppose an art teacher were teaching a pupil to emulate Raphael. To begin, and based upon the passage, which of the following lessons would be most fundamental to this emulation?

    A. Learning how to artfully and effectively arrange many human figures

    B. Learning how to channel the complexity of joy without complicated effects

    C. Learning how to use complicated effects without them seeming complicated

    D. Learning how to understand other people, like mothers, through conversation

12. According to the passage, all of the following are features of Raphael's work EXCEPT:

    A. brooding quiet.

    B. masterful composition.

    C. vigorous idealism.

    D. simple joy.

13. Which of the following statements would the author of this passage definitely believe?

    I. Raphael was the greatest artist of the Renaissance.

    II. Raphael's most technically masterful works are the ones he is remembered for most.

    III. People do not have to think or work hard in order to enjoy Raphael's work.

    A. II only

    B. III only

    C. I and II only

    D. I, II, and III

Passage 3 (Questions 14 – 19)

Beneath and very remote from scientific revolutions, which generate the progress of civilizations, are the religious and political revolutions, which have no kinship with them. While scientific revolutions derive solely from rational elements, political and religious beliefs are sustained almost exclusively by affective and mystic factors. Reason plays a feeble part in their genesis.

I have insisted at some length on the affective and mystic origin of beliefs, showing that a political or religious belief constitutes an act of faith elaborated in unconsciousness, over which, in spite of appearances, reason has no hold. I also showed that belief often reaches such a degree of intensity that nothing can be opposed to it. The man hypnotized by his faith becomes an Apostle, ready to sacrifice his interests, his happiness, and even his life for the triumph of his faith. The extremity of his belief matters little; for him it is a burning reality. Certitudes of mystic origin possess the marvelous power of domination over thought, and can only be affected by time. By the very fact that it is regarded as an absolute truth a belief necessarily becomes intolerant. This explains the violence, hatred, and persecution which were the habitual accompaniments of the great political and religious revolutions, notably of the Reformation and the French Revolution.

Certain periods of French history remain incomprehensible if we forget this affective and mystic origin of beliefs, their necessary intolerance, the impossibility of reconciling them when they come into mutual contact, and, finally, the power conferred by mystic beliefs upon the sentiments which place themselves at their service. Events such as the Reformation, which overwhelmed France for a period of fifty years, were in no wise determined by rational influences. Yet rational influences are always invoked in explanation, even in the most recent works. Thus, in the General History of Lavisse and Rambaud, we read the following explanation of the Reformation: "It was a spontaneous movement, born here and there amidst the people, from the reading of the Gospels and the free individual reflections which were suggested to simple persons by an extremely pious conscience and a very bold reasoning power." Contrary to the assertion of these historians, we may say with certainty that such movements are never spontaneous, and secondly, that reason takes no part in their elaboration. The force of the political and religious beliefs which have moved the world resides precisely in that fact.

Political revolutions may result from beliefs established in the minds of men, but many other causes produce them. The word discontent sums them up. As soon as discontent is generalized a party is formed which often becomes strong enough to struggle against the Government. Discontent must generally have been accumulating for a long time in order to produce its effects. For this reason, a revolution does not always represent a phenomenon in the process of termination followed by another which is commencing but rather a continuous phenomenon, having somewhat accel-erated its evolution. All the modern revolutions, however, have been abrupt movements, entailing the instantaneous overthrow of governments. Such, for example, were the Brazilian, Portuguese, and Chinese revolutions.

Lastly, to the contrary of what might be supposed, it is important to note that very conservative peoples are the individuals most addicted to violent revolutions. Being conservative, they are not able to evolve slowly, or to adapt themselves to variations of environment, so that when the discrepancy becomes too extreme they are bound to adapt themselves suddenly. This sudden evolution constitutes a revolution, and it arrives with violent behavior. Peoples able to adapt themselves progressively, however, do not escape revolution altogether. It was only by means of a revolution that the English, in 1688, were able to terminate the struggle which had dragged on for a century between the monarchy, which sought to make itself absolute, and the nation, which claimed the right to govern itself through the medium of its representatives.

14. Which of the following defines affective beliefs, according to the passage?

    A. Beliefs affected by rational thought

    B. Beliefs affected by negative emotional stimuli

    C. Beliefs elaborated within the subconscious

    D. Beliefs that affect change

15. Which of the following can be inferred from the passage regarding the author's beliefs on revolutions?

    A. All revolutions spring from affective and mystic beliefs that aren't influenced by rational thought.

    B. All revolutions spring from beliefs based upon rational thought.

    C. The French Revolution can only be understood from a rational context.

    D. Religious revolutions can occur as continuous phenomena.

16. Based on the passage, it can be inferred that the author believes which of the following stand in opposition to one another?

    A. Discontent and revolution

    B. Political beliefs and tolerance

    C. Scientific revolutions and rationality

    D. Conservative ideology and revolution

17. Which of the following findings, if true, would most challenge one of the author's arguments?

    A. Atheistic individuals are found to be more tolerant of other religious beliefs than religious practitioners.

    B. Scientific progress is found to leap forward in sudden shifts as opposed to a continuous progression.

    C. Rational thought is found to more powerfully motivate individuals to action than subconscious beliefs.

    D. Political affiliation is found to negatively correlate with religious affiliation.

18. It can be inferred that the author supports all of the following statements, EXCEPT:

    A. scientific revolutions are more beneficial than religious revolutions.

    B. in equal environments, conservative groups of people are more prone to violence.

    C. rational beliefs are more powerful than affective and mystic beliefs.

    D. English citizens were historically more rationally driven than French citizens.

19. The author most likely introduces the Brazilian, Portuguese, and Chinese revolutions in order to:

    A. provide evidence that qualifies his primary claim in the paragraph.

    B. transition the reader to the next topic of discussion.

    C. provide evidence that counters the preceding sentence.

    D. provide evidence that supports the main idea of the passage.

Passage 4 (Questions 20 – 26)

If we remove the notion of the universe and the notion of good and evil from scientific philosophy, it may be asked, and justifiably so, what specific problems remain for the philosopher that the scientist cannot answer? It is difficult to give an entirely precise answer to this question, but there are certain characteristics that may be noted that distinguish the province of philosophy from that of the sciences.

First, a philosophical proposition must necessarily be general: it must not deal with specific things on the surface of the earth, with the solar system, or with any other specific segment of space and time. It is this very need for generality that has led to the widely held belief that philosophy deals with the universe as a whole. While I do not believe that this belief is justified, I do believe that any philosophical proposition must be readily applicable to everything that exists, existed, or may exist. One might say that this admission is impossible to separate from the view that I actually wish to reject, however, that would be an error, and an important one at that.

The traditional view frames the universe itself as the subject of various predicates that cannot be applied to any particular thing in the universe. In this view, the attribution of these peculiar predicates to the universe is the special business of philosophy. On the contrary, I maintain that there are no propositions of which the "universe" is the subject. In other words, there is no such thing as the "universe." Moreover, I maintain that there are general propositions that can be asserted about each individual thing, like the propositions of logic. This does not mean that all things form a whole that can be regarded as another, independent thing that can be made the subject of predicates. Rather, it means that there are properties that belong to each individual, separate thing, not that there are properties belonging to the entirety of things collectively.

The philosophy for which I am advocating can be called logical atomism or absolute pluralism, because while it maintains that there are many things, it denies that these things come together to compose a whole. Therefore, we will see that in this way, philosophical propositions are not concerned with the whole of things collectively, but rather, they are concerned with all things distributively. Furthermore, they must not only be concerned with all things, but they must also be concerned with such properties of all things so as not to depend upon the accidental nature of things that there happen to be. They must be concerned with the properties of things that are true of any possible world or iteration of the universe, independent of the facts that can only be discovered via sensation.

This brings us right to the second characteristic of philosophical propositions: they must be *a priori*. A philosophical proposition must be of such a nature that it can neither be proved nor disproved by empirical evidence. All too often, we find philosophy books filled with arguments based upon the course of history, the convolutions of the brain, the eyes of shellfish, and etc. Special, accidental facts of this kind are simply irrelevant to philosophy, which ideally only ought to make assertions that would be equally true no matter what specific way the world was actually constituted.

We can synthesize these two characteristics of philosophical propositions into one statement: philosophy is the science of the possible. Of course, this statement, if unexplained, is liable to be misleading as it may be thought that the possible is something other than the general. In reality, two are indistinguishable.

20. Which of the following statements most accurately reflects what the author means when he writes in the third paragraph that " . . .there is no such thing as the 'universe'?"

    A. The whole of existence cannot be taken as a single unit.

    B. There are too few propositions of which the "universe" is the subject.

    C. The existence of the universe as a whole can neither be proved or disproved.

    D. Philosophy must deal not in specifics, but in generalities.

21. Which of the following statements best reflects why the author provides his two labels for the philosophy that he advocates in the fourth paragraph?

    A. To underscore the importance of his argument

    B. To put his argument into a more relatable context

    C. To concisely address two sides of his argument

    D. To highlight his contention with the traditional view

22. Based upon the passage, it can be implied that the author believes which of the following statements?

    A. Philosophy is more important than science.

    B. Like philosophy, science ought to ignore accidental facts.

    C. Philosophy deals with the possible and science deals with the factual.

    D. Logic is more similar to science than it is to philosophy.

23. Which of the following contrasts would the author consider to be most confusing and most important for his readers?

    A. The possible vs the general

    B. The specific vs the general

    C. Philosophy vs logic

    D. The traditional vs the modern

24. Say there is a young student who begins taking private lessons in philosophy with the author. Which of the following pursuits would the author most recommend to his new pupil?

    A. The study of that which may happen in alternate realities

    B. The study of that which has happened in alternate realities

    C. The study of that which will happen in alternate realities

    D. The study of that which could not happen in alternate realities

25. According to the passage, which of the following statements about philosophical propositions is NOT true?

    A. They can neither be proved or disproved by empirical evidence.

    B. They must be general.

    C. They must take only reality into account.

    D. They are often general propositions about individual things.

26. Which of the following statements about the author's brand of philosophy are true?

    I. It has no concern with good and evil.

    II. It has no concern with the universe as a whole.

    III. It attributes peculiar predicates to the universe.

    A. I only

    B. III only

    C. I and II only

    D. I and III only

Passage 5 (Questions 27 – 33)

Political parties ought to have, in addition to their more distant goals, more proximate or short-term aims that they will carry out in the near future. The Marxian socialism of Germany suffered for lack of them: though the party was powerful in numbers, it had no minor aims or measures to demand while waiting for the revolution, and was therefore politically weak. When finally the movement was seized by those who desired more practical policy, the change that occurred was the wrong kind: they yielded to bad policies such as militarism and imperialism instead of advocating for partial reforms, which in themselves may have been inadequate, but still would have been steps in the right direction.

French syndicalism, as it existed before the war, had a similar defect. Everything was waiting for the general strike: the day, after much preparation, when the whole proletariat would rise up as one and refuse to work, causing the property owners to admit defeat and agree to forfeit all of their privileges rather than starve. This is an excellent dramatic conception, but the love of drama is one of true vision's greatest enemies. Except under very rare conditions, men simply cannot be trained to do some sudden thing that is very different from what they have done before.

If this general strike were to succeed, the victors would, despite their penchant for anarchy, be compelled to form an administration, to create a police force to stave off looting and destruction of property, to establish a provisional government that would end up issuing dictatorial orders to certain revolutionaries. Because the syndicalists are opposed to all political action, in taking these necessary, practical steps, they would feel as if they had abandoned their raison d'être. Moreover, they would be without training and practice due to their previous aversion to politics. Therefore, even after a successful syndicalist revolution, power would be assumed by people who are not actually syndicalists.

Here is another objection to these sorts of movements: enthusiasm always wanes when there is nothing to do or no partial successes to enjoy while waiting. The only way a movement can succeed like this is if the motivating sentiment and the program itself are very simple, as in the case of oppressed nations rebelling. Whereas the line dividing an Englishman and a native of India is very clear, the line between capitalist and laborer is less so. Advocates of social revolutions often do not realize how many people there are whose interests and sympathies genuinely lay half on the side of labor and half on the side of capital. This obviously would make clear-cut, revolutionary politics quite difficult to manage.

Given all this, those who aim for an economic reconstruction that will likely not happen in the near future must be able to approach their lofty goal by degrees if they hope to have any success. They ought to take small measures that are useful of themselves, even if they will not directly lead to the end goal. These will help them to train for the policy measures they will inevitably have to carry out if their loftier ambitions come to fruition. Moreover, there must be possible achievements to reach in the near future, not just the hazy vision of utopia at the end of the tunnel.

Though I believe all this to be true, I also believe that truly vital reform requires a vision that reaches beyond the near future, a vision of ideal humanity. Without such lofty hope, the people will lack the energy and enthusiasm necessary to trudge onwards against popular opinion and against physical opposition. Any person who truly wants to change the world for the better will face ridicule, persecution, cajolery, and potential corruption. If anyone is to make it through these ordeals (and truly it is rare that they do), the ultimate goal must be vivid and alive in their minds.

27. According to the author, which of the following is the only way that a political movement with a strong long-term goal and no short-term goals can succeed?

    A. If it has the support of the majority of a populace

    B. If its motivating sentiment and execution are simple

    C. If its ultimate aim is strong and vivid in each person's mind

    D. If the opposing sides can be divided into social classes

28. In the case of Marxian socialism in Germany, what was the ultimate fault of those who seized control of the movement?

    A. They lost the enthusiasm of the people by instituting overbearing policy.

    B. They abandoned the initial motivating factor of the movement, muddling its zeal.

    C. They overcorrected the movement's lack of practical policy to its detriment.

    D. They made the movement into something resembling the system they sought to topple.

29. Based upon the passage, it can be inferred that the author believes which of the following types of political movements to be best?

    A. The one that has a strongly envisioned long-term goal and moderate short-term goals.

    B. The one that has a moderately envisioned long-term goal and zealous short-term goals.

    C. The one that has a strongly envisioned long-term goals and zealous short-term goals.

    D. The one that has a zealously envisioned long-term goal and weak short-term goals.

30. Which of the following best describes why the author introduces French syndicalism as an example?

    A. In order to further show the importance of practical policy in political movements

    B. In order to demonstrate how the inabilities of man affect the central problem

    C. In order to heighten his own credibility with another historical example

    D. In order to prove that the problem extends beyond Marxian socialism in Germany

31. Suppose a new political party has formed with the distant goal of closing the income and wealth gap in America. Also suppose that the author of the passage has been hired as a consultant for the political party. Which of the following immediate advice is the author most likely to give?

    A. Use all resources to aggressively pursue the closing of the income gap

    B. Propose legislation in the current term that would increase taxes on the wealthy

    C. Develop a well-trained militia to help achieve the closing of the income gap

    D. Develop ways to ridicule, persecute, and corrupt the opposition

32. All of the following are objections the author raises to the idea of a political party with only long-term goals EXCEPT:

    A. they will have very little to do until those long-term goals are achieved.

    B. they can be powerful in purpose but are often politically weak.

    C. their members will likely lack a strong purpose to help them face opposition.

    D. it is hard for them to maintain an adequate amount of enthusiasm.

33. Which of the following statements reflect things that ultimately made the French syndicalism movement ineffective even if they had been able to take power?

    I. Its aversion to politics

    II. The need to establish rule of law

    III. They could only be successful after a well-executed general strike.

    A. I only

    B. I and II only

    C. II and III only

    D. I and III only

Passage 6 (Questions 34 – 40)

Referring to some newspaper reports which he knew to be without foundation, Bismarck once said, "Newspapers are simply a union of printer's ink and paper." Omitting the implied slur we might say the same of printed music and printed criticism; therefore, in considering printed music we must, first of all, remember that it is the letter of the law which kills. We must look deeper, and be able to translate sounds back into the emotions which caused them. There is no right or wrong way to give utterance to music. There is but one way, namely, through the living, vital expression of the content of the music; all else is not music but mere pleasure for the ear, a thing of the senses. For the time being we must see through the composer's eyes and hear through his ears. In other words, we must think in his language. The process of creating music is often, to a great extent, beyond the control of the composer, just as is the case with the novel- ist and his characters. The language through which musical thought is expressed, however, is a different thing, and it is this process of developing musical speech until it has become capable of saying for us that which, in our spoken language, must ever remain unsaid, that I shall try to make clear in our consideration of form in music.

Until the very end of the fifteenth century, music, so far as we know, had no language of its own, that is to say, it was not recognized as a medium for expressing thought or emotion. Josquin des Prés (born at Conde in the north of France in 1450, died 1521) was the first to attempt the expression of thought in sound. Luther, in rebelling against Rome, also overturned the music of the church in Germany. He incor- porated many folk songs into the music of the Protestant church and discarded the old Gregorian chant (which was vague in rhythm, or, rather, wholly without rhythm), calling it asinine braying.

While Luther was paving the way for Bach by encouraging church music to be something more than merely the singing of certain melodies according to prescribed rules, in Italy (at the time of his death in 1546) the Council of Trent was already trying to decide upon a style of music proper for the church. The matter was definitely settled in 1562 or 1563 by the adoption of Palestrina's style. Thus, while in Germany ecclesiastical music was being broadened and an opening offered for the development of the dramatic and emotional side of music, in Italy, on the contrary, the emotional style of music was being neglected and an absolutely serene style of what may be called "impersonal" music encouraged. Italy, however, soon had opera on which to fall back, and thus mu- sic in both countries developed rapidly, although on differ- ent lines.

Now this new art was first particularly evident in the dances of these different peoples. These dances gave the music *form*, and held it down to certain prescribed rhythms and dura- tion. Little by little the emotions, the natural expression of which is music, could no longer be restricted to these dance forms and rhythms; and gradually the latter were modi- fied by each daring innovator in turn. The modifications of dance forms led up to our sonata, symphony, and symphon- ic poem, as I hope to show. Opera was a thing apart, and, being untrammelled either by dance rhythms or church laws, developed gradually and normally.

34. Based on the passage, the development of music in Italy was retarded by:

    A. Palestrina's style.

    B. The Council of Trent.

    C. Luther.

    D. Opera.

35. It can be inferred from the passage that Luther was important to the development of music due to his:

    A. focusing wholly on rhythm as the element which best expresses emotion through sound.

    B. restructuring of what was considered appropriate ecclesiastical music.

    C. linking of the church to previously underappreciated forms of music.

    D. transforming the power of Rome to Germany to reform previous systems and styles.

36. Which of the following most closely approximates the author's claim about the language of music?

    A. It is the means by which music can express thought and emotion.

    B. It is the means by which opera articulates its living expression of emotion.

    C. It opposes the pure passion expressed by dance.

    D. It transcends national and religious boundaries.

37. The author discusses Bismarck in order to:

    A. compare the control of a printer over the emotional reactions of readers to that of a composer over the emotional reactions of listeners.

    B. argue that written language is always inferior to live performances.

    C. trace a historical shift towards greater accuracy in recording music.

    D. suggest that written form can sometimes have little to do with the meaning of content.

38. Suppose that a music review came out about a new adaptation of a Bach concerto that argued that, while the performance took liberties with the score and intentions of the piece, it was successful because it created great pleasure and engaged the senses. Based on the passage, the author would most likely respond to this review by:

    A. arguing that such a performance failed due to its inaccuracy to the content of the music as laid out by the written document.

    B. praising the innovation evidenced by the creativity of the performance, suggesting that there is no right or wrong way to interpret a score.

    C. contrasting the composer's ideas and intentions with the modern world in which the work is being performed.

    D. defining the difference between utterances and intentions through an analysis of the intents of the performance.

39. Based on the passage, the contrast between German and Italian music, respectively, in the 16th century prior to the development of opera was MOST like the following:

    A. a painting full of vivid colors and intense interactions vs one that employed soft colors and nondescript images.

    B. a pop song by a young female singer vs a rap song by an older male.

    C. an orderly and restrained ballet performance vs a passionate and overwrought modern dance movement.

    D. a novel following prescribed rules vs a genre-bending short story collection.

40. Which of the following is true of opera, based on the passage?

    I. It developed independently of some other musical forms.

    II. It was defined by strictly defined rhythms and tempos.

    III. It was crucial in the development of Italian music.

    A. I only

    B. III only

    C. I and II only

    D. I and III only

Passage 7 (Questions 41 – 45)

Consumers' needs and demands are constantly evolving, so companies have begun to focus on reaching the most influential consumers in the market. Recent research suggests that market influencers are growing in importance primarily due to the proliferation of product choice in today's marketplace, and an associated growing need among consumers for help in dealing with more choices. The concepts of mavenism and opinion leadership underscore that these individuals are an indispensable target market as they spread the word about multiple product categories and new product introductions. An understanding of these innovative consumers is a crucial issue for marketers to develop more effective strategies.

With their general marketplace expertise and communication skills, influential consumers are the persons that can start word-of-mouth epidemics. The new ideas that are propagated by these consumers are communicated to connectors who know a large group of people, most of them outside the community of the mavens. It should also be highlighted that the message that is transmitted by influential consumers tends to have a stickiness factor that is memorable and appealing for the masses. As such, the quality of both the messengers, as well as the content of the message, matters upon spreading the information.

Rogers (1995) studied how innovation occurs, arguing that innovation consists of four stages, which are invention, diffusion, time, and consequences. Diffusion is the process by which an innovation is communicated through certain channels over a period of time among the members of a social system. The diffusion of innovations model demonstrates that, while the media diffuse most new ideas, audiences heavily rely on the recommendations and opinions that (originally) come from opinion leaders or mavens to decide if they adopt the innovation. Once the innovators and early adopters have the time to test the new product, the popularity of that innovation will grow rapidly as consumers start to communicate and are influenced by their word-of-mouth more substantially.

Consumer innovativeness has been defined as the tendency for consumers to have extensive technical knowledge and willingness to understand technological innovations in the market (Saaksjarvi, 2003). This means that innovators adopt innovations quickly compared to other members of the social system (Rogers, 2003). Like early adopters, opinion leaders are an attractive target for marketers as they are capable of influencing other consumers not just at the moment of the purchase decision, but earlier in the consumer buying process. But opinion leaders' primary goal is to deliberately influence other consumers (and their purchase behavior), which sets them apart from innovators.

Although market mavens have similar demographic characteristics as opinion leaders and early adopters/innovators, they differ from the opinion leaders and early adopters/purchasers on the higher levels of general knowledge about the marketplace and product marketing mix characteristics. This trait makes mavens an attractive target market and change agent for retailers and other large industries that produce and/or sell a wide range of durable and fast-moving consumer goods (FMCG). This contrasts sharply with the opinion leaders and early adopters who are more knowledgeable and want to share information about a specific range of products within a product category, or specific market environment characteristics.

Market mavens are "smart shoppers". They demonstrate very high levels of value consciousness by utilizing coupons, grocery lists, advanced budgeting tactics, together with planning their purchases using advertising (Chelminski & Coulter, 2007). Relatedly, market mavens are thought to be an important segment of consumers owing to the disproportionate influence they have on other consumers via word-of mouth (Wangenheim, 2005), viral marketing (Goldsmith et al., 2003) and coupon distribution (Goodey & East, 2008). These consumers are a vital promotional agent for small businesses relying on word-of-mouth, rather than large advertising budgets.

41. Which of the following is most likely the primary goal for a consumer innovator?

    A. To be a frontrunner with new products and innovations

    B. To be labeled as a good shopper by other consumers

    C. To fulfill a desire to influence other consumers

    D. To be known as a credible source of knowledge and experience

42. Which of the following communication theories best explains how mass media messages are transmitted in relation to the concepts of mavenism and opinion leadership?

    A. The magic bullet theory that posits the messages of mass media are fired directly into the audience's heads by the media (magic gun) without their notice or knowledge causing instant reaction from the audience minds, without hesitation.

    B. The two-step flow theory that posits opinion leaders initially consume media content, interpret it in terms of their own values and beliefs and then pass it on to opinion followers who have very little contact with media.

    C. The multi-step flow model that posits information from the mass media can flow directly to and through different types of consumers, including opinion leaders and opinion seekers, and that audiences are active and send feedback to the media.

    D. The hypodermic needle theory that posits that mass media has a powerful and direct influence on the public, which is composed of isolated individuals.

43. Which of the following is NOT a potential implication for marketing theory and marketing practice based on this passage?

    A. Marketers should integrate individuals with a tendency toward mavenship and opinion leadership as powerful sources in the context of co-producing products and services.

    B. Marketers should target only one of the three identified influential consumer groups if they hope to get the most value for their advertising dollars.

    C. Marketers with smaller budgets have the most to gain from tapping into influential consumer groups, word of mouth, viral marketing and coupon distribution.

    D. Marketing theory needs to account for the role of word of mouth and the multidirectional influence of mass media messages.

44. Given that market-mavens demonstrate high levels of value consciousness, which of the following media sources would they be most likely to read?

    I. Direct mail advertisements

    II. Trade journals

    III. Retail magazines

    A. I only

    B. I and II only

    C. I and III only

    D. I, II, and III

45. Which of the following is most likely to also spread in the same manner as word of mouth advertising?

    A. Malaria

    B. An idiom

    C. Food poisoning

    D. A meme

Passage 8 (Questions 46 – 49)

That all our knowledge begins with experience there can be no doubt. For how is it possible that the faculty of cognition should be awakened into exercise otherwise than by means of objects which affect our senses, and partly of themselves produce representations, partly rouse our powers of understanding into activity, to compare to connect, or to separate these, and so to convert the raw material of our sensuous impressions into a knowledge of objects, which is called experience? In respect of time, therefore, no knowledge of ours is antecedent to experience, but begins with it..

But, though all our knowledge begins with experience, it by no means follows that all arises out of experience. For, on the contrary, it is quite possible that our empirical knowledge is a compound of that which we receive through impressions, and that which the faculty of cognition supplies from itself (sensuous impressions giving merely the occasion), an addition which we cannot distinguish from the original element given by sense, till long practice has made us attentive to, and skillful in separating it. It is, therefore, a question which requires close investigation, and not to be answered at first sight, whether there exists a knowledge altogether independent of experience, and even of all sensuous impressions? Knowledge of this kind is called a priori, in contradistinction to empirical knowledge, which has its sources a posteriori, that is, in experience.

But the expression, "a priori", is not as yet definite enough adequately to indicate the whole meaning of the question above started. For, in speaking of knowledge which has its sources in experience, we are wont to say, that this or that may be known a priori, because we do not derive this knowledge immediately from experience, but from a general rule, which, however, we have itself borrowed from experience. Thus, if a man undermined his house, we say, "he might know a priori that it would have fallen"; that is, he needed not to have waited for the experience that it did actually fall. But still, a priori, he could not know even this much. For, that bodies are heavy, and, consequently, that they fall when their supports are taken away, must have been known to him previously, by means of experience. By the term "knowledge a priori", therefore, we shall in the sequel understand, not such as is independent of this or that kind of experience, but such as is absolutely so of all experience. Opposed to this is empirical knowledge, or that which is possible only a posteriori, that is, through experience. Knowledge a priori is either pure or impure. Pure knowledge a priori is that with which no empirical element is mixed up. For example, the proposition, "Every change has a cause", is a proposition a priori, but impure, because change is a conception which can only be derived from experience.

The question now is as to a criterion, by which we may securely distinguish a pure from an empirical cognition. Experience no doubt teaches us that this or that object is constituted in such and such a manner, but not that it could not possibly exist otherwise. Now, in the first place, if we have a proposition which contains the idea of necessity in its very conception, it is a if, moreover, it is not derived from any other proposition, unless from one equally involving the idea of necessity, it is absolutely a prior I. Secondly, an empirical judgment never exhibits strict and absolute, but only assumed and comparative universality (by induction); therefore, the most we can say is—so far as we have hitherto observed, there is no exception to this or that rule. If, on the other hand, a judgment carries with it strict and absolute universality, that is, admits of no possible exception, it is not derived from experience, but is valid absolutely a priori.

46. According to the author, all of the following are examples of impure, "a priori" knowledge, EXCEPT:

    A. An individual predicts the results of a midterm election.

    B. An individual takes a shortcut in order to avoid traffic at an intersection she has seen get congested every day at this time.

    C. A child burns his hand on a hot stove.

    D. An individual anticipates that an object will sink in water based on its perceived heft.

47. The author would most likely agree with which of the following statements?

    A. Nearly all knowledge is derived from empirical observation.

    B. Pure a priori knowledge is superior to impure a priori knowledge.

    C. Knowledge derived from scientific reasoning is inadequate.

    D. Pure a priori knowledge is more fundamental than knowledge gained through experience.

48. Based on the passage, the author uses the example "Every change has a cause" to:

    A. indicate how knowledge can be derived independently of experience.

    B. counter an argument made earlier in the passage.

    C. argue that it is impossible to separate knowledge from empirical observation.

    D. indicate how seemingly a priori knowledge can be derived from empirical observation.

49. Which of the following statements, if true, would support the arguments made by the author?

    I. Empirical observations can only be made based on an understanding of the consistency of the laws of nature.

    II. To experience objects you must have the mechanism to understand what an object is in the first place.

    III. When deprived of stimulus, individuals show no measurable brain activity

    A. II only

    B. I and II only

    C. I and III only

    D. I, II and III

Passage 9 (Questions 50 – 53)

That the end of life should be death may sound sad: yet what other end can anything have? The end of an evening party is to go to bed; but its use is to gather congenial people together, that they may pass the time pleasantly. An invitation to the dance is not rendered ironical because the dance cannot last for ever; the youngest of us and the most vigorously wound up, after a few hours, has had enough of sinuous stepping and prancing. The transitoriness of things is essential to their physical being, and not at all sad in itself; it becomes sad by virtue of a sentimental illusion, which makes us imagine that they wish to endure, and that their end is always untimely; but in a healthy nature it is not so. What is truly sad is to have some impulse frustrated in the midst of its career, and robbed of its chosen object; and what is painful is to have an organ lacerated or destroyed when it is still vigorous, and not ready for its natural sleep and dissolution. We must not confuse the itch which our unsatisfied instincts continue to cause with the pleasure of satisfying and dismissing each of them in turn. Could they all be satisfied harmoniously we should be satisfied once for all and completely. Then doing and dying would coincide throughout and be a perfect pleasure.

This same insight is contained in another wise myth which has inspired morality and religion in India from time immemorial: I mean the doctrine of Karma. We are born, it says, with a heritage, a character imposed, and a long task assigned, all due to the ignorance which in our past lives has led us into all sorts of commitments. These obligations we must pay off, relieving the pure spirit within us from its accumulated burdens, from debts and assets both equally oppressive. We cannot disentangle ourselves by mere frivolity, nor by suicide: frivolity would only involve us more deeply in the toils of fate, and suicide would but truncate our misery and leave us for ever a confessed failure. When life is understood to be a process of redemption, its various phases are taken up in turn without haste and without undue attachment; their coming and going have all the keenness of pleasure, the holiness of sacrifice, and the beauty of art. The point is to have expressed and discharged all that was latent in us; and to this perfect relief various temperaments and various traditions assign different names, calling it having one's day, or doing one's duty, or realizing one's ideal, or saving one's soul. The task in any case is definite and imposed on us by nature, whether we recognize it or not; therefore we can make true moral progress or fall into real errors. Wisdom and genius lie in discerning this prescribed task and in doing it readily, cleanly, and without distraction. Folly on the contrary imagines that any scent is worth following, that we have an infinite nature, or no nature in particular, that life begins without obligations and can do business without capital, and that the will is vacuously free, instead of being a specific burden and a tight hereditary knot to be unraveled.

Some philosophers without self-knowledge think that the variations and further entanglements which the future may bring are the manifestation of spirit; but they are, as Freud has indicated, imposed on living beings by external pressure, and take shape in the realm of matter. Deep and dark as a soul may be when you look down into it from outside, it is something perfectly natural; and the same understanding that can unearth our suppressed young passions, and dispel our stubborn bad habits, can show us where our true good lies. Nature has marked out the path for us beforehand; there are snares in it, but also primroses, and it leads to peace.

50. Which of the following best describes the relationship between "the end of an evening party" described in paragraph 1, and "the doctrine of Karma" described in paragraph 2?

   A. The example of the party describes something frivolous, and is contrasted with the solemn doctrine of Karma.

   B. Both describe situations in which we will be happiest if we accept a necessary and prescribed path.

   C. Although the party has a natural and inevitable end, the doctrine of Karma explains that life is endless.

   D. Both examples focus on the sadness that is inevitable in life.

51. A proponent of the doctrine of free will believes that each individual has the power to control his or her own life as he or she desires. What would a person of that belief most likely think of the point of view put forth in this passage?

   A. Like the author of the passage, he would agree that we are born with a destiny.

   B. Unlike the author of the passage, he would believe that the transitoriness of life is innately sad.

   C. Like the author of the passage, he would agree that everything has an inevitable end.

   D. Unlike the author of the passage, he would disagree with the notion that life unfolds according to a predetermined path.

52. Of the following, which would the author most likely agree is one's duty in life?

   A. Understanding one's true nature and following one's given path

   B. Following whatever is most interesting at any given time

   C. Atoning for errors of past lives

   D. Accepting that we are transitory and insignificant

53. The author describes all of the following as "folly" EXCEPT:

   A. thinking that we should follow our whims.

   B. imagining that we are born without nature or obligations.

   C. trying to untangle the mystery of our obligations and destiny.

   D. assuming that our potential in life is limitless.

This page intentionally left blank.

SECTION 9

Answer Key

1	D	12	C	23	B	34	A	45	D
2	D	13	B	24	A	35	B	46	C
3	B	14	C	25	C	36	A	47	A
4	A	15	D	26	C	37	D	48	D
5	C	16	B	27	B	38	A	49	B
6	B	17	C	28	C	39	A	50	B
7	B	18	B	29	A	40	D	51	D
8	B	19	A	30	B	41	A	52	A
9	D	20	A	31	B	42	C	53	C
10	C	21	C	32	C	43	B		
11	A	22	C	33	B	44	C		

Passage 1 (Questions 1 – 6)

Put shortly, there are **two views**. One, that man is **intrinsically good**, spoilt by circumstance; and the other that he is **intrinsically limited**, but disciplined by order and tradition to something fairly decent. To the one party man's nature is like a well, to the other like a bucket. The view which regards man as a well, a reservoir full of possibilities, I call the **romantic**; the one which regards him as a very finite and fixed creature, I call the **classical**.

Key terms: two views, romantic, classical

Contrast: classical view sees human nature as limited, like a bucket; romantic view sees it as infinite, like a well

I must now **shirk the difficulty** of saying exactly what I mean by romantic and classical in **verse**. I can only say that it means the result of these two attitudes towards the cosmos, towards man, in so far as it gets reflected in verse. The **romantic**, because he thinks man **infinite**, must always be talking about the infinite; and as there is always the bitter contrast between what you think you **ought** to be able to do and what man **actually** can, it always tends to be **gloomy**.

Key terms: verse, romantic, infinite

Opinion: Author says romantic verse often talks about the infinite

Cause and effect: because the romantic view looks to infinity, when confronted with man's actual limitations it tends to become gloomy

What I mean by **classical** in verse is this. That even in the most imaginative flights there is **always** a **holding back**, a reservation. The classical poet never forgets this **finiteness**, this limit of man. He remembers always that he is mixed up with earth. He may **jump**, but he **always returns** back; he never flies away into the circumambient gas. You might say if you wished that the whole of the romantic attitude seems to crystallize in verse round metaphors of flight. Hugo is always flying, flying over abysses, flying up into the eternal gases. The word infinite in every other line.

Key terms: classical, finiteness

Opinion: author says classical verse is restrained and considers man's limits

In the **classical** attitude you never seem to swing right along to the infinite nothing. If you say an **extravagant thing** which does **exceed the limits** inside which you know man to be fastened, yet there is **always** conveyed in some way at the end an impression of **yourself** standing outside it, and **not quite believing it**, or consciously putting it forward as a flourish. You never go blindly into an atmosphere more than the truth, an atmosphere too rarefied for man to breathe for long. You are always faithful to the **conception of a limit**. It is a question of pitch; in romantic verse you move at a certain pitch of rhetoric which you know, man being what he is, to be a little high-falutin. The kind of thing you get in

Hugo or Swinburne. For an example of the opposite thing, a verse written in the proper classical spirit, take the song from *Cymbeline*. Take the last two lines:

'Golden lads and girls all must,

Like chimney sweepers come to dust.'

The thing that I think quite classical is the word "**lad**". Your modern **romantic** could never write that. He would have to write "**golden youth**", and take up the thing at least a couple of notes in pitch.

Key terms: classical, conception of a limit, lad

Opinion: the tone of classical verse, as well as the topic, reflects the conception of limits

Contrast: the more colloquial word "lad" is used as an example of classicism, whereas a romantic would use the word "youth"

The **essence of poetry** to most people is that it must lead them to a **beyond** of some kind. Verse strictly confined to the earthly and the definite (Keats is full of it) might seem to them to be excellent writing, excellent craftsmanship, but not poetry. So much has **romanticism debauched us**, that, without some form of vagueness, we deny the highest. The thing has **got so bad now** that a poem which is all dry and hard, a **properly classical poem**, would **not be considered poetry** at all.

Key terms: beyond, romanticism debauched us

Opinion: author says that most people have gotten so used to the excesses of romanticism that few would appreciate a proper classical poem

In the classic it is always the **light of ordinary day**, never the light that never was on land or sea. It is always **perfectly human and never exaggerated** man is always man and never a god. But the **awful result of romanticism** is that, accustomed to this strange light, you can never live without it. Its effect on you is that of a **drug**.

Key terms: light of ordinary day, strange light drug

Opinion: we have gotten so used to the romantic viewpoint that we are almost addicted to seeing the world in this light

Main idea: Classical verse and thought are restrained and accept human limits, while romantic verse and thought use overblown language to describe the infinite and the author thinks that a negative effect of romantic verse is that the audience has gotten accustomed to romanticism's overblown poetry and now can't appreciate classical verse.

1. D is correct. Although the author starts out simply describing the two types of verse, by paragraph 3 it becomes clear that he is critical of the romantic point of view and romantic verse. He's bothered by its focus on the infinite and its lack of moderation.

   A: It's classicism, not romanticism, that is the more orderly.

   B: This is a point of criticism, not one of approval, for the author.

   C: It's not the craftsmanship that the author objects to – it's the topics and tone.

2. D is correct. Although you'd think that a dry, hard poem would be something the author criticizes, it isn't: he suggests that such a poem is a good thing – a properly classical poem that is not overblown.

   A: The author criticizes the view that poetry must address the transcendent – which is what romantic poetry does.

   B: The author likes earth-bound poems.

   C: Such a poem is illuminated by the light of the ordinary, which the author appreciates.

3. B is correct. This poem features lofty language and plenty of references to the infinite, which makes it clearly of the romantic tradition.

   A: Although this choice correctly labels the poem as romantic, it is not the common sense of the word romantic – related to a love relationship – that the author uses.

   C: No – such a theme would make it more likely to be classical, not romantic.

   D: The poem does indeed fit the romantic tradition rather well.

4. A is correct. The author makes the analogy to describe two different views of human nature: good and limitless (romantic) versus pretty good with some work, and limited (classical).

   B: In paragraph 1 the author simply describes; his views come out a little later on.

   C: No – the philosophical viewpoints are sort of a basis for the poetic styles.

   D: In paragraph 3, the author points to metaphors of flight as hallmarks of romantic poetry; he never compares that to the analogy regarding the bucket and the well.

5. C is correct. You can find the answer to this in the first line of paragraph 5: people assume that poetry needs to take them to the beyond. The author obviously sees this as a problem.

6. B is correct. The "strange light" to which the author refers is the exaggeration of romantic poetry, with its focus on the infinite. The problem, he says, is readers who become accustomed to that cease to appreciate the restrained beauty of classical poetry.

   A: Readers of romantic verse get used to the particular focus and language of romantic verse, not pleasure in general.

   C: There's nothing that says that readers think of themselves as idealized – it's that they get used to poetry as idealizing.

   D: The notion of romantic poetry as a drug is metaphorical, not literal.

Passage 2 (Questions 7 – 13)

None of the **Italian masters** has ever taken such a firm hold of the **popular imagination** as **Raphael**. While others wax and wane in esteem as they are praised by one generation and disparaged by the next, Raphael continues to be held as **the most favored painter in Christendom**. Though his work is subjected to **severe criticism**, the passing centuries do not dim his fame. Rather, he remains, as he began, the **first love of the people**.

Opinion: author thinks Raphael is the most popular and loved painter by Christian people

Cause and effect: because of Raphael's firm hold on the popular imagination, his esteem does not wax and wane

His subjects are nearly all **cheerful**, for he mostly exercised his skill on scenes that were **agreeable to contemplate**. As such, he was preeminently **the artist of joy**, so **pain** and **ugliness** were strangers to his work. This quality in him can be attributed not only to his **pleasure-loving nature**, but also to the **great influence** made upon him by the **rediscovery of the Greeks**, which happened in his day, for the Greeks dealt instinctively with **objects of delight**.

Contrast: joy vs pain and ugliness, pleasure-loving nature vs influence of the Greeks

Cause and effect: because he used his skills on scenes that are agreeable to contemplate, his subjects are nearly all cheerful

Just as Raphael's work is **compassionate** to our **hearts**, it is equally so to our **minds**, requiring neither strenuous feelings nor too much thinking. Just like his subjects do not overtax our **sympathies** with harrowing emotions, his art does not overtax our **understanding** with **complicated effects**. His works appear so simple that they seem to require no significant **intellectual effort** and no **technical knowledge** to enjoy. He does all the work for us. It was not his way to show what **difficult things** he could with his work, but rather, he made great art seem to be the **easiest thing** in the world. Of course, this ease was the result of **pure mastery**, the mastery that enabled him to arrange the fifty-two figures of *The School of Athens* and the three figures of *The Madonna of the Chair* so simply and unobtrusively that we are lead to imagine such undertakings as **mundane**. Yet in both cases, he solves essentially difficult **problems of composition** with a success scarcely paralleled.

Key terms: *The School of Athens, The Madonna of the Chair,* problems of composition

Contrast: showing he can do difficult things vs making great art seem easy, *The School of Athens* (52 figures) vs *The Madonna of the Chair* (3 figures), the making of art being mundane vs it solving difficult problems of composition

Cause and effect: because he does all the work for us, his works appear so simple that they seem to require no significant effort

Even Raphael rarely achieved the **same kind of success** twice: *The Parnassus* lacks the **variety** of *The School of Athens*, though the individual figures have a similar **grace**, and *The Fire in the Borgo* possesses parts equal in beauty to any in the previous two works, but lacks the **unity** of either. Moreover, though *The Parnassus* and *The Liberation of Saint Peter* show a **masterly adaptation** to a **severely awkward space**, *The Transfiguration* fails to solve a much easier **composition problem**.

Key terms: *The Parnassus, The Fire in the Borgo, The Liberation of Saint Peter, The Transfiguration*

Cause and effect: even Raphael rarely achieved the same kind of success twice

Though he instinctually preferred the **Greek style** of **statuesque repose** to the **portrayal of action**, Raphael showed himself capable of both. The **charge of avenging spirits** upon Heliodorus is just as impressive as the **Hellenic calm** of his Parnassus. The **vigorous realism** of Peter when he is called from his fishing to the apostleship matches the **visionary idealism** of the angel-led Peter. The **alert activity** of the swiftly moving *Sistine Madonna* perfectly complements the **brooding quiet** of *The Madonna of the Chair*.

Key terms: *Sistine Madonna*

Contrast: statuesque repose vs portrayal of action, avenging spirits vs Hellenic calm

Cause and effect: because he was capable of his preferred style of statuesque repose, and also the portrayal of action, his active works are just as good as his calmer paintings

Great though Raphael's **achievements** were in a **many directions**, he is most remembered for his **Madonnas**, those works which best expressed the **individuality of his genius**. He never ceased to be fascinated by the **sweet mystery** of **motherhood**, and so he plumbed **the depths of maternity** time and time again, always making some new discovery.

Contrast: having great achievements in many directions vs being most remembered for one type of work

Cause and effect: because they most express the individuality of his genius, Raphael's Madonnas are his most remembered works

The Madonna of the Chair most emphasizes the **physical instincts** of maternity. As Taine wrote, "She bends over the child with the **beautiful action** of a **wild animal**." Like a mother creature instinctively protecting her young, she gathers him in **her embrace** as if to shield him from some **imminent danger**. On the other hand, the *Sistine Madonna* is the most spiritual of Raphael's works, a **perfect embodiment of womanhood**, her love **transfigured** by **the spirit of sacrifice**. Forgetful of **self** and obedient to heaven, she bears her son forth for **the good of humanity**.

Contrast: human mother vs wild animal, her embrace vs imminent danger, *The Madonna of the Chair* vs *Sistine Madonna*

Cause and effect: because *Madonna of the Chair* features a mother protecting her child in her embrace, it emphasizes the physical instincts of maternity; because the woman of the *Sistine Madonna* is seemingly transfigured by sacrifice and is obedient to heaven and forgetful of self, this painting is the most spiritual of Raphael's works

Main Idea: The author expresses exactly how Raphael has maintained his hold of the popular imagination; the reasons for this success include his cheerfulness and his simplicity; his best works seem to be his Madonnas.

7.   B is correct. The Heliodorus is the only one of these choices that is not actually mentioned in the passage.

    A, C, D: These are all paintings specifically mentioned in the passage.

8.   B is correct. As the author writes in the fourth paragraph, "Even Raphael rarely achieved the same kind of success twice: The Parnassus lacks the variety of The School of Athens, though the individual figures have a similar grace..." The School of Athens is a masterwork, with 52 figures arranged simply and unobtrusively. Essentially, the masterfulness of this work was not entirely present in The Parnassus. Raphael's greatest successes were sometimes not even repeatable to the master.

    A: The giveaway here may be "often": though it does seem that Raphael may have some inconsistency in his work, it cannot be said that he was often inconsistent.

    C: He displayed mastery of craft outside of his Madonnas.

    D: The author writes this in the third paragraph about all of his paintings, and never says otherwise about another work.

9.   D is correct. In the sixth paragraph: "He is most remembered for his Madonnas, those works which best expressed the individuality of his genius." We already have the given that Raphael is a popular artist so it's likely that his "most remembered" worked refers to his "most popular" work.

10.   C is correct. As the author writes in the fifth paragraph, "Though he instinctually preferred the Greek style of statuesque repose to the portrayal of action, Raphael showed himself capable of both. The charge of avenging spirits upon Heliodorus is just as impressive as the Hellenic calm of his Parnassus." In this comparison, the "charge of avenging spirits" corresponds to the "portrayal of action," so the "Hellenic calm" refers back to the "Greek style of statuesque repose."

11.   A is correct. Raphael was able to arrange human figures masterfully, for example in his work The School of Athens.

B: It seems rather that joy, at least in the context of this passage, is simple.

C: Rather, Raphael "does not overtax our understanding with complicated effects." He didn't use them.

D: We get no mention of conversation with subjects here.

12.   C is correct. Rather, in the fifth paragraph, the author writes of the "vigorous realism" of Peter called from his fishing and the "visionary idealism" of the angel-led Peter. Choice C mixes these features and is therefore the only choice that is not a feature of his work.

13.   B is correct. Item III is true because he "does all the work for us".

    I: This is never said. We get no comparison with another individual artist. Raphael is the most popular, but not that he is the best.

    II: This is untrue because the question asks about which of these statements the author would "definitely believe". We cannot know definitely if the author believes the Madonna paintings to be Raphael's most technically masterful (though they do best express the individuality of his genius).

Passage 3 (Questions 14 – 19)

Beneath and very remote from **scientific revolutions**, which generate the progress of civilizations, are the **religious and political revolutions**, which have no kinship with them. While scientific revolutions derive solely from **rational elements**, political and religious beliefs are sustained almost exclusively by **affective and mystic factors**. Reason plays a feeble part in their genesis.

Opinion: the author believes scientific revolutions are more important than religious and political revolutions, and furthermore that the latter two revolutions are not driven by rational thought

Contrast: scientific revolutions vs religious and political revolutions

I have insisted at some length on the **affective and mystic origin** of beliefs, showing that a **political or religious belief** constitutes an act of faith elaborated in **unconsciousness**, over which, in spite of appearances, reason has no hold. I also showed that belief often reaches such a degree of intensity that nothing can be opposed to it. The man hypnotized by his faith becomes an **Apostle**, ready to sacrifice his interests, his happiness, and even his life for the triumph of his faith. The extremity of his belief matters little; for him it is a burning reality. Certitudes of mystic origin possess the marvelous power of domination over thought, and can only be affected by time. By the very fact that it is regarded as an absolute truth a belief necessarily becomes intolerant. This explains the violence, hatred, and persecution which were the habitual accompaniments of the great political and religious revolutions, notably of the **Reformation** and the **French Revolution**.

Opinion: the author believes political or religious beliefs are acts of faith determined by the subconscious brain and are held as absolute truths

Cause and effect: political and religious beliefs are held so fervently that they are intolerant

Contrast: subconscious vs rational thoughts

Certain periods of **French history** remain incomprehensible if we forget this **affective and mystic** origin of beliefs, their necessary intolerance, the impossibility of **reconciling** them when they come into mutual contact, and, finally, the power conferred by mystic beliefs upon the sentiments which place themselves at their service. Events such as the **Reformation**, which overwhelmed France for a period of fifty years, were in no wise determined by rational influences. Yet rational influences are always invoked in explanation, even in the most recent works. Thus, in the General History of **Lavisse** and **Rambaud**, we read the following explanation of the Reformation: "It was a spontaneous movement, born here and there amidst the people, from the reading of the Gospels and the free individual reflections which were suggested to simple persons by an extremely pious conscience and a very bold reasoning power." Contrary to the assertion of these

historians, we may say with certainty that **such movements are never spontaneous**, and secondly, that **reason takes no part** in their elaboration. The force of the political and religious beliefs which have moved the world resides precisely in that fact.

Key terms: French history, affective and mystic, reconciling, Reformation, Lavisse and Rambaud

Opinion: Lavisse and Rambaud incorrectly describe the French Revolution and Reformation as based out of rational thought

Cause and effect: Revolutions derive their power because they are not based upon reason

Political revolutions may result from beliefs established in the minds of men, but many other causes produce them. The word **discontent** sums them up. As soon as discontent is generalized **a party** is formed which often becomes strong enough to struggle against the **Government**. Discontent must generally have been accumulating for a long time in order to produce its effects. For this reason a revolution does not always represent a phenomenon in the process of termination followed by another which is commencing but rather a **continuous phenomenon**, having somewhat accelerated its evolution. All the modern revolutions, however, have been abrupt movements, entailing the instantaneous overthrow of governments. Such, for example, were the **Brazilian**, **Portuguese**, and **Chinese revolutions**.

Key terms: discontent, Brazilian, Portuguese, Chinese revolutions

Opinion: author believes that general discontent accumulated for a long time causes revolutions

Cause and effect: given that revolutions are sparked by the long term accumulation of discontent, they can form a continuous phenomenon, not a stop-and-start event sparked by single moments of frustration and anger

Lastly, to the contrary of what might be supposed, it is important to note that very **conservative peoples** are the individuals **most addicted to violent revolutions**. Being conservative, they are **not able to evolve slowly**, or to adapt themselves to variations of environment, so that when the discrepancy becomes too extreme they are bound to adapt themselves suddenly. This sudden evolution constitutes a revolution, and it arrives with violent behavior. Peoples able to adapt themselves **progressively**, however, do not escape revolution altogether. It was only by means of a revolution that the **English**, in **1688**, were able to terminate the struggle which had dragged on for a century between the **monarchy**, which sought to make itself absolute, and the **nation**, which claimed the right to govern itself through the medium of its representatives.

Opinion: the author believes that conservative peoples are most prone to violent revolutions

Cause and effect: conservative peoples do not adapt to change gradually thus they are more prone to violent revolutions

Contrast: conservative vs progressive

Main Idea: Political and religious beliefs have no basis in rationality, and therefore political revolutions cannot be understood within the context of reason. The absence of a rational backing explains many of the characteristics of such revolutions.

14. C is correct. The author believes that reason has no hold over affective and mystic beliefs, and furthermore that such beliefs are an act of faith "elaborated within the unconscious mind".

    A: This is the opposite of the author's definition.

    B: It can't be inferred from the passage that affective beliefs spring from negative emotional stimuli, as many other potential sources are possible.

15. D is correct. Religious and political revolutions are both motivated by the same factors. The author describes political revolutions as continuous phenomena so we can infer that religious revolutions would behave in the same manner.

    A, B: This does not apply to scientific revolutions.

    C: The author states that the French Revolution was devoid of rationality.

16. B is correct. The author states that "by the very fact that [a belief] is regarded as an absolute truth a belief necessarily becomes intolerant".

    A: The author states that the accumulation of discontent is the motivating factor for revolutions.

    C: The author states that scientific revolutions are guided by rational thought.

    D: The author believes that conservative peoples do not adapt gradually to change over time, but rather change builds around them until they break and adapt rapidly, causing revolutions.

17. C is correct. One of the author's main contentions is that religious and political beliefs are formulated in the unconscious, specifically in the absence of rational thought. The author furthermore states that "the force of the political and religious beliefs which have moved the world resides precisely in that fact", meaning that he believes that such beliefs directly derive their power due to that lack of a rational basis. A study that indicates that rational thought is a more powerful motivator than emotional responses would stand in direct opposition to the assumptions of his argument.

    A: This would support the author's argument that religious and political beliefs create intolerance.

    B: The author states that scientific revolutions are driven by rational thought; however the manner in which progress occurs is not addressed by the passage.

18. B is correct. While the author argues that conservative peoples are more prone to creating more violent revolutions, when placed in the same environment (i.e. absence of revolution or the same revolution) no inferences can be made based on the passage.

    A: The author states that political and religious revolutions are "beneath and very remote from scientific revolutions".

    C: This is in contrast to one of the author's main contentions

    D: This is tricky, but the structure of the last paragraph indicates that the example of the English people is being employed by the author of an example of a progressive people that still were compelled into a revolution.

19. A is correct. The author's point in the paragraph is to establish that revolutions can often be continuous phenomena, but rather a gradual progression from one idea to another. The Brazilian, Portuguese and Chinese revolutions are established abrupt changes, however, and the author uses them to provide evidence that modern revolutions have not behaved in a similar fashion. The examples serve to qualify his main point in the paragraph, by indicating that the phenomenon he described is not as frequent.

    B: The examples do not help transition the reader to the next paragraph (which addresses conservative vs progressive peoples).

    C: The example supports the claims made in the preceding sentence (that modern revolutions have not been the aforementioned continuous phenomenA..

    D: The abrupt nature of modern revolutions does not support the main idea of the passage.

Passage 4 (Questions 20 – 26)

If we remove the notion of the **universe** and the notion of **good and evil** from scientific philosophy, it may be asked, and justifiably so, **what specific problems remain for the philosopher** that the scientist cannot answer? It is difficult to give an entirely precise answer to this question, but there are **certain characteristics** that may be noted that distinguish the **province of philosophy** from that of the sciences.

Opinion: author thinks that philosophy has its own specific questions that remain for it, even if many questions have been taken over by the sciences

First, a philosophical proposition must **necessarily be general**: it must not deal with specific things on the surface of the earth, with the solar system, or with any other specific segment of space and time. It is this very need for generality that has led to the widely held belief that philosophy **deals with the universe as a whole**. While I do **not** believe that this belief is **justified**, I do believe that any philosophical proposition must be readily **applicable to everything** that exists, existed, or may exist. One might say that this admission is impossible to separate from the view that I actually wish to reject, however, that would be an error, and an important one at that.

Contrast: some think that philosophy applies to the universe as a whole because it is necessarily general vs the author thinks that philosophy does not apply to the universe as a whole but it is still very general

Opinion: author thinks philosophy applies to everything that exists and even everything that may exist

The traditional view frames the universe itself as the subject of various predicates that cannot be applied to any particular thing in the universe. In this view, the attribution of these peculiar predicates to the universe is the special business of philosophy. On the contrary, I maintain that **there are no propositions** of which the "universe" is the subject. In other words, **there is no such thing as the "universe."** Moreover, I maintain that there are general propositions that can be asserted about each individual thing, like the propositions of logic. This does not mean that all things form a whole that can be regarded as another, independent thing that can be made the subject of predicates. Rather, it means that there are **properties** that **belong to each individual**, separate thing, **not** that there are **properties belonging to the entirety** of things collectively.

Opinion: author thinks there's no such separate thing as the universe; author thinks there are general statements you can apply to each individual thing, but that those statements don't also apply to the entire collective of things

The philosophy for which I am advocating can be called **logical atomism** or **absolute pluralism**, because while it maintains that **there are many things**, it denies that these things come together to compose a whole. Therefore, we will see that in this way, philosophical propositions are not con-

cerned with the whole of things collectively, but rather, they are concerned with **all things distributively**. Furthermore, they must not only be concerned with all things, but they must also be concerned with such properties of all things so as **not** to depend upon the **accidental nature** of things that there happen to be. They must be concerned with the properties of things that are true of any possible world or iteration of the universe, **independent of the facts** that can only be discovered via **sensation**.

Key terms: logical atomism, absolute pluralism

Opinion: author's view is that there are many things but that they are separate; they do not come together to make a whole; author thinks philosophical statements must be general and not depend on facts that can be discovered

This brings us right to the second characteristic of **philosophical propositions: they must be *a priori*.** A philosophical proposition must be of such a nature that it can **neither be proved nor disproved by empirical evidence**. All too often, we find philosophy books filled with arguments based upon the course of history, the convolutions of the brain, the eyes of shellfish, and etc. Special, **accidental facts** of this kind are simply **irrelevant** to philosophy, which ideally only ought to make assertions that would be equally true no matter what specific way the world was actually constituted.

Key terms: *a priori*

Opinion: author thinks philosophical propositions must not depend on experience (which is what *a priori* means)

We can synthesize these two characteristics of philosophical propositions into one statement: philosophy is the science of the possible. Of course, this statement, if unexplained, is liable to be misleading as it may be thought that the **possible** is something other than the **general**. In reality, two are **indistinguishable**.

Opinion: author ends by saying that possible and general mean the same thing

Main Idea: The author sets out to answer the question he poses in the first sentence: if we removed the notion of the universe and good and evil from philosophy, what can a philosopher answer that a scientist cannot? By employing the two characteristics of the philosophical propositions, the author reveals that philosophy of the possible and it seeks to answer general questions about life, not specific ones that a scientist could answer; philosophy must be general and it must not be based upon provable or disprovable facts.

20.   A is correct. As the author writes at the end of the third paragraph, "This does not mean that all things form a whole that can be regarded as another, independent thing that can be made the subject of predicates. Rather, it means that there are properties that belong to each individual, separate thing, not that there are properties belonging to the entirety of things collectively." That whole formed by all things is not an independent thing. It is not a unit.

   B: Rather, there are none.

   C: This may be true, but the author never puts the author up to this a priori test. Rather, it is more likely that the author believes the existence of the universe to be provable.

   D: This is true, but choice A is a more appropriate answer regarding the quote in the question.

21.   C is correct. The term "logical atomism" gets at the many individual things part and the term "absolute pluralism" gets at there being many things but them not coming together to form a whole.

   A: The terms don't serve to make his argument seem more important.

   B: This is not necessarily so, especially if the reader is unfamiliar with these terms.

   D: Of course he has contention with the traditional view, but these terms don't serve to highlight it.

22.   C is correct. As the author sums up his argument in the last paragraph, ". . . philosophy is the science of the possible." It is concerned not only with what is but what could be in any possible reality. On the other hand, science is more concerned with facts. This is the answer to the primary question of the passage: what's the difference between a philosopher and a scientist? It's generalities vs specifics.

   A: This is never said.

   B: Rather, it ought not to ignore them.

   D: As the author writes in the third paragraph, "I maintain that there are general propositions that can be asserted about each individual thing, like the propositions of logic." Logic would then seem to be closer to philosophy than science.

23.   B is correct. The passage sets out to elucidate this contrast and answer the question of what differentiates a philosopher from a scientist. It is generalities vs specifics.

   A: These are indistinguishable.

   C: The author seems to think logic is closely related to philosophy, not contrasted with it.

   D: This contrast is made, but not as thoroughly as the specific vs the general.

24.   A is correct. As we know, the author believes philosophy must be concerned with "the properties of things that are true of any possible world or iteration of the universe."

   B: Choice A is better because it is more broad. That, and to say "that which has happened" implies specifics.

   C: Again, specifics.

   D: Rather, he is concerned with the possible, not the impossible.

25.   C is correct. Reality includes all of the accidental happenings that specifically make up the world. More accurately, the author thinks they must take "truth" into account. Reality is just one iteration of the possible.

   A, B, D: These are true.

26.   C is correct. I is true, given the first sentence of the passage. II is true, also given the first sentence, and the author's insistence that the universe cannot be taken as a whole.

   III: This is not true because, rather, it does not attribute peculiar predicates to the universe.

Passage 5 (Questions 27 – 33)

Political parties ought to have, in addition to their more **distant** goals, more **proximate or short-term aims** that they will carry out in the near future. The **Marxian** socialism of **Germany** suffered for lack of them: though the party was powerful in numbers, it had **no minor aims or measures to demand while waiting for the revolution**, and was therefore politically weak. When finally the movement was seized by those who desired more practical policy, the change that occurred was the wrong kind they yielded to **bad policies such as militarism and imperialism** instead of advocating for partial reforms, which in themselves may have been inadequate, but still would have been steps in the right direction.

Opinion: author thinks political parties need both short term goals and long term ones

Cause and effect: German socialist party lacked strength because it had no achievable short term goals

French syndicalism, as it existed before the war, had a **similar defect. Everything was waiting for the general strike**: the day, after much preparation, when the whole proletariat would rise up as one and refuse to work, causing the property owners to admit defeat and agree to forfeit all of their privileges rather than starve. This is an excellent dramatic conception, but the **love of drama is one of true vision's greatest enemies**. Except under very rare conditions, **men** simply **cannot** be trained to do **some sudden thing that is very different** from what they have done before.

Opinion: French syndicalism also suffered due to lack of achievable short term goals

Cause and effect: love of big dramatic moments is a weakness because you can't get people to do big sudden difficult things

If this **general strike were to succeed**, the **victors** would, despite their penchant for anarchy, be **compelled to form an administration**, to create a police force to stave off looting and destruction of property, to establish a provisional government that would end up issuing dictatorial orders to certain revolutionaries. Because the syndicalists are opposed to all political action, in taking these necessary, practical steps, they would feel as if they had abandoned their raison d'être. Moreover, **they would be without training and practice** due to their previous aversion to politics. Therefore, even after a successful syndicalist revolution, power **would be assumed by people who are not actually syndicalists**.

Cause and effect: the success of a movement whose members hate government would end up failing because, by success they would have to become the government

Here is another **objection** to these sorts of movements: **enthusiasm always wanes** when there is nothing to do or **no partial successes** to enjoy while waiting. The only way a movement can succeed like this is if the motivating sentiment and the program itself are very simple, as in the case

of oppressed nations rebelling. Whereas the line dividing an Englishman and a native of India is very clear, the **line between capitalist and laborer is less so**. Advocates of social revolutions often do not realize **how many people there are whose interests and sympathies genuinely lay half on the side of labor and half on the side of capital**. This obviously would make clear-cut, revolutionary politics quite difficult to manage.

Opinion: author thinks two problems with these socialist movements is people lose interest when there are no short-term goals and that many have sympathies for both the capitalist and the worker

Given all this, those who aim for an economic reconstruction that will likely not happen in the near future must be able to **approach their lofty goal by degrees** if they hope to have any success. They ought to **take small measures** that are useful of themselves, even if they will not directly lead to the end goal. These will help them to train for the policy measures they will inevitably have to carry out if their loftier ambitions come to fruition. Moreover, there must be **possible achievements to reach in the near future**, not just the **hazy vision of utopia** at the end of the tunnel.

Opinion: author reiterates the importance of political movements having small, achievable goals that can be reached in the near term rather than just a vision of the distant future

Though I believe all this to be true, I also believe that **truly vital reform requires a vision that reaches beyond the near future**, a vision of ideal humanity. Without such lofty hope, the people will lack the energy and enthusiasm necessary to trudge onwards against popular opinion and against physical opposition. Any person who **truly wants to change the world** for the better will **face ridicule, persecution**, cajolery, and potential corruption. If anyone is to make it through these ordeals (and truly it is rare that they do), the ultimate goal must be vivid and alive in their minds.

Contrast: despite everything said previously about short term goals the author thinks long term visionary goals are also essential to the success of anyone attempting to really change the world

Main Idea: The author's primary point here is that political parties will not be successful if they only have long-term goals: they must also have shorter-term goals to help them along the way, to keep morale high, and to train the people for how to function after the anticipated revolutions; he also notes that no movement can succeed without strong vision.

27. B is correct. In the second sentence of the fourth paragraph, the author writes, "The only way a movement can succeed like this is if the motivating sentiment and the program itself are very simple, as in the case of oppressed nations rebelling." In choice B, the word "program" has been substituted for "execution."

    A: This is not said.

    C: Without partial reforms and small successes along the way, it will flounder.

    D: Capitalist and laborer are social classes, and yet the division between them does not make the revolution simple.

28. C is correct. As the author writes in the first paragraph, "When finally the movement was seized by those who desired more practical policy, the change that occurred was the wrong kind: they yielded to bad policies such as militarism and imperialism instead of advocating for partial reforms, which in themselves may have been inadequate, but still would have been steps in the right direction." Basically, they went too far: they over-corrected the previous lack of practical policy.

    A: It is never said that they lost the enthusiasm of the people. In fact, the opposite may be true.

    B: This is never said in the passage.

    D: This is not said. It can be inferred that the brands of imperialism and militarism they brought with them were new to the country.

29. A is correct. It sums up the point of the passage: that any successful political movement must have a long-term goal that is solidly envisioned and motivating, and moderate short-term goals which keep the people in practice and keep morale high.

    B: The long-term goal must be strong and short-term goals not zealous.

    C: Again, short-term goals should not be zealous.

    D: A zealously envisioned long-term goal is probably good, but weak short-term goals will not be enough to keep up morale and keep the people in practice.

30. B is correct. At the end of the second paragraph, which is devoted to the example of French syndicalism, the author writes, "Except under very rare conditions, men simply cannot be trained to do some sudden thing that is very different from what they have done before." The first paragraph's aim was to show how a movement without short-term goals could be politically weak. The second seeks to show another facet of the central problem, that being this problem of training to do some sudden thing that one has never done before.

    A: This argument is not central to the second paragraph.

    C: He is perhaps doing this, but the primary point here is to reach that last sentence, which is another problem with political movements with only long-term goals.

    D: This could be argued as true, but is not as strong an answer. There is no sense that the author needs to prove the point made in the first paragraph again.

31. B is correct. This is a partial reform, which in itself is inadequate, but which represents a step in the right direction, as the author writes short-term policies must be.

    A: This neglects the important short-term goals.

    C: Likewise. Moreover, it reflects the militarism that developed in the German socialism movement, which the author believed to be problematic.

    D: Rather, members of a political party seeking a big change in the future can expect to face these obstacles, as the author writes in the last paragraph.

32. C is correct. Rather, this may be the only thing that such a party really has, as that long-term goal will lend a strong sense of purpose.

    A, B, D: These are true and all discussed explicitly in the passage.

33. B is correct. As the movement was opposed to all political action, its members would have to give up their motivating drive in order to successfully establish rule of law. Because of this, the movement was doomed, and even if it could succeed, a non-syndicalist would of necessity have to run the show.

    III: Even if the general strike did succeed, the two other problems would keep the movement from being successful.

Passage 6 (Questions 34 – 40)

Referring to some **newspaper** reports which he knew to be **without foundation**, **Bismarck** once said, "Newspapers are simply a union of printer's ink and paper." Omitting the implied slur we might say the same of printed music and printed criticism; therefore, in considering printed music we must, first of all, remember that it is the **letter of the law which kills**. We must look deeper, and be able to translate sounds back into the emotions which caused them. There is no right or wrong way to give utterance to music. **There is but one way**, namely, through **the living, vital expression** of the content of the music; all else is not music but mere pleasure for the ear, a thing of the senses. For the time being we must see through the composer's eyes and hear through his ears. In other words, we must think in his language. The **process of creating** music is often, to a great extent, **beyond the control of the composer**, just as is the case with the novelist and his characters. The language through which musical thought is expressed, however, is a different thing, and it is this process of **developing musical speech** until it has become capable of saying for us that which, in our spoken language, must ever remain unsaid, that **I shall try to make clear** in our consideration of form in music.

Key terms: printed music, Bismarck

Contrast: performance of music vs intent of composer; language of musical thought vs spoken language

Cause and effect: printed music does not necessarily convey emotion, but the language of music has become clearer and better at expressing emotion

Until the **very end of the fifteenth century**, music, so far as we know, had **no language of its own**, that is to say, it was not recognized as a **medium** for expressing **thought or emotion**. Josquin des **Prés** (born at Conde in the north of France in 1450, died 1521) was the first to attempt the expression of thought in sound. **Luther**, in rebelling against Rome, also overturned the music of the church in Germany. He **incorporated many folk songs** into the music of the Protestant church and discarded the old Gregorian chant (which was vague in rhythm, or, rather, wholly without rhythm), calling it asinine braying.

Key terms: fifteenth century, Prés, Luther

Contrast: music before and after fifteenth century; music before and after Luther

Cause and effect: When Luther rebelled against Rome, he changed how music functioned

While **Luther** was **paving the way for Bach** by encouraging church music to be something more than merely the singing of certain melodies according to prescribed rules, in Italy (at the time of his death in 1546) the **Council of Trent** was already trying to decide upon a style of **music proper for the church**. The matter was definitely settled in 1562 or 1563 by the adoption of **Palestrina's** style. Thus, while in **Germany**

ecclesiastical music was being broadened and an opening offered for the development of the dramatic and emotional side of music, in **Italy**, on the contrary, the **emotional style of music** was being **neglected** and an absolutely serene style of what may be called "impersonal" music encouraged. Italy, however, **soon** had **opera** on which to fall back, and thus music in both countries developed rapidly, although on different lines.

Key terms: Bach, Council of Trent, Palestrina, Germany, Italy

Contrast: dramatic and emotional style of German music vs impersonal style of Italian music

Cause and effect: Luther's reformations led to dramatic and emotional music, Palestrina's to impersonal, serene music; the development of opera led to greater development of music in Italy

Now this new art was first particularly evident in the dances of these different peoples. These **dances gave the music form**, and held it down to certain **prescribed rhythms** and duration. **Little by little the emotions**, the natural expression of which is music, could no longer be restricted to these dance forms and rhythms; and gradually the latter were modified by each daring innovator in turn. The modifications of dance forms **led up to our sonata**, symphony, and symphonic poem, as I hope to show. **Opera was a thing apart**, and, being untrammelled either by dance rhythms or church laws, **developed gradually and normally**.

Key terms: form

Contrast: opera vs dance rhythms or church laws

Cause and effect: dance gave music form, but the emotions of music modified set forms and led to new forms of music.

Main Idea: The author traces the development of music, arguing that when it began to be understood as a medium for thought and emotion in the early 16th century, it developed a language of its own; the author suggests that changes in the church and the development of dance forms and opera all contributed to the development of music in different parts of Europe.

34. A is correct. The passage discusses the development of music in Italy in the third paragraph, It states that due to "the adoption of Palestrina's style … in Italy… the emotional style of music was being neglected and an absolutely serene style of what may be called "impersonal" music encouraged. Italy, however, soon had opera on which to fall back, and thus music in both countries developed rapidly, although on different lines." This implies that Palestrina's style was a detriment to the development of music in Italy.

    B: The Council of Trent is noted as trying to create standards in church music, but not directly linked to Italy's music.

    C: Luther's influence is discussed in terms of Germany.

    D: Opera caused music in Italy to develop, not falter.

35. B is correct. According to the passage, "Luther, in rebelling against Rome, also overturned the music of the church in Germany. He incorporated many folk songs into the music of the Protestant church" and "pav[ed] the way for Bach by encouraging church music to be something more than merely the singing of certain melodies according to prescribed rules".

    A: While the passage does discuss Luther's dismissal of non-rhythmic music, it does not say he focused wholly on rhythm.

    C, D: There is no discussion of unappreciated forms or the power of Rome in the passage.

36. A is correct. In the passage, the author argues that the language of music developed as a medium for thought and emotion.

    B, C: The passage discusses music's language in general, not just in opera or dance.

    C: The ability to transcend boundaries is not discussed in the passage.

37. D is correct. After introducing the quotation from Bismarck, the author states "we might say the same of printed music and printed criticism; therefore, in considering printed music we must, first of all, remember that it is the letter of the law which kills. We must look deeper, and be able to translate sounds back into the emotions which caused them." In arguing that the emotions can be overshadowed by the letter of the law, he is contrasting the emotional content to the written form.

38. A is correct. In the passage, the author states that "there is no right or wrong way to give utterance to music. There is but one way, namely, through the living, vital expression of the content of the music; all else is not music but mere pleasure for the ear, a thing of the senses. For the time being we must see through the composer's eyes and hear through his ears." Thus the passage argues for accuracy to the composer's intentions.

    B: The passage argues there is only "one way" to "give utterance to music," thus arguing against interpretation of musical works.

    C: The author does not discuss the modern world.

    D: The passage does not try to differ between utterance and intention.

39. A is correct. In the third paragraph, the passage states that around the 1560s, "while in Germany ecclesiastical music was being broadened and an opening offered for the development of the dramatic and emotional side of music, in Italy, on the contrary, the emotional style of music was being neglected and an absolutely serene style of what may be called "impersonal" music encouraged." "Vivid colors and intense interactions" would be in line with "dramatic and emotional music," while "soft colors and nondescript images" can be associated with "serene" and "impersonal" music.

    B, D: The passage does not emphasize gender, age, or rule following.

    C: This choice gets the relationship backwards. Since German music was "dramatic and emotional," it would not be compared to an "orderly and restrained" performance.

40. D is correct. Statement I is correct because the passage states that "opera was a thing apart, and, being untrammelled either by dance rhythms or church laws, developed gradually and normally." This suggests it developed independently of many musical forms. Statement III is correct because it is stated that "Italy, however, soon had opera on which to fall back, and thus music in both countries developed rapidly, although on different lines".

    II: We are told opera developed independently of dance rhythms, but not that it was defined by any rules.

Passage 7 (Questions 41 – 45)

Consumers' needs and demands are **constantly evolving**, so companies have begun to **focus on reaching the most influential consumers** in the market. Recent research suggests that market influencers are growing in importance primarily due to the proliferation of product choice in today's marketplace, and an associated growing need among consumers for help in dealing with more choices. The concepts of **mavenism** and **opinion leadership** underscore that these individuals are an indispensable target market as they spread the word about multiple product categories and new product introductions. An understanding of these innovative consumers is a crucial issue for marketers to develop more effective strategies.

Key terms: market influencers, mavenism, opinion leadership

Opinions: author thinks marketers need to understand innovative consumers to have effective marketing strategies

With their general **marketplace expertise and communication skills**, influential consumers are the persons that can start **word-of-mouth epidemics**. The new ideas that are propagated by these consumers are communicated to connectors who know a large group of people, most of them outside the community of the mavens. It should also be highlighted that the **message** that is transmitted by influential consumers tends to have a **stickiness** factor that is memorable and appealing for the masses. As such, the quality of both the **messengers**, as well as the **content** of the message, matters upon spreading the information.

Cause and effect: some factors that make mavens effective in influencing other consumers

Rogers (1995) studied how innovation occurs, arguing that innovation consists of four stages, which are invention, diffusion, time, and consequences. **Diffusion** is the process by which an **innovation is communicated** through certain channels over a period of time among the members of a social system. The diffusion of innovations model demonstrates that, which the media diffuse most new ideas, audiences **heavily rely on the recommendations** and opinions that (originally) come from **opinion leaders or mavens** to decide if they adopt the innovation. Once the innovators and early adopters have the time to test the new product, the popularity of that innovation will grow rapidly as consumers start to communicate and are influenced by their word-of-mouth more substantially.

Key terms: Rogers, innovation stages

Cause and effect: the mavens, opinion leaders, and early adopters decide if they like the innovation and their opinion then spreads and influences consumers through word of mouth

Consumer innovativeness has been defined as the tendency for consumers to have extensive **technical knowledge** and

willingness to understand technological innovations in the market (Saaksjarvi, 2003). This means that innovators adopt innovations quickly compared to other members of the social system (Rogers, 2003). Like early adopters, opinion leaders are an **attractive target for marketers** as they are capable of influencing other consumers not just at the moment of the purchase decision, but earlier in the consumer buying process. But **opinion leaders' primary goal** is to **deliberately influence other consumers** (and their purchase behavior), which **sets them apart from innovators**.

Key terms: consumer innovativeness, opinion leaders, early adopters

Contrast: innovators adopt innovations more quickly; innovators' primary goal is different from that of opinion leaders who deliberately seek to influence consumers' decisions.

Although **market mavens** have similar demographic characteristics as opinion leaders and early adopters/innovators, they differ from the opinion leaders and early adopters/purchasers on the **higher levels of general knowledge about the marketplace** and product marketing mix characteristics. This trait makes mavens an attractive target market and change agent for retailers and other large industries that produce and/or sell a wide range of durable and fast-moving consumer goods (FMCG). This contrasts sharply with the **opinion leaders and early adopters** who are more knowledgeable and want to share information about a **specific** range of **products** within a product category, or specific market environment characteristics.

Contrast: mavens have higher levels of general knowledge about the marketplace than early adopters, who know more about a specific range of products

Market mavens are "**smart shoppers**" They demonstrate **very high levels of value consciousness** by utilizing coupons, grocery lists, advanced budgeting tactics, together with planning their purchases using advertising (Chelminski & Coulter, 2007). Relatedly, market mavens are thought to be an important segment of consumers owing to the disproportionate influence they have on other consumers via word-of mouth (Wangenheim, 2005), viral marketing (Goldsmith et al., 2003) and coupon distribution (Goodey & East, 2008). These consumers are a **vital promotional agent** for small businesses relying on word-of-mouth, rather than large advertising budgets.

Key terms: value consciousness

Contrast: mavens also differ from others in their demonstration of a high level of value consciousness

Main Idea: The passage discusses how word of mouth marketing is strongly affected by market mavens, consumer innovators, early adopters, and opinion leaders; the passage also discusses some differences between mavens (broad market knowledge and value-conscious), opinion leaders (goal of influencing others), and others.

41. A is correct. Consumer innovators tend to have extensive technical knowledge and are most likely to adopt innovations quickly compared to other members of the social system. The high level of technical knowledge suggests that these consumers are interested in the technology for the sake of the technology and because they like to be on the cutting edge of new innovations.

     B, D: Nowhere is it indicated that consumer innovators are aware of or care about what other consumers think about them.

     C: The author indicates that opinion leaders' primary goal is influence.

42. C is correct. This accounts for the communication that occurs between influential consumers and other consumers (WOM) and is also realistic about the reach of media messages to all consumers.

     A, D: These do not account for communication between consumers, which is a required aspect of market mavenism.

     B: Although some media messages may be distilled to opinion seekers through opinion leaders, this theory makes the assumption that the opinion seekers have very little contact with the media. It would be a naïve communication theory to assume that consumers have very little contact with the media, even if they are opinion seekers, and that their only source of information would be opinion leaders.

43. B is correct. Nothing in the passage suggests that targeting only one group of influential consumers is most cost-effective for advertisers. The article suggests that marketing budgets, the type of goods sold, etc. are factors that would determine which type of influential consumer would be the most influential for a company/product.

     A: This is a potential implication for marketing practice. The article says an understanding of these innovative consumers is a crucial issue for marketers to develop more effective strategies. Those strategies could include working with influential consumers as co-producers.

     C: This is a potential implication for marketing practice. Marketers with large marketing budgets may gain from word of mouth, viral marketing and coupon distribution, but they are less likely to depend on these avenues as their primary methods of marketing. So, a marketer with a smaller budget would likely have the most to gain from influential consumer groups.

     D: This is a potential implication for marketing theory.

44. C is correct. Value consciousness, in this context, means that the market maven is interested in getting a good deal, by using promotions, coupons, etc. The passage has contrasted the type of knowledge consumer innovators have (specific/technical) with the type of knowledge market mavens have (general/non-technical). The correct choice is choice C because the market maven will likely read both direct mail advertisements (I) and retail magazines (III) because they are most like to be include promotional information and to include more general information about the products.

     II: It is less unlikely that market mavens would read trade journals as trade journals tend to be more specific, in depth, and technical, and are less likely to include information about promotions.

45. D is correct. The author likens the spread of word of mouth to the spread of an epidemic. A meme spreads when one person posts it to an internet site, others see the meme and then repost the original or their own derivations of the meme to other sites. People tell or show others the meme, increasing its spread until it has "gone viral."

     A, C: These choices are not the correct choice because they cannot be transmitted from person to person, so they cannot spread like an epidemic or like word of mouth.

     B: Although idioms may be spread from person to person, they are more widely known and established within a culture. They don't tend to "flare up" or catch on and spread quickly and widely.

Passage 8 (Questions 46 – 49)

That **all our knowledge begins with experience** there can be no doubt. For how is it possible that the faculty of cognition should be awakened into exercise otherwise than by means of **objects which affect our senses**, and partly of themselves produce representations, partly **rouse our powers of understanding into activity**, to compare to connect, or to separate these, and so to convert the raw material of our sensuous impressions into a knowledge of objects, which is called experience? In respect of time, therefore, **no knowledge of ours is antecedent to experience, but begins with it.**

Opinion: the author believes that all knowledge begins with experience

Cause and effect: the experience of objects awakens the faculty of our cognition

But, though all our knowledge begins with experience, it by **no** means follows that **all arises out of experience**. For, on the contrary, it is quite possible that our **empirical knowledge** is a compound of that which we **receive** through **impressions**, and that which the faculty of **cognition** supplies from **itself** (sensuous impressions giving merely the occasion), an addition which we cannot distinguish from the original element given by sense, till long practice has made us attentive to, and skillful in separating it. It is, therefore, a question which requires close investigation, and not to be answered at first sight, whether there exists a **knowledge altogether independent of experience**, and even of all sensuous impressions? Knowledge of this kind is called **a priori**, in contradistinction to **empirical knowledge**, which has its sources **a posteriori**, that is, in experience.

Key terms: empirical knowledge, a priori, a posteriori

Opinion: the author believes that although all knowledge begins with experience, it is possible that there are aspects of knowledge that are derived completely independently of it

Contrast: a priori knowledge which is independent of experience vs a posteriori empirical knowledge which is based on experience

But the expression, "a priori," is not as yet definite enough adequately to indicate the whole meaning of the question above started. For, in speaking of knowledge which has its sources in experience, we are wont to say, that this or that may be known a priori, because we do not derive this knowledge immediately from experience, but from a general rule, which, however, we have itself borrowed from experience. Thus, if a man undermined his house, we say, "he might know a priori that it would have fallen"; that is, he needed not to have waited for the experience that it did actually fall. But still, a priori, he could not know even this much. For, that bodies are heavy, and, consequently, that they fall when their supports are taken away, must have been known to him previously, by means of experience. By the term **"knowledge a priori"**, therefore, we shall in the sequel understand, not such as is **independent** of this or that kind of experience,

but such as is **absolutely so of all experience**. Opposed to this is empirical knowledge, or that which is possible only a posteriori, that is, through experience. Knowledge a priori is either pure or impure. **Pure knowledge a priori** is that with which **no empirical element is mixed up**. For example, the proposition, **"Every change has a cause"**, is a proposition a priori, but **impure**, because **change** is a conception which can only be **derived from experience**.

Contrast: the author establishes the contrast between impure a priori knowledge, which is still rooted in experience, and pure a priori knowledge, which he defines to be independent of any experience

Cause and effect: seemingly a priori knowledge, such as a prediction that an event will occur, can actually be rooted in experience, and therefore defined by the author to be impure

The question now is as to a **criterion**, by which we may securely distinguish a **pure from an empirical cognition**. Experience no doubt teaches us that this or that object is constituted in such and such a manner, but not that it could not possibly exist otherwise. Now, in the first place, if we have a **proposition which contains the idea of necessity in its very conception**, it is a if, moreover, it is not derived from any other proposition, unless from one equally involving the idea of necessity, it is absolutely a priori. Secondly, an **empirical judgment never exhibits strict and absolute**, but only assumed and comparative universality (by induction); therefore, the most we can say is—so far as we have hitherto observed, there is no exception to this or that rule. If, on the other hand, a judgment carries with it **strict and absolute universality**, that is, admits of no possible exception, it is not derived from experience, but **is valid absolutely a priori**.

Opinion: the author argues that empirical knowledge is never absolute, because we can only assume universality by induction. (i.e. we have never observed it to be otherwise, therefore this must be universal); a priori knowledge, on the other hand, the author argues, is absolutely universal and independent of experience

Cause and effect: empirical judgment is derived from only from experience, and therefore cannot be judged to be absolutely universal

Main Idea: Empirical knowledge begins with experience, however it is possible for a priori knowledge (knowledge completely independent of empirical observation) to exist, and such a priori knowledge must be considered universal, whereas empirical observations can never be similarly absolute.

46. C is correct. According to the author, impure a priori knowledge is defined as knowledge that seemingly precedes the actual experience, but in fact is based on knowledge derived from previous experiences. Choices A, B, and D are all examples of such knowledge, where an individual has knowledge that precedes the occurrence of an event (the results of an election, traffic down the road, or the sinking of an object), however that prediction could have only been acquired through prior experience with similar instances. Choice C, however, indicates an experience where no knowledge has preceded the event, and therefore it is not an example of a priori knowledge, impure or otherwise.

47. A is correct. The author argues that all knowledge begins with experience, and furthermore that the majority of seemingly a priori knowledge is actually impure, or rooted in experience as well. Therefore while he is arguing that pure a priori knowledge can exist, he also acknowledges that the vast majority of our knowledge is derived from empirical observation.

    B, D: The author argues that pure a priori knowledge is universal and absolute in comparison to knowledge derived from experience (which can never be proved to be universal), however he never claims that one is superior or more fundamental than the other.

    C: The author argues that not all knowledge is derived from empirical observation, however he never claims that scientific knowledge is inadequate.

48. D is correct. In the third paragraph the author states "For example, the proposition, 'Every change has a cause,' is a proposition a priori, but impure, because change is a conception which can only be derived from experience."

    A: The author uses the example to indicate how seemingly a priori knowledge is actually based in experience, and therefore is not derived independently of it.

    B: The author is not countering an earlier argument made in the passage, but clarifying how certainly knowledge can seem to be a priori when it is really not.

    C: The main idea of the passage is that it is possible to separate certain types of knowledge from empirical observation.

49. B is correct. I: This would support the argument made by the author. The understanding of the consistency of the laws of nature is an assumption necessary for empirical observation, but no single experience could inform us of that knowledge. The assumption must therefore be based on an a priori understanding.

    II: This also supports the arguments of the author, and is actually a key point made later in the author's essay. If an underlying understanding is necessary to obtain experiential information from an object, it would indicate that such learning requires an a priori knowledge base.

    III: This neither supports nor challenges the author's argument. While brain activity in the absence of stimulus could be interpreted to be thoughts in the absence of experience, that connection is not clear or simple by and extent.

Passage 9 (Questions 50 – 53)

That the **end of life should be death may sound sad** yet what other end can anything have? The end of an evening party is to go to bed; but its use is to gather congenial people together, that they may pass the time pleasantly. An **invitation to the dance is not rendered ironical because the dance cannot last for ever**; the youngest of us and the most vigorously wound up, after a few hours, has had enough of sinuous stepping and prancing. The **transitoriness of things is essential to their physical being**, and not at all sad in itself; it becomes sad by virtue of a sentimental illusion, which makes us imagine that they wish to endure, and that their end is always untimely; but in a healthy nature it is not so. **What is truly sad is to have some impulse frustrated in the midst of its career**, and robbed of its chosen object; and what is painful is to have an organ lacerated or destroyed when it is still vigorous, and not ready for its natural sleep and dissolution. **We must not confuse the itch which our unsatisfied instincts continue to cause with the pleasure of satisfying and dismissing each of them in turn**. Could they all be satisfied harmoniously we should be satisfied once for all and completely. Then doing and dying would coincide throughout and be a perfect pleasure.

Opinion: death and endings are essential parts of life

Contrast: natural endings are not sad, but interrupted efforts are

This same insight is contained in another **wise myth** which has inspired morality and religion in India from time immemorial: I mean the doctrine of **Karma**. We are born, it says, with a heritage, a character imposed, and a long task assigned, all due to the ignorance which in our past lives has led us into all sorts of commitments. These obligations we must pay off, relieving the pure spirit within us from its accumulated burdens, from debts and assets both equally oppressive. We cannot disentangle ourselves by mere frivolity, nor by suicide: frivolity would only involve us more deeply in the toils of fate, and suicide would but truncate our misery and leave us for ever a confessed failure. When life is understood to be a **process of redemption**, its **various phases are taken up in turn** without haste and without undue attachment; their coming and going have all the keenness of pleasure, the holiness of sacrifice, and the beauty of art. The point is to have **expressed and discharged all that was latent in us**; and to this perfect relief various temperaments and various traditions assign different names, calling it having one's day, or doing one's duty, or realizing one's ideal, or saving one's soul. The task in any case is definite and imposed on us by nature, whether we recognize it or not; therefore we can make true moral progress or fall into real errors. Wisdom and genius lie in discerning this prescribed task and in doing it readily, cleanly, and without distraction. Folly on the contrary imagines that any scent is worth following, that we have an infinite nature, or no nature in particular, that life begins without obligations and can do business without capital, and that the will is vacuously

free, instead of being a specific burden and a tight hereditary knot to be unraveled.

Key terms: Karma, obligations, process of redemption, folly

Opinion: the doctrine of Karma says we are born into a heritage which we must understand and accept

Cause and effect: not recognizing our obligations – thinking we have none, or that life means utter freedom – is folly

Some philosophers without self-knowledge think that the variations and further entanglements which the future may bring are the manifestation of spirit; but they are, as Freud has indicated, imposed on living beings by external pressure, and take shape in the realm of matter. Deep and dark as a soul may be when you look down into it from outside, it is something perfectly natural; and the same **understanding that can unearth our suppressed young passions, and dispel our stubborn bad habits, can show us where our true good lies**. Nature has **marked** out the path for us **beforehand**; there are snares in it, but also primroses, and it leads to peace.

Key terms: philosophers, true good, peace

Opinion: those philosophers who think future events are the manifestation of spirit are mistaken

Cause and effect: understanding and following one's true path leads to peace

Main Idea: Everything has a determined path; we need to accept this and follow that path, understanding that the end of the path, death, is not inherently sad.

50.   B is correct. Think of the example in paragraph 1 as a more accessible way of saying that everything has its end, that things happen the way they happen. If we accept that the party will end, we'll be happy. Similarly, in paragraph 2, Karma is described as accepting that we are born into a path, and happiness lies in recognizing this and living that out. Choice B captures the similarity between the two.

51.   D is correct. The author of the passage believes that our lives have some predetermined path; a proponent of free will would disagree with this, so choice D is correct.

   A: No – proponents of free will believe that we choose our action, not that we're born into a destiny.

   B: We have no idea whether or not the proponent of free will believes transitoriness is sad, or not.

   C: We are told the free will believers believe in self-determination, but we don't know whether or not they believe everything inevitably must end.

52.   A is correct. While karma does give us a burden that needs to be processed and released (like in choice C. and we are, of course, transitory (as in choice D., ultimately our goal is to find and follow the path that fate and our karma have laid out for us.

   B: The author would find this to be folly – "any scent is worth following" is foolish according to the author.

53.   C is correct. What is "folly" is described at the end of paragraph 2, where the author says that following any scent (or whim) (choice A), thinking life begins without obligations (choice B), and assuming we have an infinite nature (choice D) all are folly, or foolishness. That leaves choice C as the correct answer.

SECTION 10

53 Questions, 90 Minutes

Use an answer grid from the back of the book to record your answers

Passage 1 (Questions 1 – 6)

In a typical year, nearly 1,100,000 people devote part or all of their working time to provide medical care for the people of the United States and earn their livelihood thereby. The total number is about equally divided between those who serve for fees from individuals or families, and those who are engaged by medical institutions such as hospitals, public health agencies, or clinics. There are 550,000 independent practitioners, of whom 121,000 are physicians; 57,000 are dentists; approximately 118,000 are graduate nurses and 150,000 are practical nurses; secondary or sectarian healers, midwives, chiropodists, optometrists, osteopaths, chiropractors, naturopaths or similar groups, and faith healers are approximately 110,000 in number. The institutions of the United States – hospitals clinics, public health agencies, and drug stores – employ approximately 530,000 physicians, dentists, nurses, pharmacists, social service workers, medical technicians, and lay employees.

Medical care is an esoteric economic commodity concerning which the buyer has no basis for critical judgment of quality or value. The patient does not know whether he should purchase a particular type of medical service and is frequently unable to determine whether or not the medical service has been satisfactory after its receipt. The physician, therefore, is judge both of the patient's need for the service which he has to offer, as well as of the time and conditions under which it shall be purchased. Moreover, inasmuch as medical care involves life or death (or at least the risk of death), the patient frequently believes that only one individual practitioner holds the commodity which he needs. It therefore seems impossible to search for another purveyor of medical service, as he would do if the forces of economic supply and demand operated in medicine as in the majority of business transactions. The conditions surrounding the delivery of medical care are therefore unique and are unlike those which characterize ordinary economic phenomena, because there is but one buyer and one seller and because the commodity itself is of priceless value if received.

Traditionally and inherently medical care is a personal service rendered by a professional person to an ailing or to a potential patient. Economic efficiency cannot change medical care in this respect. The patient is ultimately and inevitably the personal recipient of medical service, and he derives benefit from the medical service in proportion to the degree to which his particular medical needs are met. Just as medical service has been regarded as a personal affair, the payment for medical service has also been considered a personal obligation. Community responsibility has been accepted only in those cases where the nature of the illness involves danger to other persons or requires isolation, or where it entails long periods of treatment which cannot ordinarily be financed by the individual or his family, or where a patient is an avowed indigent and is unable to pay for medical care from his own resources. The personal nature of medical service has been the cornerstone for the evolution of present-day medicine. Each patient has exercised his right to engage a practitioner who suited his real or supposed needs, without regard to the wishes of other members of the community or the profession. Increasingly, however, this scheme of things has developed incongruities. Especially for economic reasons, the advancing perfection of medical science and art have carried medical care out of the reach of millions of families. Their voices raised in protest have made imperative an understanding of the problems and a search for practical solutions. During many centuries the economic structure within which the system of medical service has operated has reflected the views of the times. Society has been changing rapidly in the last few decades; but adjustments between the need for medical care and its effective provision have not kept pace. The newer architecture of society calls for changes in the temple of Aesculapius.

1. Based on the passage, it can be inferred that the author believes:

   A. medical professionals have worked to adjust to changing societal demands, but more is needed.

   B. the medical profession is well prepared to adjust to changing economic demands.

   C. that the esoteric nature of medicine places too much control in the hands of physicians.

   D. the economic nature of healthcare is inconsistent with normal conditions of supply and demand.

2. According to the passage, which of the following proposed changes would be most closely aligned with the author's viewpoint?

   A. Healthcare reform that distributes the responsibility for the cost of care at the state or national level.

   B. Healthcare reform that carefully sets nationwide standards for the cost of medical care.

   C. Healthcare reform that enables patients to easily switch between physicians based on the cost of medical care.

   D. Healthcare reform that assigns medical professionals to focus on community based care, rather than individual care.

3. Which of the following examples of issues within health care is NOT discussed by the author?

   A. A novel cancer treatment is discovered, but it is too expensive for low income patients to afford.

   B. A patient is aware that the treatment she has received is inadequate but is unable to seek an effective second opinion.

   C. A patient is set on seeking medical care from a specific provider regardless of potentially cheaper options.

   D. A patient agrees to pay for an expensive procedure, without an understanding of the actual cost of the treatment.

4. The statistics in the first paragraph of the passage function to:

   A. establish the complexity and size of the medical profession.

   B. give context to arguments made at the end of the first paragraph.

   C. emphasize the relatively small percentage of the medical profession accounted for by physicians.

   D. emphasize the economic inefficiency of the current medical profession.

5. In response to changing societal factors, which of the following statements are consistent with the author's belief?

   I. Healthcare must move away from individual-centered care.

   II. Healthcare must shift focus to fully educating patients on the care they receive.

   III. Healthcare economics must shift in order to cover the rising costs of advancing medical technology.

   A. II only

   B. III only

   C. I and III only

   D. II and III only

6. Which of the following, if true, would most strengthen one of the author's arguments?

   A. A study indicates that patients do not want to be informed of the cost of the procedure prior to making decisions.

   B. A study indicates that a decreasing number of families have access to the most advanced medical care due to rising costs.

   C. A study indicates that even with access to the costs of competing health services, patients tend to remain with their physicians.

   D. A study indicates that health care reform has created a market more closely driven by supply and demand.

Passage 2 (Questions 7 – 11)

Although the theatrical ballet dance is comparatively modern, the elements of its formation are of the greatest antiquity; the chorus of dancers and the performances of the men in the Egyptian chapters represent without much doubt public dancing performances. We get singing, dancing, mimicry and pantomime in the early stages of Greek art, and the development of the dance rhythm in music is equally ancient.

The Alexandrine Pantomime, introduced into Rome about 30 B.C. by Bathillus and Pylades, appears to have been an entertainment approaching the ballet. In Italy there appears to have been a kind of ballet in the 14th century, and from Italy, under the influence of Catharine de Medici, came the ballet. Balthasar di Beaujoyeulx produced the first recorded ballet in France, in the Italian style, in 1582. This was, however, essentially a Court ballet.

The theatre ballet apparently arose out of these Court ballets. Henry III and Henry IV, the latter especially, were very fond of these entertainments, and many Italians were brought to France to assist in them. Pompeo Diabono, a Savoyard, was brought to Paris in 1554 to regulate the Court ballets. At a later date came Rinuccini, the poet, a Florentine, as was probably Caccini, the musician. They had composed and produced the little operetta of "Daphne," which had been performed in Florence in 1597. Under these last-mentioned masters the ballet in France took somewhat of its present form. This passion for Court ballets continued under Louis XIII and Louis XIV.

Louis XIII as a youth danced in one of the ballets at St. Germain, it is said at the desire of Richelieu, who was an expert in spectacle. It appears that he was encouraged in these amusements to remedy fits of melancholy. Louis XIV, at seven, danced in a masquerade, and afterwards not only danced in the ballet of "Cassandra," in 1651, but did all he could to raise the condition of the dance and encourage dancing and music. His influence, combined with that of Cardinal Richelieu, raised the ballet from gross and trivial styles to a dignity worthy of music, poetry and dancing. His uncle, Gaston of Orleans, still patronized the grosser style, but it became eclipsed by the better. Lulli composed music to the words of Molière and other celebrities; amongst notable works then produced was the "Andromeda" of Corneille, a tragedy, with hymns and dances, executed in 1650, at the Petit Bourbon.

The foundation of the theatrical ballet was, however, at the instigation of Cardinal Mazarin, to prevent a lowering of tone in the establishment of the Académie de Danse under thirteen Academicians in 1661. This appears to have been merged into the Académie Royale de Musique et de Danse in 1669, which provided a proper training for débutants, under MM. Perrin and Cambert, whilst Beauchamp, the master of the Court ballets, had charge of the dancing. The first opera-ballet, the "Pomona" of Perrin and Cambert, was produced in 1671. To this succeeded many works of Lulli, to whom is attributed the increased speed in dance music and dancing, that of the Court ballets having been slow and stately.

The great production of the period appears to have been the "Triumph of Love" in 1681, with twenty scenes and seven hundred performers; amongst these were many of the nobility, and some excellent ballerine, such as Pesaut, Carré, Leclerc, and Lafontaine.

7. According to the passage, which of the following is NOT a similarity between Louis XIII and Louis XIV?

   A. They were both interested in ballet.

   B. They both performed dancing at a young age.

   C. They were both influenced by Richelieu.

   D. They both danced in ballets.

8. Based on the information in the passage, which of the following is the most reasonable assumption?

   A. Louis XIV preceded Louis XIII as king.

   B. Cardinal Richelieu was the mentor of cardinal Mazarin.

   C. Gaston of Orleans was a friend of Molière.

   D. the Italians were masters of ballet through the end of the 17th century.

9. According to the author, which of the following is most likely to be regarded as a ballet most similar to the modern style?

   A. Andromeda

   B. Alexandrine Pantomime

   C. Daphne

   D. Pomona

10. Suppose it was discovered that there were more French ballet producers than Italian in the year 1550, would this support the ideas expressed in the passage?

    A. Yes, the author states that the development of theatrical ballet took place in France.

    B. Yes, the author states that the French monarchs were important patrons of ballet and cultivated its production in France.

    C. No, the author states that Italians were brought into France during that time period to produce ballets for the French monarchs.

    D. No, the author states that ballet was developed in Italy and that only the Italians were capable of producing respectable ballets in the 16th century.

11. Which of the following is most plausible?

    A. Lulli wrote Andromeda and Triumph of Love.

    B. Perrin and Cambert wrote Andromeda.

    C. Perrin and Cambert wrote during the time of Louis XIII.

    D. Pompeo Diabono wrote ballets for both Louis XIII and Louis XIV.

Passage 3 (Questions 12 – 18)

For the groundwork of their philosophy, people generally take either too much from a few topics or too little from many. In either case, their philosophy is founded on too narrow a basis and decides upon things with insufficient grounds. The theoretic philosopher observes a few common happenings by experiment, without examining them or reducing them to certainty. For the rest, he relies upon meditation and his wit. Other philosophers have very diligently and precisely attended to a few experiments, and from these have presumed to deduce and invent entire systems of philosophy, bringing all things into conformity with them. A third type, driven by faith and religious reverence, introduces theology and tradition: some of them have gone so far as to derive the sciences from spirits. These are three species of false philosophy: the sophistic, empiric, and superstitious.

The best example of the first type is Aristotle, for he corrupted natural philosophy with logic. He made the world into categories and assigned to the human soul, which he considered to be the noblest of substances, a nature determined by words of secondary operation. He asserted that all bodies had a specific and proper motion, and that if they shared in any other motion, it was because of an external moving cause. In general he imposed countless arbitrary distinctions upon the nature of things, for he was more preoccupied with definitions in teaching and the accuracy of his wording than the actual, internal truth of things.

This can be demonstrated by comparing his philosophy with the other Greek thinkers of high repute. Motion of parts in the work of Anaxagoras, the atoms of Democritus, the heaven and earth of Parmenides, the discord and concord of Empedocles, the resolution of bodies into the common, predictable nature of fire according to Heraclitus; they all exhibit a mix of natural philosophy, the nature of things, and experiment. Meanwhile, Aristotle's physics work in merely logical terms. Moreover, we ought not to lay too much stress on his frequent recourse to experiment, for it seems he had already decided upon things before consulting experience. After he decided something, he dragged experiment along as his captive and made it accommodate itself to the decision. As such, he is to be blamed even more than his modern followers, who have abandoned experiment altogether.

The empiric school's dogmas are even more deformed, as they come not from the light of common notions, but rather, from the confined obscurity of a few experiments. This philosophy seems highly probable to those who daily practice such experiments (and have thus corrupted their imaginations), but futile and incredible to others. The best examples of this are the alchemists and their dogmas. We would be remiss if we did not warn against this school, for we can already foresee that if people are to be induced to apply seriously to experiments, and thus bid farewell to the sophistic doctrines, the empirics will pose an imminent danger, owing to their forward haste and their propensity to jump to generalities.

Lastly, the corruption of philosophy by comingling it with superstition and theology is the most injurious of the three. The sophistic and empiric schools entrap the understanding, but this fanciful, bombastic, and poetical school rather flatters it. To philosophy, this evil introduces abstracted forms and final and first causes, often neglecting the intermediate. We must exercise great caution against it, for the deification of error is the greatest evil of all: it is a plague upon understanding.

And yet, some moderns have indulged this folly so thoroughly that they have built a system of natural philosophy around the first chapter of Genesis and the book of Job, effectively seeking the dead among the living [ed note: the author here uses "dead" to refer to the concerns of mortals and "living" to refer to immortals/gods]. This ought to be restrained, for not only does fantastical philosophy spring from the mixture, but heretical religion as well. Therefore, it is wise to only render unto faith the things that are faith's.

12. According to the passage, which of the following Greek thinkers explored topics most similar to the ones Aristotle did?

   A. Parmenides

   B. Heraclitus

   C. Anaxagoras

   D. Empedocles

13. Based upon the passage, which of the following statements would the author most likely believe?

   A. The superstitious school is more troublesome than the empiric, but less so than the sophistic.

   B. The superstitious school is more troublesome than both the empiric and sophistic school.

   C. The sophistic school is more troublesome than the superstitious school, but less so than the empiric.

   D. The empiric school is more troublesome than both the sophistic and superstitious schools.

14. Based upon the passage, which of the following represents the most likely reason why the author gives a much more in depth example of the sophistic school of philosophy than he does the other two schools?

   A. Because the sophistic school is most troublesome and therefore requires the most attention.

   B. Because the author finds the sophistic school to be correct in its construction of natural philosophy

   C. Because Aristotle exemplifies the sophistic school more than anyone else embodies the other schools.

   D. Because the author himself is actually a practitioner of the sophistic school of philosophy.

15. Based upon the passage, which of the following statements accurately explains why people who don't subscribe to it find the dogmas of the empiric school to be futile and incredible?

   A. Because they likely subscribe to the sophistic or superstitious schools and are less interested in experiments

   B. Because they, like the author, understand that most philosophy is founded on too narrow a basis

   C. Because their imaginations have not been corrupted by engaging in the practice of modern philosophy

   D. Because their imaginations have not been corrupted by drawing broad concepts from a few experiments

16. Suppose there is a devoutly religious man who wants to decide which of the three schools of philosophy he primarily belongs to. He is a meditative person who tends to enjoy conducting experiments. His process for drawing philosophical conclusions is to distill a specific idea, decide upon the most efficient wording for it, and then to test it experientially. Based upon this description, which of the following schools does the man most belong to?

   A. Sophistic

   B. Empiric

   C. A mix of sophistic and empiric

   D. A mix of empiric and superstitious

17. According to the passage, all of the following statements about Aristotle are true EXCEPT:

   A. his devotion to teaching was perhaps a detriment to his philosophy.

   B. he believed that all bodies have a particular motion specific to them.

   C. he rarely mentioned experimentation in his books.

   D. his take on physics is defined in the context of logic.

18. According to the passage, which of the following statements about the superstitious school of philosophy are true?

   I. Metaphorically, it often is concerned with a point A and a point B, but not in the process of getting from A to B.

   II. It often seeks to understand mortal things within the context of immortal things.

   III. It often seeks to understand immortal things within the context of mortal things.

   A. I only

   B. I and II only

   C. I and III only

   D. I, II, and III

Passage 4 (Questions 19 – 24)

In the old days quadrupeds, birds, fishes, and insects could all talk, and they and the human race lived together in peace and friendship. But as time went on the people increased so rapidly that their settlements spread over the whole earth and the poor animals found themselves beginning to be cramped for room. This was bad enough, but to add to their misfortunes man invented bows, knives, blowguns, spears, and hooks, and began to slaughter the larger animals, birds and fishes for the sake of their flesh or their skins, while the smaller creatures, such as the frogs and worms, were crushed and trodden upon without mercy, out of pure carelessness or contempt. In this state of affairs the animals resolved to consult upon measures for their common safety.

The deer held a council under their chief, the Little Deer, and after some deliberation resolved to inflict rheumatism upon every hunter who should kill one of their number, unless he took care to ask their pardon for the offense. They sent notice of their decision to the nearest settlement of Indians and told them at the same time how to make pro-pitiation when necessity forced them to kill one of the deer tribe. Now, whenever the hunter brings down a deer, the Little Deer, who is swift as the wind and cannot be wound-ed, runs quickly up to the spot and bending over the blood stains asks the spirit of the deer if it has heard the prayer of the hunter for pardon. If the reply be "Yes" all is well and the Little Deer goes on his way, but if the reply be in the negative he follows on the trail of the hunter, guided by the drops of blood on the ground, until he arrives at the cabin in the settlement, when the Little Deer enters invisibly and strikes the neglectful hunter with rheumatism, so that he is rendered on the instant a helpless cripple. No hunter who has regard for his health ever fails to ask pardon of the deer for killing it, although some who have not learned the prop-er formula may attempt to turn aside the Little Deer from his pursuit by building a fire behind them in the trail.

Finally the birds, insects, and smaller animals came togeth-er for a like purpose, and the Grubworm presided over the deliberations. It was decided that each in turn should express an opinion and then vote on the question as to whether or not man should be deemed guilty. Seven votes were to be sufficient to condemn him. One after another denounced man's cruelty and injustice toward the other animals and voted in favor of his death. The Frog spoke first and said "We must do something to check the increase of the race or people will become so numerous that we shall be crowded from off the earth. See how man has kicked me about because I'm ugly, as he says, until my back is covered with sores;" and here he showed the spots on his skin. Next came the Bird, who condemned man because "he burns my feet off," alluding to the way in which the hunter barbecues birds by impaling them on a stick set over the fire, so that their feathers and tender feet are singed and burned. Oth-ers followed in the same strain. The Ground Squirrel alone ventured to say a word in behalf of man, who seldom hurt him because he was so small; but this so enraged the others that they fell upon the Ground Squirrel and tore him with

their teeth and claws, and the stripes remain on his back to this day.

The assembly then began to devise and name various dis-eases, one after another, and had not their invention finally failed them not one of the human race would have been able to survive. The Grubworm in his place of honor hailed each new malady with delight, until at last they had reached the end of the list, when someone suggested that it be arranged so that menstruation should sometimes prove fatal to wom-an.

When the plants, who were friendly to man, heard what had been done by the animals, they determined to defeat their evil designs. Each tree, shrub, and herb, down, even to the grasses and mosses, agreed to furnish a remedy for some one of the diseases named, and each said "I shall appear to help man when he calls upon me in his need." Thus did medicine originate, and the plants, every one of which has its use if we only knew it, furnish the antidote to counter-act the evil wrought by the revengeful animals. When the doctor is in doubt what treatment to apply for the relief of a patient, the spirit of the plant suggests to him the proper remedy.

19. Which of the following actions would have been necessary for the humans to avoid rheumatism?

   I. Be more respectful of deer killed

  II. Be more considerate toward all animals killed

 III. Cease hunting deer

  A. I only

  B. I and II only

  C. I and III only

  D. II and III only

20. Which of the following best explains why the ground squirrel was able to avoid the carelessness and contempt of the humans?

  A. He was too big to have been stepped on or kicked.

  B. He was big enough to avoid being stepped on, and small enough to avoid being hunted.

  C. He was too small to have been hunted.

  D. He was the only animals that was kind towards the humans, and thus was spared.

21. According to the passage, which of the following motivated the animals to action?

  A. A spirit of vengeance

  B. Their evil nature

  C. The grubworm influenced the other animals to action

  D. A sense of desperation

22. Which of the following most likely motivated the plants to action?

  A. Indebtedness

  B. Gratitude

  C. Compassion

  D. Justice

23. How might a member of this Native American tribe view hunting?

  A. As something immoral

  B. With indifference toward animal life

  C. As their natural right

  D. As a necessary evil

24. What is the author's apparent attitude toward the passage material?

  A. Objective

  B. Reverent

  C. Patronizing

  D. Critical

Passage 5 (Questions 25 – 29)

There is a principle, supposed to prevail among many, which is utterly incompatible with all virtue or moral sentiment; and as it can proceed from nothing but the most depraved disposition, so in its turn it tends still further to encourage that depravity. This principle is, that all benevolence is mere hypocrisy, friendship a cheat, public spirit a farce, fidelity a snare to procure trust and confidence; and that while all of us, at bottom, pursue only our private interest, we wear these fair disguises, in order to put others off their guard, and expose them the more to our wiles and machinations. What heart one must be possessed of who possesses such principles, and who feels no internal sentiment that belies so pernicious a theory, it is easy to imagine: and also what degree of affection and benevolence he can bear to a species whom he represents under such odious colors, and supposes so little susceptible of gratitude or any return of affection. Or if we should not ascribe these principles wholly to a corrupted heart, we must at least account for them from the most careless and precipitate examination. Superficial reasoners, indeed, observing many false pretenses among mankind, and feeling, perhaps, no very strong restraint in their own disposition, might draw a general and a hasty conclusion that all is equally corrupted, and that men, different from all other animals, and indeed from all other species of existence, admit of no degrees of good or bad, but are, in every instance, the same creatures under different disguises and appearances.

There is another principle, somewhat resembling the former; which has been much insisted on by philosophers, and has been the foundation of many a system; that, whatever affection one may feel, or imagine he feels for others, no passion is, or can be disinterested; that the most generous friendship, however sincere, is a modification of self-love; and that, even unknown to ourselves, we seek only our own gratification, while we appear the most deeply engaged in schemes for the liberty and happiness of mankind. By a turn of imagination, by a refinement of reflection, by an enthusiasm of passion, we seem to take part in the interests of others, and imagine ourselves divested of all selfish considerations: but, at bottom, the most generous patriot and most greedy miser, the bravest hero and most abject coward, have, in every action, an equal regard to their own happiness and welfare.

Whoever concludes from the seeming tendency of this opinion, that those, who make profession of it, cannot possibly feel the true sentiments of benevolence, or have any regard for genuine virtue, will often find himself, in practice, very much mistaken. Probity and honour were no strangers to Epicurus and his sect. Atticus and Horace seem to have enjoyed from nature, and cultivated by reflection, as generous and friendly dispositions as any disciple of the austerer schools. And among the modern, Hobbes and Locke, who maintained the selfish system of morals, lived irreproachable lives; though the former lay not under any restraint of religion which might supply the defects of his philosophy.

The most obvious objection to the selfish hypothesis is, that, as it is contrary to common feeling and our most unprejudiced notions, there is required the highest stretch of philosophy to establish so extraordinary a paradox. To the most careless observer there appear to be such dispositions as benevolence and generosity; such affections as love, friendship, compassion, gratitude. These sentiments have their causes, effects, objects, and operations, marked by common language and observation, and plainly distinguished from those of the selfish passions. And as this is the obvious appearance of things, it must be admitted, until some hypothesis be discovered, which by penetrating deeper into human nature, may prove the former affections to be nothing but modifications of the latter.

25. Which of the following best describes the differences between the two theories put forth in the first and second paragraphs?

    A. The first describes actions taken consciously while the second describes forces pushing people to actions without their conscious awareness.

    B. The first describes qualities developed in humans by society, while the second describes qualities inherent in everyone.

    C. The first describes qualities and actions that are part of human nature, while the second describes human qualities that are nurtured by society.

    D. The first assumes the conscious participation of the offenders, while the second describes qualities possessed by all, whether they are aware of it or not.

26. Which of the following describes the obvious objection to the selfish hypothesis?

    A. That it goes contrary to everyday experience

    B. That the burden of proof lies on those who advocate the hypothesis because it is new

    C. That everyone is born with a capacity for compassion without consciousness of it

    D. That the burden of proof lies on those who advocate the hypothesis because it is radical

27. Which of the following would the author most likely present as evidence against the theories presented in the passage?

    A. A boss applauding the work of one of his or her employees

    B. A worker complimenting his or her boss

    C. One friend helping another in a difficult financial situation

    D. A mother who cares for her dying infant at the expense of her own health

28. Suppose there arose a new theory of ethics stating that every action taken by an individual stems from an evolutionary desire to ensure the best propagation of his or her own genes. How would the author receive this theory?

    A. Accept it for its value in predicting the outcome of human interactions

    B. Reject it based on a pre-inclination to believe that humans can act indifferently to their own welfare

    C. Accept it based on the science backing the theory

    D. Reject it based on a lack of evidence

29. To which of the following theories would the author lend his or her support?

    A. It is impossible to know whether anything exists beyond ourselves.

    B. It is impossible to know anything beyond that which we experience in our minds.

    C. There is no reason to believe things are so because they appear so.

    D. Truth can be found without the aid of formal evidence.

Passage 6 (Questions 30 – 35)

Dr. Donald Andrews and colleagues have been developing a body of research aimed at generating principles of effective correctional treatment—that is, treatment that can reduce rearrests and reincarcerations and can help offenders reintegrate into society. Andrews and colleagues argue that correctional programs that follow three principles related to risk, criminogenic needs, and responsivity produce the best outcomes. Numerous studies and meta-analyses support the importance of these principles. Developed for correctional populations, the principles apply to the large portion of the drug-abusing population that is involved in the criminal justice system.

The risk principle consists of two elements: (i) clients who are assessed as being at higher risk for reoffending are more likely to benefit from treatment than lower risk clients; and (ii) higher risk clients should receive more intensive services than lower risk clients. In the work of Andrews and colleagues, "risk" refers to the likelihood of future criminal behavior, but it is reasonable to assume that the principle also holds for drug abuse—that is, offenders with more severe drug problems should receive higher intensity treatment, while those at lower risk of relapse should be referred to less intensive programs, such as drug education, monitoring through drug testing, or self-help. Apart from ensuring optimal outcomes, matching problem severity to treatment approach makes for efficient use of scarce treatment resources. What constitutes high and low risk depends on whether the patient is a probationer or parolee and what treatment resources are available. The guidelines for designating clients as at high risk will be tighter in systems where intensive services are in short supply than in systems where they are more available.

According to the criminogenic needs principle, offenders have many needs, and correctional treatment should focus on those related to recidivism. Andrews and colleagues have identified the following targets as the most promising for correctional treatment: procriminal attitudes, procriminal associates, impulsivity, risk taking, limited self-control, poor problem-solving skills, poor educational and employment skills, and drug and alcohol dependence. These problems are all associated with drug abuse as well as recidivism. Offenders also have other needs that may require attention for various reasons, but are not associated with criminal behavior and have little or no impact on recidivism. These include enhancing self-esteem, improving living conditions, and addressing vaguely defined personal or emotional problems. Although correctional treatment should not focus on these needs, addiction treatment might benefit from such focus. Determining risk levels and needs requires assessment instruments suitable for identifying crime factors and drug use factors.

Andrews and colleagues describe the responsivity principle as concerned with "the selection of styles and modes of service that are (A) capable of influencing the specific types of intermediate targets that are set with offenders and (B)

appropriately matched to the learning styles of offenders." This principle speaks both to the types of treatment that are most appropriate for offenders and to the characteristics of staff who deliver the treatment. The Andrews group argues that the approaches most appropriate to the learning styles of offenders include behavioral and social learning techniques such as "modeling, graduated practice, role playing, reinforcement, resource provision, and detailed verbal guidance and explanations (making suggestions, giving reasons, cognitive restructuring)." As for treatment staff, the responsivity principle recommends that they relate to their clients with warmth, flexibility, and enthusiasm, but with clear messages about the unacceptability of procriminal attitudes, behaviors, and associations.

Andrews and colleagues developed the risk/needs/responsivity principles from research on treatments for the general population of criminal offenders. In more recent work, the responsivity principle has been extended to apply to the distinctive needs of women, racial/ethnic groups, and clients of different ages. With specific reference to drug-abusing offenders, NIDA recently published research-based principles of treatment for this population. The NIDA principles are consistent with the Andrews principles; together, they provide a framework for establishing programs and other interventions that have a high likelihood of reducing drug abuse and its consequences, including associated crime and further involvement in the criminal justice system.

30. Which of the following would the author advocate as a treatment for higher risk drug-problem parolees?

    A. Administration of antidepressants

    B. A course that teaches about the dangers of drug abuse

    C. Monthly drug testing

    D. Group therapy

31. Which of the following is most likely the title of the article from which the passage was taken?

    A. Proposition of Policy Changes for Reduced Violence Among Prisoners

    B. Proposition of Policy Changes for Reduced Drug Abuse Among Prisoners

    C. Interventions to Promote Successful Re-Entry Among Drug-Abusing Parolees

    D. Interventions to Promote Successful Re-Entry Among Female Parolees

32. Suppose it were discovered that the people a former inmate associates with is the greatest factor in determining whether the former inmate will be rearrested. How would the author view this information?

    A. The author would agree with the finding because he or she mentions that personal associations are the biggest factor in determining relapse rates for drug abusers.

    B. The author would deny the finding as it disagrees with the information in the passage.

    C. The author would probably be skeptical as to the validity of the finding.

    D. The author would probably believe the finding as it would not disagree with the passage.

33. Which of the following ideas is expressed in the passage?

    A. Higher risk clients should receive more intensive care because they are more likely to benefit from treatment than lower risk clients.

    B. Higher risk clients should receive more intensive care because society is more likely to benefit from their treatment.

    C. Higher risk clients are more likely to benefit from treatment than lower risk clients because they receive more intensive care.

    D. Higher risk clients are more likely to relapse into drug abuse because they are less likely to receive sufficient care.

34. Which of the following is an example of the responsivity principle?

    A. A parolee with a history of drug abuse should receive higher intensity drug intervention than another parolee with less history of drug abuse.

    B. If a health care provider is warm, flexible, and enthusiastic, he will be able to treat any prisoner as effectively as another staff member.

    C. The type of drug rehabilitation treatment for a mentally handicapped patient will be different from that of a patient without such a condition.

    D. If a health care provider is warm, flexible, and enthusiastic, he will be able to treat any prisoner effectively.

35. Dr. Andrews is most likely a:

    A. politician.

    B. psychologist.

    C. economist.

    D. criminal justice worker.

Passage 7 (Questions 36 – 42)

There are many who acknowledge Love to be the oldest of the gods, and also the greatest source of benefits to man. I know no greater blessing to a young man at the beginning of his life than a virtuous lover, and in the case of the lover, than a beloved youth. For when we talk about the principle which ought to guide men that would live noble lives, neither kindred, nor honor, nor wealth, nor any other motive is so able to implant itself as love is.

I am speaking of the sense of honor and dishonor that both states and individuals rely upon to do good or great work. I believe that a lover who is observed in doing something dishonorable or else in cowardly submitting when dishonor is done to him, will be more pained when observed by his beloved than his father, his friends, or anyone else. The beloved also feels this way.

Therefore, if there were some way of making a state or army made up of lovers, they would be the best rulers of their own state, avoiding all dishonor and emulating each other in honorable activities, and when fighting alongside each other, even if few in number, they could conquer the world. If he were to abandon his post or throw down his arms, what lover would not rather have the whole world observe him than his beloved? Or who would desert his beloved in a dangerous situation? The world's most cowardly coward would become an inspired hero in such a situation, for Love would inspire him. As Homer says, the god breathes courage into the soul of the hero, so too does Loves infuse his own nature into the soul of the lover.

Love will make both men and women dare to die for their beloved. Alcestis is a monument of this, for she was willing to lay down her life for her husband when no one else would. Though he had a living mother and father, the tenderness of her love far exceeded theirs and by comparison made them seem to be strangers to their own blood. Her action was so noble that the gods granted her, of all those who have done virtuous deeds, the rare privilege of returning alive to earth: such is the honor the gods pay to the devotion and virtue of love.

On the other hand, they sent Orpheus away empty-handed, presenting him only with an apparition of the woman he sought. They would not give her back because he showed no spirit: he did not dare to die for love like Alcestis, but rather, planned how he might enter and exit Hades alive. Later, he died at the hands of women, the gods' punishment for his cowardice.

Different again was the reward from the gods for the true love of Achilles towards his lover Patroclus. Achilles was well aware, as he had been told by Thetis, his mother, that he might avoid death, return home, and live well into old age, if he were to abstain from killing Hector. Despite this, he gave his life to revenge Patroclus, daring to die not only in Patroclus's defense, but after Patroclus's death as well. For this, the gods honored him even more than Alcestis, sending him to the Islands of the Blest.

For these reasons, I affirm that Love is the oldest, noblest, and mightiest of the gods, as well as the greatest giver of virtue in life and of happiness in death.

36. According to the passage, which of the following is the greatest honor the gods can bestow on a person?

    A. Infusing love into the soul of the lover

    B. Breathing courage into the soul of the hero

    C. Allowing him or her to return to earth alive

    D. Sending him or her to the Islands of the Blest

37. Based upon the passage, it can be inferred that the author believes which of the following statements about love?

    A. Anyone can be inspired to greatness by love.

    B. Love is primarily responsible for making men into heroes.

    C. Dishonorable actions are more excusable when not observed by a lover.

    D. Achilles is the greatest of all heroes.

38. Which of the following is the most likely reason why the author introduces the story of Orpheus?

    A. To further illustrate the idea that women can love as well or better than men

    B. To provide a contrast to how the gods reward the devotion and virtue of love

    C. To depict how planning and manipulation are despised by the gods

    D. To make the case the Orpheus is not actually in love with his beloved

39. According to the passage, how is it exactly that Love is the greatest source of benefits to man?

    A. It can cause people to gloriously sacrifice their lives.

    B. It can help to create the ideal state or army.

    C. It is the god with the most power to bestow rewards.

    D. It causes people to behave honorably and avoid dishonor.

40. If a small sovereign state has come into existence in which all of the governors of the state are lovers, according to the passage, which of the following reasons best explains why the governors of this state would be the best rulers in all of politics?

    A. Because they would be inspired by Love to make the best practical decisions for the state

    B. Because they would constantly be observed by their lovers and therefore act only honorably

    C. Because they would be guided by the gods, for the gods favor and honor Love above all else

    D. Because they would be motivated to end all hatred and dishonorable activities in the name of love

41. According to the passage, all of the following statements are true EXCEPT:

    A. Orpheus's love of his life was lesser than his love of his beloved.

    B. Achilles's love of Patroclus was greater than his fear of death.

    C. Alcestis's love of her husband was greater than that of his parents.

    D. Achilles chose death over dishonor in deciding to kill Hector.

42. According to the passage, which of the following are qualities of a noble life?

    I. Acting dishonorably only when not observed by a lover

    II. Being guided and inspired by love in one's actions and behavior

    III. That which would make someone dare to die for love

    A. I and II only

    B. I and III only

    C. II and III only

    D. I, II, and III

Passage 8 (Questions 43 – 49)

Roman law defined property as the right to use and abuse one's own within the limits of the law - *jus utendi et abutendi re sua, guatenus juris ratio patitur*. Of course there have been those to attempt the justification of the word abuse, on the grounds that it signifies absolute domain rather than senseless and immoral abuse. What a vain distinction! It is a distinction made as an excuse for property and it is powerless against the frenzy of possession, which it neither can prevent nor restrain. If he so chooses, the proprietor may allow his crops to rot, he may sow his fields with salt, milk his cows on sand, transform his vineyard into desert, and use his vegetable-garden as a park. Do these things constitute abuse? In terms of property, use and abuse are inevitably indistinguishable.

According to the Declaration of Rights that serves as a preface to the Constitution of '93, property is "the right to enjoy and dispose at will of one's goods, one's income, and the fruit of one's labor and industry." Moreover, as Code Napoleon, article 544 reads, "Property is the right to enjoy and dispose of things in the most absolute manner, provided we do not overstep the limits prescribed by the laws and regulations." These two definitions do not differ at all from that of Roman law: they give the proprietor absolute right over a thing, and as for the restriction imposed by these codes, provided the limits prescribed by laws and regulations are not overstepped, its purpose is not to limit property, but rather, to prevent the domain of one proprietor from interfering with that of another. As such, this law serves not as a limitation of the principle, but rather, a confirmation of it.

There are two types of property. The first is property pure and simple, the dominant power over a thing, sometimes referred to as naked property. The second is possession. As Duranton says, "Possession is a matter of fact, not of right." Toullier agrees: "Property is a right, a legal power; possession is a fact." The tenant, the farmer, and the usufructuary are possessors. The owner who lets and lends for use and the heir who will come into possession upon the death of a usufructuary are proprietors. If I may venture a comparison to assist in understanding: a lover is a possessor and a spouse is a proprietor. This double definition of property, domain versus possession, is of the highest importance and it must be understood clearly in order to comprehend what is to follow.

From this notable distinction arise two kinds of rights. The jus in re is the right in a thing, the right by which one may reclaim the property one has acquired from whatever hands one finds it in. The jus ad rem is the right to a thing, giving one a claim to become a proprietor. Therefore, the right of married partners over each other's person is the jus in re, while that of two who are betrothed is the jus ad rem. In the former, possession and property are one in the same, but the latter includes only possession. As I am a laborer, I have the right to possession of the products of nature and my own industry, and as I am a proletaire, I enjoy none of them. As such, it is by virtue of the jus ad rem that I demand access to the jus in re.

43. Those who think it appropriate to use the word "abuse" in reference to property likely believe that:

    A. it is morally defensible to treat an object with reckless abandon.

    B. one who has absolute domain over a thing need not treat it senselessly or immorally.

    C. those who would use or abuse a piece of property only have jus ad rem.

    D. the frenzy of possession cannot be restrained by the law.

44. Which of the following is the most likely reason why the author quotes Duranton and Toullier in the third paragraph?

    A. To define possession within the context of property

    B. To provide outside evidence for the two types of property

    C. To lend credibility to a seemingly very personal argument

    D. To define naked property within the context of possession

45. Based upon the passage, which of the following statements would the author be most likely to believe?

    A. The jus ad rem is more desirable than the jus in re.

    B. The jus in re is more desirable than the jus ad rem.

    C. Both the jus ad rem and the jus in re are equally desirable.

    D. Neither the jus ad rem nor the jus in re are necessary.

46. According to the passage, why is the distinction made in the first paragraph a vain one?

    A. Roman law was fundamentally flawed.

    B. No one challenges that abuse is senseless and immoral.

    C. French law is just as flawed as Roman law.

    D. Use and abuse are indistinguishable.

47. Suppose the heir to a major mustard producing corporation has just married his longtime girlfriend. Based upon the passage, which of the following most accurately describes the rights the husband and wife have over each other?

    A. The rights they have over each other derive from the jus ad rem.

    B. The rights they have over each other derive from the jus in re.

    C. The rights they have over each other derive from both the jus ad rem and the jus in re.

    D. The husband's rights derive from the jus in re and the wife's from the jus ad rem.

48. According to the passage, all of the following statements about the limits of property are true EXCEPT:

    A. they are prescribed by laws and regulations that are not to be overstepped.

    B. they can protect property from the abuse of a proprietor in only a few instances.

    C. they protect the property of one person from interfering with that of another.

    D. they do not limit the acquisition of property, but rather, confirm its validity.

49. Given the definitions of property as set forth by the Declaration of Rights and the Code Napoleon, article 544, which of the following can a proprietor legally do?

    I. Take vegetables from the garden of a man who stole from him

    II. Intentionally set fire to part of his grape vines in order to lower supply

    III. Marry the wife of a man who set fire to his entire tomato crop

    A. I only

    B. II only

    C. I and II only

    D. I, II, and III

Passage 9 (Questions 50 – 53)

In its early days, socialism was a revolutionary movement of which the object was the liberation of the wage-earning classes and the establishment of freedom and justice. The passage from capitalism to the new régime was to be sudden and violent: capitalists were to be expropriated without compensation, and their power was not to be replaced by any new authority.

Gradually a change came over the spirit of socialism. In France, socialists became members of the government, and made and unmade parliamentary majorities. In Germany, social democracy grew so strong that it became impossible for it to resist the temptation to barter away some of its intransigence in return for government recognition of its claims. In England, the Fabians taught the advantage of reform as against revolution, and of conciliatory bargaining as against irreconcilable antagonism.

The method of gradual reform has many merits as compared to the method of revolution, and I have no wish to preach revolution. But gradual reform has certain dangers, to wit, the ownership or control of businesses hitherto in private hands, and by encouraging legislative interference for the benefit of various sections of the wage-earning classes. I think it is at least doubtful whether such measures do anything at all to contribute toward the ideals which inspired the early socialists and still inspire the great majority of those who advocate some form of socialism.

Let us take as an illustration such a measure as state purchase of railways. This is a typical object of state socialism, thoroughly practicable, already achieved in many countries, and clearly the sort of step that must be taken in any piecemeal approach to complete collectivism. Yet I see no reason to believe that any real advance toward democracy, freedom, or economic justice is achieved when a state takes over the railways after full compensation to the shareholders.

Economic justice demands a diminution, if not a total abolition, of the proportion of the national income which goes to the recipients of rent and interest. But when the holders of railway shares are given government stock to replace their shares, they are given the prospect of an income in perpetuity equal to what they might reasonably expect to have derived from their shares. Unless there is reason to expect a great increase in the earnings of railways, the whole operation does nothing to alter the distribution of wealth. This could only be effected if the present owners were expropriated, or paid less than the market value, or given a mere life-interest as compensation. When full value is given, economic justice is not advanced in any degree.

There is equally little advance toward freedom. The men employed on the railway have no more voice than they had before in the management of the railway, or in the wages and conditions of work. Instead of having to fight the directors, with the possibility of an appeal to the government, they now have to fight the government directly; and experience does not lead to the view that a government depart-

ment has any special tenderness toward the claims of labor. If they strike, they have to contend against the whole organized power of the state, which they can only do successfully if they happen to have a strong public opinion on their side. In view of the influence which the state can always exercise on the press, public opinion is likely to be biased against them, particularly when a nominally progressive government is in power. There will no longer be the possibility of divergences between the policies of different railways. Railway men in England derived advantages for many years from the comparatively liberal policy of the North Eastern Railway, which they were able to use as an argument for a similar policy elsewhere. Such possibilities are excluded by the dead uniformity of state administration.

And there is no real advance toward democracy. The administration of the railways will be in the hands of officials whose bias and associations separate them from labor, and who will develop an autocratic temper through the habit of power. The democratic machinery by which these officials are nominally controlled is cumbrous and remote, and can only be brought into operation on first-class issues which rouse the interest of the whole nation. Even then it is very likely that the superior education of the officials and the government, combined with the advantages of their position, will enable them to mislead the public as to the issues, and alienate the general sympathy even from the most excellent cause.

I do not deny that these evils exist at present; I say only that they will not be remedied by such measures as the nationalization of railways in the present economic and political environment. A greater upheaval, and a greater change in men's habits of mind, is necessary for any really vital progress.

50. Which of the following describes the change that came over the socialist movement as described in the passage?

    A. The socialist movement was brought about through small reforms rather than a violent revolution.

    B. Socialists began to be more involved in legislative parties than executive branches of government.

    C. Socialists began to adopt their ideals to fit with established governments.

    D. The socialist movement began to flourish only in countries with a long tradition of capitalism.

51. Which of the following does the author suggest?

    A. That the state's purchase of private businesses will decrease the profitability of those businesses

    B. That the state's purchase of private businesses will increase the profitability of those businesses

    C. That the state's purchase of private business can only advance economic justice if the original owners are compensated fairly

    D. That state purchasing of a private railway can only advance the ideals of socialism if the shareholders are undercompensated in the purchase

52. Suppose it were discovered that the state purchase of the railways resulted in improved conditions for railway workers, how would this affect the author's arguments in the passage?

    A. It would support the author's arguments that it is harder for workers to argue for reform from a private railway director than the government.

    B. It would disagree with the author's argument that a socialist government department has no special tenderness toward the claims of labor.

    C. It would support the author's statement that socialist government leaders are more educated than the people they lead.

    D. It would disagree with the author's statement that the object of socialism is to liberate the wage-earning class.

53. Which of the following is a benefit that the author would see in revolution over gradual reform?

    A. A revolution would be shorter and result in less harm to the people.

    B. A revolution would better protect the rights and freedoms of the lowest poverty-stricken classes.

    C. Wealth can be more evenly distributed when a revolution strips the capitalists of their wealth.

    D. A revolution would lead to better establishment of democratic principles.

This page intentionally left blank.

SECTION 10

Answer Key

1	D	12	C	23	D	34	C	45	B
2	A	13	B	24	A	35	B	46	D
3	B	14	C	25	D	36	D	47	B
4	A	15	D	26	A	37	A	48	B
5	B	16	A	27	D	38	B	49	B
6	B	17	C	28	D	39	D	50	A
7	C	18	B	29	D	40	B	51	D
8	B	19	A	30	D	41	A	52	B
9	D	20	B	31	C	42	C	53	C
10	C	21	A	32	D	43	B		
11	A	22	C	33	A	44	A		

Passage 1 (Questions 1 – 6)

In a typical year, nearly **1,100,000 people** devote part or all of their **working** time to **provide medical care** for the people of the **United States** and earn their livelihood thereby. The total number is about equally divided between those who **serve for fees** from individuals or families, and those who are engaged by **medical institutions** such as hospitals, public health agencies, or clinics. There are 550,000 independent practitioners, of whom 121,000 are physicians; 57,000 are dentists; approximately 118,000 are graduate nurses and 150,000 are practical nurses; secondary or sectarian healers, midwives, chiropodists, optometrists, osteopaths, chiropractors, naturopaths or similar groups, and faith healers are approximately 110,000 in number. The **institutions** of the United States – hospitals clinics, public health agencies, and drug stores – **employ approximately 530,000** physicians, dentists, nurses, pharmacists, social service workers, medical technicians, and lay employees.

Contrast: one million people work in healthcare split between work for fee vs work for institutions

Medical care is an **esoteric economic commodity** concerning which the **buyer has no basis for critical judgment** of quality or value. The patient does not know whether he should purchase a particular type of medical service and is frequently unable to determine whether or not the medical service has been satisfactory after its receipt. The physician, therefore, is judge both of the patient's need for the service which he has to offer, as well as of the time and conditions under which it shall be purchased. Moreover, inasmuch as **medical care involves life or death** (or at least the risk of death), the patient frequently believes that **only one individual practitioner** holds the commodity which he needs. It therefore seems **impossible to search for another** purveyor of medical service, as he would do if the forces of economic supply and demand operated in medicine as in the majority of business transactions. The conditions surrounding the delivery of medical care are therefore **unique** and are **unlike** those which characterize **ordinary economic phenomena**, because there is but one buyer and one seller and because **the commodity** itself is of **priceless value** if received.

Key terms: esoteric economic commodity

Contrast: normal economic conditions of supply and demand vs medical care economics

Opinion: author believes that medical care does not follow other economic models

Cause and effect: patients' ignorance does not let them exercise judgment in buying health care services; the priceless value of health care puts it outside normal economic interactions

Traditionally and inherently **medical care is a personal service** rendered by a professional person to an ailing or to a potential patient. Economic efficiency cannot change medical care in this respect. The patient is ultimately and inevitably the personal recipient of medical service, and he derives benefit from the medical service in proportion to the degree to which his particular medical needs are met. Just as medical service has been regarded as a personal affair, the **payment for medical service** has also been **considered a personal obligation. Community** responsibility has been accepted **only in those cases** where the nature of the illness involves danger to other persons or requires isolation, or where it entails long periods of treatment which cannot ordinarily be financed by the individual or his family, or where a patient is an avowed indigent and is unable to pay for medical care from his own resources. The personal nature of medical service has been the cornerstone for the evolution of present-day medicine. Each patient has exercised his right to engage a practitioner who suited his real or supposed needs, without regard to the wishes of other members of the community or the profession. Increasingly, however, **this scheme of things has developed incongruities**. Especially for economic reasons, the advancing perfection of medical science and art have carried **medical care out of the reach of millions** of families. Their voices raised in protest have made imperative an understanding of the problems and a search for practical solutions. During many centuries the economic structure within which the system of medical service has operated has reflected the views of the times. **Society has been changing** rapidly in the last few decades; but **adjustments** between the need for **medical care** and its effective provision have **not kept pace**. The newer architecture of society calls for changes in the temple of Aesculapius.

Opinion: author argues that although the practice of medicine is inherently a personal service, the rapid progression of society and medicine has rendered the "personal obligation" payment strategy to be ineffective

Contrast: personal obligation to pay vs community payment

Cause and effect: the rapid advancement of medical care has made medical care out of reach of many, therefore changes must be made to the current system

Main idea: Healthcare is an enormous industry in the US, but given the esoteric and personal nature of medicine, the economics of medical care do not follow traditional supply and demand models; to keep up with the rapid progression of society and medical advancements, changes to the current economic model must be made.

1. D is correct. The main idea of the passage is that the esoteric nature of medicine, coupled with the inherently personal nature of providing and receiving medical care, causes the economics of health care to deviate from the normal conditions of supply and demand.

   A: The passage does not describe whether or not any adjustments have already been made.

   B: The author never states whether or not he believes the medical community is prepared to make what he finds to be necessary adjustments in the face of a changing society and medical field.

   C: The author never suggests that the physician has too much control. It could instead be what the author views to be an inherent component of medical care.

2. A is correct. One of the author's main points in the passage is that the 'personal obligation' payment system has been rendered insufficient advancements in the medical field. It can be inferred that the author therefore believes that the economics of medical care must be shifted to a more community-based payment approach.

   B, C: While setting nationwide standards for cost and allowing patients to switch between providers would allow health care to more closely resemble supply and demand economics, it can't be inferred from the passage that the author believes that approaching a supply and demand model is the best strategy moving forward.

   D: The author believes that a community-based approach to handle the costs of medical care will be necessary, but he states that care is inherently personal.

3. B is correct. The author states that medical care is inherently esoteric, and therefore the average patient is unaware of whether or not he or she received satisfactory care. Furthermore the author never states that options for a second opinion aren't available to patients, but rather that patients do not have the knowledge to seek them out or that patients feel a specific connection with their physician. Answer choice B is therefore NOT an example discussed by the author, and it is the correct answer.

   A, C, D: The rising cost of medical care, patient attachment to a specific care provider, and a lack of understanding regarding medical treatments are all examples discussed by the author.

4. A is correct. The first paragraph serves to provide background information regarding the large number of individuals working within the medical field. Given the focus of the passage on the economics of health care, it can be inferred that this is to give the reader an appreciation for the number of workers and the complexity of the field.

   B: No arguments are made by the author in the first paragraph.

   C: The author never emphasizes the percentage of physicians relative to overall health care workers, nor can any meaningful conclusions be drawn in that regard based on the information in the passage.

   D: The number of health care workers does not highlight the inefficiencies of the system, rather it highlights the number of moving parts within it.

5. B is correct. Statement III is accurate. The author states that medical advancements have left millions of families without access to medical care, and therefore adjustments to the current system must be made.

   I: The author believes that providing and receiving medical care is inherently personal, and therefore individual-centered. It is the *cost* of medical care that the author argues must be distributed away from the individual.

   II: While the author argues that the esoteric nature of medical care causes it to be difficult for a patient to understand if he or she is receiving satisfactory care, it cannot be inferred that the author believes that fully educating patients on the care they receive is the best course of action.

6. B is correct. The author argues that due to the rapid advancements of the medical field, millions of families are losing their access to medical care. The study presented in answer choice B would directly support that argument, and therefore it is the correct answer.

   A: The author doesn't address whether or not patient's desire to know the price of their care, therefore it is not directly relevant to his arguments.

   C: The author states that patients perceive, particularly in matters of life and death, that only one physician is capable of providing their care, but does not address what patients would do if they were made aware of their options.

   D: The author argues that health care economics aren't currently governed by the principles of supply or demand, but that position wouldn't be strengthened by a study regarding health care reform.

Passage 2 (Questions 7 – 11)

Although the **theatrical ballet dance** is comparatively **modern**, the **elements** of its formation are of the **greatest antiquity**; the chorus of dancers and the performances of the men in the **Egyptian** chapters represent without much doubt public dancing performances. We get singing, dancing, mimicry and pantomime in the early stages of **Greek** art, and the development of the dance rhythm in music is equally ancient.

Key terms: Egyptian, Greek

Contrast: modern nature of theatrical ballet vs ancient origins of its various elements

The **Alexandrine Pantomime**, introduced into Rome about 30 B.C. by **Bathillus** and **Pylades**, appears to have been an entertainment approaching the ballet. In Italy there appears to have been a kind of ballet in the 14th century, and from Italy, under the influence of **Catharine de Medici**, came the ballet. **Balthasar di Beaujoyeulx** produced the **first recorded ballet in France**, in the Italian style, in 1582. This was, however, essentially a Court ballet.

Key terms: Alexandrine Pantomime, Bathillus, Pylades, Catharine de Medici, Balthasar di Beaujoyeulx

Opinion: author presents several examples of performances that approach the modern theatrical ballet

The theatre ballet apparently arose out of these Court ballets. **Henry III** and **Henry IV**, the latter especially, were very fond of these entertainments, and many Italians were brought to France to assist in them. Pompeo **Diabono**, a **Savoyard**, was brought to Paris in 1554 to regulate the Court ballets. At a later date came **Rinuccini**, the poet, a Florentine, as was probably **Caccini**, the musician. They had composed and produced the little operetta of "**Daphne**," which had been performed in Florence in 1597. Under these last-mentioned masters the ballet in France took somewhat of its present form. This passion for Court ballets continued under **Louis XIII** and **Louis XIV**.

Key terms: Henry III, Henry IV, Diabono, Savoyard, Rinuccini, Caccini, Daphne, Louis XIII, Louis XIV

Opinion: author thinks the development of Court ballets led to the modern theatrical ballet

Louis XIII as a youth danced in one of the ballets at St. Germain, it is said at the desire of **Richelieu**, who was an expert in spectacle. It appears that he was encouraged in these amusements to **remedy fits of melancholy**. Louis XIV, at seven, danced in a masquerade, and afterwards not only danced in the ballet of "**Cassandra**," in 1651, but **did all he could to raise the condition of the dance** and encourage dancing and music. His influence, combined with that of Cardinal Richelieu, **raised** the ballet from gross and trivial styles to a **dignity worthy of music**, poetry and dancing. His uncle, **Gaston of Orleans**, still patronized the grosser style, but it became eclipsed by the better. **Lulli** composed music

to the words of **Molière** and other celebrities; amongst notable works then produced was the "**Andromeda**" of Corneille, a tragedy, with hymns and dances, executed in 1650, at the **Petit Bourbon**.

Key terms: Richelieu, Cassandra, Gaston, Lulli, Molière, Andromeda

Opinion: author thinks that Louis XIV and Cardinal Richelieu brought dance from a "gross and trivial" style to a dignified art on par with music and poetry

The **foundation of the theatrical ballet** was, however, at the instigation of Cardinal **Mazarin**, to prevent a lowering of tone in the establishment of the **Académie de Danse** under thirteen Academicians in 1661. This appears to have been merged into the Académie Royale de Musique et de Danse in 1669, which provided a proper training for débutants, under **MM. Perrin** and **Cambert**, whilst **Beauchamp**, the master of the Court ballets, had charge of the dancing. The first opera-ballet, the "**Pomona**" of Perrin and Cambert, was produced in 1671. To this succeeded many works of **Lulli, to whom is attributed the increased speed in dance music and dancing**, that of the Court ballets having been slow and stately.

Key terms: Cardinal Mazarin, Perrin, Cambert, Beauchamp, Pomona, Perrin, Cambert

Cause and effect: the real foundation of theatrical ballet came from the work of Cardinal Mazarin; Lulli took the dances and sped up the pace of the music and dancing

The **great production** of the period appears to have been the "**Triumph of Love**" in 1681, with twenty scenes and seven hundred performers; amongst these were many of the nobility, and some excellent ballerine, such as **Pesaut**, **Carré**, **Leclerc**, and **Lafontaine**.

Key terms: Pesaut, Carré, Leclerc, Lafontaine

Opinion: author thinks Triumph of Love was the greatest production of the time

Main Idea: The theatrical ballet is a relatively modern form with ancient roots that saw its development come out of the Court ballets popular under various monarchs and reaching its modern form in the late 1600's.

7.	C is correct. The passage states that Louis XIII was encouraged to dance in the ballet at St. Germain by Richelieu but there is no mention of Louis XIV being influenced by Richelieu. The passage does state that Richelieu and Louis XIV helped make ballet more dignified.

	A, B, D: These are all stated in the passage.

8.	B is correct. Cardinal Mazarin appears to have been in power in 1661, but Cardinal Richelieu was a contemporary of Louis XIV even after 1651. This implies that the two cardinals were likely contemporary and that Richelieu was older because he was around during the reign of Louis XIII as well.

	A: This would be unlikely, since the king after the thirteenth would be named the fourteenth.

	C: Gaston of Orleans promoted the grosser style of ballet, while Molière was apparently writing for the newer more dignified style. The two may have lived at the same time but there is absolutely no reason to think they were friends.

	D: The Italians invented ballet but by the end of the 17th century, theatrical ballet had flourished in France apparently more so than in Italy. While this may be true, it is simply unsupported by the passage.

9.	D is correct. Pomona was an opera ballet produced in 1671, two years after the formation of the Academie Royale de Musique et de Danse, which represented the institutionalization of theatrical ballet, which the author states is the direct ancestor of modern ballet.

	A, B, C: These were all written earlier and are thus court ballets or something less similar to modern ballet.

10.	C is correct. The author states that Italians had to be brought into France to support French ballet

	A: This is true but is not related to the statement in the question.

	B: The French monarchs did support ballet in France by importing Italian ballet producers.

	D: This is not mentioned in the passage.

11.	A is correct. The passage states that Lulli was writing when Andromeda was produced and that he wrote ballets after 1671 during the time of Triumph of Love. Among the answer choices, it is most reasonable to assume that his name can be connected with these works as they are mentioned directly after mentioning him.

	B: Perrin and Cambert are mentioned to have written opera-ballets after the discussion of Andromeda. This is not likely.

	C: Louis XIII was likely before their time.

	D: Pompeo Diabono was too early for Louis XIV.

Passage 3 (Questions 12 – 18)

For the **groundwork** of their philosophy, people generally take either **too much** from a few topics **or too little** from many. In either case, their philosophy is founded on too narrow a basis and decides upon things with insufficient grounds. The theoretic **philosopher observes a few common happenings** by experiment, without examining them or reducing them to certainty. For the rest, he relies upon **meditation** and his **wit**. Other philosophers have very diligently and **precisely attended to a few experiments**, and from these have presumed to deduce and **invent entire systems** of philosophy, bringing all things into conformity with them. A third type, driven by faith and religious reverence, introduce **theology** and tradition: some of them have gone so far as to derive the sciences from spirits. These are three species of **false philosophy**: the **sophistic**, **empiric**, and **superstitious**.

Contrast: three types of philosophers: sophistic, empiric, superstitious

Opinion: author thinks these three types of thinkers create a false philosophy

The best example of the **first type is Aristotle**, for he **corrupted natural philosophy with logic**. He made the world into categories and assigned to the human soul, which he considered to be the noblest of substances, a nature determined by words of secondary operation. He asserted that all bodies had a specific and proper motion, and that if they shared in any other motion, it was because of an external moving cause. In general he **imposed countless arbitrary distinctions** upon the nature of things, for he was more preoccupied with **definitions** in teaching and the accuracy of his **wording** than the **actual**, internal **truth** of things.

Opinion: author thinks Aristotle is a sophistic philosopher who was more hung up on definitions and wording than actually studying the truth

This can be demonstrated by comparing his philosophy with the **other Greek thinkers** of high repute. Motion of parts in the work of **Anaxagoras**, the atoms of **Democritus**, the heaven and earth of **Parmenides**, the discord and concord of **Empedocles**, the resolution of bodies into the common, predictable nature of fire according to **Heraclitus**; they all exhibit a **mix of natural philosophy**, the nature of things, and **experiment**. Meanwhile, Aristotle's physics work in merely logical terms. Moreover, we ought not to lay too much stress on his frequent recourse to experiment, for it seems he had **already decided upon things before consulting experience**. After he decided something, he dragged experiment along as his captive and made it accommodate itself to the decision. As such, **he is to be blamed even more** than his modern followers, who have abandoned experiment altogether.

Key terms: Anaxagoras, Democritus, Parmenides, Empedocles, Heraclitus

Contrast: other Greek thinkers included experiments in their construction of natural philosophy vs Aristotle just decided in advance what he believed

Opinion: author really doesn't like the way Aristotle did things

The **empiric school's** dogmas are even more deformed, as they come not from the light of common notions, but rather, from the **confined obscurity of a few experiments**. This philosophy seems highly probable to those who daily practice such experiments (and have thus corrupted their imaginations), but futile and incredible to others. The best examples of this are the **alchemists** and their dogmas. We would be remiss if we did not warn against this school, for we can already foresee that if people are to be induced to apply seriously to experiments, and thus **bid farewell to the sophistic doctrines**, the **empirics** will pose an **imminent danger**, owing to their forward haste and their **propensity to jump to generalities**.

Opinion: author thinks alchemists are even more wrong than Aristotle because they do a few experiments and then jump to generalities

Lastly, the corruption of philosophy by comingling it with **superstition and theology** is the **most injurious** of the three. The sophistic and empiric schools entrap the understanding, but this fanciful, bombastic, and poetical school rather flatters it. To philosophy, this evil introduces abstracted forms and final and first causes, often neglecting the intermediate. We must **exercise great caution against it**, for the **deification of error** is the greatest evil of all: it is a **plague upon understanding**.

Opinion: author thinks mixing theology or superstition with philosophy is the worst possible mistake

And yet, **some moderns** have indulged this **folly** so thoroughly that they have **built a system of natural philosophy** around the first chapter of **Genesis** and the book of Job, effectively seeking the dead among the living [ed note: the author here uses "dead" to refer to the concerns of mortals and "living" to refer to immortals/gods]. This ought to be restrained, for not only does fantastical philosophy spring from the mixture, but **heretical religion** as well. Therefore, it is wise to only **render unto faith the things that are faith's**.

Cause and effect: mixing up religion with natural philosophy can make for bad philosophy and for heretical (false) religion

Opinion: author thinks we should draw a clear line between faith and natural philosophy

Main Idea: The author demonstrates three primary ways that people approach philosophy in an erroneous way; these three erroneous approaches are sophistic (theoretical), empiric (experimental), and superstitious (religious) in nature; he describes each of these schools, proceeding from least egregious to most egregious, though he does consider all of them to be significantly problematic.

12.   C is correct. In the third paragraph, when the author introduces "the other Greek thinkers of high repute," each of them is accompanied with a respective subject matter, like Democritus's atoms, Parmenides's heaven and earth, and Anaxagoras's "motion of parts," referring back to the motion studied as a part of Aristotle's philosophy in the previous paragraph.

13.   B is correct. In the fourth paragraph, the author writes that the empiric school's dogma is "even more deformed." As this comes after the description of the sophistic school, it can be assumed that the author is saying that the empiric school is even more deformed than the sophistic school. It can also be assumed that this makes it more troublesome. Moreover, as the author writes at the beginning of the sixth paragraph, "the corruption of philosophy by comingling it with superstition and theology is the most injurious of three." The term "most injurious" likely qualifies this school as the most troublesome as well.

14.   C is correct. Aristotle stands preeminently among philosophers, and in particular, sophistic philosophers. Examples for the other two schools are less specific, perhaps because a more specific example is not as plainly clear as Aristotle was for the sophistic school.

   A: We have proven above that the superstitious school is most troublesome.

   B: In fact, the author thinks all three schools of philosophy are incorrect.

   D: This may or may not be true, but as he is negatively critiquing all three schools, it is likely he considers himself to be immersed in some other school of philosophy.

15.   D is correct. In the fourth paragraph: "This philosophy seems highly probable to those who daily practice such experiments (and have thus corrupted their imaginations), but futile and incredible to others." The daily practice of these experiments corrupts imaginations, and so, those who don't practice experiments still have intact imaginations.

   A, B: These are never said.

   C: It is not modern philosophy that corrupts imaginations, but rather, "the confined obscurity of a few experiments."

16.   A is correct. This question is filled with a lot of distractions. The heart of the matter rests in his process, which is to start with an idea, word it correctly, and then test it experientially. Within the context of the passage, this style is closest to Aristotle's, and he is the example of the sophistic school.

   B: An empiricist would start with experiments.

   C: Though this might be a mix of sophistic and empiric out of the context of the passage, Aristotle is described as strictly sophistic.

   D: There are no superstitious aspects to this man's process.

17.   C is correct. Rather, as the author writes in the third paragraph, "We ought not to lay too much stress on his frequent recourse to experiment..." This frequent recourse can be taken as frequent mention. So, he mentioned experimentation, but the author doesn't think we ought to take it seriously.

   A: "...he was more preoccupied with definitions in teaching and the accuracy of his wording..."

   B: "He asserted that all bodies had a specific and proper motion."

   D: "...Aristotle's physics work in merely logical terms."

18.   B is correct. I: This is true because, as the author writes, this philosophy introduces "final and first causes, often neglecting the intermediate." Also note that it shows up in all four answer choices, so it has to be true. II: This is true because the building of a system of natural philosophy compares to "seeking the dead among the living." III: This is false. As the note points out, the dead is synonymous with mortal concerns and the living is synonymous with immortal concerns.

Passage 4 (Questions 19 – 24)

In the old days **quadrupeds**, **birds**, **fishes**, and **insects** could all talk, and they and the **human race** lived together in **peace** and friendship. But as time went on the people increased so rapidly that their settlements spread over the whole earth and the poor animals found themselves beginning to be cramped for room. This was bad enough, but to add to their misfortunes man invented bows, knives, blowguns, spears, and hooks, and began to **slaughter** the larger animals, birds and fishes for the sake of their flesh or their skins, while the smaller creatures, such as the frogs and worms, were crushed and trodden upon without mercy, out of pure **carelessness** or **contempt**. In this state of affairs the animals resolved to consult upon measures for their common safety.

Key terms: quadrupeds, birds, fishes, insects, human race

Contrast: the human relationship with animals changes from one of peace to slaughter

Cause and effect: because of their carelessness or contempt, humans step on small animals and killed larger ones

The deer held a council under their chief, the **Little Deer**, and after some deliberation resolved to inflict **rheumatism** upon every hunter who should kill one of their number, unless he took care to ask their pardon for the offense. They sent notice of their decision to the nearest settlement of **Indians** and told them at the same time how to make propitiation when necessity forced them to kill one of the deer tribe. Now, whenever the hunter brings down a deer, the Little Deer, who is swift as the wind and cannot be wounded, runs quickly up to the spot and bending over the blood stains asks the spirit of the deer if it has heard the prayer of the hunter for pardon. If the reply be "Yes" all is well and the Little Deer goes on his way, but if the reply be in the negative he follows on the trail of the hunter, guided by the drops of blood on the ground, until he arrives at the cabin in the settlement, when the Little Deer enters invisibly and strikes the neglectful hunter with rheumatism, so that he is rendered on the instant a helpless cripple. No hunter who has regard for his health ever fails to ask pardon of the deer for killing it, although some who have not learned the proper formula may attempt to turn aside the Little Deer from his pursuit by building a fire behind them in the trail.

Key terms: Little Deer, rheumatism, Indians

Contrast: the difference between those who ask pardon for killing deer and those who do not is described

Cause and effect: if you don't ask pardon for killing a deer, you'll be struck with rheumatism

Finally the birds, insects, and smaller animals came together for a like purpose, and the **Grubworm** presided over the deliberations. It was decided that each in turn should express an opinion and then vote on the question as to whether or not man should be deemed guilty. Seven votes

were to be sufficient to condemn him. One after another denounced man's cruelty and injustice toward the other animals and voted in favor of his death. The **Frog** spoke first and said "**We must do something to check the increase of the race** or people will become so numerous that we shall be crowded from off the earth. See how man has kicked me about because I'm ugly, as he says, until my back is covered with sores;" and here he showed the spots on his skin. Next came the **Bird**, who condemned man because "he burns my feet off," alluding to the way in which the hunter barbecues birds by impaling them on a stick set over the fire, so that their feathers and tender feet are singed and burned. Others followed in the same strain. The Ground Squirrel alone ventured to say a word in behalf of man, who seldom hurt him because he was so small; but this so enraged the others that they fell upon the **Ground Squirrel** and tore him with their teeth and claws, and the stripes remain on his back to this day.

Key terms: grubworm, frog, bird, ground squirrel

Opinions: the birds, insects and frogs don't like humans; the ground squirrel seems to like them more

Contrast: the ground squirrel is held in contrast to the rest of the animals as the only one advocating for the humans

Cause and effect: the frog is said to have spots because he is kicked by humans; the squirrel has stripes because he was attacked by the other animals

The assembly then began to **devise** and name various **diseases**, one after another, and had not **their invention finally failed them** not one of the human race would have been able to survive. The Grubworm in his place of honor hailed each new malady with delight, until at last they had reached the end of the list, when someone suggested that it be arranged so that menstruation should sometimes prove fatal to women.

Opinions: the grubworm seems to really enjoy the idea of human suffering

Cause and effect: the cruelty of humans towards the other animals caused the animals to invent all the various maladies that plague humanity; they ran out of ideas otherwise the illnesses they invented would've been enough to wipe out all humans

When **the plants, who were friendly to man**, heard what had been done by the animals, they determined to defeat their evil designs. Each tree, shrub, and herb, down, even to the grasses and mosses, **agreed to furnish a remedy** for some one of the diseases named, and each said "I shall appear to help man when he calls upon me in his need." **Thus did medicine originate**, and the plants, every one of which has its use if we only knew it, furnish the antidote to counteract the evil wrought by the revengeful animals. When the doctor is in doubt what treatment to apply for the relief of a patient, the spirit of the plant suggests to him the proper remedy.

Opinions: the plants are friendly to man

Contrast: the plants are contrasted to the animals, the one being friendly, the other being vengeful

Cause and effect: the plants provide the remedy for each disease inflicted by the animals

Main Idea: The author is describing the origin of diseases and their remedies according to a Native American tribe; the animals felt oppressed by the humans and thus strike them with disease, while the plants were friendly to humans and provide the remedies.

19. A is correct. The passage states that the hunter need only ask for pardon when killing a deer, and they would avoid rheumatism.

   II: It is not necessary to ask pardon for killing all animals, just the deer, because it is Little Deer who gives rheumatism

   III: It is not necessary to cease hunting deer, just ask for pardon.

20. B is correct. The passage states in the first paragraph that the larger creatures were slain and the smaller ones were stepped on. The ground squirrel was not big enough to be hunted or small enough to be stepped on.

   A, C: these are each true but not the whole explanation.

   D: The squirrel was merciful toward humans as a result of the humans not hurting the squirrel.

21. A is correct. The animals were doing this because they felt they had been oppressed by the humans. It was out of revenge.

   B: The animals are said to have performed evil by bringing about their plans but they are not necessarily of an evil nature.

   C: The grubworm did not necessarily influence the other animals.

   D: The animals may have been desperate but this was not their primary motivation.

22. C is correct. The plants are friendly to the humans. They do not want them to be hurt. It makes sense that they were moved by compassion.

   A: There is no reason to think the plants were indebted toward the humans.

   B: There is no reason to think the plants were grateful to the humans.

   D: The plants seem to be acting out of concern for the humans only.

23. D is correct. It is apparent that the tribe who subscribes to this story believes hunting to be unfair to the animals. However, they continue to do it with as much respect as possible, as per the Little Deer story.

   A: Perhaps they view it as immoral but choice D is better because they will continue to hunt.

   B: The story illustrates that they respect animal life.

   C: If they had the natural right to hunt there would be no need to apologize for the activity.

24. A is correct. The author seems to be describing the events of the story as an outsider, telling the story as he or she understands it.

   B: The author never hints at being a member of the tribe in question and shows no reverence or belief in what he or she is describing.

   C, D: There is no reason to think the author has a negative attitude towards the material he is describing.

Passage 5 (Questions 25 – 29)

There is a **principle**, supposed to prevail among many, which is **utterly incompatible with all virtue** or moral sentiment; and as it can proceed from nothing but the most depraved disposition, so in its turn it tends still further to encourage that depravity. This principle is, that all **benevolence is mere hypocrisy**, friendship a cheat, public spirit a farce, fidelity a snare to procure trust and confidence; and that while all of us, at bottom, pursue only our **private interest**, we wear these fair disguises, in order to put others off their guard, and expose them the more to our wiles and machinations. What heart one must be possessed of who possesses such principles, and who feels no internal sentiment that belies so pernicious a theory, it is easy to imagine: and also what degree of affection and benevolence he can bear to a species whom he represents under such odious colors, and supposes so little susceptible of gratitude or any return of affection. Or if we should not ascribe these principles wholly to a **corrupted heart**, we must at least account for them from the most **careless and precipitate** examination. **Superficial reasoners**, indeed, observing many false pretenses among mankind, and feeling, perhaps, **no very strong restraint in their own disposition**, might draw a general and a hasty conclusion that **all is equally corrupted**, and that men, different from all other animals, and indeed from all other species of existence, admit of no degrees of good or bad, but are, in every instance, the same creatures under different disguises and appearances.

Opinion: the author presents a theory that he or she believes incompatible with all virtue or moral sentiment; the theory is that all niceness is at its base motivated by the selfish desires of the person acting nicely

Cause and effect: the author states that anyone who espouses this theory must be corrupted or careless

There is another principle, somewhat resembling the former; which has been much insisted on by philosophers, and has been the foundation of many a system; that, whatever affection one may feel, or imagine he feels for others, **no passion is**, or can be **disinterested**; that the **most generous friendship**, however sincere, is a **modification of self-love**; and that, even **unknown to ourselves**, we seek only our own gratification, while we appear the most deeply engaged in schemes for the liberty and happiness of mankind. By a turn of imagination, by a refinement of reflection, by an enthusiasm of passion, we **seem** to take part in the **interests of others**, and imagine ourselves divested of all selfish considerations: but, at bottom, the most generous patriot and most greedy miser, the bravest hero and most abject coward, have, in every action, an **equal regard to their own happiness** and welfare.

Contrast: another theory is presented, similar to the first except the offenders act out of selfishness without being conscious of it

Cause and effect: the theory implies that everyone is acting out of a desire to furnish happiness and welfare for themselves whether they know it or not

Whoever concludes from the seeming **tendency of this opinion**, that those, who make profession of it, cannot possibly feel the **true sentiments of benevolence**, or have any regard for genuine virtue, will often find himself, in practice, very much mistaken. Probity and **honour** were no strangers to **Epicurus** and his sect. **Atticus** and **Horace** seem to have enjoyed from nature, and cultivated by reflection, as generous and friendly dispositions as any disciple of the austerer schools. And among the modern, **Hobbes** and **Locke**, who maintained the selfish system of morals, **lived irreproachable lives**; though the former lay not under any restraint of religion which might supply the defects of his philosophy.

Key Terms: Epicurus, Atticus, Horace, Hobbes, Locke

Contrast: Epicurus was apparently an advocate of theories similar to those the author describes above yet acted in seeming discord with his own theories; Hobbes and Locke are similar

Cause and effect: the belief in such theories does not imply that the person will act immorally or not feel nobler emotions

The most obvious objection to the selfish hypothesis is, that, as it is contrary to common feeling and our most unprejudiced notions, there is required the highest stretch of philosophy to establish so extraordinary a **paradox**. To the most careless observer there appear to be such dispositions as **benevolence** and **generosity**; such affections as **love, friendship, compassion, gratitude**. These sentiments have their causes, effects, objects, and operations, marked by common language and observation, and plainly distinguished from those of the selfish passions. And as this is the **obvious appearance of things**, it must be admitted, until some hypothesis be discovered, which by penetrating deeper into human nature, may prove the former affections to be nothing but modifications of the latter.

Opinion: the author believes that it is obvious that benevolence and love exist

Cause and effect: those who believe that no one can act disinterested in their own welfare must account for the apparent expression of love and charity in everyday interactions between people

Main Idea: The main idea of the passage is to present two theories that the author disagrees with and then begin to present problems with the theories and support for his or her own beliefs; the passage deals with interpersonal interactions and the motives for those interactions.

25. D is correct. The first theory is that people purposely fake good will as a means of getting what they want. The second theory is that their good will is still fake and their self-interest is the primary goal but they are not conscious of it.

    A: This is close but the explanation of the second theory is not as good as that in choice D, as the second theory says that people's self-interested behavior may or may not be conscious.

    B, C: Where the qualities come from is not in question.

26. A is correct. The paragraph explains that the theory goes against everyday experience. Thus the burden of proof lies on those who advocate for a theory so seemingly inconsistent with observation.

    B, D: The author does not mention the newness or radicalness of the theory.

    C: The author makes no such argument.

27. D is correct. The question is equivalent to asking which scenario describes one person being kind to another with no apparent benefit to themselves. This is the contradiction of the theories presented.

    A, B, C: All of these can be construed as manifestations of selfish desire.

28. D is correct. This theory resembles closely that presented in the second paragraph which the author seems to reject. The primary reason that the author rejected that theory is for its apparent lack of support from real-world observation.

    A, C: The author would likely disagree with the theory as it is similar to those in the passage.

    B: The author may have this inclination but in the passage he or she does not pretend that any personal inclination is sufficient evidence to disprove a theory.

29. D is correct. The author appears to believe in that which is most apparent to him or her. The ideas surrounding the passage are embedded in simplicity and every-day experience. It is reasonable to suppose that the author would believe that truth can be found without formal evidence, just as he or she had no evidence that the theories in the passage are false but believed the truth could be found in the observation of human interactions.

    A, B: These are similar choices; there is no reason to think that the author would espouse these theories. On the contrary, he or she seems to find truth through observation.

    C: The opposite sentiment is expressed in the passage.

Passage 6 (Questions 30 – 35)

Dr. Donald **Andrews and colleagues** have been developing a body of research aimed at generating principles of effective **correctional treatment**—that is, treatment that can reduce **rearrests** and **reincarcerations** and can help offenders **reintegrate** into society. Andrews and colleagues argue that correctional programs that follow three principles related to **risk**, **criminogenic needs**, and **responsivity** produce the best outcomes. Numerous studies and meta-analyses support the importance of these principles. Developed for correctional populations, the principles apply to the large portion of the **drug-abusing population** that is involved in the criminal justice system.

Opinion: risk, criminogenic needs, and responsivity are three principles important in the correction of the drug-abusing population of prisoners

Cause and effect: Dr. Andrews' treatment will reduce rearrests

The risk principle consists of two elements: (i) clients who are assessed as being at **higher risk** for reoffending are more likely to benefit from treatment than lower-risk clients; and (ii) higher-risk clients should receive **more intensive services** than lower-risk clients. In the work of Andrews and colleagues, "risk" refers to the likelihood of future criminal behavior, but it is reasonable to assume that the principle also holds for drug abuse—that is, offenders with more severe **drug problems** should receive higher intensity treatment, while those at lower risk of relapse should be referred to less intensive programs, such as **drug education**, monitoring through **drug testing**, or **self-help**. Apart from ensuring optimal outcomes, matching problem severity to treatment approach makes for efficient use of scarce treatment resources. What constitutes high and low risk depends on whether the patient is a probationer or parolee and what treatment resources are available. The guidelines for designating clients as at high risk will be tighter in systems where intensive services are in short supply than in systems where they are more available.

Contrast: there are low-severity patients and high-severity patients; their treatments should be different

Cause and effect: higher-risk clients are more likely to benefit from treatment; higher-risk clients should receive more treatment

According to the **criminogenic needs principle**, offenders have many needs, and correctional treatment should focus on those related to **recidivism**. Andrews and colleagues have identified the following **targets as the most promising** for correctional treatment: procriminal attitudes, procriminal associates, impulsivity, risk taking, limited self-control, poor problem-solving skills, poor educational and employment skills, and drug and alcohol dependence. These problems are all **associated with drug abuse as well as recidivism**. Offenders also have **other needs** that may require attention for various reasons, but are not associated with criminal

behavior and have **little or no impact** on recidivism. These include enhancing self-esteem, improving living conditions, and addressing vaguely defined personal or emotional problems. Although **correctional treatment should not focus on these needs**, addiction treatment might benefit from such focus. Determining risk levels and needs requires assessment instruments suitable for identifying crime factors and drug use factors.

Key terms: criminogenic needs principle

Cause and effect: a series of factors are linked to recidivism

Contrast: correctional treatment need not focus on "other needs" but maybe addiction treatment should

Andrews and colleagues describe the **responsivity principle** as concerned with "the selection of styles and modes of service that are (A) **capable of influencing** the specific types of intermediate targets that are set with offenders and (B) **appropriately matched** to the learning styles of offenders." This principle speaks both to the types of treatment that are most appropriate for offenders and to the characteristics of staff who deliver the treatment. The Andrews group argues that the approaches **most appropriate to the learning styles of offenders** include behavioral and social learning techniques such as "modeling, graduated practice, role playing, reinforcement, resource provision, and detailed verbal guidance and explanations (making suggestions, giving reasons, cognitive restructuring)." As for treatment staff, the responsivity principle recommends that they relate to their clients with **warmth**, flexibility, and enthusiasm, but with clear messages about the **unacceptability of procriminal attitudes**, behaviors, and associations.

Cause and effect: the patient should be matched to the type of service that will help the most; the different learning styles of patients necessitates this; likewise, the staff treating patients should be of a certain character to be most effective

Andrews and colleagues developed the risk/needs/responsivity principles from research on treatments for the general population of criminal offenders. In more recent work, the responsivity principle has been extended to apply to the distinctive needs of **women**, **racial/ethnic groups**, and **clients of different ages**. With specific reference to drug-abusing offenders, NIDA recently published research-based principles of treatment for this population The NIDA principles are consistent with the Andrews principles; together, they provide a framework for establishing programs and other interventions that have a high likelihood of reducing drug abuse and its consequences, including associated crime and further involvement in the criminal justice system.

Key Terms: women, racial/ethnic groups, clients of different ages

Contrast: the same principles are applied to the needs of groups defined by gender, ethnicity, and age as well

Main Idea: The main idea of the passage is to present some basic ideas or the outline of some ideas as to how to reduce prisoner rearrests and relapse into drug abuse; the author outlines three concepts that will allow for improvement in this area, they are evaluation of risk, criminogenic needs, and responsivity.

30.   D is correct. The passage states that drug testing and drug education can be used for lower risk patients but higher risk patients will likely need closer attention.

   A: There is no reason to think that the author would advocate using antidepressants as a treatment for drug abuse.

   B, C: Drug testing and drug education can be used for lower risk patients.

31.   C is correct. It is apparent that the overarching theme in the article is preventing relapse of drug use among prisoners and facilitating their reintegration into society.

   A: Violence in prisons is not a main theme of the passage.

   B: Drug abuse in prisons is not as much the main idea as amongst parolees.

   D: Women as a group are not the main focus of the passage.

32.   D is correct. The passage mentions procriminal associations as a factor related to rearrests. The author would agree with the finding but did not claim the same in the passage.

   A, B: The author never states that procriminal association is the biggest factor, so he doesn't have a strong proof either way.

   C: There is no reason to think the author would be skeptical.

33.   A is correct. The paragraph about risk analysis and treatment allocation states that higher-risk clients are more likely to benefit from treatment and thus should receive more intensive services.

   B, C, D: These are all variations on this and are not mentioned directly in the passage.

34.   C is correct. Responsivity as defined by the passage is the principle that the selection of treatment for patients should be matched to the patient.

   A: This is the risk principle.

   B, D: These are not implied by responsivity.

35.   B is correct. The passage deals with a lot of psychological issues associated with prisoners, criminology, and recidivism.

   A, D: Since Dr. Andrews is a Dr. and has done extensive research, he is likely a scholar rather than a politician or criminal justice worker.

   C: There are very few economic concepts mentioned in reference to Dr. Andrews' work.

Passage 7 (Questions 36 – 42)

There are many who acknowledge **Love** to be the **oldest of the gods**, and also the greatest source of benefits to man. I know no greater blessing to a young man at the beginning of his life than a virtuous lover, and in the case of the lover, than a beloved youth. For when we talk about the principle which ought to guide men that would live noble lives, neither kindred, nor honor, nor wealth, **nor any other motive is so able to implant itself as love** is.

Opinion: the greatest blessing a young man at the beginning of his life can have is a virtuous lover, and for the lover, a beloved youth

Contrast: Love vs the rest of the gods (implied, kindred vs honor vs wealth vs love

I am speaking of the sense of honor and dishonor that both states and individuals rely upon to do good or great work. I believe that a lover who is observed in **doing something dishonorable** or else in cowardly submitting when dishonor is done to him, will **be more pained** when **observed by his beloved** then his father, his friends, or anyone else. The beloved also feels this way.

Cause and effect: because of his intimate connection to his beloved, a man who does something dishonorable will be more pained when observed by his lover than even when he is observed by his father or friends

Therefore, if there were some way of **making a state or army made up of lovers**, they would **be the best rulers** of their own state, avoiding all dishonor and emulating each other in honorable activities, and when fighting alongside each other, even if few in number, they could conquer the world. If he were to abandon his post or throw down his arms, what lover would not rather have the whole world observe him than his beloved? Or **who would desert his beloved in a dangerous situation**? The most world's most cowardly **coward** would **become an inspired hero** in such a situation, for Love would inspire him. As Homer says, the god breathes courage into the soul of the hero, so too does Loves infuse his own nature into the soul of the lover.

Contrast: the whole world observing vs the lover observing, world's most cowardly coward vs inspired hero

Cause and effect: if there were a way to make a state or army made up of lovers, they would be the best rulers of their own state, and they would be a great army, respectively; because of the inspiration of Love, the world's most cowardly coward would become an inspired hero if his beloved needed saving from a dangerous situation

Love will make both **men and women dare to die for their beloved**. **Alcestis** is a monument of this, for she was willing to **lay down her life** for her husband when no one else would. Though he had a living mother and father, the tenderness of her love far exceeded theirs and by comparison made them seem to be strangers to their own blood. Her

action was **so noble** that the gods granted her, of all those who have done virtuous deeds, the **rare privilege of returning alive to earth**: such is the honor the gods pay to the devotion and virtue of love.

Cause and effect: because she did it when no one else would, Alcestis is a monument to the fact that both men and women will dare to die for their beloveds; because of the nobility of her actions, the gods granted her the rare privilege of returning alive to earth

On the other hand, they **sent Orpheus away empty-handed**, presenting him only with an apparition of the woman he sought. They would not give her back because **he showed no spirit**: he did not dare to die for love like Alcestis, but rather, planned how he might enter and exit Hades alive. Later, he died at the hands of women, the **gods' punishment for his cowardice**.

Contrast: Orpheus vs Alcestis, planning how to enter and exit Hades alive vs daring to die for love

Cause and effect: because he lacked spirit and had planned how he might safely carry out his mission the gods send Orpheus away empty-handed

Different again was the reward from the gods for the **true love** of **Achilles** towards his lover **Patroclus**. Achilles was well aware, as he had been told by **Thetis**, his mother, that **he might avoid death**, return home, and live well into old age, if he were to **abstain from killing Hector**. Despite this, he **gave his life to revenge Patroclus**, daring to die not only his defense, but after his death as well. For this, **the gods honored him even more** than Alcestis, sending him to the Islands of the Blest.

Key terms: Achilles, Patroclus, Thetis

Cause and effect: if he were to abstain from killing Hector, Achilles would live into old age, because of his actions in the name of love, the gods honored Achilles

For these reasons, I affirm that **Love** is the oldest, noblest, and **mightiest** of the gods, as well as the greatest giver of virtue in life and of happiness in death.

Opinion: the author affirms that love is the oldest, noblest, and mightiest of gods

Main Idea: The author sets out to give anecdotal proof that Love is the oldest of the gods and provides the greatest benefits to man; using more general examples first, he explains how love causes people to act honorably and to shun dishonor; then, he introduces three specific examples, Alcestis, Orpheus, and Achilles, to depict how highly esteemed love is by the gods.

36. D is correct. As the author writes about Achilles at the end of the sixth paragraph, ". . . the gods honored him even more than Alcestis, sending him to the Islands of the Blest." Previously, Alcestis's story had been the example of how the gods honor "the devotion and virtue of love." Achilles managed to do even better.

   A: This is not so much an honor as something that happens to some people.

   B: Likewise, and the passage makes the case that Love is the greatest of the gods, not whoever is responsible for courage.

   C: This is the reward bestowed upon Alcestis, which is surpassed by Achilles.

37. A is correct. As the author writes in the third paragraph, "The world's most cowardly coward would become an inspired hero in such a situation (if his beloved were in a dangerous situation), for Love would inspire him." Surely if the world's most cowardly coward can be inspired to become a hero, surely anyone else can as well.

   B: Rather, that is said to be courage, though there is some truth to this. Choice A is more obvious.

   C: It is not that they are inexcusable, they are just more likely to happen if no lover is observing.

   D: This may be true, but it is not clearly stated.

38. B is correct. The phrase at the beginning of paragraph five, before the introduction of Orpheus, says it all: "On the other hand . . ." His story shows that the gods not only honor the devotion and virtue of love and dislike cowardice, they punish cowardice when it takes the place of love. This story is a foil to that of Alcestis.

   A: This may be true, but the point here is to measure and compare the actions of the gods.

   C: This does become clear, that the gods do not like this behavior, but again, the point here is comparison: Choice B gets that better.

   D: First, it is not clear whether he is not in love or if he is just not deeply enough in love. Second, again, the point is comparison.

39. D is correct. In the second paragraph, the author writes, "I am speaking of the sense of honor and dishonor that both states and individuals rely upon to do good or great work." It is clear from the second and third paragraphs that having a deep love in one's life guides some towards honorable behavior and the shunning of dishonorable behavior. There is no greater blessing to a young man than a virtuous lover because this love will help guide him towards in the direction of an honorable, virtuous life.

   A: It can, but this is not the primary reason why love benefits man.

   B: It can, but again, not the essential reason.

   C: This is not clear. In the passage, it seems that all the gods bestow rewards.

40. B is correct. This is the point made in the second and third paragraphs about how love makes people avoid dishonor and emulate each other in honorable activities. He that is most pained is the man who does dishonor and is observed by his lover. To avoid pain, the man will act honorably, and in such a state, such observance would be constant.

   A: This is not his the essential reason why such a state would be ideal, that being the actual observance of each other by lovers.

   C: Again, misses the essential reason.

   D: This point is never made that this state would go so far as to make the whole world like it. Rather, it would in itself function honorably.

41. A is correct. This is not true, because Orpheus's love of his life would seem to have been greater than the love he held for his beloved, especially in comparison to Alcestis and Achilles.

   B, C, D: All are true.

42. C is correct. I: Acting honorably would seem to be always choice-worthy. Love works as a guide in making people act honorably and nobly. This is how it bestows benefits. II: This choice gets it right, as does Item III, as far as how much the gods honor daring to die for love.

Passage 8 (Questions 43 – 49)

Roman law defined **property** as the **right to use and abuse** one's own within the limits of the law - *jus utendi et abutendi re sua, guatenus juris ratio patitur*. Of course there have been those to attempt the **justification** of the word **abuse**, on the grounds that it signifies absolute domain rather than senseless and immoral abuse. What a **vain distinction**! It is a distinction made as an excuse for property and it is powerless against the frenzy of possession, which it neither can prevent nor restrain. If he so chooses, the proprietor may allow his crops to rot, he may sow his fields with salt, milk his cows on sand, transform his vineyard into desert, and use his vegetable-garden as a park. Do these things constitute abuse? In terms of property, **use and abuse are inevitably indistinguishable**.

Cause and effect: if he so chooses, the proprietor can abuse his lands, crops, or livestock as much as he so desires; because of all this, in terms of property, use and abuse are necessarily indistinguishable

According to the **Declaration of Rights** that serves as a **preface** to **the Constitution of '93**, property is "**the right to enjoy and dispose at will** of **one's goods**, **one's income**, and **the fruit of one's labor and industry**." Moreover, as **Code Napoleon, article 544** reads, "Property is the right to enjoy and dispose of things in **the most absolute manner**, provided we do not overstep **the limits prescribed by the laws and regulations**." These two **definitions** do not differ all from that of Roman law: they give the proprietor **absolute right** over a thing, and as for the **restriction** imposed by these codes, provided the limits prescribed by laws and regulations are not overstepped, its purpose is not to limit property, but rather, to prevent **the domain** of one proprietor from interfering with that of another. As such, this law serves not as a **limitation** of **the principle**, but rather, a **confirmation** of it.

Key terms: Declaration of Rights, preface, the Constitution of '93, Code Napoleon article 544

Contrast: restrictions limiting property vs preventing the domain of one proprietor from interfering with that of another, limitation of the principle vs confirmation of it

Cause and effect: because they give a proprietor absolute right over a thing and do not limit property, but prevent the domain of one proprietor from interfering with that of another, the French definitions of property do not differ from that of Roman law; because of this, law does not limit the principle of property, but rather, confirms it

There are **two types** of property. The first is property pure and simple, the **dominant power** over a thing, sometimes referred to as **naked property**. The second is **possession**. As Duranton says, "Possession is a **matter of fact**, not of **right**." Toullier agrees: "Property is a right, a **legal power**; possession is a fact." The **tenant**, the **farmer**, and the **usufructuary** are **possessors**. The **owner** who lets and lends for use and the **heir** who will come into possession upon the death of a

usufructuary are **proprietors**. If I may venture a comparison to assist in understanding: a lover is a possessor and a spouse is a proprietor. This **double definition** of property, domain versus possession, is of the highest importance and it must be understood clearly in order to comprehend what is to follow.

Contrast: naked property vs possession, matter of fact vs matter of right, legal power vs fact, tenant and farmer and usufructuary vs owner and heir

From this **notable distinction** arise **two kinds of rights**. The **jus in re** is **the right in a thing**, the right by which one may reclaim the property one has acquired from whatever hands one finds it in. The **jus ad rem** is **the right to a thing**, giving one a **claim** to **become** a proprietor. Therefore, the right of **married partners** over each other's person is the jus in re, while that of two who are **betrothed** is the jus ad rem. In the former, possession and property are one in the same, but the latter includes only possession. As I am a **laborer**, I have the right to possession of the **products of nature** and **my own industry**, and as I am a **proletaire**, I enjoy none of them. As such, it is by virtue of the jus ad rem that I demand **access** to the jus in re.

Key terms: jus in re, jus ad rem, proletaire

Contrast: jus in re vs jus ad rem, the right in a thing vs the right of a thing, the right to reclaim property that has been taken vs the right to claim to be a proprietor

Main Idea: The author sets out to demonstrate that Roman law and French law both have property laws that are troublesome, with use and abuse indistinguishable; the author divides property into two sorts: naked property and possession, the first of which being a right, accompanying the jus in re, the second of which being a fact, accompanying the jus ad rem; the author makes the case that he has the jus ad rem to his own industry and the products of nature, but is denied the jus in re due to the current system regarding property.

43. B is correct. At the start of the passage, the author tells us that some attempt to defend the word "abuse" in relation to property by noting that it signifies absolute power over a thing and does not refer to senseless, abusive treatment of the thing. They seem to acknowledge that senseless maltreatment of a thing would be a bad form of abuse, but that in this context the word doesn't mean that sort of treatment.

44. A is correct. In the third paragraph, the first type of property is defined as "property pure and simple" and "the dominant power over a thing," which is "referred to as naked property." The second type, however, is not defined by the author. Instead, the quotes from Duranton and Toullier serve to provide a definition of possession. "Possession is a matter of fact, not right." This statement contrasts possession to the first definition, which is a right. Toiler's statement poses property against possession in order to elucidate possession, as property has already been defined for us.

   B: This doesn't seem necessary. Moreover, evidence is not being given, but definitions are.

   C: The argument has not yet become as personal as it will in the very final lines of the passage.

45. B is correct. The author ends the passage by writing, "I demand access to the jus in re." He has the jus ad rem as a laborer, but not the jus in re. So, he has the right of claiming himself a proprietor, but does not get to enjoy the things he has a right to possess because he is a proletaire. The assumption is that he would be able to actually enjoy these things if he had the jus in re in addition to the jus ad rem.

   A: Vice versa

   C: In jus in re, possession and property are one and the same. In jus ad rem, there's only naked property. Therefore, jus in re is more complete, and therefore more desirable.

   D: There is never a conversation about whether these two kinds of rights are necessary or not, but the author definitely treats them as important. He doesn't wish them to go away. Rather, he desires both.

46. D is correct. The distinction mentioned refers to the attempt to justify the word "abuse," arguing that it refers to absolute domain rather than senseless abuse. However, this distinction cannot keep the frenzy of possession from wreaking havoc, examples of which are given. The author asks if these things constitute abuse (and it is seemingly a rhetorical question). The author finds use and abuse, ultimately, to be indistinguishable as far as property goes.

   A: This is never said and is much too broad.

   B: Rather, people do, calling the word "abuse" absolute domain rather than senseless misuse.

   C: This is perhaps true, but has nothing to do with why the distinction is vain.

47. B is correct. "The right of married partners over each other's person is the jus in re . . ."

48. B is correct. Choice B is false because proprietors seem to have full rein when it comes to how they abuse their property. The author describes no instance in which abuse of property can be curtailed or punished.

49. B is correct. II is true because a proprietor can do anything to his crops and possessions.

   I: This is false because there are laws and regulations that "prevent the domain of one proprietor from interfering with that of another." Basically, they protect property from others, not from proprietors.

   III: This is false because we know that spouses fall under property, domain, and jus in re. A man cannot take another man's property.

Passage 9 (Questions 50 – 53)

In its early days, **socialism** was a revolutionary movement of which the object was the liberation of the **wage-earning** classes and the establishment of freedom and justice. The passage from **capitalism** to the new régime was to be sudden and violent: capitalists were to be expropriated without compensation, and their power was not to be replaced by any new authority.

Key terms: socialism, wage-earning classes, capitalism

Opinion: some thought socialism was supposed to be a sudden and violent shift of power away from capitalism

Gradually a change came over the spirit of socialism. In France, socialists became **members of the government**, and made and unmade **parliamentary majorities**. In Germany, social democracy grew so strong that it became impossible for it to resist the temptation to **barter away some of its intransigence** in return for government recognition of its claims. In England, the Fabians taught the advantage of reform as against revolution, and of conciliatory bargaining as against irreconcilable antagonism.

Key terms: members of the government, parliamentary majorities

Contrast: there was a change made in the socialist movement towards gradual reform; socialist ideals began to take hold in legislative bodies

The method of **gradual reform** has many merits as compared to the method of **revolution**, and I have no wish to preach revolution. But gradual reform has **certain dangers**, to wit, the ownership or control of businesses hitherto in private hands, and by encouraging **legislative interference** for the benefit of various sections of the wage-earning classes. I think it is at least doubtful whether such measures do anything at all to contribute toward the ideals which inspired the early socialists and still inspire the great majority of those who advocate some form of socialism.

Key terms: gradual reform, revolution, certain dangers, legislative interference

Opinion: the author is of the opinion that gradual reform towards socialism is no better than revolution and that it will not lead to the benefit of the society

Contrast: gradual reform is contrasted to revolution

Cause and effect: gradual reform will lead to legislative interference for the benefit of some sections of the wage-earning class, but will not contribute toward the ideals which inspired early socialists

Let us take as an illustration such a measure as state **purchase of railways**. This is a typical object of state socialism, thoroughly practicable, already achieved in many countries, and clearly the sort of step that must be taken in any piecemeal approach to complete **collectivism**. Yet I see no reason to believe that any **real advance** toward **democracy, freedom,** or **economic justice** is achieved when a state takes over the railways after full compensation to the shareholders.

Key terms: purchase of railways, collectivism, real advance, democracy, freedom, economic justice

Opinion: the author believes that the state purchase of railways will lead to no advance in economic justice if the shareholders are fully compensated for it

Cause and effect: the state's purchase of railways is a clear step towards socialism

Economic justice demands a diminution, if not a total abolition, of the proportion of the national income which goes to the recipients of rent and interest. But when the holders of railway shares are given **government stock** to replace their shares, they are given the prospect of an income in perpetuity equal to what they might reasonably expect to have derived from their shares. Unless there is reason to expect a great increase in the earnings of railways, the whole operation does **nothing to alter the distribution of wealth**. This could only be effected if the present owners were expropriated, or paid less than the market value, or given a mere life-interest as compensation. When full value is given, **economic justice is not advanced** in any degree.

Key terms: government stock, nothing to alter the distribution of wealth, economic justice is not advanced

Opinion: the author believes that paying the previous railroad owners with government stock is equivalent to allowing them the economic advantage they would have had owning the railroad

Cause and effect: the author states that only if the railway shareholders are underpaid in the purchase will there be some just distribution of wealth

There is equally little advance toward **freedom**. The men employed on the railway have no more voice than they had before in the management of the railway, or in the **wages** and **conditions of work**. Instead of having to fight the directors, with the possibility of an appeal to the government, they now have to fight the government directly; and experience does not lead to the view that **a government department has any special tenderness toward the claims of labor**. If they strike, they have to contend against the whole organized power of the state, which they can only do successfully if they happen to have a strong **public opinion** on their side. In view of the influence which the state can always exercise on the press, public opinion is likely to be biased against them, particularly when a nominally progressive government is in power. There will no longer be the possibility of **divergences** between the policies of different railways. Railway men in England derived advantages for many years from the comparatively liberal policy of the North Eastern Railway, which they were able to use as an argument for a similar policy elsewhere. Such possibilities are excluded by the **dead uniformity** of state administration.

Key terms: freedom, wages, conditions of work, public opinion, divergences, dead uniformity

Opinion: the author believes that state purchase of railways will lead to more difficulties in railway workers being heard

Cause and effect: overall, when the state controls an aspect of the economy, the author would argue that the lack of divergence between competing businesses will lead to a loss of freedom and advancement, i.e. "dead uniformity"

And there is no real advance toward **democracy**. The administration of the railways will be in the hands of officials whose bias and associations **separate them from labor**, and who will develop an autocratic temper through the habit of power. The democratic machinery by which these officials are nominally controlled is cumbrous and remote, and can only be brought into operation on first-class issues which rouse the **interest of the whole nation**. Even then it is very likely that the superior education of the **officials** and the government, combined with the advantages of their position, will enable them to **mislead the public** as to the issues, and alienate the general sympathy even from the most excellent cause.

Key terms: democracy, separate them from labor, interest of the whole nation

Cause and effect: the state control of goods will not advance democracy; the government is too distant from the people and the issues they face

I do not deny that these evils exist at present; I say only that they will **not** be **remedied** by such measures as the **nationalization** of **railways** in the present economic and political environment. **A greater upheaval**, and a greater change in men's habits of mind, is necessary **for any really vital progress**.

Opinion: the author seems to think that a socialist revolution is preferable to gradual reform because "a greater upheaval" is necessary

Contrast: the author admits that the issues he or she described are not unique to socialist governments

Main Idea: The main idea of the passage is to explain the change that occurred in the socialist movement from revolution to reform and some of the results that come of gradual socialist reform; the author is arguing that socialist reform is not effective in distributing wealth, espousing freedom, or promoting democracy.

50. A is correct. The passage states that the idea of a socialist revolution gave way to gradual reform and introduction of socialist ideas into legislation.

    B: The author does not discuss, and seems to have no particular interest in the executive branch of government.

    C: The change in socialist movement was not that their ideals changed, but that the violent revolution gave way to gradual reform.

    D: The author doesn't mention how long capitalism has been around in any given country.

51. D is correct. The passage states that wealth will not be redistributed unless the original railway owners are expropriated of their property, that is, not compensated fully.

52. B is correct. The passage states that government control of industry would only lead to increased difficulties for workers in being heard. One reason that the author gives for this is that history has shown that governments have no special tenderness toward the claims of labor.

    A: The opposite is argued in the passage.

    C: There is little connection between this and the question stem.

    D: It would not disagree with this statement.

53. C is correct. The author states that in a revolution "capitalists were to be expropriated without compensation" and later states that when gradual reform occurs, the capitalists are compensated fully for their losses which means economic justice will not be served.

    A: The author never makes this argument.

    B: There is no mention of this in the discussion of the idea of socialist revolution.

    D: The author does not mention this either.

SECTION 11

53 Questions, 90 Minutes

Use an answer grid from the back of the book to record your answers

Passage 1 (Questions 1 – 5)

Obesity is a major contributor to serious health conditions in children and adults, including type 2 diabetes, cardiovascular disease, many cancers, and numerous other diseases and conditions. As rates of obesity have soared in the past three decades, it is clear that increasing the number of people who can achieve and maintain a healthy weight is a critical public health goal, although one that faces formidable challenges. Reducing the prevalence of obesity and its associated medical conditions will require broad-based efforts—by government, the private and nonprofit sectors, businesses, community organizations, healthcare professionals, schools, families, and individuals. The foundation of such efforts is research to illuminate the causes and consequences of obesity, to develop and evaluate new prevention and treatment strategies to see what works, and to determine how to implement and expand promising approaches to reach those who could most benefit.

New research will define potential candidates for new drug development, inform the development of more effective lifestyle interventions that better reflect the biologic underpinnings of people's behaviors, and open novel avenues for prevention and treatment strategies for obesity and its associated diseases. This research encompasses opportunities in genetics, neuroscience, metabolism, cell biology, and other areas that will improve our understanding of fundamental biologic pathways involved in weight regulation—and what goes awry in obesity.

A wide range of other factors may influence obesity, in addition to the biological factors addressed in the previous paragraph. Research ought to explore these behavioral, social, cultural, and environmental factors, which span multiple interacting levels. A better understanding of such factors can enhance the design of intervention, surveillance, and translation strategies. Research focused on the consequences of obesity can inform health care and policy, and identify population subgroups most affected by obesity and critical periods for weight gain, both of which can be used to target intervention and translation efforts.

An array of research opportunities are outlined that can further advance obesity prevention and management through carefully designed and evaluated interventions. These research areas encompass behavioral and environmental approaches to lifestyle change, from individual- and family-based to community-wide strategies, as well as surgical interventions. Because no single approach is likely to be appropriate for everyone, research to evaluate multiple and diverse approaches in many different settings will yield a broader empirical basis for individual and public health changes. In addition to identifying successful interventions for achieving a healthier weight, this research may also reduce the onset or severity of obesity-associated conditions and improve quality of life.

Advances in obesity research depend on accurate tools and measurements to enhance understanding of etiology and allow for evaluation of interventions. Examples of research opportunities include the development of biomarkers; designing tools to better assess food intake, fitness, functional status, and thermogenesis; improving imaging methods; advancing technologies for determining body composition; and developing objective measurement systems to better evaluate changes in policy and environments. Also highlighted are emerging methodologies to enable researchers to better capture and model complex relationships in obesity.

1.   Which of the following is LEAST likely to be advocated by the author?

   A. Research into the biological foundations of obesity

   B. Research into the behavioral and sociological triggers of obesity

   C. Research into the development of weight-loss medication

   D. Research into obesity interventions and their implementation in society

2.   With which of the following statements would the author most likely agree?

   A. The fight against obesity must begin with individuals and families.

   B. The fight against obesity must be spearheaded by a better understanding of the biological underpinnings of obesity.

   C. The fight against obesity will be most successful when approached from the top down, with government taking the lead.

   D. The sociological, preventative, and educational sides of obesity intervention are the most important in the fight against obesity.

3.   Suppose it were discovered that where someone lives is the biggest social determining factor of whether or not they are obese. How would the author react to this information?

   A. The author would doubt its authenticity because it goes against reason.

   B. The author would welcome the information and attempt to implement it into social interventions.

   C. The author would bemoan receiving the information and advocate that people move out of high obesity areas.

   D. The author would doubt its authenticity because it contradicts his own research.

4.   Suppose it were discovered that the leading cause of diabetes is not obesity. How would this affect the author's claims and the validity of the author's ideas?

   A. It would not weaken the argument that obesity is a major contributor to serious health conditions.

   B. It would weaken the argument that obesity is a major contributor to serious health conditions.

   C. It would weaken the argument that reducing the prevalence of obesity and its associated medical conditions will require broad-based efforts.

   D. It would strengthen the argument that reducing the prevalence of obesity and its associated medical conditions will require broad-based efforts.

5.   Which of the following is most likely a statement the author would make?

   A. Because obesity is a multifaceted problem, the plan outlines a multifaceted research agenda.

   B. We must aim all our efforts at studies focusing on populations at disproportionate risk for obesity and its consequences.

   C. Through the efforts of similar research plans in the past 30 years, the average American BMI has decreased.

   D. Obesity is an common medical disorder with what can be uncommonly mild consequences.

Passage 2 (Questions 6 – 10)

In August 2013, a group of protesters gathered in Los Angeles to rally against the Listening and Spoken Language Symposium, an event sponsored by the Alexander Graham Bell Institute for the Deaf and Hard of Hearing. The protesters were deaf, and many of the exhibitors at the symposium represented or were affiliated with companies that sold cochlear implants; a recent technological development, cochlear implants are surgically-implanted electronic devices that can provide a deaf or hard of hearing person with some degree of hearing. Cochlear implants can be implanted in babies, children, and adults. While the implants cannot restore normal hearing, they can give many users increased ability to receive auditory signals.

The protest reflected a deeply controversial subject among deaf people: the promotion of "oralism," an educational stance which supports the teaching of lip-reading and oral speech to children who are deaf or hard of hearing, and de-emphasizes or eliminates the teaching of American Sign Language (ASL). To the people at the rally – Deaf activists and their supporters – proponents of oralism are guilty of what Deaf activists call "audism" – the belief that it is inherently better to hear than to be deaf, and that deafness is a disability rather than a difference. Cochlear implants, they believe, promote the idea that deaf people need "fixing." At root is whether one sees deafness as a disability or as a culture; some people describe this as self-identifying as deaf, with a small "d," or as Deaf, with a capital "D." Some deaf or hard of hearing people note that it is difficult for hearing people to understand why a deaf or hard of hearing person would not embrace the opportunity to hear and participate as fully as possible in the oral world. But to those who identify as Deaf, ASL use is a key part of their culture. Deaf people who use ASL share a language, history, social framework, and community identity. Asking a deaf person, they say, to give up their Deaf identity is like asking any other person of an ethnic or cultural minority to renege on their deep cultural connections. Thus, audism is a form of cultural disrespect and discrimination.

AG Bell has a long and complex relationship with the people it serves. Its founder, Alexander Graham Bell, was important in the spread of oralism as the dominant paradigm for educating deaf children. Bell, whose mother and wife were both deaf, believed that deaf people needed to assimilate into hearing culture; he advocated that the deaf population should relinquish sign language, and eliminate separate schools, social clubs, and publications for the deaf. Deaf advocates criticize Bell's beliefs as overtly hostile, and credit his actions as leading to a lengthy dark period in which deaf children had little or no contact with other deaf people, lived with families that were non-signing, and were often presumed to be stupid – situations that were difficult and damaging. Today, though, AG Bell considers itself an advocacy group for deaf people, and asserts that providing information on cochlear implants is one aspect of that advocacy. On their website, they state that their goal is "to ensure that every child and adult with hearing loss has the opportunity to listen, talk and thrive in mainstream society." To some Deaf activists, though, assimilation in mainstream society is not the goal; more essential is having pride in and a sense of belonging to a rich, vibrant, and distinct culture.

6. Why might the author describe AG Bell's relationship with the people it serves as "complex"?

   A. Whether one considers its longstanding promotion of oralism in the best interests of deaf individuals depends on one's viewpoints on assimilation and deaf identity.

   B. AG Bell has vacillated throughout its history between promoting use of oral language and advocating for the primacy of ASL.

   C. Despite his purported advocacy for deaf people, AG Bell's founder, Alexander Graham Bell, was clearly hostile to the community he served.

   D. The majority of deaf people view AG Bell as a supportive institution, but Deaf activists criticize its promotion of oralism.

7. A person who identifies as deaf would most likely take which view of cochlear implants?

   A. The implants may represent a helpful communication tool for those who use them.

   B. Because the implants are visible, they further divide deaf users from mainstream society.

   C. The development of cochlear implants is another instance of audism.

   D. Cochlear implants, though seemingly helpful, are actually destructive to Deaf culture.

8. Suppose a secondary school had a policy of educating its deaf and hard of hearing students in bilingual ASL/English classes. What might a Deaf activist think about this education model?

   A. Most likely that it is positive, because it promotes the learning of ASL.

   B. Most likely that it is positive, because it increases the chances that students will thrive in mainstream hearing society.

   C. Most likely that it is misguided, because Deaf activists do not believe in communication through non-ASL languages.

   D. Most likely that it is misguided, since such classes tend to alienate students from both hearing and deaf communities.

9. Of the following, which best explains why Deaf refers to a unique culture?

   A. Deaf people experience discrimination in the same way that other minorities do.

   B. Unless deaf people self-advocate, they are not recognized as belonging to a valid cultural group.

   C. Deaf culture shares many features with other oppressed groups.

   D. Deaf culture has a distinct language, history, literary tradition, and shared institutions.

10. Based on information in the passage, how might a representative of AG Bell refute a Deaf activist's critique of that institution's promotion of cochlear implants?

   A. By asserting that Deaf activists represent a small minority of deaf and hard of hearing people

   B. By suggesting that use of cochlear implants is a form of advocacy and self-empowerment

   C. By denying that oralism implies the superiority of spoken language

   D. By emphasizing that only a small percentage of people eligible for cochlear implants actually get them

Passage 3 (Questions 11 – 17)

Michelangelo's Moses is seated, his body faces forward, his head, with its mighty beard, looks to the left, his right foot touches the ground, and his left leg is raised such that only the toes touch the ground. His right arm connects the Tables of the Law, which contain the Ten Commandments, with part of his beard while his left arm lies in his lap, pressing his beard against his body. At this point, if I were to give a more detailed description of the statue, I would be preempting what I want to say later on. I should mention that the descriptions of this figure given by other writers are curiously unsuitable: that which has not been understood has been perceived inaccurately.

Grimm writes that the right hand, "under whose arm the Tables rest, grasps his beard," Lübke writes, "Profoundly shaken, he grasps with his right hand his magnificent streaming beard," and Springer writes that "Moses presses the left hand against his body, and thrusts the other, as though unconsciously, into the mighty locks of his beard." On the other hand, Justi believes that the fingers of his right hand were playing with his beard "as an agitated man nowadays might play with his watch-chain." Müntz believes this as well. A further step removed, Thode writes of the "calm, firm posture of the right hand upon the Tables resting against his side." He does not sense any excitement in the statue, even in the right hand. And as Jakob Burckhardt complains, "The celebrated left arm has no other function than to press his beard to his body."

Seeing as these mere descriptions do not agree, we are not surprised to find a myriad of divergent views as to the meaning of the statute and its various features. In my opinion, the facial expression of this Moses is best characterized by Thode, who sees it as "a mixture of wrath, pain, and contempt . . . wrath in his threatening contracting brows, pain in his glance, and contempt in his protruded under lip and in the down-drawn corners of his mouth."

Of course, other admirers have seen with other eyes. As Dupaty writes, "His august brow seems to be but a transparent veil only half concealing his great mind." Lubke completely disagrees, stating that "one would look in vain in that head for an expression of higher intelligence; his down-drawn brow speaks nothing but a capacity for infinite wrath and an all-compelling energy." Differing even more, Guillaume sees no emotion in the face at all, "only a proud simplicity, an inspired dignity, a living faith. The eye of Moses looks into the future, he foresees the lasting survival of his people and the immutability of his law." Müntz agrees with Guillame, writing that "the eyes of Moses rove far beyond the race of men. They are turned towards those mysteries which he alone has seen." As Steinmann writes, this Moses is "no longer the stern Law-giver, no longer the terrible enemy of sin, armed with the wrath of Jehovah, but the royal priest, whom age may not approach, beneficent and prophetic, with the reflection of eternity upon his brow, taking his last farewell of his people."

There are even those who claim the Moses of Michelangelo says nothing at all (and who are honest enough to admit to it). As one critic wrote in the *Quarterly Review* of 1858, "There is an absence of meaning in the general conception, which precludes the idea of a self-fulfilling whole." What is more astonishing is that there are others who find nothing to admire in the statue and who actually revolt against it, complaining of its brutality and the animal cast of the head.

Did the master fashion such a vague, ambiguous script in stone such that all of these different readings could possibly be true?

11. Which of the following physical descriptions of the statue of Moses is true?

    A. Only his left hand touches his beard.

    B. His right leg is significantly raised.

    C. Only the toes of his left foot touch the ground.

    D. His right arm lies in his lap, pressing his beard to his body.

12. Based upon the passage, whch of the following is the likeliest reason why the author included opinions from so many different writers?

    A. To prove the relative ineptitude of most writers in assessing great works of art

    B. To set up the last sentence of the passage with real world examples.

    C. To demonstrate the great academic and critical vigor that Michelangelo's work inspires

    D. To make the case that Michelangelo was the greatest master of art to have lived

13. Which of the following writers believes both that Moses was playing with his beard and that he was looking beyond men towards the holy mysteries?

    A. Guillame

    B. Lübke

    C. Justi

    D. Müntz

14. Based upon the passage, which of the following statements about the statue of Moses is the author most likely to believe?

    A. The figure of the statue is characterized by a complex mix of thoughts and feelings.

    B. The figure of the statue is more preoccupied with spiritual concerns than human concerns.

    C. The figure of the statue possesses an infinite capacity for wrath and the punishment of his followers.

    D. The figure of the statue seems to lack the qualities that would make it a self-sufficing whole.

15. Suppose there are two writers that the author forgot to mention in his passage. They both believe that the statue represents Moses after returning from Mount Sinai. However, they differ in regard to how Moses is changed by this experience. The first writer believes that Moses has been calmed by the experience while the second believes that Moses has been thoroughly shaken up by his encounter with God. These two writers, respectively, are most similar to which of the following two writers that are mentioned in the passage.

    A. Steinmann and Thode

    B. Steinmann and Lübke

    C. Lübke and Steinmann

    D. Guillame and Müntz

16. All of the following are feelings attributed to the statue in the passage EXCEPT:

    A. contempt.

    B. calm.

    C. fear.

    D. beneficence.

17. Which of the following statements accurately reflect Müntz's opinions about the statue?

    I. The figure may be agitated.

    II. The figure's face betrays no emotion.

    III. The figure is preoccupied with his encounter with God.

    A. III only

    B. I and III only

    C. II and III only

    D. I, II, and III

Passage 4 (Questions 18 – 24)

How great a virtue is temperance, how important it is throughout a whole man's life! Yet God commits the management of this great trust, without specific laws or prescriptions, entirely to the demeanor of every grown man. For those actions that enter into a man and do not issue out of him, therefore defiling him not, God does not keep man captive under a perpetual childhood, but trusts him with the gift of reason to be his own chooser. There would be little need left for preaching if law were to govern those things previously governed only by moral encouragement.

Solomon informs us that reading too much is weariness to the flesh, but neither he nor any other inspired author tells us that reading is unlawful. If God had wanted to limit us in this regard, it would have been more expedient to have told us what was unlawful than what was wearisome. As far as the burning of the Ephesian books by St. Paul's converts, it is said that the books were magic tomes, used for sorcery. It was a private, voluntary act: the remorseful men burnt their own books where another man may perhaps have read them in some useful way.

We know that good and evil grow up together in this world, almost inseparably, and that the knowledge of good is so interwoven with the knowledge of evil, and in many cunning resemblances is hardly to be discerned, that those scattered seeds which Psyche was given the incessant labor of culling out and sorting were not more intermixed. From the rind of one apple, the knowledge of good and evil, as two twins cleaving together, leapt forth into the world. This is that doom that Adam fell into, knowing both good and evil, or rather, knowing good by evil. Generations hence, what wisdom can there be to chose or forbear without the knowledge of evil? The person that can apprehend and reflect upon vice, with all her seeming pleasures, and yet abstain, distinguishing and preferring that which is truly better, is a true warfaring Christian.

I cannot praise a cloistered virtue, unexercised and unbreathed, that never sets out and sees her adversary, but rather, slinks out of the race in which that immortal garland is to be run for. Certainly we do not bring innocence into the world, for we much more likely bring impurity: that which purifies us is a trial, and trial is by whatever is contrary. Therefore, that virtue which is young in the contemplation of evil, that knows not what vice promises to her followers, and rejects it, is but a blank virtue, not a pure one.

This is why our sage and serious poet Spenser, whom I would dare to claim as a better teacher than Scotus or Aquinas, described true temperance with the character of Guion, bringing him through the cave of Mammon, the bower of earthly bliss, that he might see and abstain. Because knowing vice is so necessary to the constitution of human virtue, and the scanning of error to the confirmation of truth, how can we better scout into the regions of sin and falsity than by reading all kinds of tractates and by hearing all kinds of

reason and opinion? This is the benefit afforded us by books promiscuously read.

18. Based upon the passage, which of the following statements are likely true?

   I. The "race" in the fourth paragraph refers to the pursuit of temperance.

  II. Sin and falsity are better exposed by a narrow, specific, and steadfast worldview.

 III. The warfaring Christian is truly an exemplar of temperance.

  A. III only

  B. I and III only

  C. II and III only

  D. I, II, and III

19. According to the passage, which of the following best describes the burning of the Ephesian books?

  A. The burning of the books was part of their conversion process.

  B. Paul required his converts to burn their sorcery books.

  C. People converted by Paul decided to burn their books themselves.

  D. Paul encouraged those he converted to burn their sorcery books.

20. Based upon the passage, which of the following does the author most likely believe about Solomon?

  A. He was the wisest king portrayed in the Bible.

  B. God spoke through him to the people.

  C. He thought reading was a heathenish distraction.

  D. He was as prolific a reader as he was a writer.

21. Based upon the passage, which of the following best describes a blank virtue?

  A. It is immature.

  B. It is untested.

  C. It is misguided.

  D. It is indicative of a warfaring Christian.

22. In what way does the author use the allusion to Psyche to further his argument?

  A. He describes the difficulty of differentiating good and evil by claiming it as difficult as Psyche's task.

  B. He describes the virtue of differentiating good and evil by juxtaposing it to Psyche's task.

  C. He describes the pleasure of differentiating good and evil by referencing Psyche, goddess of pleasure.

  D. He compares Psyche's task to the burning of the Ephesian books, furthering the point made at the end of the second paragraph.

23. Say the author is tutoring a new private pupil, a precocious, curious, yet troublemaking boy of 14 years old. Which of the following would the author most encourage his student to do?

  A. Expose himself to earthly pleasures like those found in the cave of Mammon.

  B. Commit himself to a task as tedious yet edifying as Psyche's.

  C. Read a vast array of books that challenge his current understanding.

  D. Read a lot, but not too much, so as not to weary the flesh.

24. Based upon the passage, all of the following statements about temperance are true EXCEPT:

  A. it may be encouraged through voracious reading.

  B. not all grown people have the potential to possess it.

  C. it must be tested by vices to be full.

  D. it is difficult to maintain.

Passage 5 (Questions 25 – 30)

Before inquiring into which type of government is best, one ought to first determine what way of living is best. Provided that no accidents interfere, it is most likely that those who enjoy the best government will also live the happiest, best lives according to their circumstances. Therefore, one ought to know what way of living is most desirable, and then afterwards, whether this best life for man in general is the same for man as citizen.

What is good in relation to man can be divided into three sorts: that which is external, that which pertains to the body, and that which pertains to the soul. All three sorts must conspire together, for no one would claim that a man was happy if he had no fortitude, no temperance, no justice, or no prudence, if he shuddered in fear from flies, if he committed a crime to satisfy his hunger or thirst, if he murdered his friend for a farthing, and if he was feeble or wanting in his mind, as a child or a madman.

Some people may dispute this, citing quantity and degree: they may think that a small amount of virtue is sufficient for happiness, but when it comes to riches, property, power, and honors, that men ought to strive to increase these things without bounds in pursuit of the best life. On the contrary, experience teaches us that external goods do not produce virtue, but virtue produces them.

As far as the happy life goes, whether it is to be found in pleasure, virtue, or both, it is certain that those whose morals are most pure, and who are most cultivated in mind and character, will enjoy more of it, even though their external fortunes are moderate next to those who possess mountains of wealth yet are deficient in the higher qualities. After thorough reflection, this is clear, for all that is external has its limit, like any instrument or machine, and all things that are external and useful are of such a nature that when there is an excess in or of them, they either do harm, or at the very best, become useless to the possessor. But for every good quality of the soul, the higher it is in degree, the more useful it is, and the more noble.

When we are comparing things with one another, the best state of each particular thing corresponds in excellence to the distance in quality between the things themselves. So, if the soul is more noble than our possessions and our bodies in both absolute and relative terms, it must be admitted that the best states of these things necessarily stand in the same relation to one another as the things do themselves. Again, it is for the sake of the soul that external and bodily goods are desirable at all, and so, the wise man chooses them for the sake of the soul, not the soul for the sake of them.

Let us accept that every person enjoys as much happiness as he or she possesses virtue and wisdom, and as much as he or she behaves according to their dictates. God himself exemplifies this, for he is completely happy, not from possessing external goods, but in himself and by virtue of his nature. Here lies the difference between good fortune and happiness: every external good owes itself in some degree to chance or fortune, but it is not from chance or fortune that someone becomes wise or just. It follows that the happiest, best city is the one that is best and acts the best, for no one does well that doesn't act well, and the deeds of both a man and a city cannot be worthy of praise without virtue and wisdom. In this way, the things that are just, wise, and prudent in a person are the same things that are just, wise, and prudent in a city.

25. All of the following statements about external goods are true EXCEPT:

   A. they are never more useful than even the most minute amount of good qualities of the soul.

   B. they are useful to their possessor until they exceed a particular limit.

   C. when they have exceeded their limit, they can only be harmful or useless.

   D. they are like instruments or machines, working properly only within limits.

26. According to the passage, the three types of goods in relation to man must conspire together to make a person happy, but those that dispute this claim say that:

   A. people ought to have more bodily goods than goods of the soul.

   B. people only need few external goods but ought to acquire more goods of the soul.

   C. people ought to have more goods of the soul than external goods.

   D. people only need few goods of the soul but ought to acquire more external goods.

27. According to the passage, why should we investigate the best way of living before investigating the best way of governing?

   A. Because it is likely that the best city is the one with the best people born into it

   B. Because it is likely that the people who live the best lives live in the best city

   C. Because a city essentially functions like a person, structurally and spiritually

   D. Because the aim of government is to create conditions for the best life possible

28. Why does the author introduce the example of God?

   A. To demonstrate the direct relationship between possessing virtue and wisdom and possessing happiness

   B. To demonstrate that what is just, prudent, and wise in a man is just, prudent, and wise in a city

   C. To demonstrate that there are no limits attached to goods of the soul like there are to external goods

   D. To demonstrate that man created the notion of God in order to represent the best life possible

29. Based upon the passage, it can be inferred that the author most believes which of the following statements about living the best life?

   A. People ought to pursue the cultivation of their mind and character only after they have acquired enough external and bodily goods to become self-sufficient.

   B. People ought to pursue the cultivation of their mind and character to a degree proportionate to their pursuit of external and bodily goods.

   C. People ought to pursue the cultivation of their mind and character without limit and worry only moderately about the pursuit of external and bodily goods.

   D. People ought to pursue the cultivation of their mind and character to a degree befitting their innate dispensation of wisdom and virtue.

30. Suppose a philosopher is interested in making an inquiry into what type of university is best. Extrapolating from the passage, which of the following most represents the best and most basic way to begin this inquiry?

   A. One ought to determine which university produces the most successful people.

   B. One ought to determine the best way of learning in general.

   C. One ought to determine the best way of living in general.

   D. One ought to determine which university has the wisest and most just teachers.

Passage 6 (Questions 31 – 35)

Amongst all the Grecian games, the Olympic held undeniably the first rank, and that for three reasons. They were sacred to Jupiter, the greatest of the gods; instituted by Hercules, the first of the heroes; and celebrated with more pomp and magnificence, amidst a greater concourse of spectators attracted from all parts, than any of the rest.

If Pausanias may be believed, women were prohibited to be present at them upon pain of death; and during their continuance, it was ordained, that no woman should approach the place where the games were celebrated, or pass on that side of the river Alpheus. One only was so bold as to violate this law, and slipt in disguise amongst those who were training the wrestlers. She was tried for the offence, and would have suffered the penalty enacted by the law, if the judges, in regard to her father, her brother, and her son, who had all been victors in the Olympic games, had not pardoned her offence, and saved her life.

This law was very conformable with the manners of the Greeks, amongst whom the ladies were very reserved, seldom appeared in public, had separate apartments, called Gynæcea, and never ate at table with the men when strangers were present. It was certainly inconsistent with decency to admit them at some of the games, as those of wrestling and the Pancratium, in which the combatants fought naked. The same Pausanias tells us in another place, that the priestess of Ceres had an honorable seat in these games, and that virgins were not denied the liberty of being present at them. For my part, I cannot conceive the reason of such inconsistency, which indeed seems incredible.

The Greeks thought nothing comparable to the victory in these games. They looked upon it as the perfection of glory, and did not believe it permitted to mortals to desire any thing beyond it. Cicero assures us, that with them it was no less honorable than the consular dignity in its original splendor with the ancient Romans. And in another place he says, that to conquer at Olympia, was almost, in the estimation of the Grecians, more great and glorious, than to receive the honour of a triumph at Rome. Horace speaks in still stronger terms of this kind of victory. He is not afraid to say that "it exalts the victor above human nature; they were no longer men but gods."

We shall see hereafter what extraordinary honors were paid the victor, of which one of the most affecting was, to date the year with his name. Nothing could more effectually stimulate their endeavors, and make them regardless of expenses, than the assurance of immortalizing their names, which, through all future ages would be enrolled in their annals, and stand in the front of all laws made in the same year with the victory. To this motive may be added the joy of knowing, that their praises would be celebrated by the most famous poets, and form the subject of conversation in the most illustrious assemblies; for these odes were sung in every house, and formed a part in every entertainment. What could be a more powerful incentive to a people, who had no other object and aim than that of human glory?

31. Which of the following would best explain why the priestess of Ceres was allowed to attend the Olympic games?

   A. The priestess of Ceres was honored and viewed as more than the average woman.

   B. The priestess of Ceres held political power over all men in the city.

   C. The priestess of Ceres lived in a different time in which Greek women were allowed to attend the games.

   D. The author is mistaken that women were not allowed to attend the games.

32. According to the passage, in ancient Rome, which honor is comparable to that which the Greeks would feel with victory in the Olympic games?

   A. Victory in the coliseum

   B. Victory at battle

   C. Being elected as a roman consul

   D. Becoming the emperor of Rome

33. Which of the following describes the attitude of the author with regards to the writings of Pausanias?

   A. Cynical

   B. Confused

   C. Angry

   D. Incredulous

34. How might the passage thesis be affected upon learning that Olympic victors were often pardoned from serious transgressions of the law?

   A. It would support the assertion that victors were held in great esteem.

   B. It would undermine the assertion that victors were not above the law.

   C. It would not affect the premise of the passage because there is no mention of this scenario in the passage.

   D. It would undermine the assertion that Grecian women were very reserved.

35. What aspects of Greek culture are highlighted by their practice of the Olympic games?

   I. Their social practices

   II. The workings of their judicial system

   III. The highest purpose of the Grecian people

   A. II only

   B. I and II only

   C. I and III only

   D. I, II, and III

Passage 7 (Questions 36 – 40)

I'll make a sharp distinction between Operative Witchcraft and Ritual Witchcraft. Under Operative Witchcraft I class all charms and spells, practised by the priests and people of every religion. They are part of the common heritage of the human race and are therefore of no practical value in the study of any one particular cult.

Ritual Witchcraft—or, as I propose to call it, the Dianic cult—embraces the religious beliefs and ritual of the people known in late mediaeval times as "Witches". The evidence proves that underlying the Christian religion was a cult practised by many classes of the community, chiefly, however, by the more ignorant or those in the less thickly inhabited parts of the country. It can be traced back to pre-Christian times, and appears to be the ancient religion of Western Europe. The god, anthropomorphic or theriomorphic, was worshipped in well-defined rites; the organization was highly developed; and the ritual is analogous to many other ancient rituals. The dates of the chief festivals suggest that the religion belonged to a race which had not reached the agricultural stage; and the evidence shows that various modifications were introduced, probably by invading peoples who brought in their own beliefs. I have not attempted to disentangle the various cults; I am content merely to point out that it was a definite religion with beliefs, ritual, and organization as highly developed as that of any other cult in the world.

The deity of this cult was incarnate in a man, a woman, or an animal; the animal form being apparently earlier than the human, for the god was often spoken of as wearing the skin or attributes of an animal. At the same time, however, there was another form of the god in the shape of a man with two faces. Such a god is found in Italy (where he was called Janus or Dianus), in Southern France, and in the English Midlands. The feminine form of the name, Diana, is found throughout Western Europe as the name of the female deity or leader of the so-called Witches, and it is for this reason that I have called this ancient religion the Dianic cult. The geographical distribution of the two-faced god suggests that the race or races, who carried the cult, either did not remain in every country which they entered, or that in many places they and their religion were overwhelmed by subsequent invaders.

The dates of the two chief festivals, May Eve and November Eve, indicate the use of a calendar which is generally acknowledged to be pre-agricultural and earlier than the solstitial division of the year. The fertility rites of the cult bear out this indication, as they were for promoting the increase of animals and only rarely for the benefit of the crops. The cross-quarter-days, February 2 and August 1, which were also kept as festivals, were probably of later date, as, though classed among the great festivals, they were not of so high an importance as the May and November Eves. To February 2, Candlemas Day, probably belongs the sun-charm of the burning wheel, formed by the whirling dancers, each carrying a blazing torch; but no special ceremony seems to be assigned to August 1, Lammas Day, a fact suggestive of a later introduction of this festival.

36. Referring to a religious organization as a cult is significant as the term implies the group is of lesser or minority status within the larger society, or heretical in the eyes of the controlling religion. Based on the passage, what is a likely reason for the passage author referring to the followers of Diana as a cult?

    A. The Dianic worshippers were of a lower, marginalized status within a Christian society.

    B. Members of the Dianic cult were leftovers of a disappearing and weakening pre-Christian religion.

    C. Animal worship was considered violent and ignorant by the larger society.

    D. Because Dianic worship was pre-agricultural, the beliefs are, by definition, pre-religious, and therefore cult-like.

37. The author implies that religions borne of agricultural societies tend to celebrate:

    A. at broadly different times each year, depending on weather and planting/harvesting seasons.

    B. on specific dates which correspond with traditionally important annual events in the agricultural calendar.

    C. on dates carried over from remembered hunting and gathering events, such as relocation to follow a herd.

    D. astronomically-determined dates which are best measured by societies aware of seasons.

38. Which of the following titles most accurately describes this passage?

    A. A Discourse on Practical Versus Ritual Witchcraft

    B. The Resurrection of Dianic Beliefs in Modern Christianity

    C. The History of the Dianic Cults

    D. Janus and Diana: New Evidence of Europe's Indigenous Religion

39. Based on the passage, which possible geographic distribution of Dianic beliefs in Western Europe would be most likely?

    A. Evidence of Dianic beliefs is found throughout countries along the southern and western borders of Western Europe, in a continuous ring along the African continent and Atlantic Ocean.

    B. Evidence of Dianic beliefs is found in a broad geographic range across Western Europe, but entirely absent in some intervening regions, resulting in some isolated pockets of Dianic tradition.

    C. Dianic belief is most prevalent near modern Italy and France, diminishing predictably in all directions (on the continent) from these epicenters, with the exception of the coast near the English Channel.

    D. Evidence of Dianic ritual is found in local Catholic and Orthodox variants throughout Western Europe to this day, except in Italy, France, and England, where the modern practice has become extinct.

40. The author would probably agree with the characterization of the Dianic belief system as:

    A. well-established and well-organized, but decentralized with many local variations.

    B. a combination of sophisticated and formalized adopted beliefs and primitive witchcraft techniques.

    C. a scattered, minor belief system from the ancient days of Western Europe.

    D. a primitive but highly-organized ancient agricultural religion, influenced by many invading peoples in history.

Passage 8 (Questions 41 – 47)

Though the world of natural phenomena seemed to man wayward and inexplicable for so long, we eventually came to perceive in it a pervasive order and uniformity. In the same way, we have found a manifest order and uniformity in the economic world, albeit of a less majestic kind. Man depends upon his fellow men for the very means of life, and yet, he takes this cooperation as if for granted, with a complacent confidence and naive unconsciousness, just as he takes the rising of tomorrow's sun. Many observers have been justifiably and notably impressed by the reliability of this unorganized cooperation.

As Bastiat exclaimed some seventy years ago, "Upon entering Paris, I said to myself -- here are a million human beings who would all die in short time if provisions suddenly ceased flowing into this great metropolis. The imagination is baffled when it attempts to appreciate the vast multiplicity of commodities that must enter the city tomorrow in order to keep the inhabitants from falling prey to the convulsions of famine, pillage, and rebellion. And yet, at this moment, all these people sleep soundly, and their peaceful slumbers are not disturbed for a single moment by the prospect of such a catastrophe. On the other hand, eighty departments have labored today, without cooperation and without any mutual understanding, in order to provide for Paris."

This theme may well excite a sense of wonder, but wonder must always be watched with a careful eye, for he is liable to bring along with him a hanger-on we know as worship. Here, in the realm of economics, this hanger-on can do nothing but mischief. There are only a few short steps between the passage quoted above, the glorification of the existing system of society, the defense of a whole slew of indefensible things, and a stubbornly contrary attitude towards all projects of reform. These are short steps, but they are ones that are quite unjustifiable to take.

The evils of our economic system are simply too obvious to be ignored: far too many people have a harsh personal experience of the wastefulness of its production, the injustice of its distribution, the sweating it necessitates, its unemployment, and its slums. When the attempt is made to brush over these evils with obsequious rhetoric about the majesty of economic law and order, we should not be surprised that the spirits of many men will revolt and retort by denying the existence of order in the economic world, declaring that the spectacle which they, the disadvantaged masses, see is one of chaos, confusion, and discord. At this point, we become absorbed by a controversy as stale, flat, and unprofitable as that general one between the "theorist" and the "practical man."

The truth is that this language of private praise and public criticism is inappropriate. First of all, it is important to note that the order that I have spoken of makes itself clear not only in those economic phenomena which are beneficial to man, but in those that are hurtful as well. Even in the alteration of good and bad trade, which causes so much unemployment and misery, there is a measurable, rhythmic regularity like that of the seasons, or like the ebb and flow of the tide. This is not an elegance to be admired. Moreover, to the extent that economic order is comprised of adjustments and tendencies that are beneficial (as is mainly true), there is no justification for assuming that these are either sufficient to secure a prosperous community, or that they are dependent upon the social arrangement that already exists. Therefore, we ought to refrain from premature polemics and embrace a spirit of detachment when we examine further aspects of this elaborate, unorganized cooperation of which so much has already been said and written.

41. According to the passage, which of the following statements about economic order is true?

 I. Not everyone believes it exists.

 II. It is made clear by the study of economics, which is comparable to science, the study of nature.

 III. Bastiat was justified in being impressed by the economic order he observed in Paris.

 A. I only

 B. II only

 C. I and II only

 D. I, II, and III

42. Within the context of the passage, what does Bastiat represent?

 A. Public criticism

 B. Private criticism

 C. Public praise

 D. Private praise

43. Based upon the passage, which of the following is the most likely reason why the author begins the passage with a mention of "the world of natural phenomena?"

 A. To demonstrate the significant influence the natural world has over economics

 B. To praise the remarkable progress that mankind has made so quickly

 C. To introduce the idea that people bring order and uniformity to their environments

 D. To contextualize humanity's ability to perceive order in the economic world

44. Based upon the passage, it is most likely that the author believes which of the following statements?

 A. The alteration of good and bad trade is inevitable.

 B. The alteration of good and bad trade is awe-inspiring in its regularity.

 C. Worship is typically always a negative phenomenon as it blocks rationality.

 D. Once an economic system is properly established, projects of reform are not necessary.

45. According to the passage, which of the following statements explains why "this language of private praise and public criticism is inappropriate?"

 A. It leads to class warfare that can inhibit society.

 B. It gives more power to the private interests.

 C. It provides no benefit to either party.

 D. It ignores the evils of our economic system.

46. Suppose that four different economists are applying for the same professorship at a certain university. Also suppose that the author of this passage is the Dean of the Economics Department at this university, and therefore has the final say on who is hired. Based upon the passage, which of the following professors is most likely to be hired by the author?

 A. The one whose research primarily consists of conducting oral histories and comparing them

 B. The one whose research primarily consists of statistics, calculus, and social science

 C. The one whose research primarily consists of historical analysis of defunct economies

 D. The one whose research primarily consists of utopian philosophy and its contemporary application

47. According to the passage, all of the following statements about the "unorganized cooperation" of the economic world are true EXCEPT:

 A. in how it is perceived, it is comparable to tomorrow's rising run.

 B. it does not require any kind of mutual understanding to function.

 C. despite our complacency and naivety, it is eminently reliable.

 D. it is helpful but not essential to modern human life.

Passage 9 (Questions 48 – 53)

Besides a good will, there is nothing that can be conceived in the world that can be called good without qualification. The talents of the mind, such as intelligence, wit, and judgment, and the qualities of temperament, such as courage, resolution, and perseverance, are unquestionably good and desirable in many ways. However, these gifts of nature have also the potential to become bad and mischievous if the will that makes use of them is not good, for it is the will and how it uses things which we call character.

Honor, power, riches, the well-being and contentment with one's condition which we know as happiness, and even health, inspire pride, and often presumption if there is no good will to correct the influence of these things upon the mind. An impartial, rational spectator will never take pleasure from seeing a person, adorned with absolutely no features of a good will, enjoying unchecked prosperity. Therefore, having a good will seems to be an essential condition even of being worthy of happiness.

There are some qualities that, despite having no intrinsic unconditional value, serve this good will and may facilitate its action. Though they are essential for a good will, thus qualifying the esteem we have for them, these qualities are not regarded as being absolutely good. For example, calm deliberation, moderation in the affections and passions, and self-control are qualities that are not only good, but even seem to make up, at least in part, the intrinsic value of a person. This being said, they do not deserve to be called good without qualification, even though the ancients praised them so unconditionally. Without the guidance of a good will, even these qualities may become bad: the coolness of a villain not only makes him more dangerous, but also makes him more loathsome than he would be without it.

A good will is not good because of what it performs or because of its aptness for the attainment of an end, but rather, it is good by virtue of volition. In other words, it is a good in itself, and considered by itself, it is esteemed far higher than all the things that can be brought about by it in favor of a particular inclination or even the sum total of all inclinations. Even if the will lacked any power to accomplish its purpose, due perhaps to a disfavor of fortune, even if its strongest efforts achieved nothing, and all that was left was the good will (to be clear, this is not merely a good wish, but the summoning of all the means in its power), then it would still shine like a jewel, by its own brilliance, as a thing which in itself contains its whole value. Therefore, its usefulness or uselessness neither adds nor subtracts from its value. So, the will's usefulness would enable us to handle it more easily in attracting to it the attention of those who are not yet connoisseurs, but not to recommend it to true connoisseurs, or to gauge its true value.

Of course, there is something odd about this idea of the absolute value of mere will, in which no real significance is given to its utility. Though even common reason may assent to this idea, a suspicion arises that this is really just the product of high concept fancy and that we have perhaps misunderstood the whole purpose of nature in claiming reason as the governor of our will. Therefore, we will further examine this idea from this point of view.

48. According to the passage, which of the following accurately describes how gifts of nature, like intelligence, wit, courage, and perseverance can become bad and mischievous?

A. The person that has received those gifts is lacking in terms of character.

B. The person that has received those gifts is lacking in terms of education.

C. The person that has received those gifts is lacking in terms of honor.

D. The person that has received those gifts is lacking in terms of happiness.

49. Which of the following is the most likely explanation of why the author introduces the three goods that presuppose a good will in the third paragraph?

A. In order to how to demonstrate how exactly a good will is said to be good in itself

B. In order to show that, like a good will, they contribute to the intrinsic value of a person

C. In order to compare them favorably against the qualities mentioned in the previous paragraph

D. In order to further prove the fact that only a good will is entirely good in itself

50. Based upon the passage, which of the following statements would the author most likely believe?

A. A person cannot possess happiness unless he or she possesses a good will.

B. Truths ought to be examined beyond their common understanding.

C. There are some qualities besides a good will that have intrinsic unconditional value.

D. The usefulness of good will is valuable to all connoisseurs of such things.

51. As the author writes in the second paragraph, "An impartial, rational spectator will never take pleasure from seeing a person, adorned with absolutely no features of a good will, enjoying unchecked prosperity." If all of the following people were to enjoy unchecked prosperity, who might the rational spectator most enjoy seeing with that prosperity?

A. The investor who used venture capital to seed a new start-up that is devoted to water desalinization

B. The woman who, with courage and perseverance, became the first person to circumnavigate the globe via sea kayak

C. The man who used his intelligence and wit to outsmart a hacker and protect a large bank from a massive security breach

D. The woman who summoned all the means in her power to care for a sick, homeless child, though the child died

52. All of the following things are necessarily essential qualities of a person with a good will EXCEPT:

A. volition.

B. calm deliberation.

C. strong inclination.

D. moderation.

53. Which of the following statements accurately address problems with the central idea of this passage?

I. The argument presupposes that reason is the ultimate governor of our will.

II. There is absolutely no importance given to the utility of will.

III. It does not seem to be scientifically provable or measurable.

A. I only

B. I and II only

C. II and III only

D. I, II, and III

This page intentionally left blank.

SECTION 11

Answer Key

1	C	12	B	23	C	34	A	45	C
2	D	13	D	24	B	35	C	46	B
3	B	14	A	25	A	36	A	47	D
4	A	15	B	26	D	37	B	48	A
5	A	16	C	27	B	38	C	49	D
6	A	17	D	28	A	39	B	50	B
7	A	18	B	29	C	40	A	51	D
8	A	19	C	30	C	41	D	52	C
9	D	20	B	31	A	42	D	53	D
10	B	21	B	32	C	43	D		
11	C	22	A	33	B	44	A		

Passage 1 (Questions 1 – 5)

Obesity is a major contributor to serious health conditions in children and adults, including **type 2 diabetes**, **cardiovascular disease**, many **cancers**, and numerous other diseases and conditions. As **rates of obesity have soared** in the past three decades, it is clear that increasing the number of people who can achieve and maintain a healthy weight is a critical public health goal, although one that faces formidable challenges. **Reducing** the prevalence of **obesity** and its associated medical conditions will require **broad-based efforts**—by government, the private and nonprofit sectors, businesses, community organizations, healthcare professionals, schools, families, and individuals. The foundation of such efforts is research to illuminate the **causes** and consequences of obesity, to develop and evaluate new prevention and **treatment strategies** to see what works, and to determine how to implement and expand promising approaches to reach those who could most benefit.

Opinion: the author states that obesity is a serious condition that needs to be approached from many angles

Cause and effect: obesity causes other illnesses like diabetes, heart disease, and cancers; the obesity epidemic can only be handled with collaboration and a wide spread effort

New research will define potential candidates for new **drug** development, inform the development of more effective **lifestyle** interventions that better reflect the biologic underpinnings of people's **behaviors**, and open novel avenues for **prevention** and treatment strategies for obesity and its associated diseases. This research encompasses opportunities in genetics, neuroscience, metabolism, cell biology, and other areas that will improve our understanding of fundamental biologic pathways involved in weight regulation—and what goes awry in obesity.

Opinion: drug development and behavioral research are important in understanding how to deal with obesity

A wide range of other **factors** may **influence obesity**, in addition to the biological factors addressed in the previous paragraph. Research ought to explore these **behavioral, social, cultural, and environmental** factors, which span multiple interacting levels. A better understanding of such factors can enhance the design of intervention, surveillance, and translation strategies. Research focused on the **consequences of obesity** can inform health care and policy, and identify population subgroups most affected by obesity and **critical periods for weight gain**, both of which can be used to target intervention and translation efforts.

Opinion: the causes and consequences of obesity should be studied

Contrast: there are other causes of obesity besides the obvious biological underpinnings

Cause and effect: an increased understanding of the causes and consequences of obesity will allow us to intervene more effectively

An array of research opportunities are outlined that can further advance obesity **prevention** and **management** through carefully designed and evaluated interventions. These research areas encompass behavioral and environmental approaches to lifestyle change, from **individual**- and family-based to **community-wide** strategies, as well as surgical interventions. Because **no single approach** is likely to be appropriate for everyone, research to evaluate multiple and diverse approaches in many different settings will yield a broader empirical basis for individual and public health changes. In addition to identifying successful interventions for achieving a healthier weight, this research may also reduce the onset or severity of obesity-associated conditions and improve quality of life.

Key terms: prevention, management

Opinion: intervention is a key in fighting obesity

Contrast: intervention can occur at the individual, family, and community-wide level

Advances in obesity research **depend on accurate tools** and measurements to enhance understanding of **etiology** and allow for evaluation of interventions. Examples of research opportunities include the development of biomarkers; designing tools to better assess food intake, fitness, functional status, and thermogenesis; improving imaging methods; advancing **technologies for determining** body composition; and developing objective measurement systems to better evaluate changes in policy and environments. Also highlighted are emerging methodologies to enable researchers to better capture and model complex relationships in obesity

Cause and effect: improved methodologies will be helpful in fighting obesity

Main Idea: the main idea of the passage is to present the author's ideas as to what is necessary in the fight against obesity and why it is necessary; the author focuses on research that needs to be done; the ideas are presented almost as a proposal or a game plan of research that will be done to address the obesity epidemic.

1. C is correct. The passage mentions medical treatments as a part of the research into prevention and management of obesity but makes no other mention of the importance of developing drugs for obesity. It seems that their focus is more on the other factors that lead to obesity.

   A, B, D: These are all directly mentioned in the passage and have paragraphs devoted to them.

2. D is correct. There is much more discussion into the sociological and preventative interventions than the biological.

   A, B, C: Although each of these various factors are brought up in the passage, none of them are discussed at length or implied to be the most important approach.

3. B is correct. The author seems to think that a lot of research remains to be done and much remains to be found. He or she would probably welcome new findings and try to find ways to implement useful information.

   A, D: There is no reason to think the author would doubt the information's authenticity.

   C: The author would probably welcome the information.

4. A is correct. The fact that obesity is not the major contributor to diabetes, however unlikely, does not mean that it is not a contributor to it and still a major contributor to other serious health conditions.

5. A is correct. The author clearly believes that obesity is a multifaceted problem.

   B: The author would not make such a strong statement.

   C: The rates of obesity have soared in the past three decades. This is not true and is thus not a good choice.

   D: The author clearly believes the consequences of obesity to be serious, not mild.

Passage 2 (Questions 6 – 10)

In August 2013, a group of **protesters** gathered in Los Angeles to rally against the Listening and Spoken Language Symposium, an event sponsored by the **Alexander Graham Bell Institute** for the Deaf and Hard of Hearing. The protesters were **deaf**, and many of the exhibitors at the symposium represented or were affiliated with companies that sold **cochlear implants**; a recent technological development, cochlear implants are surgically-implanted electronic devices that can provide a deaf or hard of hearing person with some degree of hearing. Cochlear implants can be implanted in babies, children, and adults. While the implants cannot restore normal hearing, they can give many users increased ability to receive auditory signals.

Key terms: protesters, deaf, cochlear implants

Cause and effect: deaf protesters were objecting to AG Bell's promotion of cochlear implants

The protest reflected a deeply **controversial subject** among deaf people: the promotion of "**oralism**," an educational stance which supports the teaching of lip-reading and oral speech to children who are deaf or hard of hearing, and de-emphasizes or eliminates the teaching of **American Sign Language (ASL)**. To the people at the rally – Deaf activists and their supporters – proponents of oralism are guilty of what Deaf activists call "**audism**" – the belief that it is inherently better to hear than to be deaf, and that deafness is a disability rather than a difference. Cochlear implants, they believe, promote the idea that deaf people need "fixing." At root is whether one sees deafness as a disability or as a **culture**; some people describe this as self-identifying as deaf, with a small "d," or as **Deaf**, with a capital "D." Some deaf or hard of hearing people note that it is difficult for hearing people to understand why a deaf or hard of hearing person would not embrace the opportunity to hear and participate as fully as possible in the oral world. But to those who identify as Deaf, ASL use is a key part of their culture. Deaf people who use ASL share a language, history, social framework, and community identity. Asking a deaf person, they say, to give up their Deaf identity is like asking any other person of an ethnic or cultural minority to renege on their deep cultural connections. Thus, **audism is a form of cultural disrespect** and discrimination.

Key terms: oralism, audism, Deaf, ASL

Contrast: deaf refers to auditory disability, whereas Deaf refers to a culture

Opinion: Deaf activists assert that cochlear implants are indicative of audism, the idea that hearing is better than deafness, with which they strongly disagree

AG Bell has a long and complex relationship with the people it serves. Its founder, **Alexander Graham Bell**, was important in the spread of oralism as the dominant paradigm for educating deaf children. **Bell**, whose mother and wife were both deaf, believed that deaf people needed to **assimilate into hearing culture**; he advocated that the deaf population should relinquish sign language, and eliminate separate schools, social clubs, and publications for the deaf. Deaf advocates criticize Bell's beliefs as overtly hostile, and credit his actions as leading to a lengthy dark period in which deaf children had little or no contact with other deaf people, lived with families that were non-signing, and were often presumed to be stupid – situations that were difficult and damaging. Today, though, **AG Bell considers itself an advocacy group for deaf people**, and asserts that providing information on cochlear implants is one aspect of that **advocacy**. On their Website, they state that their goal is "to ensure that every child and adult with hearing loss has the opportunity to listen, talk and thrive in mainstream society." To some Deaf activists, though, **assimilation** in mainstream society is not the goal; **more essential is having pride** in and a sense of belonging to a rich, vibrant, and distinct culture.

Key terms: Alexander Graham Bell, advocacy, assimilation

Opinion: Alexander Graham Bell was a proponent of oralism rather than of ASL use

Contrast: AG Bell's stated goal is that deaf people can thrive in mainstream society; Deaf activists are more focused on building a strong, distinct, and positive culture

Main idea: The passage describes protests regarding the promotion of cochlear implants and how they reflect differing views on oralism in the deaf community.

6. A is correct. Paragraph 3 describes AG Bell's relationship with the deaf community; the issue is that throughout their history they have promoted oralism as a way of educating and supporting deaf people, but not everyone agrees that such a stance is in the best interests of the deaf community.

    B: AG Bell has always promoted oralism.

    C: Whether Bell was hostile to deaf people is debatable; more important, the issue is not just Bell but the institution that continues today.

    D: The passage never tells us whether the majority of deaf people look favorably on AG Bell or not.

7. A is correct. A person who identifies as deaf with a small "d" most likely does not share the views of Deaf activists, so you can eliminate choices B, C, and D. Most likely, they would view the implants as a potentially helpful communication tool.

8. A is correct. Deaf activists are in favor of the teaching of ASL, and would most likely support an educational institution that promoted that.

    B: Deaf activists are not focused on students thriving in the hearing mainstream – they are more concerned with building a separate culture.

    C: We know that Deaf activists are in favor of the teaching of ASL, but the passage never implies that they believe deaf people should not be able to communicate in English as well.

9. D is correct. Look to the end of the second paragraph for your answer here. Deaf culture, says the author, has a shared language, history, and social framework.

    A: They probably do, but that is not described in the passage as the reason Deaf is its own culture.

    B: Deaf advocates are certainly pro-advocacy, but this doesn't explain why Deaf is a distinct culture.

    C: Again, probably true, but not an explanation of why Deaf is a culture and not just an auditory condition.

10. B is correct. Deaf activists say that cochlear implants promote audism, but AG Bell claims that providing information on cochlear implants is a form of advocacy and will help deaf people thrive.

    A: We don't know what percentage of deaf and hard of hearing people identify as Deaf.

    C: Oralism by definition is the promotion of spoken language.

    D: Whether many or few deaf people use cochlear implants is insignificant to whether or not they promote audism.

Passage 3 (Questions 11 – 17)

Michelangelo's Moses is seated his body faces forward, his head, with its mighty beard, looks to the left, his right foot touches the ground, and his left leg is raised such that only the toes touch the ground. His right arm connects the **Tables of the Law**, which contain the **Ten Commandments**, with part of his beard while his left arm lies in his lap, pressing his beard against his body. At this point, if I were to give a more detailed description of the statue, I would be pre-empting what I want to say later on. I should mention that the **descriptions of this figure given by other writers are curiously unsuitable**: that which has not been understood has been perceived inaccurately.

Opinion: author thinks the descriptions given by other writers are wrong

Grimm writes that the right hand, "under whose arm the Tables rest, grasps his beard," **Lübke** writes, "Profoundly shaken, he grasps with his right hand his magnificent streaming beard," and **Springer** writes that "Moses presses the left hand against his body, and thrusts the other, as though unconsciously, into the mighty locks of his beard." On the other hand, **Justi** believes that the fingers of his right hand were playing with his beard "as an agitated man nowadays might play with his watch-chain." **Müntz** believes this as well. A further step removed, **Thode** writes of the "calm, firm posture of the right hand upon the Tables resting against his side." He does not sense any excitement in the statue, even in the right hand. And as Jakob **Burckhardt** complains, "The celebrated left arm has no other function than to press his beard to his body."

Key terms: Grimm, Lübke, Springer, Justi, Müntz, Thode, Burckhardt

Contrast: different authors have varying interpretations of Moses's posture in the statue

Seeing as these **mere descriptions do not agree**, we are not surprised to find a myriad of **divergent views as to the meaning of the statute** and its various features. In **my opinion**, the facial expression of this Moses is **best characterized** by **Thode**, who sees it as "**a mixture of wrath, pain, and contempt** . . . wrath in his threatening contracting brows, pain in his glance, and contempt in his protruded under lip and in the down-drawn corners of his mouth."

Opinion: the author thinks that the facial expression of Moses is best characterized by Thode, who sees a strong mix of negative emotions

Of course, other admirers have seen with other eyes. As **Dupaty** writes, "His august brow seems to be but a transparent veil only half concealing his great mind." **Lubke** completely disagrees, stating that "one would look in vain in that head for an expression of higher intelligence; his down-drawn brow speaks nothing but a capacity for infinite wrath and an all-compelling energy." Differing even more, **Guillaume** sees no emotion in the face at all, "only a proud sim-plicity, an inspired dignity, a living faith. The eye of Moses looks into the future, he foresees the lasting survival of his people and the immutability of his law." **Müntz agrees with Guillame**, writing that "the eyes of Moses rove far beyond the race of men. They are turned towards those mysteries which he alone has seen." As **Steinmann** writes, this Moses is "no longer the stern Law-giver, no longer the terrible enemy of sin, armed with the wrath of Jehovah, but the royal priest, whom age may not approach, beneficent and prophetic, with the reflection of eternity upon his brow, taking his last farewell of his people."

Contrast: various critics have had differing interpretations as to the meaning of the expression on Moses's face

There are even those who claim the Moses of Michelangelo **says nothing at all** (and who are honest enough to admit to it). As one critic wrote in the *Quarterly Review* of 1858, "**There is an absence of meaning in the general conception**, which precludes the idea of a self-fulfilling whole." What is more **astonishing** is that there are others who find nothing to admire in the statue and who actually **revolt against it**, complaining of its brutality and the animal cast of the head.

Opinion: author seems to disagree pretty strongly with those who say that the statue is a bad one (they revolt against it) or who think it has no message at all

Did **the master** fashion **such a vague, ambiguous script** in stone such that all of these different readings could possibly be true?

Opinion: the author poses a question about whether Michelangelo's Moses could be as ambiguous as it seems from all these varying interpretations

Main Idea: The author sets out to show just how differently a great work of art like Michelangelo's statue of Moses can be viewed; not only do writers and critics disagree on the meaning of the statue, they disagree on a basic description of the figure; despite ending with an open-ended question, the author does have some set opinions about the piece, as well as the other writers.

11. C is correct. As the author writes at the end of the first sentence of the passage, ". . . his left leg is raised such that only the toes touch the ground."

    A: Both arms touch it: the right arm touches it and joins it to the Tables while the left hand presses his beard to his body, as some of the writers mention in the second paragraph.

    B: Rather, his left leg is raised.

    D: Rather, his left arm does this.

12. B is correct. The last sentence: "Did the master fashion such a vague, ambiguous script in stone such that all of these different readings could possibly be true?" Certainly this question would be ineffective if the author hadn't presented several different readings. We don't know what the author believes the answer is, though that he favors one reading of the statue's meaning in particular suggests that he may think there is a right answer.

    A: He says that many writers provide descriptions that are "curiously unsuitable", so inapt would be a better world than inept or ineptitude. Also, he does not say a similar thing about meaning. He only says it about the physical descriptions of the piece.

    C: Certainly we see in the passage how much thought and contention this statue has inspired, but it does not seem to be the author's primary point.

    D: This is never said and we have no other artist to compare him to in the passage.

13. D is correct. Justi believed that Moses was playing with his beard, and the author follows this by saying, "Müntz believes this as well." Later, in the fourth paragraph, Müntz is quoted as writing that "the eyes of Moses rove far beyond the race of men . . . turned towards those mysteries which he alone has seen."

    A: Guillame satisfies the second part but not the first.

    B: Lübke writes that Moses is profoundly shaken and is grasping his beard. Moreover, he thinks the figure's face lacks intelligence and possesses only infinite wrath and all-compelling energy.

    C: Justi does believe that Moses was playing with his beard, but does not express an opinion about what Moses is looking at.

14. A is correct. As the author writes in the third paragraph, "In my opinion, the facial expression of this Moses is best characterized by Thode, who sees it as a mixture of wrath, pain, and contempt . . ." Certainly this qualifies as a complex mix of thoughts and feelings.

15. B is correct. At the end of the fourth paragraph, Steinmann is mentioned as describing how Moses is no longer the "stern Law-giver" or "terrible enemy of sin," but rather, is "beneficent and prophetic." This seems pretty calm. And in the very beginning of the second paragraph, Lübke writes that Moses is "profoundly shaken." Hence, these two writers, of the choices given, most represent the two unnamed writers that the author forgot to include.

    A: Yes, Steinmann sees Moses as having a sense of calm, but so does Thode.

    C: This is a reverse of the correct answer.

    D: The Moses of both Guillame and Müntz is quite calm.

16. C is correct. Fear is never mentioned as a quality expressed by the figure of the statue.

    A, B, D: These qualities are all attributed to the statue in the passage.

17. D is correct. Justi writes that Moses plays with his beard "as an agitated man nowadays plays with his watch-chain." As the author adds, "Müntz believes this as well." Now, it is not necessarily true that Müntz believes Moses to be agitated, but it is possible given the comparison. Also, throw in the fact that according to Müntz, Moses is looking beyond his people, may suggest he is agitated with them. Therefore, Item I is true.

    II: Guillame sees no emotion in Moses' face at all, and the author writes that Müntz agrees with Guillame. But what about the agitation? Moses may not be expressing agitation in his face, but he may be expressing it in his body. Therefore, Item II is true.

    III: As Müntz claims, ". . . the eyes of Moses rove far beyond the race of men. They are turned towards those mysteries which he alone has seen." Therefore, Item III is true.

Passage 4 (Questions 18 – 24)

How great a **virtue** is **temperance**, how important it is throughout a whole man's life! Yet God commits the **management** of this **great trust**, without **specific laws** or **prescriptions**, entirely to **the demeanor** of **every grown man**. For those actions that enter **into** a man and do not issue **out** of him, therefore defiling him not, God does not keep man captive under a **perpetual childhood**, but trusts him with **the gift of reason** to be **his own chooser**. There would be little need left for preaching if law were to govern those things previously governed only by **moral encouragement**.

Contrast: the importance of temperance vs the fact that God grants the management of it without any specific laws or prescriptions, actions that enter into a man vs those that issue out of him

Cause and effect: because the actions that enter into a man do not defile him, God does not keep us under perpetual childhood with laws about what we can and cannot take in, but rather, gives us the gift of reason to make us our own choosers

Solomon informs us that reading **too much** is **weariness to the flesh**, but neither he nor any other **inspired author** tells us that reading is unlawful. If God had wanted to limit us in this regard, it would have been more expedient to have told us what was unlawful than what was wearisome. As far as **the burning** of the **Ephesian books** by **St. Paul's converts**, it is said that the books were **magic tomes**, used for sorcery. It was a private, **voluntary act**: the **remorseful men** burnt their own books where another man may perhaps have read them in some **useful way**.

Contrast: reading too much being weariness to the flesh vs reading being unlawful

Cause and effect: if God had wanted to limit our reading, he would have told us (through the mouth piece of Solomon) that reading was unlawful

We know that **good** and **evil** grow up together in this world, almost inseparably, and that the **knowledge** of good is so interwoven with the knowledge of evil, and in many **cunning resemblances** is hardly to be discerned, that those **scattered seeds** which **Psyche** was given the **incessant labor** of culling out and sorting were not more intermixed. From the rind of **one apple**, the knowledge of good and evil, as two twins cleaving together, leapt forth into the world. This is that **doom** that **Adam** fell into, knowing both good and evil, or rather, knowing good by evil. Generations hence, what **wisdom** can there be to chose or forbear without the knowledge of evil? The person that can apprehend and reflect upon **vice**, with all her **seeming pleasures**, and yet abstain, distinguishing and preferring that which is truly better, is **a true warfaring Christian**.

Contrast: the knowledge of good vs the knowledge of evil, apprehending and reflecting upon vice vs abstaining and preferring that which is better

Cause and effect: because good and evil grow up together, and because they are often difficult to discern from one another, it is as difficult to sort them out as it was for Psyche with her seeds; because he can see and reflect upon vice and yet abstain from it, this person is said to be a true warfaring Christian

I cannot praise a **cloistered virtue**, unexercised and unbreathed, that never sets out and sees her **adversary**, but rather, slinks out of **the race** in which that **immortal garland** is to be run for. Certainly we do not bring **innocence** into the world, for we much more likely bring **impurity**: that which purifies us is **a trial**, and trial is by whatever is **contrary**. Therefore, that virtue which is **young in the contemplation of evil**, that knows not what vice promises to her followers, and rejects it, is but a **blank virtue**, not a **pure one**.

Contrast: cloistered virtue vs uncloistered virtue (implied, virtue that is young in the contemplation of evil vs virtue that is old (implied)

Opinion: author thinks that a virtue that has been tested by a trial is a higher, purer virtue but that a "blank virtue" that has not contemplated evil is lesser

This is why our **sage and serious poet Spenser**, whom I would dare to claim as a better teacher than **Scotus** or **Aquinas**, described **true temperance** with the character of **Guion**, bringing him through the cave of Mammon, the **bower of earthly bliss**, that he might see and abstain. Because **knowing vice** is so **necessary** to the constitution of human **virtue**, and the scanning of error to the confirmation of truth, how can we better **scout** into the regions of sin and **falsity** than by **reading all kinds** of tractates and by hearing all kinds of reason and opinion? This is the benefit afforded us by **books promiscuously read**.

Contrast: Spenser vs Scotus and Aquinas, indulging in earthly bliss vs abstaining

Cause and effect: Spenser described true temperance by having his character Guion go through the cave of Mammon and abstain from its earthly bliss; because knowing vice is necessary to being virtuous, the best way to scout into regions of sin and falsity is by reading and being exposed to all kinds of different opinions

Main Idea: The author makes the case that the best way to know right from wrong is to experience wrong and know it fully, for even the person that chooses right from wrong yet does not have a full conception of wrong has a "blank virtue"; the passage is about the benefit that "books promiscuously read" offer us.

18. B is correct. "I cannot praise a cloistered virtue, unexercised and unbreathed, that never sets out and sees her adversary, but rather, slinks out of the race in which that immortal garland is to be run for." The opposite of slinking out of the race is engaging in the race, and the opposite of an unexercised virtue is an exercised virtue. As the author claims, the virtue of temperance must be worked at to become pure. So, I is true. III is true because this person "can apprehend and reflect upon vice, with all her seeming pleasures, and yet abstain."

   II: They are exposed by a wide worldview, the kind that comes "by reading all kinds of tractates and by hearing all kinds of reason and opinion."

19. C is correct. As the author writes in the last sentence of the second paragraph, "It was a private, voluntary act: the remorseful men burnt their own books where another man may perhaps have read them in some useful way." It was a voluntary act.

   A: The author refers to "the burning of the Ephesian books by St. Paul's converts," meaning they were already converts before burning them.

   B: Rather, the burning was voluntary.

   D: This may have been true, but the author gives us no inclination whether it is.

20. B is correct. The passage tells us that Solomon was an "inspired writer." Then the author writes, "If God had wanted to limit us in this regard, it would have been more expedient to have told us what was unlawful than what was wearisome." This supposes that God did tell us what was wearisome. We know that Solomon informed us what was wearisome, and that he was an inspired author, so we can assume that God spoke through Solomon.

   C: Rather, he thought it was wearisome.

   D: We know he was an "inspired author" and he must have read too as he talks about reading, but this claim is just more tenuous than the one in Choice B.

21. B is correct. As the author writes at the end of the fourth paragraph, "Therefore, that virtue which is young in the contemplation of evil, that knows not what vice promises to her followers, and rejects it, is but a blank virtue, not a pure one." This virtue is the one that has not yet been purified by trial, and even though it chooses rightly, it is not a pure and tested virtue.

   A: This is true, but the essential quality of a blank virtue isn't that it's immature, but that it's untested.

   C: Rather, it does make the right decision.

   D: Rather, a warfaring Christian, according to the end of the third paragraph, experiences vice and is able to distinguish it and prefer that which is truly better.

22. A is correct. As the author writes in the third paragraph, "The knowledge of good is so interwoven with the knowledge of evil, and in many cunning resemblances is hardly to be discerned, that those scattered seeds which Psyche was given the incessant labor of culling out and sorting were not more intermixed." So, good and evil are as intermixed as those scattered seeds. We know that Psyche had to engage in incessant labor to sort the seeds, so if good and evil are just as intermixed, they must require incessant labor as well, and thus, difficulty.

   B: First of all, this anecdote has more to do with the difficulty than the virtue. Secondly, it's not quite a juxtaposition, but rather, a comparison.

   C: Not pleasure, but difficulty.

   D: The comparison is not being made between this and that anecdote.

23. C is correct. The whole passage is dedicated to "the benefit afforded us by books promiscuously read." All anecdotes serve this purpose. Even the story of Guion is a literary one that we can experience and appreciate in Spenser's work. Reading books promiscuously can help us to make our virtue more pure, for through reading we can experience a whole manner of things, right and wrong, that help share our morality.

   A: Perhaps, but this misses the main point.

   B: Again, this misses the point. These anecdotes serve the idea of reading as many differing opinions as one can.

   D: It seems that the author does not fully support this notion of reading wearying the flesh. He believes that we ought to read all kinds of works and hear all kinds of reason and opinions.

24. B is correct. Rather, all grown people are given the management of this great trust, as the author writes in the first sentence. Here, "man" can stand for "person," as the author refers to mankind instead of just males.

Passage 5 (Questions 25 – 30)

Before inquiring into **which type of government is best**, one ought to **first** determine what way of **living** is best. Provided that no accidents interfere, it is most likely that **those who enjoy the best government** will also live the **happiest, best lives** according to their circumstances. Therefore, one ought to know **what way of living is most desirable**, and then afterwards, whether this best life for man in general is the same for man as citizen.

Opinion: author thinks that determining the best government requires first determining the best way of life

What is **good** in relation to man can be divided into **three sorts**: that which is **external**, that which pertains to the **body**, and that which pertains to the **soul**. **All three sorts must conspire together**, for no one would claim that a man was happy if he had no fortitude, no temperance, no justice, or no prudence, if he shuddered in fear from flies, if he committed a crime to satisfy his hunger or thirst, if he murdered his friend for a farthing, and if he was feeble or wanting in his mind, as a child or a madman.

Opinion: author thinks that having a good life requires the interaction of the three sorts of goods (external, body, soul)

Some people may **dispute** this, citing quantity and degree: they may think that a **small amount of virtue is sufficient** for happiness, but when it comes to **riches**, property, power, and honors, that men ought to strive to increase these things without bounds in pursuit of the best life. On the contrary, experience teaches us that **external goods do not produce virtue, but virtue produces them**.

Opinion: some think when seeking goods, people should aim for a little virtue and then unlimited riches and powers

Contrast: author's opinion contrasts, saying that virtue produces external goods, not vice versa

As far as the **happy life** goes, whether it is to be found in pleasure, virtue, or both, it is certain that those whose **morals are most pure**, and who are most cultivated in mind and character, will **enjoy more of it**, even though their external fortunes are moderate next to those who possess mountains of wealth yet are deficient in the higher qualities. After thorough reflection, this is clear, for **all that is external has its limit**, like any instrument or machine, and all things that are external and useful are of such a nature that when there is an **excess** in or of them, they either **do harm**, or at the very best, become useless to the possessor. But for every good quality of the **soul**, the **higher it is in degree, the more useful it is, and the more noble**.

Opinion: author thinks that being a more moral person means you're going to have a happier life

Contrast: external material goods are only good up to a point, after which they become useless or harmful vs. more goods of the soul are always better

When we are **comparing things** with one another, the best state of each particular thing corresponds in excellence to the distance in quality between the things themselves. So, if the **soul** is **more noble** than our **possessions** and our **bodies** in both absolute and relative terms, it must be admitted that the **best states of these things necessarily stand in the same relation** to one another as the things do themselves. Again, it is **for the sake of the soul** that external and bodily goods are desirable at all, and so, the wise man chooses them for the sake of the soul, not the soul for the sake of them.

Opinion: author thinks the soul is inherently better than the body or external things, so goods of the soul must inherently be better than goods of the body (pleasure) or external goods (material wealth)

Cause and effect: material goods are only useful when they contribute to the goods of the soul

Let us accept that every person **enjoys as much happiness as he or she possesses virtue and wisdom**, and as much as he or she behaves according to their dictates. **God himself exemplifies this**, for he is completely happy, not from possessing external goods, but in himself and by virtue of his nature. Here lies the difference between **good fortune and happiness**: every **external** good owes itself in some degree to **chance** or fortune, but it is **not from chance** or fortune that someone becomes **wise** or just. It follows that the happiest, best city is the one that is best and acts the best, for no one does well that doesn't act well, and the **deeds** of both a man and a city cannot be **worthy of praise** without **virtue** and **wisdom**. In this way, the things that are just, wise, and prudent in a person are the same things that are just, wise, and prudent in a city.

Opinion: author thinks a person's level of virtue defines how high their level of happiness can reach

Cause and effect: because God is infinitely virtuous, he can be completely happy

Contrast: external goods depend on luck vs happiness depends on wisdom and justice

Main Idea: To investigate the nature of the best possible government, we must first look to how to live the best life; because the soul is higher and better than the body or material goods, we should focus on the goods of the soul; thus the best city has justice and wisdom the way the best person does.

25. A is correct. There is a range between limits within which an external good is useful. Though the author never established a system for comparing usefulness, the "most minute amount of good qualities of soul" are not necessarily of as much value as an external good of substantial value. As the author does state that all three types of human goods conspire together, it is possible that a valuable external good is more valuable than a minute amount of a good quality of the soul.

26. D is correct. In the third paragraph, the author writes about the people who dispute this claim, " . . . they may think that a small amount of virtue is sufficient for happiness, but when it comes to riches, property, power, and honors, that men ought to strive to increase these things without bounds in pursuit of the best life." All of these things, riches, power, property, and honors, are external goods. Virtue, on the other hand, is a good of the soul.

  A: The people disputing his claim mention external goods, not bodily goods such as pleasure.

  B: This statement is more in line with the author's claim.

  C: Again, this is more akin to what the author is saying.

27. B is correct. As he writes in the first paragraph, " . . . it is most likely that those who enjoy the best government will also live the happiest, best lives according to their circumstances." Flip this statement: those who live the happiest, best lives likely enjoy the best government. In other words, they live in the best city, which has the best government.

  A: This is never said, and it can be argued that the author doesn't believe the best people are naturally so from birth. Rather, the best person acts the best and must possess virtue and wisdom and act according to their dictates. It is not from chance or fortune that someone becomes wise or just.

  C: This is never said.

  D: This may be true, but it is not the reason directly given by the author.

28. A is correct. As the sixth paragraph begins, "Let us accept that every person enjoys as much happiness as he or she possesses virtue and wisdom, and as much as he of she behaves according to their dictates." The next sentence says it all: "God himself exemplifies this . . ." It could also be argued that the example of God is also used to exemplify the difference between good fortune and happiness, for his happiness comes not from external goods, but from his nature. Indeed, the God example does introduce this argument.

  B: This happens later in the paragraph and is not directly linked to the God example.

  C: This has already been addressed.

  D: This is never said.

29. C is correct. As the author writes in the fourth paragraph, "As far as the happy life goes, whether it is to be found in pleasure, virtue, or both, it is certain that those whose morals are most pure, who are most cultivated in mind and character, will enjoy more of it, even though their external fortunes are moderate . . ." As he writes later, "for every good quality of the soul, the higher it is in degree, the more useful it is, and the more noble." Cultivation of mind and character is one of these things that, the higher it is in degree, the more useful it is. Moreover, the author writes that those with great wealth but less of the higher qualities enjoy less of the happy life by comparison.

  A: This is never said, though it is a reasonable statement.

  B: This is never said.

  D: The author claims that wisdom and virtue are not innate: "it is not from chance or fortune that someone becomes wise or just."

30. C is correct. If the best way of living is helpful in determining the best way of government, it is likely that it will be helpful in determining the best university as well, which has its own set of laws and structures like a government does. We could say that it is most likely that those who enjoy the best university will also live the happiest, best lives as students. It seems that the author believes the most basic way of understanding anything is to understand the best way of living, and to use that information to inform how the best form of something can serve that best way of living.

  A: Success here is not defined well enough: if it is financial success, we know it is flat out wrong. If it is success of behaving justly, it is a better option, but still not as strong as Choice C.

  B: This would be a good idea, but it is not the most basic way as the question asks.

  D: But what if the students are awful?

Passage 6 (Questions 31 – 35)

Amongst all the Grecian games, the **Olympic** held undeniably **the first rank**, and that for three reasons. They were **sacred** to Jupiter, the greatest of the gods; **instituted by Hercules**, the first of the heroes; and celebrated with more pomp and magnificence, amidst a greater concourse of spectators attracted from all parts, than any of the rest.

Key terms: Olympic games, first rank, sacred

Cause and effect: the games are said to be first rank (the most important to the Grecian people) for three given reasons

If **Pausanias** may be believed, **women were prohibited** to be present at them upon pain of death; and during their continuance, it was ordained, that no woman should approach the place where the games were celebrated, or pass on that side of the river Alpheus. One only was so bold as to violate this law, and slipt in disguise amongst those who were training the wrestlers. She was tried for the offence, and would have suffered the penalty enacted by the law, if the judges, **in regard to her father, her brother, and her son, who had all been victors in the Olympic games, had not pardoned her offence, and saved her life.**

Key terms: Pausanias, women, prohibited

Opinion: the author seems to be unsure as to whether Pausanias should be believed

Contrast: as contrasted to men, women were prohibited from being present and competing in the games; additionally, there is a contrast between the treatment of women and the pardon of the woman who was related to Olympic victors

Cause and effect: the woman was pardoned as a result of her being related to Olympic victors; this illustrates the respect given to said victors

This law was very **conformable with the manners of the Greeks,** amongst whom the **ladies** were very **reserved**, seldom appeared in public, had separate apartments, called **Gynæcea**, and never ate at table with the men when strangers were present. It was certainly inconsistent with decency to admit them at some of the games, as those of wrestling and the Pancratium, in which the combatants fought naked. The same Pausanias tells us in another place, that the **priestess of Ceres** had an **honorable** seat in these games, and that **virgins** were not denied the liberty of being present at them. For my part, **I cannot conceive** the reason of such inconsistency, which indeed seems **incredible**.

Key terms: reserved, gynaecea, priestess of Ceres, virgins, incredible

Opinion: the author's opinion again comes through that Pausanias' information seems inconsistent

Contrast: the priestess of Ceres is contrasted with other women who are not allowed to be at the games; she is given an honorable seat

Cause and effect: as a result of the Greek customs, women were very reserved and stayed largely separated from the men

The Greeks thought **nothing comparable** to the **victory** in these games. They looked upon it as the **perfection of glory**, and did not believe it permitted to mortals to desire any thing beyond it. Cicero assures us, that with them it was no less honorable than the **consular dignity** in its original splendor with the ancient Romans. And in another place he says, that to conquer at Olympia, was almost, in the estimation of the Grecians, more great and glorious, than to receive the honour of a triumph at Rome. Horace speaks in still stronger terms of this kind of victory. He is not afraid to say, that "it exalts the victor above human nature; they were **no longer men but gods.**"

Contrast: the honor and glory of Olympic victory is compared and contrasted to the consular dignity (the Roman consul being the highest office of government in the original ancient Roman Republic)

Cause and effect: victory in the Olympic games brings great honor and essentially elevated men to the status of god

We shall see hereafter what extraordinary **honors** were paid the victor, of which one of the most affecting was, to **date the year with his name**. Nothing could more effectually stimulate their endeavors, and make them regardless of expenses, than the assurance of immortalizing their names, which, through all future ages would be enrolled in their annals, and stand in the front of all laws made in the same year with the victory. To this motive may be added the joy of knowing, that their praises would be celebrated by the most famous **poets**, and form the subject of **conversation** in the most illustrious assemblies; for these **odes** were sung in every house, and formed a part in every entertainment. What could be a more powerful incentive to a people, who had no other object and aim than that of **human glory**?

Key terms: honors, date the year, poets, conversation, odes, human glory

Cause and effect: victory in the Olympic games brought many honors and was looked upon as the peak of human achievement

Main Idea: The main idea is that the Olympic games were of great importance to the Greeks, that the victors of the Olympic games were highly honored, and that the practice of the Olympic games illustrates many aspects of Greek culture.

31. A is correct. This question asks us to reason why a woman was allowed to attend the Olympic games when as a general rule, it seems they were not allowed. Based on the passage, women were generally treated very differently than men. Such a discrepancy most likely means that the priestess of Ceres was not viewed as the other women were viewed. Choice B through D are unfounded and unlikely the reason.

32. C is correct. The passage states that the honor of winning at the Olympic games was comparable to the "consular dignity" of ancient Rome. Even without a knowledge of the "consular dignity" one can reason that C is correct because it contains the same wording. The Roman consul was the highest elected office.

   A, B, D: These are not grounded in passage information.

33. B is correct. This question asks us to determine the author's attitude towards the writings of Pausanias. We read in the passage the author cannot conceive of reasons for some discrepancies in Pausanias' writing. The author seems unsure of what to believe. The author believes there is truth behind Pausanias' writings but is confused by discrepancies.

   A: The author is not cynical towards Pausanias' writings

   C, D: These emotions are much too strong and the author does not use any language to suggest such a strong reaction. The MCAT will rarely include passages in which the author is angry or incredulous.

34. A is correct. This question asks us to interpret additional information in the context of passage information. We learn in the passage that the relatives of Olympic victors were liable to be pardoned from offenses. It is likely that victors themselves would be held above the law as well because of the great esteem which was held for them.

35. C is correct. Statement I is true because we learn of the Greek peoples' view towards women and how they were treated differently. Thus this aspect of Greek culture was discussed. Statement III is true because we also learn that the Olympic games represent the greatest achievement in human glory, which is the highest aim of the Grecian people

   II: The workings of the Greek judicial system are not any clearer from the passage information.

Passage 7 (Questions 36 – 40)

I'll make a sharp distinction between **Operative** Witchcraft and **Ritual** Witchcraft. Under **Operative** Witchcraft I class all charms and spells, practised by the priests and people **of every religion**. They are part of the **common heritage** of the human race and are therefore of **no** practical **value** in the study of **any one particular cult**.

Contrast: operative witchcraft vs ritual witchcraft

Cause and effect: charms and spells common through all cultures and peoples, not particular to a given cult

Ritual Witchcraft—or, as I propose to call it, the **Dianic cult**—embraces the religious beliefs and ritual of the people known in late mediaeval times as "Witches". The evidence proves that **underlying the Christian** religion was a cult practised by many classes of the community, chiefly, however, by the **more ignorant** or those in the less thickly inhabited parts of the country. It can be traced back to **pre-Christian times**, and appears to be the ancient religion of Western Europe. The god, anthropomorphic or theriomorphic, was worshipped in well-defined rites; the organization was **highly developed**; and the ritual is analogous to many other ancient rituals. The **dates of** the chief **festivals** suggest that the religion belonged to a race which had **not** reached the **agricultural** stage; and the **evidence shows** that various **modifications** were introduced, probably by **invading peoples** who brought in their own beliefs. I have not attempted to disentangle the various cults; I am content merely to point out that it was a definite religion with beliefs, ritual, and organization as highly developed as that of any other cult in the world.

Key terms: Dianic cult, Witches, Christian, pre-Christian times, Western Europe

Contrast: Christian vs Dianic (more ignorant lower classes within a community, or those in more isolated communities)

Cause and effect: dates of chief festivals of Dianic cults are evidence practitioners were non-agricultural; modifications to the Dianic cult made by invading peoples

The **deity** of this cult was **incarnate** in a man, a woman, or an animal; the **animal form** being apparently **earlier** than the human, for the god was often spoken of as wearing the skin or attributes of an animal. At the same time, however, there was another form of the god in the shape of a **man with two faces**. Such a god is found in Italy (where he was called **Janus** or Dianus), in Southern France, and in the English Midlands. The feminine form of the name, **Diana**, is found **throughout Western Europe** as the name of the **female deity** or leader of the **so-called Witches**, and it is for this reason that I have called this ancient religion the Dianic cult. The geographical distribution of the two-faced god suggests that the race or races, who carried the cult, **either did not remain** in every country which they entered, or that in many places they and their religion **were overwhelmed** by subsequent invaders.

Key terms: Janus, Diana

Contrast: male Janus vs female Diana, animal vs human form of the god

Cause and effect: geographic distribution suggests something happened to Dianics in certain regions

The **dates of the two chief festivals**, **May** Eve and **November** Eve, indicate the use of a calendar which is generally acknowledged to be **pre-agricultural** and earlier than the solstitial division of the year. The fertility rites of the cult bear out this indication, as they were for promoting the increase of animals and only rarely for the benefit of the crops. The **cross-quarter-days, February 2 and August 1**, which were also kept as festivals, were probably of later date, as, though classed among the great festivals, they were **not of so high an importance** as the May and November Eves. To February 2, **Candlemas** Day, probably belongs the sun-charm of the burning wheel, formed by the whirling dancers, each carrying a blazing torch; but no special ceremony seems to be assigned to August 1, **Lammas** Day, a fact suggestive of a later introduction of this festival.

Key terms: cross-quarter-days, Candlemas, Lammas

Contrast: May and November holidays were more important than the February and August ones

Cause and effect: author concludes that the dates of the holidays shows a focus that is not on agriculture

Main Idea: The passage serves to discuss the origins, beliefs, and history of the Dianic cult including its contrast with Christianity and its geographic distribution.

36. A is correct. In the second paragraph, the author tells us that the Dianic cult was practiced primarily by those who were among the more ignorant classes in the larger Christian society.

37. B is correct. The author suggests that the specific dates of festivals implies a non-agricultural origin, which also implies that specific dates in other societies reveal an agricultural origin.

   A, C: These contradict the passage as it implies that they would celebrate dates that important with respect to agriculture, rather than carrying over holidays from hunter-gatherer days.

   D: This is very likely true, but the passage author makes no mention of the astronomical connection, so this answer choice is not really implied by the author.

38. C is correct. Though "Cult" would be better than "Cults" (the passage briefly mentions there are many individual groups but otherwise treats it as one homogenous religion), but the passage does provide a broad overview of the history and spread of these beliefs throughout Europe.

   A: This is a close match for some of the main ideas found in the introductory paragraph, but although the first paragraph often reveals the main idea or thesis of a passage, in this case it merely lays out some definitional groundwork before jumping into the real point of the text.

   B: This is not supported by the passage, which says very little to suggest significant mingling between Dianic and Christian beliefs.

   D: This is somewhat tempting, as the passage does suggest Dianic cults (and the unnamed Janus/Dianus equivalents) as Western Europe's ancient religion, but the passage author does not emphasize that "new evidence" has come up, instead making more of a survey and summary of what is currently known.

39. B is correct. If the (unspecified) geographic distribution is evidence that Dianic worshippers either did not remain or were conquered by invaders of a different religious stripe, what could that distribution be? There must be regions where Dianics logically would have been expected to be, but somehow aren't. For example, regions which are in-between known Dianic regions would also be expected to have Dianic worshippers, as the spread of the people would have necessitated crossing that intermediate region. Gaps in such intervening regions, as suggested in answer choice B, would indeed serve as evidence of either a deliberate choice not to settle or conflict with other groups, as described in the passage

40. A is correct. The second paragraph describe the rituals as well-defined, and multiple parts of the passage establish the religion as ancient and therefore long-lived and well-established. The passage author also mentions that there are, in fact, many different Dianic cults, stating elsewhere that other cultural practices, perhaps from invaders or neighbors, have also been absorbed by Dianic cults in different regions.

   B: This does not work as the author makes clear in the first paragraph that practical witchcraft is not unique to Dianic cults but common everywhere, and never describes these techniques as primitive.

   C: This does not work as this was the original religion in ancient Western Europe and did not become scattered or fringe (if indeed it has done so) until later beliefs like Christianity came in.

   D: This is incorrect, as the religion was not originally agricultural in nature.

Passage 8 (Questions 41 – 47)

Though the **world of natural phenomena** seemed to man wayward and inexplicable for so long, we eventually **came to** perceive in it a pervasive **order** and uniformity. In the same way, we have **found a manifest order** and uniformity in the **economic world**, albeit of a less majestic kind. **Man depends upon his fellow men** for the very means of life, and yet, he takes this cooperation as if for granted, with a complacent confidence and naive unconsciousness, just as he takes the rising of tomorrow's sun. Many observers have been justifiably and notably **impressed by the reliability** of this **unorganized cooperation**.

Contrast: taking social cooperation for granted vs taking the rising of tomorrow's sun for granted

Cause and effect: because we were able to find uniformity in the seemingly wayward natural world, we were also able to do so in the economic world; because of its reliability, many observers have been impressed

As **Bastiat** exclaimed some seventy years ago, "Upon entering **Paris**, I said to myself -- here are a **million human beings** who would all die in short time if **provisions** suddenly ceased **flowing into** this great metropolis. The imagination is baffled when it attempts to appreciate the **vast multiplicity of commodities that must enter the city tomorrow** in order to keep the inhabitants from falling prey to the convulsions of famine, pillage, and rebellion. And yet, at this moment, all these people sleep soundly, and their peaceful slumbers are not disturbed for a single moment by the prospect of such a catastrophe. On the other hand, eighty departments have labored today, without cooperation and without any mutual understanding, in order to provide for Paris."

Contrast: a million human beings surviving with provisions vs dying in short time without them, peaceful slumber vs the prospect of such a catastrophe

Cause and effect: if provisions stopped coming into Paris, a million people would die in short order or fall prey to the convulsions of famine, pillage, and rebellion

This theme may well excite a **sense of wonder**, but wonder must always be watched with a **careful** eye, for he is liable to bring along with him a hanger-on we know as **worship**. Here, in the realm of economics, this hanger-on can do nothing but mischief. There are only a few short steps between the passage quoted above, the **glorification of the existing system** of society, the **defense of** a whole slew of **indefensible things**, and a stubbornly contrary attitude towards all projects of reform. These are short steps, but they are ones that are quite unjustifiable to take.

Cause and effect: because wonder is liable to bring along the hanger-on worship, we ought to watch wonder with a careful eye; the wonder of the quoted passage leads to the glorification of the existing system which can lead to defense of indefensible things

The **evils of our economic system are simply too obvious to be ignored** far too many people have a harsh personal experience of the wastefulness of its production, the injustice of its distribution, the sweating it necessitates, its unemployment, and its slums. When the attempt is made to **brush over these evils with obsequious rhetoric about the majesty of economic law and order**, we should not be surprised that the spirits of many men will revolt and retort by denying the existence of order in the economic world, declaring that the spectacle which they, **the disadvantaged masses, see is one of chaos, confusion, and discord**. At this point, we become absorbed by a controversy as **stale**, flat, and unprofitable as that general one between the "**theorist**" and the "**practical man**."

Contrast: evils vs obsequious rhetoric about the majesty of economic law and order, spirits of many men vs the existence of order in the economic world, the spectacle seen by someone like Bastiat vs the spectacle seen by the disadvantaged masses

Cause and effect: because the evils of our economic system are obvious, they cannot be ignored; if the attempt is made to brush over these evils, it will cause the spirits of men to revolt and to retort by denying the existence of order in the economic world

The truth is that this language of private praise and public criticism is inappropriate. First of all, it is important to note that the **order** that I have spoken of makes itself clear not only in those **economic phenomena** which are **beneficial** to man, but in those that are **hurtful as well**. Even in the alteration of good and bad trade, which causes so much unemployment and misery, there is a measurable, rhythmic regularity like that of the seasons, or like the ebb and flow of the tide. This is not an elegance to be admired. Moreover, to the extent that economic order is comprised of adjustments and tendencies that are beneficial (as is mainly true), there is no justification for assuming that these are either sufficient to secure a prosperous community, or that they are dependent upon the social arrangement that already exists. Therefore, we ought to refrain from premature polemics and **embrace a spirit of detachment** when we **examine** further aspects of this elaborate, **unorganized cooperation** of which so much has already been said and written.

Contrast: economic phenomena that are beneficial to man vs those that are hurtful, tendencies that are beneficial vs those that are sufficient to secure a prosperous community

Cause and effect: if economic order is comprised of beneficial tendencies, this does not mean that these are sufficient for a prosperous community or that they depend on social arrangement (rather, they may create social arrangement), because of all this, we should refrain from premature polemics and embrace a sense of detachment when we talk about economics

Main Idea: After comparing it to nature that once seemed inexplicable but now seems ordered, the author says we ought to approach economics with a wary eye; he explains the evils of our economic system and believes a sense of detachment will be beneficial to us when we discuss economics.

41. D is correct. I is true because many men will revolt against rhetoric about the majesty of economic law and order by denying its existence. II is true because of the comparison drawn in the first two sentences of the passage. III is true because the system actually is impressive. The author warns against a sense of wonder that can lead to worship. He never claims we ought to not be impressed.

42. D is correct. Bastiat's perspective, presented in the long quote in the second paragraph, introduces the notion of a sense of wonder that brings the hanger-on worship. This type of wonder that Bastiat typifies is the foil to the disillusionment felt by those who suffer harsh experiences under the economic system. These many represent public criticism while Bastiat, an individual, represents private praise.

43. D is correct. The key here is the phrase "in the same way" at the beginning of the second sentence, which introduces the economic world. Just as the natural world seemed wayward and inexplicable at first, so too did the economic world. And just as we were eventually able to find order in the natural world, we did so as well in the economic world.

  A: This may be true, but is never clearly stated.

  B: The tone is distinctly not expressive of praise.

  C: We didn't invent it, we found it.

44. A is correct. In the fifth paragraph, the author writes that in the alteration of good and bad trade "there is a measurable, rhythmic regularity like that of the seasons, or like the ebb and flow of the tide." We can assume that the author, in comparing the ups and downs of trade to the seasons and the tide (which are inevitable), and in describing its regularity, believes that it is inevitable, at least within the economic system

  B: The author believes "this is not an elegance to be admired."

  C: He never writes that worship does mischief or is problematic anywhere else outside economics.

  D: The author believes having a "stubbornly contrary attitude towards all projects of reform" is not a desirable thing, this seems to imply that he believes reform is still necessary in a fully established economy.

45. C is correct. This controversy, between private praise and public criticism, is stale, flat, and unprofitable, just like that general debate between the "theorist" and the "practical man." The author believes this kind of debate does nothing for either side, it is "unprofitable." The author's intention here is to advocate for detachment in studying economics as he believes that will be more useful.

  A: Though perhaps alluded to or suggested, class warfare is not mentioned directly.

  B: It is more likely true that private interests already have more power. This debate actually seems even: few with more power = more with less power. The controversy is stale and flat because it goes nowhere.

  D: Rather, the public criticism side of the debate is all about the evils of the economic system.

46. B is correct. The professor B is the one most representative of a "spirit of detachment," using objective mathematics and science.

  A: This would bring in personal tastes (i.e attachment).

  C: The phrase at the end of the passage, "of which so much has already been said and written," seems to carry with it some disdain. The author calls upon us to "examine further aspects" of economic systems, suggesting a forward-looking thrust and avoiding wasting time by looking backwards.

  D: Utopian philosophy seems to be indicative of a kind of attachment, perhaps to wishful thinking.

47. D is correct. In the first paragraph: "Man depends upon his fellow men for the very means of life." The flow of provisions into Paris is indelibly linked to the "unorganized cooperation" of the economic system. Therefore, this unorganized cooperation seems to be essential.

  A, B, C: These statements are all true and stated in the passage.

Passage 9 (Questions 48 – 53)

Besides a **good will**, there is nothing that can be conceived in the world that can be called **good without qualification**. The talents of the mind, such as intelligence, wit, and judgment, and the qualities of temperament, such as courage, resolution, and perseverance, are unquestionably good and desirable in many ways. However, these **gifts of nature** have also the **potential to become bad** and mischievous if the will that makes use of them is not good, for it is the will and how it uses things which we call character.

Contrast: a good will can be called good without qualification vs nothing else can be called good without qualification

Cause and effect: if the will that makes use of them is not good, gifts of nature, which seem to be good things, could become bad and mischievous

Honor, power, riches, the well-being and contentment with one's condition which we know as happiness, and even health, inspire **pride**, and often presumption **if there is no good will** to correct the influence of these things upon the mind. An impartial, rational spectator will never take pleasure from seeing a person, adorned with absolutely no features of a good will, enjoying unchecked prosperity. Therefore, having a good will seems to be an **essential** condition **even of being worthy of happiness**.

Cause and effect: seemingly good things, without the influence of good will, can lead to pride and presumption, having a good will seems to be an essential condition of being worthy of happiness

There are **some qualities** that, despite having no intrinsic unconditional value, **serve this good will and may facilitate its action**. Though they are always essential for a good will, thus qualifying the esteem we have for them, these qualities are **not regarded as being absolutely good**. For example, **calm deliberation**, moderation in the affections and passions, and self-control are qualities that are not only good, but even seem to make up, at least in part, the intrinsic value of a person. This being said, they do not deserve to be called good without qualification, even though the ancients praised them so unconditionally. Without the guidance of a good will, **even these qualities may become bad the coolness of a villain not only makes him more dangerous, but also makes him more loathsome** than he would be without it.

Cause and effect: these seemingly good qualities can become bad without the guidance of a good will, because the coolness of a villain makes him more dangerous and more loathsome, it is clear that these goods cannot be called good without qualification

A good will is not good because of what it performs or because of its aptness for the attainment of an end, but rather, it is **good by virtue of volition**. In other words, it is a **good in itself**, and considered by itself, it is esteemed far higher than all the things that can be brought about by it in favor of a particular inclination or even the sum total of all inclina-

tions. Even if the will lacked any power to accomplish its purpose, due perhaps to a disfavor of fortunate, **even if** its strongest efforts **achieved nothing**, and all that was left was the good will (to be clear, this is not merely a good wish, but the summoning of all the means in its power), then it **would still shine like a jewel**, by its own brilliance, as a thing which in itself contains its whole value. Therefore, its **usefulness or uselessness neither adds nor subtracts from its value**. So, the will's usefulness would enable us to handle it more easily in attracting to it the attention of those who are not yet connoisseurs, but not to recommend it to true connoisseurs, or to gauge its true value.

Cause and effect: if the will lacked any power to accomplish goals, it would still shine like a jewel and be a good in itself, for it contains its whole value

Of course, there is **something odd about this idea** of the absolute value of mere will, in which no real significance is given to its utility. Though even common reason may assent to this idea, a suspicion arises that this is really just the product of **high concept fancy** and that we have **perhaps misunderstood** the whole purpose of nature in claiming reason as the governor of our will. Therefore, we will further examine this idea from this point of view.

Opinion: although the author favors the view of a good will as good in itself, he acknowledges that there's something odd about that point of view and that it's worth examining further the possibility that this view has gotten it wrong

Main Idea: The author makes the case that the only thing that can be considered good without qualification is a good will; the author explores exactly what it is about a good will that makes it good, that being the act of volition; even without the ability to achieve its ends, a good will is still inherently good; the author does acknowledge that this conception of good will may perhaps be the product of a high concept fancy and a misunderstanding of reason and will in the first place.

48. A is correct. As the author writes at the end of the first paragraph, " . . . these gifts of nature have also the potential to become bad and mischievous if the will that makes use of them is not good, for it is the will and how it uses things which we call character." So, if a person has a bad will that does not use things well, he or she has a bad character. Therefore, this person is lacking in this regard.

B: Education is not mentioned here.

C, D: Not necessarily so. Both of these are given as qualities that must be kept in check, just like those described in the question. Character is essential to the regulation of all of these qualities.

49. D is correct. The author is making the point that even these three goods, which seem to be, on first consideration, good in themselves, may become bad. "Without the guidance of a good will, even these qualities may become bad . . . " He is continuing the argument begun in the first paragraph about seemingly good qualities that can become bad without the guidance of the will. He is attempting to prove that no quality, no matter how good it seems, is entirely good in itself. Rather, the only thing that can be said to be good in itself is a good will.

A: This happens in the fourth paragraph, with the introduction of "volition."

B: They do, but the author's primary point is to further the argument he has already begun.

C: They are compared favorably, but this point is secondary to the actual comparison: all of these qualities, though they seem different, share in the fact that they are not good in themselves.

50. B is correct. Choice B is drawn from the intriguing fifth paragraph, in which the author questions the point he has been making for the previous four. Because suspicions arise (and rightfully so he might say), we ought to further examine the problem from this suspicious point of view.

A: This is not true, because the author writes that someone who is happy must have a good will to correct the influence of happiness. This means that someone without a good will can still be happy, but won't have the influence of that happiness corrected.

C: This is not true, according to the passage.

D: Rather, it is only valuable in attracting people to become connoisseurs.

51. D is correct. Choice D is most directly representative of a person with a good will, particularly as it is described in the fourth paragraph. No inclination is mentioned. None of the qualities that can potentially be bad are mentioned. Rather, this seems to be a sheer act of

goodness, and even though she failed, her act was driven by good will and therefore the outcome can not affect the goodness of the act, for good will is good in itself and shines "like a jewel" even if the will lacks the power to accomplish its purpose due to a disfavor of fortune.

A: The word investor immediately implies that the man is seeking returns on this venture seeding.

B: First of all, those qualities, courage and perseverance are not necessarily good. Second of all, this woman is not displaying a good will as directly as the woman of Choice D.

C: Again, the words intelligence and wit. He may have a good will, but it is not as obviously clear as it is in choice D.

52. C is correct. As the author writes of the good will, " . . . it is a good in itself, and considered by itself, it is esteemed far higher than all the things that can be brought about by it in favor of a particular inclination or even the sum total of all inclinations." So, even if someone had the sum total of all inclinations possible and worked on behalf of them, a good will would still be esteemed higher than the things brought about by those inclinations. So, it seems that inclinations, in this sense, are not necessarily essential to having a good will.

A: A good will is good by virtue of its volition.

B, D: These are two of the qualities that are essential to a good will.

53. D is correct. I: As the author writes in the penultimate sentence of the passage, " . . . a suspicion arises that this is really just the product of high concept fancy and that we have perhaps misunderstood the whole purpose of nature in claiming reason as the governor of our will." How exactly does this second part of the sentence relate? The author implies it as a general misunderstanding that may perhaps undermine the argument of the passage. Therefore, Item I is true. II: As the author writes of good will, or "mere will" as he calls it in this context, " . . . no real significance is given to its utility." This makes Item II true. III: This is perhaps a bit more tenuous. If this idea about good will is really just "the product of high concept fancy," it is based not in reality, but in fancy, or fantasy. It potentially has no basis in reality. For measuring things with a basis in reality, we use science, to either measure them or attempt to prove them. The will, something intangible and perhaps even invented, does not seem to have qualities that would make it scientifically measurable (i.e. physical existence). So, Item III is true as well.

SECTION 12

53 Questions, 90 Minutes

Use an answer grid from the back of the book to record your answers

Passage 1 (Questions 1 – 6)

In 1988, a British surgeon and medical researcher named Andrew Wakefield published a paper in the medical journal *The Lancet* postulating a link between administration of the measles, mumps, and rubella vaccine (MMR) and the appearance of autism, as well as certain gastroenterological conditions, in children. Written with twelve co-authors, Wakefield's paper identified a syndrome they called "autistic enterocolitis," and linked the MMR vaccine to autism and bowel disease. The study on which the paper was based – of twelve children with behavioral symptoms consistent with Autism Spectrum Disorder, or ASD – claimed that eight of the twelve children developed "behavioral symptoms" within two weeks of receiving the MMR vaccine.

The paper was immediately and enormously controversial, in the UK and worldwide. Although Wakefield *et al* did not make a definitive connection between the vaccine and autism in the Lancet paper, Wakefield had held a press conference prior to the paper's publication, at which he called for the suspension of the triple vaccine until further research proved it safe. At the press conference, Wakefield stated that speaking out against the vaccine was a "moral issue."

In the wake of the Lancet article, subsequent studies were unable to support Wakefield's results. Concerns were raised that a study of twelve children was too small to be statistically valid. However, the article – or, more specifically, Wakefield's press conference – created near panic for many parents. The number of parents who opted not to give their children the MMR vaccine jumped tremendously, and consequently, incidence of measles increased. One report suggested that in England alone, MMR vaccination rates dropped from 92% to 73% as a result of concerns about MMR and autism.

Nonetheless, the anti-vaccine movement has continued to grow, particularly as the incidence of autism and autism spectrum disorders continues to rise. Thousands of parents believe vaccines – and, most specifically, the MMR vaccine – caused their child's disability. Doubters say that such belief is based on anecdotal evidence and cannot be supported; yet many parents have no doubt that the regression and skill loss typical in the emergence of autism undeniably followed vaccination.

Wakefield was accused by a *Sunday Times* reporter of conflict of interest in 2004; the reporter said that some of the children in Wakefield's study had been recruited by a lawyer preparing a lawsuit against MMR vaccine manufacturers. Two years later, it was reported that Wakefield was paid over $500,000 by the lawyers involved in the suit, a fact that he had not previously disclosed. In February 2010, *The Lancet* formally withdrew Wakefield's paper, calling it fraudulent. Shortly after that, the British General Medical Council permanently revoked Wakefield's license to practice medicine. Wakefield continues to protest his innocence, and claims that he was targeted by public health officials and pharmaceutical companies.

No further studies have documented a clear link between the MMR vaccine and regressive autism. However, in 2013, the federal Vaccine Injury Compensation Program, or vaccine court, as it is commonly known, awarded millions of dollars in compensation to the families of two children who attested that the debilitating encephalopathy their children suffered was directly attributable to vaccines. While the children have autism-like symptoms, the ruling is scrupulous in not directly linking autism with the vaccines. Most of the documents pertaining to the case are sealed, and not available to the public. Those who see clear correlation between the MMR vaccine and ASD see this as admission that there is a link. Those who do not view the ruling as just compensation for vaccine-related injuries – but not as proof of the role of the MMR vaccine in the development of autism.

1. A supporter of Wakefield's theory might assert:

    A. even if Wakefield's study was flawed, there remains a possibility of a link between the vaccine and autism.

    B. it is more important to address the vaccine as a likely cause of autism than it is to prevent measles.

    C. although the link between the vaccine and autism was disproved, the connection between the vaccine and bowel disease remains valid.

    D. anecdotal evidence is sufficient to establish a link between the vaccine and autism.

2. What might Wakefield have meant in saying that speaking out against the MMR vaccine was for him a "moral issue"?

    A. He felt he was ethically obligated to disclose a pubic health risk.

    B. Unlike the manufacturers of the MMR vaccine, he was motivated by an ethical code, rather than financial gain.

    C. His motive to address a serious public health risk overrode his unorthodox methodology.

    D. He could be more effective as a public advocate than as a medical researcher.

3. Detractors of the theory that the MMR vaccine is related to the development of autism might be likely to believe:

    A. although clear evidence of the cause of autism has not been established, it is still possible that the MMR vaccine is a factor.

    B. anecdotal evidence is not enough to establish a link between the vaccine and ASD.

    C. Wakefield was motivated by profit rather than by his purported moral code.

    D. the connection between the vaccine and autism is wholly a result of scare tactics by the media.

4. Which of the following is analogous to the "anecdotal evidence" mentioned in Paragraph 4?

    A. Suggesting that an outbreak of measles is related to decreased MMR vaccination rates

    B. Studying the relationship between students' study habits and post-college income

    C. Data supporting that vaccines have low incidences of side effects

    D. A man with greying hair pointing to a stressful event as the cause of the grey hair

5. According to the passage, all of the following accusations were made against Wakefield EXCEPT:

    A. he was compensated inappropriately for his study.

    B. he was not in reality motivated by moral issues.

    C. his choice of subjects was biased.

    D. the results of his study were statistically invalid.

6. Which of the following scenarios would likely support the hypothesis that no clear causal connection exists between the MMR vaccine and ASD?

    A. Children with autism received additional vaccines at the same time the MMR vaccine was administered.

    B. Children with autism are unlikely to be awarded compensation in vaccine court.

    C. Children with autism may also have gastroenterological health issues.

    D. Children with autism exhibited symptoms of ASD prior to receiving the MMR vaccine.

Passage 2 (Questions 7 – 13)

The Diagnostic and Statistical Manual of Mental Disorders, or DSM, is used to diagnose mental and behavioral disorders. Published by the American Psychiatric Association (APA), the DSM has been revised several times over the past six decades to reflect changes in psychiatric research and practice. The most recent edition, *DSM-5*, was released in 2013. One of the greatest changes from *DSM-IV* to *DSM-5* is in revisions to the definition of autism and related neuro-developmental disorders. *DSM-5* officially eliminates several autism spectrum diagnoses. Gone are Asperger's syndrome, a diagnosis which usually was applied to individuals without language deficit or intellectual disability; pervasive developmental disorder, not otherwise specified, or PPD-NOS, which typically applied to higher-functioning people who did not meet all the criteria for autism; and childhood disintegrative disorder, which referred to children who exhibited severe regression after the age of three. These diagnoses are now incorporated into one single diagnosis – autism spectrum disorder, or ASD.

The APA states that the goal of the revision was to overcome inconsistencies in how autism is diagnosed. According to a member of the APA task force that addressed autism-related diagnoses, even among clinicians with expertise in diagnosing autism spectrum disorders, there was significant variation in diagnoses within the spectrum. The single, overarching ASD diagnosis is meant to address that; its intention is to provide a single framework for parents, educators, doctors, and other service providers to use and language to discuss people on all parts of the spectrum. Furthermore, the APA asserts that the *DSM-5* is meant to be a "living document." (Hence the change from Roman numerals to Arabic numbers; "5" is meant to signify 5.0, and the expectation of ongoing updates as psychiatric understanding and practice are refined.)

The new diagnosis still differentiates qualifiers, such as language ability, intellectual disability, and regression, and rates severity levels from one to three. One significant change is that in order to receive an autism spectrum disorder diagnosis, a child must exhibit deficits in social communication, as well as restricted or repetitive behavior, each of which is rated in severity. A child who exhibits communication deficit but not restricted or repetitive behavior will be given a new diagnosis: social communication disorder. How insurance companies deal with this new diagnosis remains to be seen: while 37 states have laws that regulate insurance coverage of children with autism, such laws would not apply to social communication disorder.

Although the change in the DSM has been greeted with enthusiasm by many psychiatrists and behavioral health providers – some of who felt that the *DSM-IV* made it harder for people with Asperger's and PPD-NOS to receive services – not everyone shares this belief. Some parents and patients have expressed a concern that the new criteria would be more, not less, exclusionary, particularly for people with Asperger's and PDD-NOS. Although the APA autism task force

estimated that fewer than 10 percent of people currently diagnosed with autism would not meet the new *DSM-5* standards, other studies suggest that over 75% of people with Asperger's would not receive a diagnosis under the new standards – and would not qualify for needed services. Some advocates assert that the revision represents an effort for schools and insurance companies to control costs. Others have expressed the concern that if a significant number of higher functioning individuals are not diagnosed, the prevalence rate of autism will be unrealistically decreased. One other issue: to some, a diagnosis of autism carries a stigma that a diagnosis of Asperger's does not; will higher-functioning individuals and their families avoid the autism label – and thus refuse support that could be truly helpful?

7. According to the passage, what issue did the APA hope to address in its revisions to the diagnostic criteria and categories for autism and related disorders in the DSM in 2013?

   A. The inaccurately high prevalence rate of autism spectrum disorders

   B. The stigma of an autism diagnosis

   C. The overrepresentation of individuals with social communication disorders without repetitive behaviors

   D. The complexities in diagnosing autism spectrum disorders

8. Which of the following represents a diagnosis that exists in *DSM-5* but not *DSM-IV*?

   A. Social communication disorder

   B. PPD-NOS

   C. Asperger's syndrome

   D. Restrictive or repetitive behavior

9. Suppose a child receives a behavioral evaluation in 2014 and is found to exhibit Level 2 communication deficit, and no repetitive behavior. Which diagnosis is she likely to receive?

   A. Asperger's syndrome

   B. PPD-NOS

   C. Social communication disorder

   D. Autism spectrum disorder

10. Which of the following best captures the author's view on changes regarding autism qualifiers in the *DSM-5*?

   A. While the changes are intended to simplify and clarify the diagnostic process, they may have unintended consequences.

   B. Although the APA has stated that their goal is to simplify the diagnostic process, the changes will actually create more confusion than clarity.

   C. Parents and patients are at odds with behavioral health providers regarding the accuracy of the new diagnostic qualifiers.

   D. Although the new qualifiers may seem sound, in actuality they will disqualify the majority of individuals with autism from receiving appropriate support services.

11. According to the passage, critics of the *DSM-5* point to all of the following as potential problems in diagnosing or providing support to people with autism spectrum disorders EXCEPT:

   A. it is unclear whether insurance companies will extend coverage to people diagnosed with social communication disorder, but who under the *DSM-IV* would have received services with a diagnosis of autism.

   B. people with Asperger's may feel stigmatized, and thus be less likely to pursue helpful services, by the new ASD diagnosis.

   C. a significant number of people who qualified for services under the *DSM-IV* criteria would not receive benefits under the new system.

   D. because clinicians and educators are likely to be unfamiliar with the new qualifiers, some individuals will be misdiagnosed and thus not qualify for support services.

12. Suppose that in 2016, the APA recognizes a study documenting that the majority of children who would have received an autism spectrum disorder diagnoses under the *DSM-IV* will no longer qualify for autism-related services under the *DSM-5*. According to the passage, what might the APA's response to this study be?

   A. To recognize the flaws in *DSM-5* and begin preparation of *DSM-6*

   B. To revise and update, since *DSM-5* is a "living document" that can incorporate new research

   C. To take no action, since qualification for services is not the focus of the DSM

   D. To take no action, because the study documents the over-reporting of ASD that *DSM-5* intended to address.

13. Based on the passage, which of the following represents a benefit of the *DSM-5*, according to some clinicians?

   A. *DSM-5* helps to shift the focus away from higher functioning individuals, who were over-reported under *DSM-IV* criteria.

   B. *DSM-5* represents an equitable means for service providers to control costs.

   C. *DSM-5* does away with distinctions that divided the autism community.

   D. *DSM-5* gives clinicians, teachers, parents, and patients a clearer diagnostic framework and better serves people on all parts of the spectrum.

Passage 3 (Questions 14 – 18)

The question as to what we mean by truth and falsehood, which we considered in the preceding chapter, is of much less interest than the question as to how we can know what is true and what is false. This question will occupy us in the present chapter. There can be no doubt that some of our beliefs are erroneous; thus we are led to inquire what certainty we can ever have that such and such a belief is not erroneous. In other words, can we ever know anything at all, or do we merely sometimes by good luck believe what is true? Before we can attack this question, we must, however, first decide what we mean by "knowing", and this question is not so easy as might be supposed.

At first sight we might imagine that knowledge could be defined as "true belief". When what we believe is true, it might be supposed that we had achieved a knowledge of what we believe. But this would not accord with the way in which the word is commonly used. To take a very trivial instance: If a man believes that the late Prime Minister's last name began with a B, he believes what is true, since the late Prime Minister was Sir Henry Campbell Bannerman. But if he believes that Mr. Balfour was the late Prime Minister, he will still believe that the late Prime Minister's last name began with a B, yet this belief, though true, would not be thought to constitute knowledge. If a newspaper, by an intelligent anticipation, announces the result of a battle before any telegram giving the result has been received, it may by good fortune announce what afterwards turns out to be the right result, and it may produce belief in some of its less experienced readers. But in spite of the truth of their belief, they cannot be said to have knowledge. Thus it is clear that a true belief is not knowledge when it is deduced from a false belief.

In like manner, a true belief cannot be called knowledge when it is deduced by a fallacious process of reasoning, even if the premises from which it is deduced are true. If I know that all Greeks are men and that Socrates was a man, and I infer that Socrates was a Greek, I cannot be said to know that Socrates was a Greek, because, although my premises and my conclusion are true, the conclusion does not follow from the premises.

But are we to say that nothing is knowledge except what is validly deduced from true premises? Obviously we cannot say this. Such a definition is at once too wide and too narrow. In the first place, it is too wide, because it is not enough that our premises should be true, they must also be known. The man who believes that Mr. Balfour was the late Prime Minister may proceed to draw valid deductions from the true premise that the late Prime Minister's name began with a B, but he cannot be said to know the conclusions reached by these deductions. Thus we shall have to amend our definition by saying that knowledge is what is validly deduced from known premises. This, however, is a circular definition: it assumes that we already know what is meant by 'known premises'. It can, therefore, at best define one sort of knowledge, the sort we call derivative, as opposed to intuitive knowledge. We may say: "Derivative knowledge is what is validly deduced from premises known intuitively". In this statement there is no formal defect, but it leaves the definition of intuitive knowledge still to seek.

Leaving on one side, for the moment, the question of intuitive knowledge, let us consider the above suggested definition of derivative knowledge. The chief objection to it is that it unduly limits knowledge. It constantly happens that people entertain a true belief, which has grown up in them because of some piece of intuitive knowledge from which it is capable of being validly inferred, but from which it has not, as a matter of fact, been inferred by any logical process.

14. The author states that the definition of knowledge as logical deductions from true beliefs is too narrow for which of the following reasons?

  A. We are able to know things without them being inferred by logical deductions.

  B. We are able to know things that are deduced from false beliefs.

  C. We are able to know things that are deduced from knowledge.

  D. Not everything deduced from true beliefs is knowledge.

15. Which of the following is an example of intuitive knowledge?

  A. Identifying a smell without knowing the source

  B. A mathematical theorem proven true by axioms assumed to be true

  C. A mathematical axiom taken to be true, upon which proofs of theorems are developed

  D. Identifying the source of a sound without seeing the source

16. Which of the following is NOT a reason that a certain true belief cannot be considered knowledge?

  A. The belief is arrived at from illogical reasoning.

  B. The belief is deduced from another true belief.

  C. The belief is true but founded on a valid deduction from a false belief.

  D. The belief is a savvy guess about the future that turns out to be right.

17. Which of the following is a line of reasoning most similar to that given in the third paragraph?

  A. If the streets are wet when it is raining and the streets are wet, then it is raining.

  B. If all dogs are mammals and my pet skipper is a mammal, then skipper is a dog.

  C. If the streets are wet when it is raining and it is raining, then the streets are wet.

  D. If all dogs are mammals and my pet skipper is a dog, then skipper is a mammal.

18. The purpose of the example of the prime minister whose name begins with "b" is to show that:

  A. people often espouse false beliefs.

  B. a true belief does not always equate with true knowledge.

  C. people often espouse true beliefs inferred from false beliefs.

  D. people often espouse false beliefs inferred from true beliefs.

Passage 4 (Questions 19 – 24)

Alfred Lord Tennyson's *In Memoriam*, perhaps the most extended exploration of internalized grief in the English language, seemingly argues against the mere existence of time. Anniversaries, Christmases, weddings, all serve as a slight to the mourning speaker, who "long[s] to prove/ no lapse of moons can canker Love/whatever fickle tongues may say" (XXVI, 2-4). Affronted by the way the outside world regains its equilibrium after the death of Arthur Henry Hallam, Tennyson/the Narrator withdraws within his self, eschewing both the natural passing of time and the "fickle tongues" of societal soothing. In doing so, he enacts lyric poetry's prime directive to travel within.

Northrop Frye, paraphrasing John Stuart Mill's categorization of poetry as an "overheard" utterance (80), deems lyric poetry "preeminently the utterance that is overheard… the individual communing within himself" (249-50). This intense self-reflexivity means that the lyric poem necessarily engages with, by strenuously placing itself out of, time: Kenneth Burke terms lyric poetry as caught in a "state of arrest" (245). Lyric poetry is thus, in some ways, a protest against temporality and, as such, must grapple with time to defeat it. Yet Tennyson's poem makes time a character even more central, in some ways, than Hallam himself. The poet grapples not just with the quotidian passing of time which affronts the mourner, not just with the disjunct between the time of the living and the eternal time of the after-life with which he struggles to believe, but with the vast immensity of time on earth. In his most famous treatment of time and geology, stanza LXVI, Tennyson contemplates the "scarped cliff" which hold within it "a thousand types," now extinct (2;3). It is after facing the material reality of the many fossilized types embodied within the cliffs that Tennyson confronts not just the reality of "nature, red in tooth and claw" (15), but also the way that human subjectivity, be it "blown about the desert dust,/Or seal'd within the iron hills" is, in some ways, erased by the passage of long geological time (19-20).

The "futil[ity]" of life, for Tennyson, is emphasized by coming face to face with "A monster then, a dream,/A discord. Dragons of the prime" (21-22). Literally a fossilized dinosaur, the dragon affronts Tennyson because of its temporal "discord," a tangible artifact of the passage of time which so offends him. Yet at the same time, the "dragon'" serves as an instance of frozen time, and the ability to capture items out of time, as it were, slowly begins to comfort the narrator. In the following cantos, he slowly begins to envision Hallam in an analogous position to the dragon, "richly shrined" (LVII 7), and is ultimately able to envision him as one that "canst not die" because of his a-temporality, or rather, simul-temporality: like the fossil, a material object in the now that is the literal trace of a long past time, Hallam inheres within the "past, present, and to be" (CXXIX 11,13). Tennyson casts this as a return to faith if not traditional religion: be Hallam a second coming or an evolutionary "closer link" to a new biological "type" (Epilogue 127,138), by finding a way for Hallam to exist in simultaneous versions of time, Tennyson finds a way to resume his enmeshment in earthly time (the

word "time" appears four time in the epilogue, "hours" and "now" three each). However, Hallam's transcendence is only understandable to the narrator when he roots himself within actuality: the will to live and believe rises "out of the dust" from a "spiritual rock" (CXXXI 5,3). Ultimately, lyric poetry does allow Tennyson to master, or at least come to terms with time, but only by merging with the material: rooted in the now, speaking of the past, fossils and, ultimately Hallam, allow Tennyson to accept his own unidirectional trudge through a temporality that suddenly blooms with multiple, asynchronous paths.

19. Based on the passage it can be assumed that Tennyson likened Hallam to a dragon in order to do which of the following?

    A. Argue that fossils are the strongest indicators of past time

    B. Set up a model of frozen time that offers an alternative to death

    C. Symbolize a monster against which a hero struggles in order to develop religious resonance

    D. To imagine a relationship to time that is both a reminder of the past and in existence now

20. The author brings up Frye and Mill in order to:

    A. enumerate the various writers who influenced Tennyson's poetry.

    B. contrast their ideas to those of Burke.

    C. suggest that all great poets protest temporality.

    D. emphasize the interiority and self-examination that lyric poetry entails.

21. Suppose that it was discovered that the epilogue was not written by Tennyson, but rather by another friend. Based on the passage, the author would most likely assert that:

    A. Tennyson was too overcome by grief to write after Hallam's death.

    B. Tennyson was not fully over the continuation of everyday time in contrast to the eternal time indicated by Hallam's death.

    C. Tennyson had originally written a grimmer ending that repudiated the idea of traditional religion, but his friend realized it would not be well received.

    D. Tennyson lost interest in the project after a short time.

22. Based on the passage, in his poetry, Tennyson addresses which of the following questions about time?

    I. The long stretch of time for which the earth has existed

    II. Belief in an afterlife with an unending, rather than limited, time span

    III. The everyday passing of time, despite the sorrow of death

    A. I only

    B. II only

    C. I and III only

    D. I, II, and III

23. Based on the passage, which of the following is the best definition of lyric poetry?

    A. A form in which interiority and singular moments are emphasized

    B. A musical form which features repetition and upbeat tempos

    C. A form centered about protests and legal matters

    D. A poetic form that emphasizes the passing of time

24. Based on the passage, *In Memoriam* was written to commemorate the passing of:

    A. Northrop Frye

    B. Alfred Lord Tennyson

    C. Arthur Henry Hallam

    D. John Stuart Mill

Passage 5 (Questions 25 – 31)

I suppose that humans have reached the point at which the obstacles to their survival in a natural state possess a greater power of resistance than the resources each individual has available for their own defense and survival in that state. Therefore, this primitive state can no longer subsist, and if humans could not change their manner of existence, the human race would perish. Because people cannot generate new forces, but rather, can only direct and unite existing ones, they have no other choice for survival than to form an aggregate of forces great enough to overcome the obstacles of the natural world. These forces must be gathered around a single motive power, and they must act cooperatively.

This sum of forces requires many people to come together, and here a significant question arises: because the force and liberty of every person are the primary drives for their own self-preservation, how might they pledge them to the collective whole while maintaining their own interests and without neglecting the care that they owe to themselves? This conundrum is concisely defined by the following terms:

"The problem is to find a form of association which will defend and protect the person and goods of each associate with the whole common force, and in which, each person, while uniting themselves with all, may still obey themselves alone, and remain as free as before." This is the essential problem of human civilization for which the social contract is the solution.

The clauses of the social contract are so finely determined by the nature of this act of unification that the smallest change to them would make the whole ineffective. For this reason, though they have perhaps never been formally recorded, they are the same in all civilized societies and all people tacitly recognize them; that is, until the social contract is violated and each person regains their original rights and resumes their natural liberty, all the while losing the conventional liberty for which they renounced that natural liberty.

Properly understood, these clauses may be reduced to one: the social contract requires the total surrender of each person, along with all their rights, to the whole community, for if each person, without exception, gives themselves absolutely, the conditions are the same for all. If this is so, no person will have any interest in making the contract and its clauses burdensome to others.

And if the surrender is thorough and unreserved, the union will be as perfect as it can be, for no person will have anything more to demand. If some individuals were able to retain certain rights, and because there would be no common superior to decide between them and the rest of the public, each of these individuals, being on one certain point his or her own judge, would ask to be so on all points. In this case, the state of nature would continue on, rendering the group at best dysfunctional and at worst tyrannical.

In giving themselves to all, each person really gives himself or herself to nobody. Because there is no one person over whom they do not have the same rights as those they yield to others over themselves, they gain an equivalent for everything they lose in the initial surrendering, and an increase of force for the preservation of what belongs to them, their life and their resources. So, if we ignore for a moment those parts of the social contract that are not essential, we may reduce it to this: "Each of us puts our person and all our powers in common under the supreme direction of the general will, and, in our collective capacity, we receive each member and power as an indivisible part of the whole."

25. According to the passage, the most important clause of the social contract is that:

   A. All people must totally surrender themselves and their rights to the community.

   B. The sum of the forces of the community must be greater than natural obstacles to survival.

   C. All people must engage in the social contract for their own individual good.

   D. All people must reserve some part of their rights to maintain individual liberty.

26. According to the passage, the clauses of the social contract are:

   A. heavily adaptable.

   B. slightly adaptable.

   C. strictly rigid.

   D. loosely structured.

27. Based upon the passage, it can be inferred that the author believes which of the following statements about the social contract?

   A. Once initiated, it is very rare that it ever fails.

   B. It is one of the means for creating society.

   C. It exists in slightly different forms across the world.

   D. It is universal to all civilized societies.

28. The statement made after the colon in the fifth paragraph is most likely employed to:

   A. demonstrate the costs and benefits of the social contract.

   B. demonstrate the rigidity of the social contract.

   C. demonstrate how difficult the social contract is to achieve.

   D. demonstrate that there is only one clause of the social contract.

29. Say that a community of people is going to engage in a social contract. One of these people wants to retain his right to take crops as he pleases, whether they belong to him or not. Which of the following results is most likely to happen first?

   A. He will amass an unfair amount of property and become the most powerful citizen in the newly formed society.

   B. The social contract will fall apart, rendering the group at best dysfunctional and at worst tyrannical.

   C. There will be no one to judge him on this point but himself, and he'll judge himself on other points as well.

   D. The community will convene and decide by a majority vote to either banish or murder him.

30. All of the following are qualities of the social contract EXCEPT:

   A. one violation of the social contract voids it in entirety.

   B. it is almost never formally recorded.

   C. people lose more than they gain, but it is necessary.

   D. natural liberty is traded for conventional liberty.

31. According to the passage, which of the following statements are true of the clauses of the social contract?

   I. Ideally they are understood explicitly.

   II. Violating one violates the whole contract.

   III. They are determined by the scholars of a group.

   A. I only

   B. II only

   C. I and II only

   D. II and III only

Passage 6 (Questions 32 – 37)

Mr. Wittgenstein's *Tractatus Logico-Philosophicus*, whether or not it proves to give the ultimate truth on the matters with which it deals, certainly deserves, by its breadth and scope and profundity, to be considered an important event in the philosophical world. Starting from the principles of Symbolism and the relations which are necessary between words and things in any language, it applies the result of this inquiry to various departments of traditional philosophy, showing in each case how traditional philosophy and traditional solutions arise out of ignorance of the principles of Symbolism and out of misuse of language.

In order to understand Mr. Wittgenstein's book, it is necessary to realize the problem that concerns him. In the part of his theory which deals with Symbolism, he is concerned with the conditions that would have to be fulfilled by a logically perfect language. There are various problems as regards language. First, there is the problem of what actually occurs in our minds when we use language with the intention of meaning something by it; this problem belongs to psychology. Secondly, there is the problem of the relation subsisting between thoughts, words, or sentences, and what it is they refer to or mean; this problem belongs to epistemology. Thirdly, there is the problem of using sentences to convey truth rather than falsehood; this belongs to the special sciences dealing with the subject-matter of the sentences in question. Fourthly, there is the question: what relation must one fact (such as a sentence) have to another in order to be capable of being a symbol for that other? This last is a logical question, and is the one with which Mr. Wittgenstein is concerned. He is concerned with the conditions for accurate Symbolism, i.e. for Symbolism in which a sentence "means" something quite definite. In practice, language is always more or less vague, so that what we assert is never quite precise. Thus, logic has two problems to deal with in regard to Symbolism: (1) the conditions for sense rather than nonsense in combinations of symbols; (2) the conditions for uniqueness of meaning or reference in symbols or combinations of symbols. A logically perfect language has rules of syntax that prevent nonsense, and has single symbols which always have a definite and unique meaning. Mr. Wittgenstein is concerned with the conditions for a logically perfect language—not that any language is logically perfect, or that we believe ourselves capable, here and now, of constructing a logically perfect language, but that the whole function of language is to have meaning, and it only fulfills this function in proportion as it approaches the ideal language which we postulate.

The essential business of language is to assert or deny facts. Given the syntax of a language, the meaning of a sentence is determinate as soon as the meaning of the component words is known. In order that a certain sentence should assert a certain fact there must, however the language may be constructed, be something in common between the structure of the sentence and the structure of the fact. This is perhaps the most fundamental thesis of Mr. Wittgenstein's theory. That which has to be in common between the sentence

and the fact cannot, so he contends, be itself in turn said in language. It can, in his phraseology, only be shown, not said, for whatever we may say will still need to have the same structure.

32. Based on the passage, symbolism is the study of:

    A. the principles that drive philosophical inquiry.

    B. relations between language and objects.

    C. how the senses are portrayed through language.

    D. visual images as stand-ins for ideas.

33. Based on the passage which of the following best describes the relationship between sentence and fact?

    A. Syntax arranges facts so sentences can express them.

    B. Language can be used to describe the connection.

    C. The two must share structural congruities.

    D. Symbolism links the two to prevent nonsense.

34. Which of the following assumptions best supports the author's assessment of the value of Wittgenstein's work?

    A. Not understanding a principle may result in the invalidation of previous beliefs.

    B. It is necessary to understand the relations between words and things in all languages.

    C. There is no such thing as a logically perfect language.

    D. Syntax and subject matter must be logically linked.

35. Based on the passage, Wittgenstein interrogates traditional philosophy through his focus on:

    A. the failure of traditional solutions.

    B. the method to create an ideal language.

    C. the uncoupling of fact and syntax.

    D. the relation between language and meaning.

36. Suppose that a scientist processed MRIs of speakers when they were trying to lie about a subject as opposed to when they were saying what they believed to be true about it. Based on the passage, this would be a study in the field of:

    A. psychology.

    B. epistemology.

    C. neurology.

    D. subject-matter.

37. Wittgenstein would agree that all of the following were true of a logically perfect language EXCEPT that:

    A. its ultimate purpose is the production of sense.

    B. its syntactical structures prevent nonsense.

    C. one could never construct such a language.

    D. each symbol within it has exclusive meaning.

Passage 7 (Questions 38 – 43)

"Then, too," the dancer went on, "it is quite evident that one must study art. But most of the study of art for dancing is not in learning its technique but in seeing the beautiful old pictures and sculpture and studying their composition, their posturing. You see it needs travel to be a dancer—one must see the beautiful old pictures, and get their beauty"—Miss Wihr laughed and spread out her arms in a graceful inclusive gesture—"into one's self. The same is true of sculpture, which is necessary if one is to do the Greek dances. One of the most famous dancers of the present time takes almost all her poses straight from the old statues—studies the Greek postures, and makes them flow together. As for color, and the other branches of art," Miss Wihr went on, "they are not absolutely required even for creative work. But they are often desirable: every form of beauty is.

Of course a dancer must know literature, especially legend and poetry. Out of the old legends and folk-tales come many of the most beautiful dances and dance-pictures. Poetry is necessary as a rhythmic form of beauty that must go along with what is exquisite in the dance. A dance must be a picture. It must also be a poem. When I have students here for lessons I always read a poem to them before the formal 'work' begins."

"You see," the dancer went on earnestly, "you must study up, study up, all the time, if you are to master dancing as a creative art. You must be a thoroughly well-educated person. And to begin with, you must have a good mind—not merely a sense of beauty and artistry, but a good, sturdy, hard-working brain. And then the dance itself comes from within. I tell my pupils that they cannot learn to dance by imitating me. They must think things out, and they must dance by themselves. If the dance is not in you, you can never get it from anything outside. Someone else may make you a dancing machine, but a dancer you yourself must be."

"The actual exercises that one has in dancing are not so different from those of the gymnasium." The dancer stretched out her arms and took one of the familiar one-two-three-four motions of early school days—arms out, elbows bent, hands at shoulders, then out again. It was a quick, muscular, strong, and jerky exercise. Then she did it again. But the second time there was no jerkiness, no sudden stop; the positions seemed to flow into each other; there was the suggestion of a gentle river in the slow movement of the dancer's arms. "You see," she said, "those exercises are exactly the same. The one is simply softened. The emphasis is not on muscular force, but on grace. Yet they are equally healthful. That is why so many women take dancing lessons as a sort of gymnastic course to strengthen their bodies and at the same time make them more graceful."

38. Based on the passage, many women take dancing lessons in order to:

    A. develop health and grace.

    B. become softer and more pleasing.

    C. escape the tedious routines of the gymnasium.

    D. develop greater muscular force and definition.

39. Based on the passage it can be assumed that which of the following is a valid way of creating a dance?

    A. Ignoring color for a greater focus on other branches of art, such as sculpture

    B. Studying techniques of different areas carefully in order to create true beauty

    C. Being open to all forms of art as a means of increasing one's self awareness

    D. Stringing together the poses from the art of a culture to create a dance

40. In arguing that a dancer must know legend, Wihr is assuming which of the following?

    A. Literature is the highest branch of art and thus ought to inform dance.

    B. The contrast between picture and poem is bridged in legends.

    C. Understanding the basis of the content of a dance leads to richer art.

    D. Legends are a prime way to get beauty into one's self.

41. Based on the passage, which would be the most useful educational experience for a dancer?

    A. A trip around Europe, studying the art and literature of each country

    B. A trip around the world, observing the different dances in each country

    C. A trip around Europe, watching the performances of national ballets of each country

    D. A trip around the world, gaining bodily strength to complete particular postures

42. Suppose Wihr attended a recital in which a young dancer performed several pieces that were identical in gesture, movement, and form to pieces by older, famous dancers. Based on the passage, Wihr's response would be:

    A. negative due to the fact that such a dancer was not respecting the boundaries of others' creative work.

    B. negative due to the fact that such a dancer was drawing upon external resources rather than internal ones.

    C. positive due to the fact that a young artist must absorb as much of her art form as possible to develop.

    D. positive due to the fact that the only way to absorb composition and posturing is through active imitation.

43. Based on the passage, Wihr means which of the following in describing a "dancing machine"?

    A. One who is hyper-intellectual in their approach, analyzing dance rather than feeling beauty

    B. One who knows the steps and gestures of a dance, but has no internal reasoning as to why

    C. One who is a master of the form, having studied art, sculpture, literature, and music in order to understand the root of dance

    D. One who is too concerned with imitating others rather than developing a new style that reflects a unique viewpoint and knowledge

Passage 8 (Questions 44 – 49)

Giotto was the first of the great personalities in Florentine painting, and though he provides no exception to the rule that the great Florentines used the arts in their endeavor to express themselves, he, renowned as an architect, sculptor, wit, and versifier, differed from the majority of his Tuscan successors in possessing a peculiar aptitude for the essential in painting *as an art*. Yet, before we may appreciate his real value, we ought to come to an agreement on what constitutes the essential in the art of figure-painting, for this form was not only the primary interest of Giotto, but of the entire Florentine school.

Scientists have discovered that sight alone cannot give us an accurate sense of the third dimension. In our infancy, and long before we are conscious of it, the sense of touch and the muscular sensations of movement teach us to appreciate depth in both objects and space. This is what is referred to as the third dimension. Then, still in infancy, we learn to make touch and the third dimension the test of reality. As children, we are still somewhat aware of the close connection between touch and the third dimension. For example, a child of five cannot persuade herself of the unreality of a trick mirror until she has touched the mirror. Beyond childhood, we forget this connection. However, every time our eyes recognize reality, we actually give tactile value to retinal impressions.

As an art form, painting aims to give us a lasting and realistic impression of artistic reality with only two dimensions. Therefore, the painter must do consciously what we all do unconsciously: construct the perception of the third dimension. He must accomplish this objective in the same way we all do, by giving tactile value to retinal impressions. So, his first act is to rouse the tactile sense in his viewers, for we must have the illusion of being able to touch a figure, we must have the illusion of muscular sensations inside our hands corresponding to the figure of the painting, before we take the work for granted as real and therefore let it affect us lastingly.

Therefore, it follows that the essential in the art of figure-painting is to somehow stimulate our consciousness of tactile values with a work that has at least as much power to appeal to our tactile imagination as the actual object represented. In this way, as he realized the essential in painting and stimulated our tactile consciousness better than all others, Giotto was the supreme master. It is this quality that will make him a source of the highest kind of aesthetic delight for at least as long as traces of his work remain on decaying panels and crumbling walls. For though he was a great poet, an enthralling story-teller, and a splendid composer, superior to the many masters who painted between the decline of the antique and the birth of the modern which he ignited, he was superior in these qualities by degree only. None of these many masters possessed the power to stimulate the tactile imagination, and therefore, they never painted a figure with true artistic existence. Their works have value as elaborate, highly intelligible symbols, capable of communicating meaning, and yet they lose all higher value the moment this meaning is delivered.

On the other hand, Giotto's paintings not only possess as much power to appeal to the tactile imagination as the objects they represent (human figures in particular), but they actually possess more. In this way, his work conveyed a keener sense of reality than both that of his contemporaries and that of the very objects he represented in his paintings.

44. Which of the following is the most likely reason why the author mentions infants and children?

   A. To parallel the development of an artist, from fledgling and curious to unconsciously adept

   B. To make a case for the sense of touch having an innate connection to the appreciation of all art

   C. To give an in-depth illustration of the development of artistic taste and sensibility

   D. To further describe the quality in humans that the essential in figure painting aims to satisfy

45. Based upon the passage, which of the following statements is most likely to be believed to be true by the author?

   A. Sight is the most important sense for the appreciation of art.

   B. Touch is the most important sense for the appreciation of art.

   C. The best art offers us a heightened perception of reality.

   D. Giotto was the greatest artist to come out of the Renaissance.

46. According to the passage, why exactly must the artist arouse our tactile imaginations? Because we must feel like we can touch a figure in order for us to:

   A. allow it to affect us lastingly

   B. understand its purpose or meaning

   C. imagine its life outside of the work

   D. fully appreciate its closeness to reality

47. Suppose one of Giotto's contemporaries is trying his very best to match or surpass the skill of the master. Unfortunately, he is constantly frustrated. Which of the following fundamental problems is most likely to be afflicting this artist?

   A. His sense of touch and movement is not as finely tuned as Giotto's is.

   B. As an infant and child he experimented less with his sense of touch than Giotto did.

   C. He views painting more as a form of expression than as a craft.

   D. For the most part, he does not work as hard as Giotto does.

48. According to the passage, all of the following statements about Giotto are true EXCEPT:

   A. his special ability rested in his aptitude for the craft of making art.

   B. he was uninterested in his work as a means for expression.

   C. his human figures were perhaps his most impressive.

   D. he was, for the most part, interested in figure-painting.

49. Based upon the passage, which of the following statements are true?

   I. There is a distinct difference between art for expression's sake and art for art's sake.

   II. Giotto is superior to all artists between the fall of the antique and the height of the modern.

   III. The conscious process of figure-painting mirrors the unconscious process of seeing in three dimensions.

   A. I only

   B. III only

   C. I and II only

   D. I and III only

Passage 9 (Questions 50 – 53)

Herbart's great service lay in taking the work of teaching out of the region of routine and accident. He brought it into the sphere of conscious method; it became a conscious business with a definite aim and procedure, instead of being a compound of casual inspiration and subservience to tradition. Moreover, everything in teaching and discipline could be specified, instead of our having to be content with vague and more or less mystic generalities about ultimate ideals and speculative spiritual symbols. He abolished the notion of ready-made faculties, which might be trained by exercise upon any sort of material, and made attention to concrete subject matter, to the content, all-important. Herbart undoubtedly has had a greater influence in bringing to the front questions connected with the material of study than any other educational philosopher. He stated problems of method from the standpoint of their connection with subject matter: method having to do with the manner and sequence of presenting new subject matter to insure its proper interaction with old.

The fundamental theoretical defect of this view lies in ignoring the existence in a living being of active and specific functions which are developed in the redirection and combination which occur as they are occupied with their environment. The theory represents the Schoolmaster come to his own. This fact expresses at once its strength and its weakness. The conception that the mind consists of what has been taught, and that the importance of what has been taught consists in its availability for further teaching, reflects the pedagogue's view of life. The philosophy is eloquent about the duty of the teacher in instructing pupils; it is almost silent regarding his privilege of learning. It emphasizes the influence of intellectual environment upon the mind; it slurs over the fact that the environment involves a personal sharing in common experiences. It exaggerates beyond reason the possibilities of consciously formulated and used methods, and underestimates the role of vital, unconscious, attitudes. It insists upon the old, the past, and passes lightly over the operation of the genuinely novel and unforeseeable. It takes, in brief, everything educational into account save its essence—vital energy seeking opportunity for effective exercise. All education forms character, mental and moral, but formation consists in the selection and coordination of native activities so that they may utilize the subject matter of the social environment. Moreover, the formation is not only a formation of native activities, but it takes place through them. It is a process of reconstruction, reorganization.

A peculiar combination of the ideas of development and formation from without has given rise to the recapitulation theory of education, biological and cultural. The individual develops, but his proper development consists in repeating in orderly stages the past evolution of animal life and human history. The former recapitulation occurs physiologically; the latter should be made to occur by means of education. The alleged biological truth that the individual in his growth from the simple embryo to maturity repeats the history of the evolution of animal life in the progress of forms from the simplest to the most complex (or expressed technically, that ontogenesis parallels phylogenesis) does not concern us, save as it is supposed to afford scientific foundation for cultural recapitulation of the past. Cultural recapitulation says, first, that children at a certain age are in the mental and moral condition of savagery; their instincts are vagrant and predatory because their ancestors at one time lived such a life. Consequently (so it is concluded) the proper subject matter of their education at this time is the material—especially the literary material of myths, folk-tale, and song—produced by humanity in the analogous stage. Then the child passes on to something corresponding, say, to the pastoral stage, and so on till at the time when he is ready to take part in contemporary life, he arrives at the present epoch of culture.

50. The author discusses Herbart in order to:

   A. argue against the concept of the "Schoolmaster" and his absolute power in education.

   B. justify the recapitulation theory of education and its stages of educational fitness.

   C. emphasize his importance in accentuating the material of study for the student.

   D. contrast an emphasis on pedagogy and content with one on process and environment.

51. Suppose that an education class focused primarily on the ways in which students interacted with new information and applied it to their larger environment. This approach would be closest to:

   A. the author's, because it focused on biological elements as opposed to imposing the standards of culture.

   B. the author's, because it focused on students and their process as opposed to the duties of the instructor.

   C. Herbart's, because he de-emphasized routine and accident in developing pedagogy.

   D. Herbart's, because he de-emphasized the environment versus common experiences.

52. All of the following would be valid educational techniques under the theory of cultural recapitulation EXCEPT:

   A. saving modern works of culture for teenagers who have completed much of their development.

   B. asking children to analyze folk tales in order to trace the various stages of development they embody.

   C. furnishing older children with simple romances and visions of country life as reading material.

   D. thinking about the subject matter of education in terms of the cultural stages through which mankind has advanced.

53. Which of the following best describes the attitude of the author toward the recapitulation theory of education?

   A. Disdain

   B. Skepticism

   C. Implicit belief

   D. Careful consideration

This page intentionally left blank.

SECTION 12

Answer Key

1	A	12	B	23	A	34	A	45	C
2	A	13	D	24	C	35	D	46	A
3	B	14	A	25	A	36	A	47	C
4	D	15	C	26	C	37	C	48	B
5	B	16	B	27	D	38	A	49	D
6	D	17	B	28	B	39	D	50	D
7	D	18	B	29	C	40	C	51	B
8	A	19	D	30	C	41	A	52	B
9	C	20	D	31	B	42	B	53	B
10	A	21	B	32	B	43	B		
11	D	22	D	33	C	44	D		

Passage 1 (Questions 1 – 6)

In 1988, a British surgeon and medical researcher named Andrew **Wakefield** published a paper in the medical journal *The Lancet* postulating a link between administration of the measles, mumps, and rubella **vaccine (MMR)** and the appearance of **autism**, as well as certain **gastroenterological conditions**, in children. Written with twelve co-authors, Wakefield's paper identified a syndrome they called "**autistic enterocolitis**," and linked the MMR vaccine to autism and bowel disease. The **study** on which the paper was based – of **twelve children** with behavioral symptoms consistent with Autism Spectrum Disorder, or ASD – claimed that **eight** of the twelve children developed "**behavioral symptoms**" within two weeks of receiving the MMR vaccine.

Key terms: Andrew Wakefield, MMR vaccine, Autism Spectrum Disorder

Cause and effect: Researcher Andrew Wakefield thinks he found a link between the MMR vaccine and autism

The paper was immediately and enormously **controversial**, in the UK and worldwide. Although Wakefield *et al* did not make a definitive connection between the vaccine and autism in the Lancet paper, **Wakefield** had held **a press conference** prior to the paper's publication, at which he called for the **suspension of the triple vaccine** until further research proved it safe. At the press conference, Wakefield stated that speaking out against the vaccine was a "**moral issue**."

Key terms: controversial, moral issue

Opinion: Wakefield called for suspending the vaccine

In the wake of the Lancet article, **subsequent studies** were **unable to support Wakefield's results**. Concerns were raised that a study of twelve children was too small to be statistically valid. However, the article – or, more specifically, **Wakefield's press conference** – created near **panic** for many parents. The number of parents who opted not to give their children the MMR vaccine jumped tremendously, and consequently, incidence of **measles increased**. One report suggested that in England alone, MMR vaccination rates dropped from 92% to 73% as a result of concerns about MMR and autism.

Key terms: statistically valid, near panic, incidence of measles

Cause and effect: the public panicked as a result of the study; MMR vaccination rates dropped; incidence of measles rose

Opinion: some said the study was too small to be valid

Nonetheless, the **anti-vaccine movement** has continued to **grow**, particularly as the incidence of autism and autism spectrum disorders continues to rise. Thousands of parents believe vaccines – and, most specifically, the MMR vaccine – caused their child's disability. **Doubters** say that such belief is based on **anecdotal evidence** and cannot be supported; yet many parents have no doubt that the regression and skill loss typical in the emergence of autism undeniably followed vaccination.

Key terms: anti-vaccine movement, parents, anecdotal evidence

Contrast: many parents of children with autism believe the MMR vaccine was responsible; critics say this is based solely on anecdotal evidence

Wakefield was accused by a *Sunday Times* reporter of **conflict of interest** in 2004; the reporter said that some of the children in Wakefield's study had been recruited by a **lawyer** preparing a **lawsuit against MMR vaccine manufacturers**. Two years later, it was reported that Wakefield was paid over $500,000 by the lawyers involved in the suit, a fact that he had not previously disclosed. In February 2010, *The Lancet* **formally withdrew Wakefield's paper**, calling it **fraudulent**. Shortly after that, the **British General Medical Council** permanently **revoked Wakefield's license** to practice medicine. Wakefield continues to protest his innocence, and claims that he was targeted by public health officials and pharmaceutical companies.

Key term: conflict of interest

Cause and effect: Wakefield was accused of fraud and lost his license to practice medicine

Opinion: Wakefield maintains he is innocent

No further studies have **documented a clear link** between the MMR vaccine and regressive autism. However, in 2013, the federal Vaccine Injury Compensation Program, or **vaccine court**, as it is commonly known, **awarded millions of dollars** in compensation to the families of two children who attested that the debilitating encephalopathy their children suffered was directly attributable to vaccines. While the children have autism-like symptoms, **the ruling** is scrupulous in **not directly linking autism with the vaccines**. Most of the **documents** pertaining to the case are **sealed**, and not available to the public. Those who see clear correlation between the MMR vaccine and ASD see this as admission that there is a link. Those who do not view the ruling as just compensation for vaccine-related injuries – but not as proof of the role of the MMR vaccine in the development of autism.

Key terms: vaccine court, encephalopathy

Contrast: a US federal program compensated children with autism injured by the MMR vaccine, but still does not link the vaccine with autism.

Main Idea: Andrew Wakefield raised a controversy regarding whether the MMR vaccine is a cause of autism; though he was discredited, many still suspect a link.

1.   A is correct. Wakefield's supporter might admit that there were issues surrounding the study, but still see the possibility of a link.

   B: Even if a supporter thought it were crucial to investigate the cause of autism, he wouldn't necessarily say that was more important than preventing measles.

   C: Wakefield's supporter would likely say the link between the MMR vaccine and autism was not disproved.

   D: The supporter doesn't necessarily believe that anecdotal evidence is enough.

2.   A is correct. Use elimination here.

   B: Wakefield never says the MMR vaccine manufacturers are motivated by financial gain and not ethics so choice B is out.

   C: We aren't told nor is it suggested that Wakefield's methodology was based on ethical or moral motives.

   D: He was a medical researcher doing research, not a public advocate.

   We're left with choice A; he felt his study was addressing a serious health issue.

3.   B is correct. A detractor of the MMR/ASD link would likely say the only "evidence" is anecdotal – which is not enough to prove the connection.

   A, C: These would represent views of a supporter, not a detractor, of the theory.

   D: Perhaps a detractor would believe this, but not "wholly"; the choice is worded too strongly.

4.   D is correct. Anecdotal evidence is based on individual reports rather than driven by data.

5.   B is correct. Wakefield was accused of being paid for his research, choice A; by being provided with subjects involved in a lawsuit, choice C; and reporting on a study that was too small to be valid, choice D. But nowhere in the passage is he accused of not being motivated by moral issues, as he claimed – choice B.

6.   D is correct. If a child had symptoms of autism prior to receiving the MMR vaccine, that would weaken the causal connection between administration of the vaccine and the emergence of autism symptoms.

   A: If a child received other vaccines at the time of the MMR, it would not disprove the connection between the MMR vaccine and autism symptoms, though it certainly would add another factor to consider.

   B: Not getting financially compensated would not prove or disprove a connection.

   C: They might have other issues, but that would not prove (or disprove) that no clear causal connection exists between the MMR vaccine and autism.

Passage 2 (Questions 7 – 13)

The **Diagnostic and Statistical Manual of Mental Disorders**, or DSM, is used to diagnose mental and behavioral disorders. Published by the **American Psychiatric Association** (APA), the DSM has been revised several times over the past six decades to reflect changes in psychiatric research and practice. The most recent edition, **DSM-5**, was released in 2013. One of the greatest changes from DSM-IV to DSM-5 is in **revisions to the definition of autism and related neurodevelopmental disorders**. DSM-5 officially eliminates several autism spectrum diagnoses. **Gone are Asperger's syndrome**, a diagnosis which usually was applied to individuals without language deficit or intellectual disability; pervasive developmental disorder, not otherwise specified, or **PPD-NOS**, which typically applied to higher-functioning people who did not meet all the criteria for autism; and **childhood disintegrative disorder**, which referred to children who exhibited severe regression after the age of three. These diagnoses are now incorporated into one single diagnosis – **autism spectrum disorder**, or ASD.

Key terms: DSM, APA, DSM-5, Asperger's, autism spectrum disorder

Contrast: the DSM-5 incorporates the numerous autism spectrum disorders that were previously differentiated under the DSM-IV under one, single diagnosis

The APA states that the goal of the revision was to **overcome inconsistencies** in how autism is **diagnosed**. According to a member of the APA task force that addressed autism-related diagnoses, even among clinicians with expertise in diagnosing autism spectrum disorders, there was **significant variation in diagnoses** within the spectrum. The single, overarching ASD diagnosis is meant to address that; its intention is to provide a **single framework** for parents, educators, doctors, and other service providers to use and language to discuss people on all parts of the spectrum. Furthermore, the APA asserts that the DSM-5 is meant to be a "**living document**." (Hence the change from Roman numerals to Arabic numbers; "5" is meant to signify 5.0, and the expectation of ongoing updates as psychiatric understanding and practice are refined.)

Key terms: inconsistencies, single framework, living document

Opinion: the APA says that the new single diagnosis will help accurately diagnose autism and will aid people on all parts of the spectrum vs the previous situation with inconsistent diagnoses made even by trained specialists

The new diagnosis **still** differentiates **qualifiers**, such as language ability, intellectual disability, and regression, and rates severity levels from one to three. One significant change is that in order to receive an autism spectrum disorder diagnosis, a child must exhibit deficits in **social communication**, as well as **restricted or repetitive behavior**, each of which is rated in severity. A child who exhibits communication deficit but not restricted or repetitive behavior will be given a new

diagnosis: **social communication disorder**. How insurance companies deal with this new diagnosis remains to be seen: while 37 states have laws that regulate insurance coverage of children with autism, such laws would not apply to social communication disorder.

Key terms: qualifiers, social communication deficits, restrictive or repetitive behavior

Contrast: under the new system, a person must exhibit restricted or repetitive behavior, not just communication deficits, to receive an ASD diagnosis

Although the change in the DSM has been greeted with enthusiasm by many psychiatrists and behavioral health providers – some of who felt that the DSM-IV made it harder for people with Asperger's and PPD-NOS to receive services – not everyone shares this belief. Some parents and patients have expressed a **concern that the new criteria would be more, not less, exclusionary**, particularly for people with Asperger's and PDD-NOS. Although the APA autism task force estimated that fewer than 10 percent of people currently diagnosed with autism would not meet the new DSM-5 standards, other **studies suggest that over 75% of people with Asperger's** would **not** receive a **diagnosis** under the new standards – and would not qualify for needed services. Some **advocates** assert that the revision represents an effort for **schools** and **insurance** companies to **control costs**. Others have expressed the concern that if a significant number of higher functioning individuals are not diagnosed, the prevalence rate of autism will be unrealistically decreased. One other issue: to some, a diagnosis of autism carries a stigma that a diagnosis of Asperger's does not; will higher-functioning individuals and their families avoid the autism label – and thus refuse support that could be truly helpful?

Opinion: some advocates for people with autism are concerned that the new standards will prevent some people with autism from receiving support services and blame schools and insurance companies trying to cut costs

Cause and effect: the new criteria may disqualify up to 10% of those with an autism spectrum diagnosis (such as Asperger's) from a diagnosis under the new criteria

Main idea: The DSM-5 revision updated how autism and related disorders are diagnosed in an effort to clarify the diagnosis of autism, but some fear it may cause rather than solve problems.

7.   D is correct. Look to paragraph 2 for the answer to this one. The problem, according to the APA, was that diagnosis among the different autism spectrum disorders was inconsistent and difficult even for experienced clinicians; the new qualifiers and diagnoses were meant to address that.

A: Prevalence rate is an issue brought up by advocates in paragraph 4; according to the passage, it's not a concern of the APA.

B: The stigma of an autism diagnosis (in contrast to an Asperger's diagnosis) is another issue brought up by advocates in paragraph 4; it's not a factor in revamping the DSM.

C: Again, this is not mentioned as the APA's concern.

8.   A is correct. One of the salient features of the DSM-5 is that it eliminates the distinct diagnoses of Asperger's syndrome (choice C) and PPD-NOS (choice B). Restricted or repetitive behavior (choice D) is a qualifier, not a diagnosis, under the new DSM. But social communication disorder, choice A, is a diagnosis that is new to DSM-5.

9.   C is correct. In paragraph 3, we're told that the DSM-5 (released in 2013) has two new qualifiers: social communication deficits, and restrictive or repetitive behavior. A person must exhibit both to some degree to receive an autism spectrum disorder diagnosis. In this question, a child with communication deficit but no repetitive behavior would receive the new diagnosis of social communication disorder.

A, B: These both represent diagnoses eliminated in the 2013 revision.

D: Without restrictive or repetitive behavior, a child would not be diagnosed with autism spectrum disorder.

10.   A is correct. The author describes the changes, explains the position of the APA, but also raises concerns by some clinicians and advocates. Choice A best captures this.

B: Some advocates might believe this, but the author neither supports nor challenges this position.

C: There is disagreement, but it's not as simple as parents and patients vs providers. "Advocates" may include providers.

D: This concern is raised but the author does not present it as his point of view, and the word "majority" is too strong.

11.   D is correct. Concerns over coverage of social communication disorder (choice A) is mentioned at the end of paragraph 3; stigmatization (choice B) and disqualification (choice C) are both mentioned as potential problems in paragraph 4. Only choice D – concern that service providers are not familiar with the new qualifiers – is not discussed as a potential issue.

12.   B is correct. Paragraph 2 discusses the APA's goals in revising the DSM, and their assertion that the new version is a "living document" that will continue to evolve and be revised as needed.

13.   D is correct. Look to paragraph 4 for your answer. Proponents of the new DSM say it clarifies the diagnostic process, and perhaps gives higher functioning patients a greater chance of receiving appropriate services than they had under DSM-IV.

A: Actually, it seems like some proponents think higher functioning individuals were underserved under DSM-IV.

B: Concerns that DSM-5 represents a cost-cutting effort is raised by critics, not proponents, of the new system.

C: DSM-5 does away with some fundamental distinctions, but no mention that they divided the autism community.

Passage 3 (Questions 14 – 18)

The question as to what we mean by **truth** and **falsehood**, which we considered in the preceding chapter, is of much less interest than the question as to **how we can know** what is true and what is false. This question will occupy us in the present chapter. There can be no doubt that **some of our beliefs are erroneous**; thus we are led to inquire what certainty we can ever have that such and such a belief is not erroneous. In other words, **can we ever know anything** at all, or do we merely sometimes by good luck believe what is true? Before we can attack this question, we must, however, first decide what we mean by **"knowing"**, and this question is not so easy as might be supposed.

Opinions: the author questions whether it is possible to truly know anything

Contrast: the author states that the question of how to tell what is true and false is more interesting than the question of what is meant by truth and falsehood

Cause and effect: if we are able to understand what is meant by knowing, we will be able to better answer whether we can know anything at all

At first sight we might imagine that **knowledge** could be defined as **"true belief"**. When what we believe is true, it might be supposed that we had achieved a knowledge of what we believe. But this would not accord with the way in which the word is commonly used. To take a very trivial instance: If a man believes that the late **Prime Minister's last name began with a B**, he believes what is true, since the late Prime Minister was Sir Henry Campbell Bannerman. But if he believes that Mr. Balfour was the late Prime Minister, he will still believe that the late Prime Minister's last name began with a B, yet this belief, though true, would not be thought to constitute knowledge. If a newspaper, by an intelligent anticipation, announces the result of a battle before any telegram giving the result has been received, it may by good fortune announce what afterwards turns out to be the right result, and it may produce belief in some of its less experienced readers. But in spite of the truth of their belief, they cannot be said to have knowledge. Thus it is clear that a true belief is **not knowledge** when it is **deduced from a false belief**.

Key terms: Prime Minister's last name

Contrast: a true belief and false belief are obviously different; even a true belief does not imply possession of knowledge

Cause and effect: holding a true belief that is deduced from a false belief is not knowledge

In like manner, a true belief **cannot** be called **knowledge** when it is **deduced by a fallacious process of reasoning**, even if the premises from which it is deduced are true. If I know that all Greeks are men and that Socrates was a man, and I infer that Socrates was a Greek, I cannot be said

to know that Socrates was a Greek, because, although my **premises** and my **conclusion** are **true**, the conclusion does not follow from the premises.

Cause and effect: true belief based on true facts but deduced by faulty logic cannot be knowledge

But are we to say that nothing is **knowledge** except what is **validly deduced from true premises**? Obviously we cannot say this. Such a definition is at once **too wide** and **too narrow**. In the first place, it is too wide, because it is not enough that our premises should be true, they must also be known. The man who believes that Mr. Balfour was the late Prime Minister may proceed to draw valid deductions from the true premise that the late Prime Minister's name began with a B, but he cannot be said to know the conclusions reached by these deductions. Thus we shall have to amend our definition by saying that knowledge is what is validly deduced from **known premises**. This, however, is a **circular definition**: it assumes that we already know what is meant by "known premises". It can, therefore, at best define one sort of knowledge, the sort we call **derivative, as opposed to intuitive** knowledge. We may say: **"Derivative knowledge** is what is validly deduced from premises known intuitively". In this statement there is no formal defect, but it leaves the definition of **intuitive knowledge** still to seek.

Contrast: the premises need not only be true, but known; derivative knowledge is different from intuitive; intuitive knowledge will lead us to derivative knowledge

Cause and effect: once we know a piece of intuitive knowledge, we can use the definition of derivative knowledge as a logical deduction from premises known intuitively

Leaving on one side, for the moment, the question of intuitive knowledge, let us consider the above suggested definition of derivative knowledge. The chief objection to it is that it unduly **limits knowledge**. It constantly happens that people **entertain a true belief**, which has grown up in them because of some piece of intuitive knowledge from which it is **capable of being validly inferred**, but from which it **has not**, as a matter of fact, **been inferred** by any logical process.

Opinion: author believes there are other ways to know something than by logical inference

Cause and effect: the statement that knowledge must be logically deduced from known premises is said to be too narrow because people may have knowledge that *could* be inferred but hasn't

Main Idea: The passage develops a definition of derivative knowledge requiring that such knowledge is a true belief that has been correctly deduced from premises that are known to be true, and the author notes that the premises can be known intuitively.

14. A is correct. The passage states that the definition is too narrow because "It constantly happens that people entertain a true belief, which has grown up in them because of some piece of intuitive knowledge from which it is capable of being validly inferred, but from which it has not, as a matter of fact, been inferred by any logical process."

    B: This is false according to the author.

    C: This is true but does not explain why the statement is too narrow because all knowledge is necessarily a true belief.

    D: This is true but does not explain why the statement is too narrow.

15. C is correct. The author states that a piece of intuitive knowledge would provide a sort of base upon which other derivative knowledge could be known. From that derivative knowledge you could arrive at more and more knowledge. The construction of the tower of knowledge would begin with a single piece of intuitive knowledge, much like mathematical theory is built upon simple axioms taken to be true.

    A, D: The author never addresses sense perceptions in the discussion of knowledge.

    B: This would be derivative knowledge.

16. B is correct. The scenario where the premises are true and the belief deduced from them is true but not knowledge is possible. However, a belief deduced from another true belief may be knowledge, whereas options A, C, and D preclude the possibility that the belief is knowledge.

    A, C, D: These imply that the belief is not knowledge, because it is based on bad reasoning, false beliefs, or a lucky guess.

17. B is correct. Consider carefully the example "all Greeks are men and that Socrates was a man, and I infer that Socrates was a Greek". This follows the pattern "All X are Y. Q is a Y. Therefore Q is an X." Only choice B matches this and is correct.

18. B is correct. The example of the prime minister goes to show that a true belief can be held which does not constitute knowledge. This is stated directly in the second paragraph.

    A: This contradicts the passage, since the prime minister's name did, in fact, start with a "b".

    C, D: These are just distractor answer choices because they are not associated with the prime minister example. The author never discusses what people "often" do or don't do.

Passage 4 (Questions 19 – 24)

Alfred Lord Tennyson's *In Memoriam*, perhaps the **most** extended exploration of **internalized grief** in the English language, seemingly argues against the mere existence of time. Anniversaries, Christmases, weddings, all serve as a slight to the mourning speaker, who "long[s] to prove/ no lapse of moons can canker Love/whatever fickle tongues may say" (XXVI, 2-4). Affronted by the way the outside world regains its equilibrium after the death of Arthur Henry **Hallam**, Tennyson/the Narrator withdraws within his self, eschewing both the natural passing of time and the "fickle tongues" of societal soothing. In doing so, he enacts **lyric poetry**'s prime directive to **travel within**.

Key terms: Alfred Lord Tennyson, *In Memoriam*, Arthur Henry Hallam

Contrast: outside world continuing on vs the narrator's grief

Cause and effect: because the outside world continues after the death of Hallam, the narrator turns inward in the poem

Northrop **Frye**, paraphrasing John Stuart **Mill's** categorization of poetry as an "overheard" utterance (80), deems **lyric poetry** "preeminently the utterance that is overheard... the individual **communing within himself**" (249-50). This intense self-reflexivity means that the lyric poem necessarily engages with, by strenuously placing itself **out of, time**: Kenneth **Burke** terms lyric poetry as caught in a **"state of arrest"** (245). Lyric poetry is thus, in some ways, a protest against temporality and, as such, must grapple with time to defeat it. Yet **Tennyson's** poem makes **time a character** even more central, in some ways, than Hallam himself. The **poet grapples** not just with the **quotidian passing of time** which affronts the mourner, not just with the disjunct between the time of the living and the **eternal time of the after-life** with which he struggles to believe, but with **the vast immensity of time on earth**. In his most famous treatment of time and geology, stanza LXVI, Tennyson contemplates the "scarped cliff" which hold within it "a thousand types," now extinct (2;3). It is after facing the material reality of the many fossilized types embodied within the cliffs that Tennyson confronts not just the reality of "nature, red in tooth and claw" (15), but also the way that **human subjectivity**, be it "blown about the desert dust,/Or seal'd within the iron hills" is, in some ways, **erased by** the passage of long **geological time** (19-20).

Key terms: Northrop Frye, John Stuart Mill, Kenneth Burke

Opinion: Frye and Mill emphasize poetry as being an internal idea "overheard" by the reader; Kenneth Burke says lyric poetry is in a "state of arrest"

Cause and effect: because lyric poetry is about internal private moments, it must escape time and thus is heavily engaged with it; in envisioning the "scarped cliff," Tennyson deals with both extinction and the way geological time makes human time seem insignificant

The **"futil[ity]"** of life, for Tennyson, is emphasized by coming face to face with "A monster then, a dream,/A discord. Dragons of the prime" (21-22). Literally a **fossilized dinosaur**, the dragon affronts Tennyson because of its temporal "discord," a tangible artifact of the passage of time which so offends him. Yet at the same time, the "dragon'" serves as an instance of frozen time, and the ability to **capture items out of time**, as it were, slowly begins to **comfort the narrator**. In the following cantos, he slowly begins to envision **Hallam** in an analogous position to the dragon, "richly shrined" (LVII 7), and is ultimately able to envision him as one that **"canst not die"** because of his a-temporality, or rather, simul-temporality: like the fossil, a material object in the now that is the literal trace of a long past time, Hallam inheres within the "past, present, and to be" (CXXIX 11,13). Tennyson casts this as a **return to faith** if not traditional religion: be Hallam a second coming or an evolutionary "closer link" to a new biological "type" (Epilogue 127,138), by finding a way for Hallam to exist in simultaneous versions of time, Tennyson finds a way to resume his enmeshment in earthly time (the word "time" appears four time in the epilogue, "hours" and "now" three each). However, Hallam's transcendence is only understandable to the narrator when he roots himself within actuality: the will to live and believe rises "out of the dust" from a "spiritual rock" (CXXXI 5,3). Ultimately, **lyric poetry** does allow **Tennyson** to master, or at least **come to terms with time**, but only by merging with the material: rooted in the now, speaking of the past, fossils and, ultimately Hallam, allow Tennyson to accept his own unidirectional trudge through a temporality that suddenly blooms with multiple, asynchronous paths.

Contrast: the dragon/dinosaur represents both the passage of time and the ability to freeze time

Cause and effect: by addressing material objects that deal with the passing of time, the narrator is able to deal with the death of Hallam and the many relations to time which he encounters

Main Idea: The passage examines how the narrator of Tennyson's poem moves through his grief about the death of Arthur Henry Hallam, using lyric poems, which are focused on internal, private moments; it suggests that the passage of time even after Hallam's death is what affects Tennyson the most, and he works through it by finding material objects that both show the passage of time and are, in a sense, timeless.

19. D is correct. The passage states that "the 'dragon' serves as an instance of frozen time, and the ability to capture items out of time, as it were, slowly begins to comfort the narrator... the fossil [is] a material object in the now that is the literal trace of a long past time." Choice D focuses on time in the present and past.

   A, B, C: the passage does not address questions of what best indicates past time, is an alternative to death, or what develops religious resonance.

20. D is correct. The second paragraph introduces Frye and Mill and discusses the way in which they stress "intense self-reflexivity".

   A: There is no indication Tennyson knew of Frye and Mill.

   B: Burke's argument about a "state of arrest" is painted as a response to self-reflexivity.

   C: The passage does not address poets besides Tennyson.

21. B is correct. The passage suggests that the fact that words about time appear frequently in the epilogue means that "by finding a way for Hallam to exist in simultaneous versions of time, Tennyson finds a way to resume his enmeshment in earthly time," so if he did not write the epilogue, it might suggest that he was not over the issues about time with which the poem struggled.

   A: The poem was written after Hallam's death, so choice A is not correct.

   C: The passage does not suggest that Tennyson questioned religion overtly, as in choice C.

   D: There is no indication about how long Tennyson focused on the project.

22. D is correct. The first paragraph states that "the poet grapples not just with the quotidian passing of time," which is the everyday passing of time, as in choice III, "the disjunct between the time of the living and the eternal time of the after-life," as in choice II, and "the vast immensity of time on earth," as in choice I.

23. A is correct. The second paragraph discusses various definitions of lyric poetry, including the idea of "the individual communing within himself" and that it is caught in a "state of arrest".

   B, C: There is no discussion of music or protests.

   D: While the passage suggests Tennyson used the lyric form to interrogate questions of form, it does not suggest the form focused on time.

24. C is correct. The first paragraph states that the poem has a "mourning speaker" who is "affronted by the way the outside world regains its equilibrium after the death of Arthur Henry Hallam," meaning it is about the passing of Hallam.

   A, D: These are critics of poetry.

   B: Tennyson is the author of the poem.

Passage 5 (Questions 25 – 31)

I suppose that humans have reached the point at which the **obstacles to their survival** in a natural state possess a **greater** power of resistance than the **resources each individual** has available for their own defense and survival in that state. Therefore, this primitive state can no longer subsist, and if humans could not change their manner of existence, the human race would perish. Because people cannot generate new forces, but rather, can only direct and unite existing ones, they have **no other choice** for survival than to form an **aggregate** of forces great enough to overcome the obstacles of the natural world. These forces must be gathered around a single motive power, and they **must act cooperatively**.

Opinion: humans have reached the point at which the obstacles to survival possess more resistance than the resources that each individual has

Contrast: obstacles to survival vs resources available for defense, generating new forces vs directing and uniting existing ones

Cause and effect: because people cannot generate new forces, but can only direct existing ones, they have no other choice for survival but to form an aggregate of forces great enough to overcome nature's obstacles

This sum of forces requires many people to come together, and here a significant question arises: because the force and liberty of every person are the primary drives for their own self-preservation, how might they **pledge them to the collective whole** while **maintaining** their **own interests** and without neglecting the care that they owe to themselves? This conundrum is concisely defined by the following terms:

Contrast: the collective whole vs self-interest

Cause and effect: because the individual liberty of every person is the drive for self-preservation, a question arises: how can a person pledge themselves to the whole while maintaining their own interests?

"The problem is to find a form of **association** which will **defend** and protect the **person** and goods of each associate with the whole common force, and in which, each person, while uniting themselves with all, may still obey themselves alone, and **remain as free as before**." This is the essential problem of human civilization for which **the social contract** is the solution.

Contrast: each person uniting vs still maintaining his or her freedom

Cause and effect: because the problem with aggregating forces together is that every person wants to remain free and is interested in their own self-preservation, the social contract is the proper solution

The clauses of the social contract are so finely determined by the nature of this act of unification that **the smallest change** to them would make the whole **ineffective**. For this reason,

though they have perhaps **never been formally recorded**, they are the **same in all civilized societies** and all people tacitly recognize them; that is, until the social contract is violated and each person regains their original rights and resumes their natural liberty, all the while losing the conventional liberty for which they renounced that natural liberty.

Contrast: the clauses never being recorded vs being tacitly recognized in all societies, original rights and natural liberty vs conventional liberty

Cause and effect: because the social contract is so finely determined by social unification, the smallest change to them will make the whole thing ineffective

Properly understood, these clauses may be reduced to one: the social contract requires the **total surrender of each person**, along with all their rights, **to the whole community**, for if each person, without exception, gives themselves absolutely, the **conditions are the same for all**. If this is so, no person will have any interest in making the contract and its clauses burdensome to others.

Key terms: total surrender, whole community

Contrast: each person vs whole community, each person vs every other person

Cause and effect: if each person totally surrenders all their rights to the community, the conditions will be the same for all, and no one will have any interest in making the contract and its clauses burdensome

And **if the surrender is thorough and unreserved**, the union will be as perfect as it can be, for no person will have anything more to demand. If some individuals were able to **retain certain rights**, and because there would be no common superior do decide between them and the rest of the public, each of these individuals, being on one certain point his or her **own judge**, would ask to **be so on all points**. In this case, the state of nature would continue on, rendering the group at best **dysfunctional** and at worst tyrannical.

Contrast: all people surrendering all things thoroughly vs some individuals retaining certain rights, these individuals vs the rest of the public,

Cause and effect: if some people retain certain rights, they will be their own judges on these certain rights, and will ask to be so on all points; if this were to happen, tyranny results

In giving themselves to all, each person really **gives himself** or herself to **nobody**. Because there is no one person over whom they does not have the same rights as those they yield to others over themselves, they **gain an equivalent for everything** they lose in the initial **surrendering**, and an **increase of force** for the preservation of what belongs to them, their life and their resources. So, if we ignore for a moment those parts of the social contract that are not essential, way may reduce it to this: "Each of us puts our person and all our powers in common under the **supreme direction of the**

general will, and, in our collective capacity, we receive each member and power as an indivisible part of the whole."

Contrast: giving themselves to all vs giving themselves to nobody, rights over other people vs rights yielded to other people

Cause and effect: because there is no person over whom an individual does not have the same rights as those that the individual yields to others over themselves, the individual gains an equivalent for everything he or she surrenders and actually gains an increase of force

Main Idea: The passage sets out to define the social contract: by surrendering themselves to the community, people can actually better their ability to protect themselves; if all people engage in the contract equally, those rights that are given up have equivalents in the newly formed society.

25.   A is correct. As the author writes in the fifth paragraph, "Properly understood, these clauses may be reduced to one: the social contract requires the total surrender of each person, along with all their rights, to the whole community, for if each person, without exception, gives themselves absolutely, the conditions are the same for all." As these clauses can be reduced to one clause if understood, we may assume that this one clause is the most important, foundational clause.

26.   C is correct. As the author writes in the fourth paragraph, "The clauses of the social contract are so finely determined by the nature of this act of unification that the smallest change to them would make the whole ineffective." As they cannot be changed by one iota, they are strictly rigid.

   A, B: These clauses are not adaptable.

   D: The social contract is rigid, not loose.

27.   D is correct. The author writes, "though they have perhaps never been formally recorded, they are the same in all societies and all people tacitly recognized them." The social contract's clauses are the same for all civilized societies. Therefore, the idea of the social contract is universal to all civilized societies.

   A: This is never said. And, the failure of the social contract is mentioned in paragraph six.

   B: This is possibly true, but never clearly stated.

   C: This is false, according to the author.

28.   B is correct. The social contract requires total surrender of each person and all their rights with no exception. Certainly this is a rigid system.

   A: The cost and benefit of the social contract is more clearly stated by the quotation in the seventh paragraph, accounting for both what goes in and what each member receives from it.

C: It is implied that the social contract is difficult as it is a rigid system, but never said directly.

D: Rather, all the clauses can be distilled into one.

29.   C is correct. As the author writes in paragraph six, "If some individuals were able to retain certain rights, and because there would be no common superior to decide between them and the rest of the public, each of these individuals, being on one certain point his or her own judge, would ask to be so on all points." This is the author's direct answer to this question.

   A, B: These may happen but Choice C will happen first and cause the dissolution of the social contract.

   D: This is never said or implied.

30.   C is correct. Rather, people would seem to gain more than they lose. As the seventh paragraph makes clear, people gain an equivalent for everything they lose in the surrendering, and they actually gain an increase in force for preservation of themselves and their property. This represents a net gain, not a net loss.

   A, B, D: These statements are true and are made in the passage.

31.   B is correct. II is true, as violating one part of the contract, however small, violates the whole contract.

   I: This is false because they author writes that they are understood tacitly, the opposite of explicitly.

   III: This is false because these clauses are actually "determined by the nature of this act of unification." They innately arise from the need for humans to come together and amass the sum of their forces.

Passage 6 (Questions 32 – 37)

Mr. Wittgenstein's *Tractatus Logico-Philosophicus*, whether or not it proves to give the ultimate truth on the matters with which it deals, certainly deserves, by its **breadth** and **scope** and **profundity**, to be considered an **important event** in the philosophical world. Starting from the principles of **Symbolism** and the relations which are necessary between words and things in any language, it applies the result of this inquiry to various departments of traditional philosophy, showing in each case how traditional philosophy and traditional solutions arise out of **ignorance** of the **principles** of **Symbolism** and out of **misuse of language**.

Key terms: Mr. Wittgenstein's Tractatus Logico-Philosophicus, Symbolism

Opinion: author believes that Tractatus Logico-Philosophicus has to be considered an important event in philosophical world

Cause and effect: using principles of symbolism can show how traditional philosophy and its solutions are based on ignorance and misuse of language

In order to understand Mr. Wittgenstein's book, it is necessary to **realize the problem that concerns him**. In the part of his theory which deals with Symbolism, he is concerned with the conditions that would have to be fulfilled by a **logically perfect language**. There are various problems as regards language. First, there is the problem of what actually occurs in our minds when we use language with the intention of meaning something by it; this problem belongs to **psychology**. Secondly, there is the problem of the relation subsisting between thoughts, words, or sentences, and what it is they refer to or mean; this problem belongs to **epistemology**. Thirdly, there is the problem of using sentences to convey truth rather than falsehood; this belongs to the special sciences dealing with the **subject-matter** of the sentences in question. Fourthly, there is the question: what relation must one fact (such as a sentence) have to another in order to be capable of being a symbol for that other? This last is a **logical** question, and is the one with which Mr. Wittgenstein is concerned. He is concerned with the conditions for accurate Symbolism, i.e. for **Symbolism in which a sentence "means" something quite definite**. In practice, language is always more or less vague, so that what we assert is never quite precise. Thus, logic has two problems to deal with in regard to Symbolism: (1) the conditions for **sense rather than nonsense** in combinations of symbols; (2) the conditions for **uniqueness of meaning** or reference in symbols or combinations of symbols. A logically perfect language has rules of syntax that prevent nonsense, and has single symbols which always have a definite and unique meaning. Mr. Wittgenstein is concerned with the conditions for a logically perfect language—not that any language is logically perfect, or that we believe ourselves capable, here and now, of constructing a logically perfect language, but that the whole function of language is to have meaning, and it only

fulfills this function in proportion as it approaches the ideal language which we postulate.

Key terms: psychology, epistemology, subject-matter, logical, sense, uniqueness of meaning

Contrast: sense vs nonsense in combining symbols; unique meaning vs multiple meanings; ideal language with sense and uniqueness vs actual imperfect language with which we deal

Cause and effect: focusing on various problems of language leads to being dealt with by different fields; focusing on symbolism, or relation between sentences as symbolic of facts, raises two problems: conditions for sense and uniqueness of meaning

The **essential business of language is to assert or deny facts**. Given the **syntax** of a language, the **meaning** of a sentence is determinate as soon as the **meaning of the component words** is known. In order that a certain sentence should assert a certain fact there must, however the language may be constructed, be something in common between the structure of the sentence and the structure of the fact. This is perhaps the most fundamental thesis of Mr. Wittgenstein's theory. That which has to be **in common between the sentence and the fact cannot**, so he contends, be **itself in turn said in language**. It can, in his phraseology, only be **shown, not said,** for whatever we may say will still need to have the same structure.

Opinion: writer argues that the most fundamental element of Wittgenstein's theory is that the structure of a sentence is related to the structure of fact and thus cannot be said, only shown

Cause and effect: because the structure of a sentence depends on the structure of the fact it symbolizes, one can only show the connection between the two, not say it

Main Idea: The passage addresses a work by Wittgenstein, Tractatus Logico-Philosophicus, stating that its focus on symbolism, or the relation between words and what they represent, makes it a work of huge philosophical importance, as it raises questions about the various assumptions and conclusions of philosophy.

32. B is correct. The first paragraph introduces "Symbolism and the relations which are necessary between words and things in any language".

  A: Symbolism is a principle that affects traditional philosophy, but not what drives it as in choice A.

  C, D: Neither senses nor visual images are mentioned in the passage.

33. C is correct. The third paragraph states that part of Wittgenstein's theory identifies "that which has to be in common between the sentence and the fact" can "only be shown, not said, for whatever we may say will still need to have the same structure." Thus the two share structure.

  A: The passage does not directly explain how syntax relates to facts, eliminating choice A.

  B: The passage states that language cannot express the connection, since it is a connection of language.

  D: According to the passage, syntax, not symbolism, "prevent[s] nonsense," eliminating choice D.

34. A is correct. The first paragraph states that Wittgenstein's work is "an important event in the philosophical world" because, whether it is right or not, it applies "the principles of Symbolism…to various departments of traditional philosophy, showing in each case how traditional philosophy and traditional solutions arise out of ignorance of the principles of Symbolism and out of misuse of language." Thus it suggests that applying a newly understood principle may change how philosophy is assessed.

  B: The passage does not address understanding all languages, but rather understanding how language form affects philosophy.

  C, D: Neither the existence of a logically perfect language nor syntax are discussed in terms of the overall value of Wittgenstein's work.

35. D is correct. The passage focuses on how symbolism, or the relation between words and things may change how we assess certain philosophical issues.

  A: It is stated that "traditional philosophy and traditional solutions arise out of ignorance of the principles of Symbolism and out of misuse of language," not that the failure of these traditional solutions may change how we think about philosophy, as in choice A.

  B: How to create an ideal language is not discussed in the passage.

  C: Fact and syntax are linked in the final paragraph, but are not described as Wittgenstein's major focus, as in choice C.

36. A is correct. The second paragraph divides issues of language into several disciplines, and states that "the problem of what actually occurs in our minds when we use language with the intention of meaning something by it . . . belongs to psychology." Thus a study of the activities of the mind would be psychology.

  B, D: Epistemology and subject-matter are described as having other foci.

  C: Neurology is not discussed in the passage.

37. C is correct. A logically perfect language is described as having "rules of syntax which prevent nonsense," as in choice B and being composed of "single symbols which always have a definite and unique meaning," as in choice D. Further, "the whole function of language is to have meaning," or to produce sense, as in choice A. Thus the credited answer is C. While it is stated that we are not "capable, here and now, of constructing a logically perfect language," that does not mean that such a feat would never be possible.

Passage 7 (Questions 38 – 43)

"Then, too," the dancer went on, "it is quite evident that one must **study art**. But most of the study of art for dancing is not in learning its technique but in seeing the beautiful old pictures and sculpture and studying their **composition**, their **posturing**. You see it needs **travel** to be a dancer—one must see the beautiful old pictures, and get their beauty"—**Miss Wihr** laughed and spread out her arms in a graceful inclusive gesture—"into one's self. The same is true of sculpture, which is necessary if one is to do the **Greek dances**. One of the most famous dancers of the present time takes almost all her poses straight from the old statues—studies the Greek postures, and makes them flow together. As for **color**, and the other branches of art," Miss Wihr went on, "they are not absolutely required even for creative work. But they are often **desirable**: every form of beauty is.

Key terms: Miss Wihr; Greek dances

Contrast: studying for technique vs studying for beauty

Cause and effect: by immersing oneself in art and sculpture, one learns the composition and posturing necessary for dance

Of course a dancer must know **literature**, especially **legend and poetry**. Out of the old legends and folk-tales come many of the most beautiful dances and dance-pictures. Poetry is necessary as a **rhythmic form of beauty** that must go along with what is exquisite in the dance. A dance must be a picture. It must also be a poem. When I have students here for lessons I always read a poem to them before the formal 'work' begins."

Contrast: old legends and folk tales create content and poetry offers a rhythmic form of beauty

Cause and effect: reading a poem before dancing can heighten awareness of rhythm

"You see," the dancer went on earnestly, "you must **study up, study up, all the time**, if you are to master dancing as a creative art. You must be a **thoroughly well-educated person**. And to begin with, you must have a **good mind**—not merely a sense of beauty and artistry, but a good, sturdy, hard-working brain. And then the dance itself comes from within. I tell my pupils that they cannot learn to dance by imitating me. They must think things out, and they must dance by themselves. If the dance is not in you, you can never get it from anything outside. **Someone else may make you a dancing machine, but a dancer you yourself must be.**"

Contrast: knowing the moves of a dance vs dancing from within

Cause and effect: when a person is well educated and has studied creative arts, the dance comes from within and makes them a true dancer

"The actual **exercises** that one has in dancing are not so different from those of the **gymnasium**." The dancer stretched out her arms and took one of the familiar one-two-three-four motions of early school days—arms out, elbows bent, hands at shoulders, then out again. It was a quick, muscular, **strong, and jerky** exercise. Then she did it again. But the second time there was no jerkiness, no sudden stop; the **positions seemed to flow** into each other; there was the suggestion of a gentle river in the slow movement of the dancer's arms. You see," she said, "those **exercises** are exactly the **same**. The one is simply softened. The emphasis is not on muscular force, but on grace. Yet they are **equally healthful**. That is why so many women take dancing lessons as a sort of gymnastic course to strengthen their bodies and at the same time make them more graceful."

Contrast: jerky gymnasium-style exercises vs graceful dancer ones

Cause and effect: while dance and gymnasium exercises differ, they are equally healthful and thus many women take dance for both strength and health

Main Idea: The passage consists of a series of statements from an interview with Miss Wihr about what a dancer needs to be successful. She stresses familiarity with a number of types of art, including sculpture and literature, so that the mind is active and knowledgeable about beauty, as well as the ability to complete motions with grace.

38. A is correct. The fourth paragraph focuses on dance as exercise: Wihr states that exercises from the gymnasium and dance are "exactly the same. The one is simply softened. The emphasis is not on muscular force, but on grace. Yet they are equally healthful. That is why so many women take dancing lessons as a sort of gymnastic course to strengthen their bodies and at the same time make them more graceful." Thus they take classes for grace and health.

   B, D: Dance has softer movements, eliminating choice D, but it is the movement, not the people who are softened.

   C: There is no mention of how tedious or exciting any routines are.

39. D is correct. In the passage, Wihr suggests that one great dancer creates her Greek dances by studying Greek sculptures and making their poses flow together.

   A: While Wihr says color may be less important than other elements, she does not say to ignore it altogether.

   B: Wihr suggests that dancers should study other art forms, not specific techniques.

   C: The passage does not discuss all forms of art.

40. C is correct. In discussing legend, Wihr states "out of the old legends and folk-tales come many of the most beautiful dances and dance-pictures." Thus she implies that legends suggest the content of many dances.

   A, D: The author does not suggest that literature is the "highest branch of art," nor that legends are necessarily one of the best ways to achieve beauty.

   B: The author discusses poems for their rhythmic content, not as something linked to pictures.

41. A is correct. Throughout the passage, Wihr focuses on the need for a dancer to be well educated in various art forms.

   B, C: In the third paragraph, Wihr argues against imitation of other people's dances, stating a dance must come from within.

   D: While Wihr suggests many turn to dance to gain bodily strength, she does not stress dancers' need for strength, as in choice D.

42. B is correct. In the passage, Wihr argues against imitation because dancers "must think things out, and they must dance by themselves."

   A: There is no discussion of ownership of creative work in the passage.

   C, D: Wihr is against imitation, eliminating the positive responses of choices C and D.

43. B is correct. In the third paragraph, Wihr states that "the dance itself comes from within. I tell my pupils that they cannot learn to dance by imitating me. They must think things out, and they must dance by themselves. If the dance is not in you, you can never get it from anything outside. Someone else may make you a dancing machine, but a dancer you yourself must be".

   A: Wihr does not specifically mention overthinking dance.

   C: The description of a dance machine is negative, whereas Wihr admires those who know a lot about various art forms.

   D: Wihr does not emphasize unique viewpoints, just having an internal sense of beauty.

Passage 8 (Questions 44 – 49)

Giotto was the first of the **great personalities** in **Florentine painting**, and though he provides no exception to **the rule** that the great Florentines used the arts in their **endeavor to express themselves**, he, renowned as an architect, sculptor, wit, and versifier, differed from **the majority** of his Tuscan successors in possessing a **peculiar aptitude** for **the essential** in painting *as an art*. Yet, before we may appreciate his **real value**, we ought to come to an agreement on what constitutes the essential in the art of **figure-painting**, for this form was not only the **primary interest** of Giotto, but of the entire **Florentine school**.

Key terms: Giotto, Florentine painting

Contrast: painting as a means for expression vs painting as an art; appreciating his real value vs agreeing on what constitutes the essential figure-painting

Cause and effect: because he possessed a peculiar aptitude for the essential in painting Giotto differed from the majority of his Tuscan successors

Scientists have discovered that **sight** alone cannot give us an accurate sense of the **third dimension**. In our **infancy**, and long before we are conscious of it, the **sense of touch** and the **muscular sensations of movement** teach us to appreciate **depth** in both objects and space. This is what is referred to as the third dimension. Then, still in infancy, we learn to make touch and the third dimension the **test of reality**. As **children**, we are still somewhat aware of the **close connection** between touch and the third dimension. For example, a child of five cannot persuade herself of the unreality of a trick mirror until she has touched the mirror. Beyond childhood, we forget this connection. However, every time our eyes recognize reality, we actually give **tactile value** to **retinal impressions**.

Contrast: consciously forgetting the connection of touch and reality vs unconsciously giving tactile value to retinal impressions

Cause and effect: because the sense of touch and muscular sensations of movement teach us to appreciate depth, we learn to make touch and the third dimension the test of reality

As an art form, painting aims to give us a **lasting and realistic impression** of **artistic reality** with only **two dimensions**. Therefore, the painter must **do consciously what we all do unconsciously**: construct the perception of the third dimension. He must accomplish this objective in the same way we all do, by giving tactile value to retinal impressions. So, his **first act** is to rouse the tactile sense in his **viewers**, for we must have **the illusion** of being able to touch a figure, we must have the illusion of muscular sensations inside our hands corresponding to the figure of the painting, before we take the work **for granted as real** and therefore let it affect us lastingly.

Cause and effect: because the aim of painting is to give us a lasting and realistic impression of artistic reality with only two dimensions, the painter must consciously construct the perception of the third dimension, something we all do unconsciously; in order to achieve this, he must give tactile value to retinal impressions

Therefore, it follows that the essential in the art of figure-painting is to somehow stimulate our consciousness of tactile values with **a work** that has at least as much **power** to appeal to our **tactile imagination** as **the actual object represented**. In this way, as he realized the essential in painting and stimulated our tactile consciousness better than all others, Giotto was **the supreme master**. It is this quality that will make him a source of the **highest kind of aesthetic delight** for at least as long as traces of his work remain on decaying panels and crumbling walls. For though he was a great **poet**, an enthralling **story-teller**, and a splendid **composer**, superior to the many masters who painted between **the decline** of **the antique** and **the birth** of **the modern** which he ignited, he was superior in these qualities **by degree only**. None of these many masters possessed the power to stimulate the tactile imagination, and therefore, they never painted a figure with **true artistic existence**. Their works have value as elaborate, highly intelligible **symbols**, capable of communicating **meaning**, and yet they lose all **higher value** the moment this meaning is delivered.

Contrast: works of art having value as symbols capable of communicating meaning vs works of art stimulating our tactile sense

Cause and effect: because of the argument made in the previous paragraph, it follows that the essential in figure-painting is to stimulate our consciousness of tactile values with a work that has at least as much power to appeal to our tactile imaginations as the actual image represented; because he realized this, Giotto was the supreme master

On the other hand, Giotto's paintings not only possess as much power to appeal to the tactile imagination as the objects they represent (human figures in particular), but they **actually possess more**. In this way, his work conveyed a **keener sense of reality** than both that of his **contemporaries** and that of the very objects he represented in his paintings.

Cause and effect: because Giotto's painting possesses more power to appeal to the tactile imagination than the objects they represent, his work conveys a keener sense of reality than both that of his contemporaries and that of the objects he represented in his work

Main Idea: The author posits that Giotto was the first great Florentine painter, because he possessed a peculiar aptitude for the essential in painting as an art form, not only a form of expression; this essential element is to stimulate the consciousness of tactile values in the viewer; the author ends by claiming that Giotto's figures were even more "life-like" than the actual objects he represented in his work, suggesting that his work possessed more reality than real objects.

44. D is correct. The second paragraph is dedicated to how our sense of the third dimension is not accounted for only by sight, but also by touch as well. The author describes how we develop our perception of third dimension, depth, through the interplay of sight and touch. This relationship, conscious during childhood, becomes unconscious afterwards. As the essential quality of figure-painting is to stimulate the sense of touch, and therefore, reality, this description of childhood experimenting serves to set up the quality in humans that the essential element of figure painting aims to satisfy.

    A: This seems like it could be true, but no such connection is ever made or even implied.

    B: Rather, the author seems to be making a case for the sense of touch having an innate connection to the appreciation of figure-painting specifically.

    C: Rather, this is an illustration of how we develop our perception of depth. As it is often said, there's no accounting for taste.

45. C is correct. According to the author, Giotto's work "conveys a keener sense of reality than . . . that of the very objects he represented in his paintings." So, his work offers a keener, or heightened sense of reality.

    A: We know that touch is important too.

    B: You cannot see art without sight.

    D: We don't know that from this passage. We know that the author believes him to have been the first great Florentine painter, and that he was superior to all artists between the end of the antique and the beginning of the modern. But the claim is never made that he is the greatest of the renaissance.

46. A is correct. As the author writes in the second half of the third paragraph, the artist's "first act is to rouse the tactile sense in his viewers, for we must have the illusion of being able to touch the figure . . . before we take the work for granted as real and therefore let is affect us lastingly"

    B: Purpose and meaning can exist without this tactile quality.

    C: The author never mentions imagining the life of the subject outside of the work.

D: This is a difficult one to weed out, but the author does write that "painting aims to give us a lasting and realistic impression of artistic reality with only two dimensions." There is a difference here between reality (actual objects) and artistic reality (painted objects). An artist's work ought to evoke tactile feelings of reality, but it need not necessarily be close to reality in its depiction. For the author, a painting will not fool someone into thinking it contains real, three-dimensional. Rather, it evokes the feeling of that.

47. C is correct. As the author writes in the first paragraph, Giotto differed from most of his compatriots in not only using painting for expression, but for artistry as well, for crafting a thing. To Giotto, it was both, and this set him apart.

    A: The passage isn't concerned with the sense of touch itself, but rather how that sense can be conveyed in paintings.

    B: Rather, it seems that all children experiment in this way. The author gives us no reason to believe some children do it more than others.

    D: This is unclear and unknowable given what we have.

48. B is correct. Rather, "he provides no exception to the rule that the great Florentines used the arts in their endeavor to express themselves . . ."

    A, C, D: These are all true in the passage.

49. D is correct. I: This is true as this is one of the qualities that separates Giotto from his contemporaries and successors. II: This is false, or at least not necessarily true, because the author writes that he was "superior to the many masters who painted between the decline of the antique and the birth of the modern . . ." We don't know about the height of the modern. III: This is true because, as the author writes in the third paragraph, "the painter must do consciously what we all do unconsciously: construct the perception of the third dimension."

Passage 9 (Questions 50 – 53)

Herbart's great service lay in taking the work of teaching out of the region of routine and accident. He brought it into the sphere of **conscious method**; it became a conscious business with a **definite aim and procedure**, instead of being a compound of casual inspiration and subservience to tradition. Moreover, everything in teaching and discipline could be **specified**, instead of our having to be content with vague and more or less mystic generalities about ultimate ideals and speculative spiritual symbols. He abolished the notion of ready-made faculties, which might be trained by exercise upon any sort of material, and made **attention to concrete subject matter, to the content, all-important**. Herbart undoubtedly has had a greater influence in bringing to the front questions connected with the material of study than any other educational philosopher. He stated problems of method from the standpoint of their connection with subject matter: method having to do with **the manner and sequence of presenting new subject matter** to insure its proper interaction with old.

Key terms: Herbart, method, subject matter

Opinion: author argues that Herbart had the greatest influence of any educational influence in terms of focusing on material of study and making teaching about conscious method

Contrast: teaching as routine, accidental vs conscious and specific

Cause and effect: Herbart shifted the attention of teaching to doing it with specific content matter and thinking about the order to present subject matter so it interacts with previous lessons

The fundamental theoretical **defect of this view** lies in **ignoring** the existence in **a living being of active and specific functions** which are developed in the redirection and combination which occur as they are occupied with their environment. The theory represents the **Schoolmaster** come to his own. This fact expresses at once its strength and its weakness. The conception that the mind consists of what has been taught, and that the importance of what has been taught consists in its availability for further teaching, reflects the **pedagogue's view of life**. The philosophy is eloquent about the duty of the teacher in instructing pupils; it is almost **silent regarding his privilege of learning**. It emphasizes the influence of intellectual environment upon the mind; it slurs over the fact that the environment involves a personal sharing in common experiences. It **exaggerates beyond reason** the possibilities of consciously formulated and used **methods**, and **underestimates** the role of **vital, unconscious, attitudes**. It insists upon the old, the past, and passes lightly over the operation of the genuinely novel and unforeseeable. It takes, in brief, everything educational into account save its essence—vital energy seeking opportunity for effective exercise. **All education** forms character, mental and moral, but formation consists in the selection and **coordination of native activities** so that they may **utilize the subject matter of the social environment**. Moreover, the formation is not only a formation of native activities, but it takes place through them. It is a process of **reconstruction, reorganization**.

Contrast: duties of instructor vs privilege in learning; emphasis on the teacher vs the vital energy and process of the learner; emphasis on past vs emphasis on the new

Cause and effect: formation of character consists of selecting and coordinating activities and the process of reorganization that takes place through them

A **peculiar combination of the ideas** of development and formation from without has given rise to the **recapitulation theory of education**, biological and cultural. The individual develops, but his proper **development consists in repeating in orderly stages the past evolution** of animal life and human history. The former recapitulation occurs physiologically; the latter should be made to occur by means of education. The alleged biological truth that the individual in his growth from the simple embryo to maturity repeats the history of the evolution of animal life in the progress of forms from the simplest to the most complex (or expressed technically, that ontogenesis parallels phylogenesis) does not concern us, save as it is supposed to afford scientific foundation for cultural recapitulation of the past. **Cultural recapitulation says**, first, that **children** at a certain age are in the mental and moral condition of **savagery**; their instincts are vagrant and predatory because their ancestors at one time lived such a life. Consequently (so it is concluded) the **proper subject matter of their education** at this time is the material—especially the literary material of **myths**, folk-tale, and song—**produced by humanity in the analogous stage**. Then the child passes on to something corresponding, say, to the pastoral stage, and so on till at the time when he is ready to take part in contemporary life, he arrives at the present epoch of culture.

Key terms: recapitulation theory

Cause and effect: believing in a recapitulation theory means that one believes certain materials from different stages of humanity's history are appropriate to children at certain stages

Main Idea: The author discusses several theories of education, including a content focused one and one based upon ideas of recapitulation, to highlight their flaws; in contrast, he emphasizes learning as a process that involves interaction with the social environment.

50. **D is correct.** The second paragraph suggests some of the problems of Herbart's philosophy, particularly his emphasis on the instructor as opposed to interaction with the social environment, which the author advocates. The third paragraph brings up another theory upon which the author casts doubt. Thus it can be inferred that Herbart's is one of the theories against which the author is comparing his.

   A, C: while these are statements made about Herbart's theory, they are not the author's primary purpose in bringing him up.

   B: The recapitulation theory is not connected to Herbart's ideas.

51. **B is correct.** In the second paragraph, the author suggests that the essence of education rests in "vital energy" and the formation of character through interaction with the social environment, so the class would be aligned with the author's ideas and emphasizing the role of the student rather than the instructor.

   A: The author argues that biological elements are not what the educational theory focuses on.

   C, D: Herbart focuses on the teacher's role, not the students.

52. **B is correct.** The author explains that the theory of "cultural recapitulation says, first, that children at a certain age are in the mental and moral condition of savagery; their instincts are vagrant and predatory because their ancestors at one time lived such a life. Consequently (so it is concluded) the proper subject matter of their education at this time is the material—especially the literary material of myths, folk-tale, and song—produced by humanity in the analogous stage. Then the child passes on to something corresponding, say, to the pastoral stage, and so on till at the time when he is ready to take part in contemporary life, he arrives at the present epoch of culture." In essence, children should be given works that correspond to the historical evolution of human culture, as in choices A, C and D.

   Choice B suggests that children should analyze cultural works to trace stages of development, which is not discussed in the passage, making that the credited choice.

53. **B is correct.** The author discusses recapitulation in the third paragraph and says it is "it is supposed to afford scientific foundation" and adds "(so it is concluded)" to the idea of what to do with that information. These phrases suggest doubt, or skepticism.

   A, C: Disdain and implicit belief both suggest strong feelings that are not supported in the passage.

   D: The "supposed" and putting "so it is concluded" in parentheses both suggest the authors has some doubts, meaning the idea is not being carefully considered, as in choice D.

APPENDIX A

CARS Performance Tracking Sheet

Date	Title	Strategy	% Correct	Confidence
12/25/2016	Full Section 1	Slow read, took notes	75%	Medium

APPENDIX B

Score Conversion Chart

Table 1 Raw Score to Scaled Score Conversion for CARS Sections

The scaled-to-percentile conversions are taken from official AAMC publications regarding the scoring of the exam for the 2015 cycle. The raw-to-scaled conversion is modeled on AAMC Practice Test (Scored) 1, but when applying this scale to the timed sections in this book, the scores should be understood only as rough estimates.

Raw Score (Number of Questions Correct)	**Scaled Score**	**Percentile**[*]
51-53	132	100
49-50	131	99
47-48	130	97
46-46	129	93
43-45	128	87
41-42	127	81
39-40	126	70
36-38	125	58
33-35	124	44
30-32	123	33
27-29	122	22
24-26	121	14
20-23	120	8
16-19	119	3
0 - 15	118	1

* Percentile rank is given in this table as an example of how percentile correlates with scaled score, taken from official AAMC sources. This is for illustration purposes only and does not represent performance of test-takers from the material on these exams.

APPENDIX C

Answer Sheets

Remove the following pages from the book to record your answers. Then score your work on the answer grid, but ***don't mark the right answers on the timed section***. That way you can come back to your work later and review the questions in the section without having all of the correct answers marked in the book already.

Answer Grid – Section 1

1		12		23		34		45	
2		13		24		35		46	
3		14		25		36		47	
4		15		26		37		48	
5		16		27		38		49	
6		17		28		39		50	
7		18		29		40		51	
8		19		30		41		52	
9		20		31		42		53	
10		21		32		43			
11		22		33		44			

Answer Grid – Section 2

1		12		23		34		45	
2		13		24		35		46	
3		14		25		36		47	
4		15		26		37		48	
5		16		27		38		49	
6		17		28		39		50	
7		18		29		40		51	
8		19		30		41		52	
9		20		31		42		53	
10		21		32		43			
11		22		33		44			

Answer Grid – Section 3

1		12		23		34		45	
2		13		24		35		46	
3		14		25		36		47	
4		15		26		37		48	
5		16		27		38		49	
6		17		28		39		50	
7		18		29		40		51	
8		19		30		41		52	
9		20		31		42		53	
10		21		32		43			
11		22		33		44			

Answer Grid – Section 4

1		12		23		34		45	
2		13		24		35		46	
3		14		25		36		47	
4		15		26		37		48	
5		16		27		38		49	
6		17		28		39		50	
7		18		29		40		51	
8		19		30		41		52	
9		20		31		42		53	
10		21		32		43			
11		22		33		44			

Answer Grid – Section 5

1		12		23		34		45	
2		13		24		35		46	
3		14		25		36		47	
4		15		26		37		48	
5		16		27		38		49	
6		17		28		39		50	
7		18		29		40		51	
8		19		30		41		52	
9		20		31		42		53	
10		21		32		43			
11		22		33		44			

Answer Grid – Section 6

1		12		23		34		45	
2		13		24		35		46	
3		14		25		36		47	
4		15		26		37		48	
5		16		27		38		49	
6		17		28		39		50	
7		18		29		40		51	
8		19		30		41		52	
9		20		31		42		53	
10		21		32		43			
11		22		33		44			

Answer Grid – Section 7

1		12		23		34		45	
2		13		24		35		46	
3		14		25		36		47	
4		15		26		37		48	
5		16		27		38		49	
6		17		28		39		50	
7		18		29		40		51	
8		19		30		41		52	
9		20		31		42		53	
10		21		32		43			
11		22		33		44			

Answer Grid – Section 8

1		12		23		34		45	
2		13		24		35		46	
3		14		25		36		47	
4		15		26		37		48	
5		16		27		38		49	
6		17		28		39		50	
7		18		29		40		51	
8		19		30		41		52	
9		20		31		42		53	
10		21		32		43			
11		22		33		44			

Answer Grid – Section 9

1		12		23		34		45	
2		13		24		35		46	
3		14		25		36		47	
4		15		26		37		48	
5		16		27		38		49	
6		17		28		39		50	
7		18		29		40		51	
8		19		30		41		52	
9		20		31		42		53	
10		21		32		43			
11		22		33		44			

Answer Grid – Section 10

1		12		23		34		45	
2		13		24		35		46	
3		14		25		36		47	
4		15		26		37		48	
5		16		27		38		49	
6		17		28		39		50	
7		18		29		40		51	
8		19		30		41		52	
9		20		31		42		53	
10		21		32		43			
11		22		33		44			

Answer Grid – Section 11

1		12		23		34		45	
2		13		24		35		46	
3		14		25		36		47	
4		15		26		37		48	
5		16		27		38		49	
6		17		28		39		50	
7		18		29		40		51	
8		19		30		41		52	
9		20		31		42		53	
10		21		32		43			
11		22		33		44			

Answer Grid – Section 12

1		12		23		34		45	
2		13		24		35		46	
3		14		25		36		47	
4		15		26		37		48	
5		16		27		38		49	
6		17		28		39		50	
7		18		29		40		51	
8		19		30		41		52	
9		20		31		42		53	
10		21		32		43			
11		22		33		44			

9 781511 766692